NEURO-ONCOLOGY

NEURO-ONCOLOGY: BLUE BOOKS OF NEUROLOGY SERIES

JEREMY H. REES, PhD, FRCP
Consultant Neurologist
National Hospital for Neurology and Neurosurgery;
Honorary Senior Lecturer
Institute of Neurology
University College London
Queen Square
London

PATRICK Y. WEN, MD
Associate Professor of Neurology
Harvard Medical School;
Director, Division of Cancer Neurology
Department of Neurology
Brigham and Women's Hospital;
Clinical Director
Center for Neuro-Oncology
Dana-Farber Cancer Institute
Boston, Massachusetts, USA

SAUNDERS
ELSEVIER

SAUNDERS
ELSEVIER

1600 John F. Kennedy Blvd.
Ste 1800
Philadelphia, PA 19103-2899

NEURO-ONCOLOGY ISBN: 978-0-7506-7516-1

Library of Congress Cataloging-in-Publication Data

Neuro-oncology / [edited by] Jeremy Rees, Patrick Y. Wen.
p. ; cm. – (Blue books of neurology series ; 36)
Includes bibliographical references.
ISBN 978-0-7506-7516-1 (alk. paper)
1. Brain–Tumors. I. Rees, Jeremy. II. Wen, Patrick Y. III. Series: Blue books of neurology ; 36.
[DNLM: 1. Brain Neoplasms. W1 BU9749 v.36 2009 / WL 358 N49354 2010]
RC280.B7N474 2010
616.99'481–dc22

2009037536

Acquisitions Editor: Adrianne Brigido
Developmental Editor: Taylor Ball
Publishing Services Manager: Hemamalini Rajendrababu
Project Manager: Gopika Sasidharan
Designer: Steven Stave

BLUE BOOKS OF NEUROLOGY

1 **Clinical Neurophysiology**
ERIC STALBERG • ROBERT R. YOUNG

2 **Movement Disorders**
C. DAVID MARSDEN • STANLEY FAHN

3 **Cerebral Vascular Disease**
MICHAEL J.G. HARRISON • MARK L. DYKEN

4 **Peripheral Nerve Disorders**
ARTHUR K. ASBURY • R.W. GILLIATT

5 **The Epilepsies**
ROGER J. PORTER • PAOLO I. MORSELLI

6 **Multiple Sclerosis**
W. IAN MCDONALD • DONALD H. SILBERBERG

7 **Movement Disorders 2**
C. DAVID MARSDEN • STANLEY FAHN

8 **Infections of the Nervous System**
PETER G.E. KENNEDY • RICHARD T. JOHNSON

9 **The Molecular Biology of Neurological Disease**
ROGER N. ROSENBERG • ANITA E. HARDING

10 **Pain Syndromes in Neurology**
HOWARD L. FIELDS

11 **Principles and Practice of Restorative Neurology**
ROBERT R. YOUNG • PAUL J. DELWAIDE

12 **Stroke: Populations, Cohorts, and Clinical Trials**
JACK P. WHISNANT

13 **Movement Disorders 3**
C. DAVID MARSDEN • STANLEY FAHN

14 **Mitochondrial Disorders in Neurology**
ANTHONY H.V. SCHAPIRA • SALVATORE DIMAURO

15 **Peripheral Nerve Disorders 2**
ARTHUR K. ASBURY • P.K. THOMAS

16 **Contemporary Behavioral Neurology**
MICHAEL R. TRIMBLE • JEFFREY L. CUMMINGS

17 **Headache**
PETER J. GOADSBY • STEPHEN D. SILBERSTEIN

18 **The Epilepsies 2**
ROGER J. PORTER • DAVID CHADWICK

19 **The Dementias**
JOHN H. GROWDON • MARTIN N. ROSSOR

20 **Hospitalist Neurology**
MARTIN A. SAMUELS

21 **Neurologic Complications in Organ Transplant Recipients**
EELCO F.M. WIJDICKS

22 **Critical Care Neurology**
DAVID H. MILLER • ERIC C. RAPS

23 **Neurology of Bladder, Bowel, and Sexual Dysfunction**
CLARE J. FOWLER

24 **Muscle Diseases**
ANTHONY H.V. SCHAPIRA • ROBERT C. GRIGGS

25 **Clinical Trials in Neurologic Practice**
JOSE BILLER • JULIEN BOGOUSSLAVSKY

26 **Mitochondrial Disorders in Neurology 2**
ANTHONY H.V. SCHAPIRA • SALVATORE DIMAURO

27 **Multiple Sclerosis 2**
W. IAN MCDONALD • JOHN H. NOSEWORTHY

CONTENTS

CONTRIBUTING AUTHORS

Ashok R. Asthagiri, MD
Surgical Neurology Branch
National Institute of Neurological Disorders and Stroke
National Institutes of Health
Bethesda, Maryland

Anthony Béhin, MD
Fédération de Neurologie Mazarin
Paris, France

Michael Brada, MD, FRCP, FRCR
Professor of Clinical Oncology
Institute of Cancer Research
The Royal Marsden Hospital
Sutton, United Kingdom

Marc C. Chamberlain, MD
Department of Neurology
Fred Hutchinson Cancer Research Center
University of Washington
Seattle, Washington
Department of Neurology
University of Southern California
Los Angeles, California

Daysi Chi, MD
Fédération de Neurologie Mazarin
Paris, France

V. Peter Collins, MD, FRCP
Department of Histopathology
University of Cambridge
Cambridge, United Kingdom

Paul R. Cooper, MD
Department of Neurosurgery
New York University Medical Center
New York, New York

Josep Dalmau, MD, PhD

Department of Neurology
University of Pennsylvania Hospital
Philadelphia, Pennsylvania

Lisa M. DeAngelis, MD

Department of Neurology
Memorial Sloan-Kettering Cancer Center
New York, New York

Jan Drappatz, MD

Division of Neuro-Oncology
Department of Neurology
Brigham and Women's Hospital
Center for Neuro-Oncology
Dana Farber/Brigham and Women's Cancer Center
Harvard Medical School
Boston, Massachusetts

James L. Fisher, PhD

Research Scientist
James Cancer Hospital
Ohio State University
Columbus, Ohio

Robin Grant, MD, FRCP

Consultant Neurologist
Edinburgh Centre for Neuro-Oncology
Western General Hospital
Edinburgh, United Kingdom

Griffith R. Harsh, MD, MBA, MA

Professor of Neurology and Neurological Sciences and Otolaryngology
Stanford University Medical Center
Stanford, California

Silvia Hofer, MD

Medical Oncology Department
University Hospital Zürich
Zürich, Switzerland;
Academic Unit of Radiotherapy and Oncology
The Institute of Cancer Research
Neuro-Oncology Unit
The Royal Marsden NHS Foundation Trust
London and Sutton, United Kingdom

Mark T. Jennings, MD

Professor of Pediatrics
Section Chief
Child Neurology University of
Illinois College of Medicine
Peoria, Illinois

Hoang-Xuan Khe, MD

AP-HP, Groupe Hospitalier Pitié-Salpêtrière
Service de Neurologie Mazarin
Paris, France

Siow Ming Lee, PhD, FRCP

Senior Lecturer in Medical Oncology
The Meyerstein Institute
Middlesex Hospital
London, United Kingdom

Srinivasan Mukundan, PhD, MD

Department of Radiology
Brigham and Women's Hospital
Boston, Massachusetts

Lakshmi Nayak, MD

Department of Neurology and Neuroscience
Weill Medical College of Cornell University;
Department of Neurology
Memorial Sloan-Kettering Cancer Center
New York, New York

Andrew D. Norden, MD

Division of Neuro-Oncology
Department of Neurology
Brigham and Women's Hospital
Center for Neuro-Oncology
Dana Farber/Brigham and Women's Cancer Center
Harvard Medical School
Boston, Massachusetts

Claudio S. Padovan, MD

Department of Neurology
Ludwig Maximilian University
Munich, Germany

Nicholas H. Post, MD

Department of Neurosurgery
New York University Medical Center
New York, New York

Nader Pouratian, MD

Department of Neurological Surgery
University of Virginia
Charlottesville, Virginia

Lawrence D. Recht, MD

Professor of Neurology
Stanford University Medical Center
Stanford, California

Jeremy Rees, PhD, FRCP

Senior Lecturer in Medical Neuro-Oncology
Honorary Consultant Neurologist
National Hospital for Neurology and Neurosurgery
London, United Kingdom

Damien Ricard, MD

Service de Neurologie
HIA du Val-de-Grâce
Paris, France

Myrna Rosenfeld, MD, PhD

Professor of Neurology
Department of Neurology
University of Pennsylvania Hospital
Philadelphia, Pennsylvania

A. Rousseau, MD

Groupe hospitalier Pitié-Salpêtrière
Laboratoire de Neuropathologie
Paris, France

Kate Scatchard, MBBS, MRCP

Medical Oncology
Middlesex Hospital
London, United Kingdom

David Schiff, MD

Department of Neurology
University of Virginia
Charlottesville, Virginia

Judith Schwartzbaum, PhD

Associate Professor
Division of Epidemiology
College of Public Health
Ohio State University
Columbus, Ohio

Jason P. Sheehan, MD, PhD

Department of Neurological Surgery
University of Virginia
Charlottesville, Virginia

Tali Siegal, MD

Director, Lesli and Michael Gaffin Center for Neuro-Oncology
Sharett Institute of Oncology
Hadassah Hebrew University Hospital
Jerusalem, Israel

Tzony Siegal, MD, DMD

Director, Chosen Specialties Clinics
Spinal Surgery Consultant
Assuta Hospital
Tel Aviv, Israel

M. Sierra del Rio, MD

Groupe Hospitalier Pitié-Salpêtrière
Service de Neurologie
Paris, France

Carole Soussain, MD

Centre René-Huguenin
Service d'Hématologie
Saint-Cloud, France

Jan Stauss, MD

Department of Radiology
Brigham and Women's Hospital
Harvard Medical School
Boston, Massachusetts

Andreas Straube, MD

Department of Neurology
Ludwig Maximilian University
Munich, Germany

Hannes Vogel, MD

Associate Chair for Neuropathology
Department of Pathology
Professor of Pathology, Pediatrics, and Neurosurgery
Stanford University Medical Center
Stanford, California

Patrick Y. Wen, MD

Associate Professor of Neurology
Harvard Medical School;
Director, Division of Cancer Neurology
Department of Neurology
Brigham and Women's Hospital;
Clinical Director
Center for Neuro-Oncology
Dana-Faber Cancer Institute
Boston, Massachusetts

Margaret R. Wrensch, PhD

Stanley D. Lewis and Virginia S. Lewis Endowed Chair in Brain Tumor Research
Professor of Neurological Surgery and Epidemiology and Biostatistics
University of California, San Francisco
San Francisco, California

Geoffrey S. Young, MD

Department of Radiology
Brigham and Women's Hospital
Harvard Medical School
Boston, Massachusetts

SERIES PREFACE

The *Blue Books of Neurology* have a long and distinguished lineage. Life began as the *Modem Trends in Neurology* series and continued with the monographs forming *BIMR Neurology*. The present series was first edited by David Marsden and Arthur Asbury, and saw the publication of 25 volumes over a period of 18 years.

The guiding principle of each volume, the topic of which is selected by the Series Editors, was that each should cover an area where there had been significant advances in research and that such progress had been translated to new or improved patient management.

This has been the guiding spirit behind each volume, and we expect it to continue. In effect, we emphasize basic, translational, and clinical research but principally to the extent that it changes our collective attitudes and practices in caring for those who are neurologically afflicted.

Tony Schapira took over as joint editor in 1999 following David's death, and together with Art oversaw the publication and preparation of a further 8 volumes. In 2005, Art Asbury ended his exceptional co-editorship after 25 years of distinguished contribution and Martin Samuels was asked to continue the co-editorship with Tony.

The current volumes represent the beginning of the next stage in the development of the Blue Books. The editors intend to build upon the excellent reputation established by the Series with a new and attractive visual style incorporating the same level of high-quality review. The ethos of the Series remains the same: up-to-date reviews of topic areas in which there have been important and exciting advances of relevance to the diagnosis and treatment of patients with neurological diseases. The intended audience remains those neurologists in training and those practicing clinicians in search of a contemporary, valuable, and interesting source of information.

ANTHONY H.V. SCHAPIRA
MARTIN A. SAMUELS
Series Editors

PREFACE

This is the first 'Blue Book' in neuro-oncology and now justifies inclusion in this illustrious Neurology series as a sign of the increasing interest and developments in this field. Indeed it is a tribute to the vision of Elsevier that such a book was commissioned, in recognition of the explosive advances in pathology, molecular biology and imaging that have transformed the landscape of neuro-oncology.

These advances, both in the clinical and scientific arena of neuro-oncology, have generated increasing optimism for our patients with these terrible diseases. As a result, a subspecialty that was only of interest to neurosurgeons and neuropathologists has now been adopted by an increasing number of disciplines to the point that clinical care is now delivered by multidisciplinary teams consisting of neurologists, radiation and medical oncologists, clinical nurse specialists, palliative care physicians, neuropsychologists and allied health professionals. It is hoped that this book will appeal to all members of the multidisciplinary team.

The book represents a collaboration between experts on both sides of the Atlantic and aims to provide a comprehensive review of the pathology, genetics, radiological and clinical features of benign and malignant tumors of the nervous system, together with chapters on metastases and the neurological complications of cancer and its treatments. Childhood brain tumors and the neurological complications of bone marrow and organ transplantation are also covered for completeness.

Most chapters have been written by one or two authors from the same institution, who have extensive experience in the management of these tumors. We have tried to recruit specialists from a number of different cancer centers to provide a variety of different viewpoints and we hope that this approach will provide a well-balanced reference for those who work in this field.

We would like to dedicate this work to those patients and their families who live every day with the daunting challenge of these diseases.

JEREMY H. REES, PhD, FRCP
PATRICK Y. WEN, MD

1 Pathology and Molecular Genetics of Common Brain Tumors

V. PETER COLLINS

Introduction

This chapter aims to provide an outline of the surgical pathology and the recognized genetic and molecular changes of common tumors of the nervous system in children and adults. The current World Health Organization (WHO) histological classification for nervous system tumors will be used as its framework.[1] The histological basis for classification and malignancy grading of the tumors is briefly presented and some of the common diagnostic problems outlined. The WHO classification is complex, listing over 120 histological entities. In the case of some of the tumors recognized, there is as yet only a histological description and no genetic information is available. The reader is referred to the fourth edition of the WHO classification of tumors of the nervous system and the specialized literature for the tumor types not addressed here.[1] The genetic and molecular information we have on the common tumors is steadily increasing, but is still rudimentary. While the genetic and molecular findings are not, as yet used, clinically, as soon as molecular targeted therapies become available and are found to be effective, histological investigation will *have* to be supplemented with molecular data.

Most classifications of brain tumors presented during the last 60 years build on the 1926 work of Bailey and Cushing.[2] In their classification, tumors were named after the recognized cell types in the developing embryo/fetus or adult that the tumor cells most resembled histologically. The cell type of origin of the majority of brain tumors is unknown, as no premalignant states are recognized. In some tumors the cells may be so dysplastic that they show no similarities to any normal cell type—thus the use of terms such as glioblastoma. In the present WHO classification (for an overview, see Table 1-1), tumors are divided up into those of neuroepithelial origin (includes the glial, glioneuronal, neuronal, pineal and embryonal tumors), tumors of cranial and paraspinal nerves, tumors of the meninges, lymphomas and hematopoetic neoplasms, germ cell tumors, tumors of the sellar region and metastases. The tumor types and their possible WHO grades are given in Table 1-1.

It is impossible to cover the histopathology and genetics of all these different tumor types in one chapter, so the focus will be on the common tumors of children (pilocytic astrocytomas, ependymomas, and medulloblastomas), and of adults (the diffuse astrocytic tumors including astrocytomas, anaplastic astrocytomas, and glioblastomas, as well as oligodendrogliomas and meningiomas). In addition, lymphomas and metastases will be very briefly considered.

GENERAL CONSIDERATIONS

Many brain tumors are morphologically heterogeneous, and many brain tumor types are known to become more malignant with time, with their progression initially being focal. Thus, for both reasons, adequate sampling of a tumor is essential to determine the correct tumor classification or type of tumor as well as the WHO grade. Classification of brain tumors is dependent on the recognition of areas with the characteristic histology for a particular tumor type, often assisted by immunocytochemical methods. Immunocytochemistry permits the demonstration of antigens associated with a particular cell type and even their subcellular location. As yet, there are no single antibodies or even panels of antibodies that unequivocally identify any of the brain tumors listed in the 2007 WHO classification.[2] Thus, the presence or absence of an antigen only adds a further piece of information, helping to indicate the tumor type.

Once a tumor has been classified, the histologically most malignant part of the tumor determines the malignancy grade (often referred to as the WHO grade when using the criteria defined by the WHO classification).[1] The histological criteria for malignancy grading are not uniform for all tumor types and thus all tumors must be classified first before a WHO malignancy grade can be determined. The WHO system recognizes four grades of malignancy; these provide an assessment of the biological aggressiveness of the untreated tumor. Grade I tumors are the biologically least aggressive and may be cured by surgery alone (e.g., pilocytic astrocytoma). Grade IV tumors are biologically highly aggressive, with rapid growth and the ability to infiltrate locally and disseminate within the central nervous system. Untreated, they are rapidly fatal (e.g., glioblastoma). General criteria for determining WHO malignancy grade include cellularity, degree of polymorphism and atypia, the incidence of mitoses, the presence of spontaneous necrosis and the degree of angiogenesis induced by the tumor (microvascular proliferation), but, as indicated above, these are not universal. The criteria for determining the WHO grade for each tumor type have been empirically derived by correlating the histology of surgically removed tumor tissue with otherwise untreated patient survival. Extrapolation from such studies provides a basis for

TABLE 1-1 Familial Syndromes Associated with Human Brain Tumors

Disorder	Gene	Location	Protein function	Tumor types associated with disorder	Involved in sporadic CNS tumors	References
Neurofibromatosis type 1	*NF1*	17p11.2	GTPase activating protein homology	Astrocytomas (brain stem, optic nerve) ependymomas, PNETs and meningiomas (pheochromocytoma), etc.	Unknown	246
Neurofibromatosis type 2	*NF2*	22q12.2	Ezrin/moesin/ radixin-like	Vestibular schwannomas, meningiomas, spinal schwannomas	Meningiomas, schwannomas	247
Turcot syndrome A	*APC*	5q21-q22	Regulates β-catenin	Medulloblastoma	Unknown	248
Turcot syndrome B	*MLH1* *MSH2* *MLH3* *PMS1* *PMS2*	3p21.3 2p22-p21 14q24 2q31-q33 7p22	Microsatellite instability (MIN+)	Glioblastoma (unknown if all germline mutations are associated with glioblastoma)	Unknown; astrocytic tumors that are MIN+ occur but are uncommon	249
Basal cell nevus syndrome/ Gorlin syndrome	*PTCH*	9q22.3	Receptor for SHH inhibits SMO	Medulloblastoma	Medulloblastoma	248
Cowden disease (multiple hamartoma syndrome, Lhermitte-Duclos, etc.)	*PTEN*	10q22-q23	Dual specificity phosphatase and tensin homology	Astrocytomas reported but tumors in other organs more common—thyroid, breast, female genitourinary tract	Glioblastoma	250
Tuberous sclerosis	*TSC1*	9q34 (40%)	Binds to pTSC2	Subependymal giant cell astrocytoma as well as various harmartomas	Unknown	251

Table continued on following page

TABLE 1-1 Familial Syndromes Associated with Human Brain Tumors (Continued)

Disorder	Gene	Location	Protein function	Tumor types associated with disorder	Involved in sporadic CNS tumors	References
	TSC2	16p13.3	GTPase activating protein homology	Subependymal giant cell astrocytoma as well as various harmartomas	?	251
von Hippel-Lindau	*VHL*	3p26-p25	Part of a transcription elongation factor inhibiting, e.g., VEGF expression	Hemangioblastoma (pheochromocytoma/ RCC, etc.)	Unknown	252
Li Fraumeni	*TP53 (only 70%)*	17p13.1	Transcription factor, apoptosis induction, etc.	Many including astrocytomas	Mainly astrocytic	253, 254
Melanoma-astrocytoma syndrome	*CDKN2A/ p14ARF*	9p21	Cell cycle control (G1-S)/p53 level control	Astrocytomas	Astrocytic	255

an assessment of prognosis, but the provision of therapy may radically alter this assessment.

Tumor type and grade generally determine the choice of conventional therapy. It is important to remember that radiation therapy or chemotherapy administered prior to histological diagnosis will alter tumor morphology, making classification and grading extremely difficult or impossible. The WHO morphological criteria have been determined for untreated tumors. In addition, WHO grading of a biopsy is always considered a minimum malignancy grading, as more anaplastic regions may be present in unbiopsied areas of the tumor.

The use of objective methods of measuring cell proliferation and cell death (apoptosis) in tumors to determine WHO malignancy grade is conceptually attractive. However, the wide variations in proliferation indices observed in different areas of individual tumors have resulted in difficulties in defining relevant proliferation levels. The same applies to the assessment of the numbers of cells undergoing apoptosis. In the WHO system, mitotic counts (mitoses per ten $0.16\,mm^2$ high power fields) are currently only used in the grading of meningiomas. The MIB-1 antibody that recognizes the same antigen as the Ki67 antibody and thus cells in the cell cycle can also be used to assess cell cycle activity. Other antibodies that identify antigens associated with proliferation (e.g., Cdc6 and Mcm5) can be applied to formalin-fixed, paraffin-embedded tissues following microwave antigen retrieval.[3,4] However, the WHO system generally only gives information on commonly observed ranges for both the mitotic index and MIB index for most tumor types and WHO malignancy grades.

Today, almost any neoplastic or nonneoplastic lesion in the CNS can be biopsied using widely available neuroradiological and stereotactic techniques. The list of potential diagnoses a neuropathologist may be expected to make, often on the basis of very small and fragmented biopsies, is vast. The importance of clinical information cannot be overemphasized. Information must be provided to the neuropathologist on age, neuroradiological findings including location of the lesion, relevant clinical and family history, and whether the patient has received *any* treatment, including steroids. In the case of stereotactic biopsies, morphology combined with immunocytochemistry may only provide a differential diagnosis with the most likely diagnosis being reached by considering all the information available at a multidisciplinary team meeting.

Most brain tumors are sporadic. However, a number of familial cancer syndromes are associated with an increased risk of brain tumors (see Table 1-1 and the references therein). Even in the case of the commonest syndromes (neurofibromatosis type 1 and neurofibromatosis type 2), the precise relative risk is difficult to define.

In contrast to many epithelial neoplasms, no lesion is recognized as a precursor for any brain tumor type and, as a result, the cell of origin of these monoclonal proliferations is unknown in all cases. Recent work in animal models provides some data supporting the idea that some brain tumors arise from neuroectodermal stem cells. They are present throughout life, have proliferative potential, are migratory and can differentiate along a number of paths—all features they have in common with brain tumor cells. Furthermore, there is some evidence that at least some of the common types of brain tumors may be made up of a smallish population of therapy-resistant tumor-initiating cells (also called tumor stem cells in some texts), with the main bulk of the tumor consisting of a progeny lacking these tumor-initiating abilities.[5–9] If this tumor-initiating cell population is not eradicated, the tumor will recur–a common experience with current therapies for many of the malignant brain tumors. Thus, much effort is currently being channeled into defining and studying this subpopulation in the hope of finding ways to specifically kill these cells.[10,11] While the genetic status (e.g., gene copy number, mutations, amplifications, etc.) of tumor-initiating cells and their progeny is likely to be identical, the epigenetic status (e.g., methylation) and the expression characteristics may differ considerably.

Childhood Tumors

PILOCYTIC ASTROCYTOMAS

The astrocytomas encompass a number of tumors of differing grade including the pilocytic astrocytomas. The majority of astrocytomas are found in adults (see following discussion). The commonest form of astrocytoma found in children is the pilocytic astrocytoma, WHO malignancy grade I. These tumors may arise anywhere from the optic nerve to the medulla oblongata. They most commonly occur in the cerebellum. They may be solid, mono- or polycystic and are generally well circumscribed. The prognosis for patients with pilocytic astrocytomas that can be excised is relatively good, with over 90% 10-year survival reported.[12] Pilocytic astrocytomas are generally biologically unaggressive, and, in contrast to the adult diffuse astrocytic tumors, maintain their grade I status over years and even decades. Only very occasionally will these tumors progress to malignant astrocytic tumors or seed the neuroaxis.[13] Pilocytic astrocytomas show a wide morphological spectrum, from pilocytic bipolar cellular areas with Rosenthal fibers (Fig. 1-1A) to less cellular protoplasmic astrocytoma-like areas with eosinophilic granular bodies and clear cells. Such clear-cell areas are reminiscent of oligodendrogliomas and, in the posterior fossa, may also be confused with clear cell ependymomas, particularly in biopsies. The presence of features typically associated with a malignant biological behavior (e.g., atypia, microvascular proliferation (Fig. 1-1B), or even mitosis) does not carry the same sinister implications as in the adult diffuse astrocytic tumors. This morphological variability can make histopathological diagnosis extremely difficult. NF1 patients have an increased incidence of pilocytic astrocytomas, particularly involving the optic nerve, and these behave in a particularly benign fashion.[14]

Many cases of pilocytic astrocytomas have been studied cytogenetically and further cases analyzed using conventional comparative genomic hybridization (cCGH). Many show normal cytogenetic and cCGH findings.[15–18] Polysomy has been found, most commonly of chromosomes 5 and 7, and, in addition, of chromosomes 6, 11, 15, and 20 (in decreasing frequency). Polysomy has been reported to be most common in adult patients with pilocytic astrocytoma.[19] Molecular genetic studies have been few; single *TP53* mutations have been reported, and loss of one allele of *NF1* has been found in pilocytic tumors from NF1 patients but not in sporadic cases.[20–24] Studies of promotor methylation of some genes known to be involved in adult diffuse astrocytic gliomas have provided inconsistent data.[25,26] There appears to be no evidence for methylation of the *NF1* gene in sporadic tumors.[27] Recently a number of groups have noted that a small region on 7q34 has

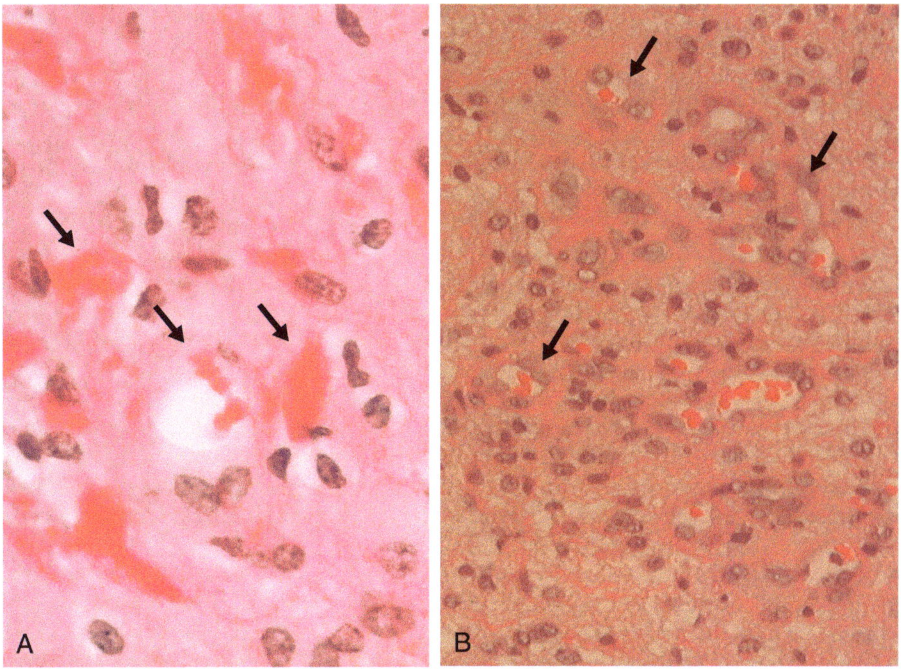

Figure 1-1 Pilocytic astrocytoma WHO grade I. A, An area with many Rosenthal fibers (arrows). **B,** This shows an area with microvascular proliferation (arrows) in an otherwise typical pilocytic astrocytoma. (H&E)

increased copy number in a high percentage of pilocytic astrocytomas.[28–30] Further studies by Jones et al. showed this to be a tandem duplication of approximately 2 Mb resulting in an in-frame fusion gene encoding the kinase domain of the *BRAF* proto-oncogene. The fusion protein was shown to have constitutive kinase activity and to transform NIH3T3 cells. This rearrangement produced a specific and unique fusion *BRAF* oncogene in 29/44 (66%) of the pilocytic astrocytomas. An additional two tumors showed the well-known *BRAF* V600E mutation and a further three tumors were in patients diagnosed with the NF1 syndrome. Thus, a total of 34/44 (77%) of the pilocytic tumors in the series showed alterations in the MAPK (mitogen-activated protein kinase) pathway.[29] This tandem duplication producing a fusion oncogene was not found in over 200 high-grade astrocytic tumors, demonstrating the specificity of the finding. As this rearrangement occurs in the majority of pilocytic astrocytomas, it provides a diagnostic marker for this tumor type as well as a potential target for molecular therapies.

EPENDYMOMA

There are four WHO malignancy grades of ependymal tumors. The grade I tumors include the subependymoma (usually found incidentally on the surface of the ventricular system in middle-aged or elderly patients) and the myxopapillary ependymoma (usually at the cauda equina and mainly in adults). The ependymoma WHO grade II accounts for about 10% of all intracranial tumors in children. It is most frequent in children under 3 years old, but is also the most common adult tumor of the spinal cord. Anaplastic ependymomas WHO grade III occur mainly intracranially, and their incidence is uncertain due to unclear histological criteria for this diagnosis. Ependymoblastoma WHO grade IV is a highly malignant tumor that in the current WHO classification is placed among the embryonal tumors, in the primitive neuroectodermal tumor subgroup. Ependymoblastoma is a rare entity occurring in neonates and very young children.

Ependymomas arise at or close to ependymal surfaces (ventricular system and the spinal canal) and very occasionally at extraneural sites. The commonest location is in the fourth ventricle, followed by the spinal canal (in adults), the lateral ventricles, and the third ventricle. The formation of ependymal rosettes and sometimes canals (Fig. 1-2), in some area of the tumor is a key histological feature. More commonly, perivascular pseudorosettes are found; however, these are not specific to ependymomas and can occur in other gliomas. As indicated above, the differentiation of ependymomas (WHO grade II) from anaplastic ependymomas (WHO grade III) is not well defined and is usually based on low mitotic rate, low levels of cellularity and nuclear polymorphism. Necrosis and microvascular proliferation do not have the same significance in this tumor type as in the adult astrocytic tumors described later in this chapter. Most ependymomas (WHO grade II) show immunoreactivity for glial fibrillary acidic protein (GFAP), S-100 protein, and epithelial membrane antigen (EMA). There have been a number of immunocytochemical studies attempting to identify prognostic markers. Some have been shown to be significant in single reports, but require confirmation.[31–33] Among these, the expression of human telomere reverse transcriptase (hTERT) has been recently reported as a predictive marker of poor outcome in pediatric intracranial ependymomas.[34] The cell of origin of these tumors has been suggested to be the radial glia cell.[35]

Classical cytogenetic, metaphase, and array CGH studies as well as molecular genetic studies have identified copy number abnormalities that affect almost all chromosomes in the majority of ependymoma types.[20,36–47] Even the often incidentally discovered and very benign subependymomas show copy number changes involving, in some cases, chromosomes 6, 7, 8, and 14 in some cases.[46] Myxopapillary ependymomas frequently show concurrent gain of chromosomes

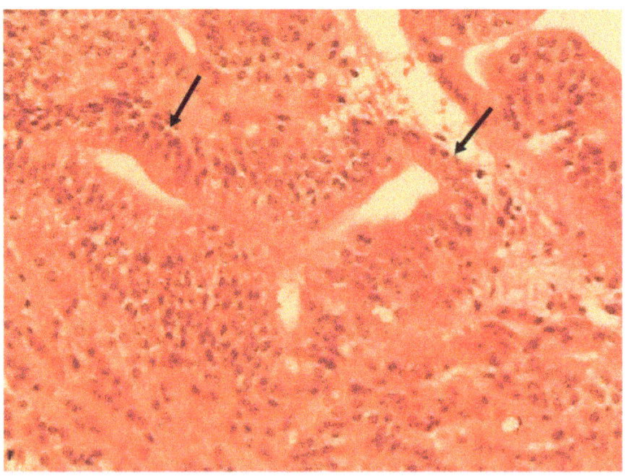

Figure 1-2 Ependymoma WHO grade II. Note the multiple ependymal canals (arrows) lined by tumor cells resembling a normal ependymal surface. Note that the tumor is relatively cellular (compare with the diffuse astrocytoma WHO grade II, Fig. 1-4A). (H&E)

9 and 18.[41] Deletions and regions of increased copy number are common in the ependymomas WHO grade II and the anaplastic ependymomas WHO grade III. Losses on chromosome 22 were an early finding (20) and this has been shown to be a frequent event, particularly in adult spinal ependymomas (over 50%). This is true both of ependymomas arising in patients with the neurofibromatosis Type 2 (NF2) syndrome as well as in sporadic cases, but is less frequent in pediatric and intracranial ependymomas.[42,48] Loss of both wild-type copies of the *NF2* gene has been demonstrated in both the sporadic and NF2 syndrome-related intramedullary spinal ependymomas of adults.[37,49,50] This occurs in the NF2 patients by loss of the single wild-type *NF2* gene with retention of the constitutively mutated copy, while in the sporadic cases it is generally by loss of most of one 22q and somatic mutation of the single retained *NF2* gene.[37,50–53] Some ependymomas have been reported to have no apparent abnormalities, but this probably reflects on the level of resolution obtained with the analytical method used. The genes targeted by the allelic losses and gains in ependymomas are in most cases unknown. Some studies have attempted to correlate chromosomal abnormalities with progression-free survival or overall survival. The findings to date indicate that gain of 1q is associated with a worse clinical outcome.[38,42,54] Gains of 7q and 9p as well as losses of 17 and 22 have been reported to occur more frequently in recurrent tumors.[55] Single cases have been reported with loss of the wild-type allele of genes such as the *MEN1* gene.[50,56] Mutations of *TP53* or genetic changes affecting the integrity of the p53 pathway are uncommon in ependymomas. This contrasts with their frequency in the diffuse astrocytic tumors.[57–60] More recently, global gene expression has been analyzed in ependymomas; preliminary findings suggest that there are specific expression profiles associated with the various histological subtypes and even patient survival.[43,61,62] Most of these studies have been done on relatively small series of tumors and much further work is required before any of the findings can be introduced into clinical practice.

MEDULLOBLASTOMA

Medulloblastomas are highly malignant tumors and are WHO graded as IV. They have a peak incidence in childhood (around 7 years of age) but can occur into late middle age. Childhood and adult medulloblastomas are histologically identical being highly cellular, malignant, invasive tumors occurring in the posterior fossa. There are a number of subtypes; these include the classic, desmoplastic/nodular, large cell, and anaplastic cell variants. The large cell and anaplastic cell variants can be difficult to differentiate, but both have a significantly poorer prognosis than the other subtypes and therefore need to be recognized. All subtypes can show production of melanin and focal myogenic differentiation. Medulloblastomas in children (particularly the large cell variant) must be differentiated histologically from atypical teratoid or rhabdoid tumors, which have an extremely poor clinical outcome and do not respond to the current relatively successful treatment protocols for medulloblastomas.[63–67] Loss of wild-type INI1/hSHF5/SMARCB1 genes is the genetic hallmark of the atypical teratoid or rhabdoid tumors.[68,69] Classical medulloblastomas consist of densely packed tumor cells with round to oval or carrot-shaped hyperchromatic nuclei with scanty cytoplasm, high mitotic and apoptotic rates, and usually neuroblastic rosettes in

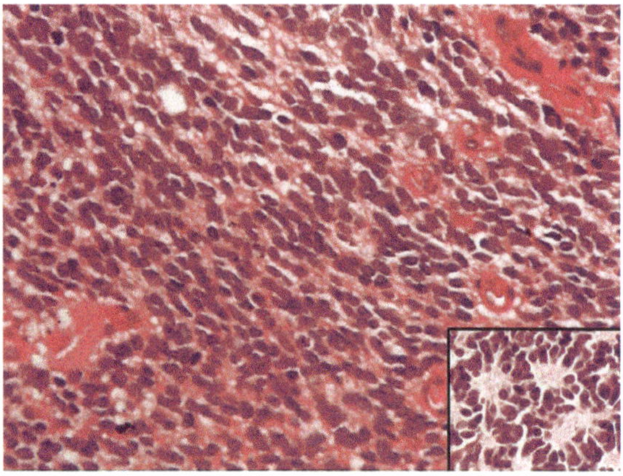

Figure 1-3 Medulloblastoma WHO grade IV with typical neuroblastic rosettes (inset). Rosettes can be difficult to find in some cases. (H&E)

some areas (Fig. 1-3). In adults, the possibility of a metastasis of a small-cell lung cancer must often be excluded. Neuronal differentiation and glial differentiation may be present, particularly in the nodular areas of the desmoplastic/nodular and medulloblastoma with extensive nodularity variants. Microvascular proliferation is uncommon. Tumors arise with similar frequency in the cerebellar vermis (mainly in children) and the cerebellar hemispheres (older patients) and often invade the fourth ventricle, with occasional brainstem involvement. There is a high risk of seeding through the subarachnoid space due to the tendency of the tumor to penetrate the ependymal surface. Many antigens can be identified focally in medulloblastomas (nestin, vimentin, neurofilament proteins, GFAP, retinal S-antigen, N-CAMs, Trk-A, -B, -C, etc.) and while most are not of any great importance in the diagnosis of classical cases, the identification of EMA and smooth muscle actin will help differentiate atypical teratoid tumors from the large cell medulloblastomas.

Immunocytochemically-identifiable prognostic markers in medulloblastoma have been reported. High nuclear expression of p53 and high expression levels of Erb-B2 (Her2) have been reported as indicators of a poor outcome.[70–77] Studies of TrkB mRNA levels have indicated that high levels are associated with a favorable outcome, however, some immunocytochemical studies of TrkB have not shown any differences between patients with tumors expressing the protein and those without.[78,79] There have also been a number of gene-expression profiling studies of medulloblastomas and these, by correlating the data with outcome, have attempted to identify expression signatures indicating a good or bad prognosis.[80,81]

At the genetic level, gain of 17q and loss of 17p are common findings. Generally, this is associated with the formation of isodicentric 17q (previously inaccurately called isochromosome 17q). Isodicentric 17q consists of two 17q with two centromeres and two small fragments of proximal 17p fused at the terminal ends of the 17p sequences.[82,83] The fusion occurs in a number ways in a region of complex repeat sequences.[82] Isodicentric 17q is observed in 30% to 50% of cases. Other frequent copy number aberrations reported are gain of the whole of 1q, gain of chromosome 7, and loss of 10q (84–89). Amplification of each of the three *MYC* genes has been found in individual cases; this is associated with a poor survival.[82,90,91] Other genes found to be amplified in individual cases include *PDGFRA*, *KIT*, OTX2 (14q21-q22), and *MYB*.[82,92,93] Various candidate genes have been examined in the common regions of loss including *TP53*, *HIC1*, and *KCTD11* on 17p and *DMBT1*, *PTEN*, and *SUFU* on 10q. Only single cases with *TP53* mutations have been found but a significant incidence of methylation of the *HIC1* gene has been reported. *DMBT1* has been identified as a deletion polymorphism in humans and the losses are therefore unlikely to be of significance. Single mutations of *PTEN* have been documented, and while constitutive *SUFU* mutations have been found in some children with medulloblastoma and seem to predispose to medulloblastoma in mice, no mutations have been identified in sporadic medulloblastomas.[94–98] Metastatic disease has been reported to be associated with elevated expression levels of PDGF receptors and ligands by tumor cells.[99,100]

The study of two familial tumor syndromes exhibiting a predisposition to medulloblastoma formation has led to major advances in our understanding of medulloblastoma biology. Gorlin syndrome (also known as hereditary nevoid basal cell carcinoma syndrome) and Turcot syndrome type A (associated with the familial adenomatous polyposis [FAP] syndrome) are due to inherited mutations of one copy of the *PTCH* (9q) and the *APC* (5q) genes respectively. The protein products of these two genes are involved in two interconnected cellular pathways that are fundamental to neural development and cell turnover. Hemizygous loss and mutation of the retained allele of *PTCH* in sporadic medulloblastomas has been demonstrated.[101,102] Mutations in other genes coding for components of the PTCH pathway have also been reported, if only in single cases. These include *SMO*[103–105] and *SUFU*.[95,98] All these mutations result in activation of the pathway, with increased transcription of a group of genes including *WNT* (see following discussion). Thus, inhibitors of this pathway could be therapeutically useful. Cyclopamine is a natural alkaloid that inhibits the PTCH pathway; this and other inhibitors are currently being investigated.[106,107] A key protein in the Wnt pathway is APC, and it is the inheritance of a mutated *APC* gene that causes FAP syndrome. In sporadic tumors, only a few *APC* mutations have been identified. APC forms a complex with at least seven proteins that bind hyperphosphorylated β-catenin, permitting its ubiquitination and thus targeting β-catenin for degradation. This mechanism is important for the control of cellular levels of β-catenin. Tumor-specific mutations affecting the region of β-catenin that is phosphorylated (a requirement for sequestration by the APC complex) and the ubiquitin-binding region have been reported.[108,109] This would allow cellular β-catenin to escape this control mechanism and to accumulate and act as a transcription factor. Mutations of *AXIN1*, a gene coding for one of the proteins in the APC complex, have also been found.[110] Thus, disruption of these complex pathways, upstream or downstream of WNT, is associated with the development of medulloblastoma. This also clearly demonstrates that a cellular mechanism can be disrupted by mutations of many different genes coding for the proteins involved, indicating that it is the pathway that is the target in oncogenesis and not a particular gene. Further examples of this will be seen later in this chapter. Despite these advances, alterations in the genes coding for components of the PTCH and WNT/APC pathways have only been found in a small percentage of sporadic tumors.[111,112] However, the WNT signaling is extremely complex and many aspects have yet to be investigated.[113]

Common Adult Tumors

DIFFUSE ASTROCYTIC TUMORS

The diffuse astrocytic tumors include the astrocytomas (WHO grade II), the anaplastic astrocytomas (WHO grade III), as well as the glioblastomas (Fig. 1-4). These tumors predominate in adults, with the most malignant form, the glioblastoma WHO grade IV being the most common. The astrocytoma WHO grade II tumors (A) have a peak incidence in people between 25 and 50 years of age, while the peak incidence of glioblastomas (GB) is in those between 45 and 70. All are commoner in males and most are located in the cerebral hemispheres. The astrocytomas (WHO grade II) and anaplastic astrocytomas have been well documented to progress to tumors of higher malignancy grade.[114,115] Glioblastomas are therefore divided into those that develop by progression from a previously diagnosed tumor of lower malignancy grade and those that appear to develop de novo.[116,117] Both clinical and molecular data support the hypothesis that although these

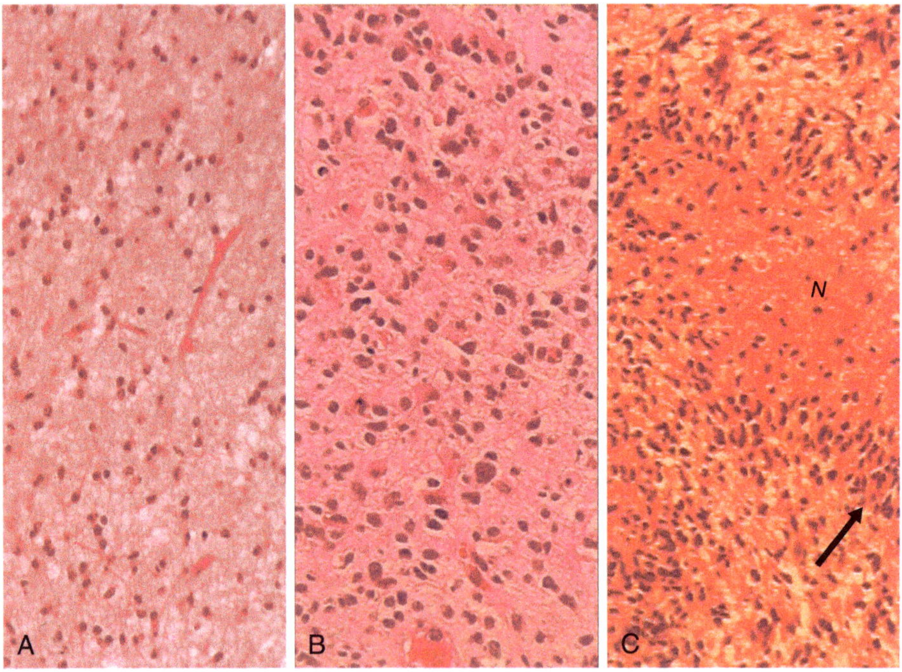

Figure 1-4 **A, Astrocytoma WHO grade II;** note the monomorphic tumor cell population with their extensions producing a loosely textured matrix. **B, Anaplastic astrocytoma WHO grade III,** with increased cellularity and polymorphism but lacking microvascular proliferation and necrosis. **C, Glioblastoma WHO grade IV.** Note high cellularity, polymorphism, with pseudopalisading (arrow) around an area of necrosis (*N*). (H&E)

tumors may arise due to the mutation of different genes, the gene mutations target and disrupt the same cellular pathways.[60,118–120] The relevance of the histologically based malignancy-grading scheme is demonstrated by its prognostic value. Patients with a diffuse astrocytoma (WHO grade II) have an median survival of between 6 and 7 years, patients with anaplastic astrocytomas (WHO grade III) have a median survival half that time,[121] while glioblastoma (WHO grade IV) patients have an average survival of a little over 1 year using the latest therapeutic regimens.[122,123] The combination of radiotherapy with temozolomide, following debulking surgery, has improved outcome from a median survival in this group of 9 to 11 months, when treated with conventional surgery followed by radiotherapy and various chemotherapy regimens, to 14.6 months.[123] As the term "diffuse astrocytoma" implies, these tumors do not have a clear border and show varying levels of infiltration into the surrounding brain (Fig. 1-5 A-D). Infiltrative ability varies widely from astrocytic tumors that are relatively well localized (rare) to gliomatosis cerebri (also rare), where there is extensive infiltration of a large region of the central nervous system.

In diffuse astrocytomas (WHO grade II) the tumor cells morphologically resemble astrocytes, generally show little nuclear atypia, and have extensions producing

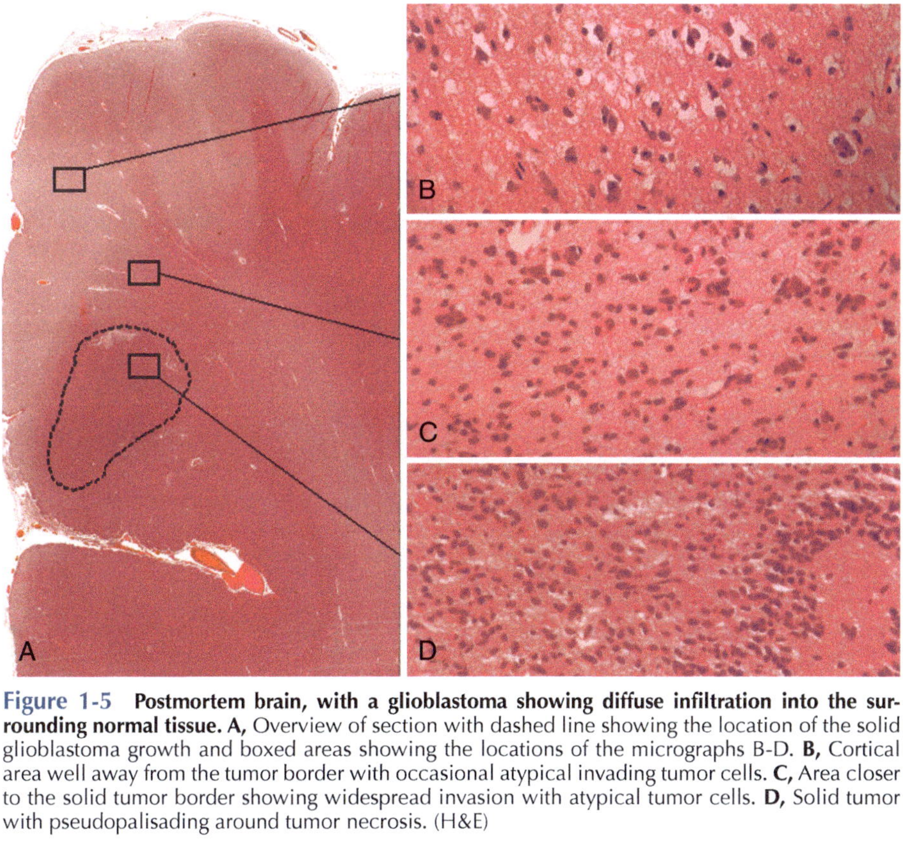

Figure 1-5 Postmortem brain, with a glioblastoma showing diffuse infiltration into the surrounding normal tissue. A, Overview of section with dashed line showing the location of the solid glioblastoma growth and boxed areas showing the locations of the micrographs B-D. **B,** Cortical area well away from the tumor border with occasional atypical invading tumor cells. **C,** Area closer to the solid tumor border showing widespread invasion with atypical tumor cells. **D,** Solid tumor with pseudopalisading around tumor necrosis. (H&E)

a loosely textured matrix (Fig. 1-4A). They usually express S-100 protein and glial fibrillary acidic protein. Anaplastic astrocytomas (WHO grade III) are more cellular, with pleomorphic tumor cells showing nuclear atypia. There is some mitotic activity, but the tumor cells generally still display the histological and immunocytochemical characteristics of astrocytes (Fig. 1-4B). No evidence of spontaneous tumor necrosis or abnormal microvascular proliferation is permitted in anaplastic astrocytomas. Glioblastomas (WHO grade IV) are more cellular than the anaplastic astrocytomas and show a wide spectrum of morphologies. They can be very pleomorphic with giant-cell forms, but generally retain some of the phenotypical characteristics of astrocytes. Mitosis, spontaneous tumor necrosis with pseudopalisading of tumor cells, as well as florid endothelial proliferation are inevitably found in some areas of a well-sampled tumor (Fig. 1-4C). A large central necrotic area with a ring-like zone of contrast enhancement, representing the viable tumor tissue, can often be identified by neuroimaging.

The following section will describe the major genetic abnormalities known in all three grades (II–IV) of diffuse astrocytomas. A simplified overview of the function of some of the proteins encoded by the genes referred to in the text is provided in Figs. 1-6 and 1-7. Cytogenetic and molecular data is limited on the

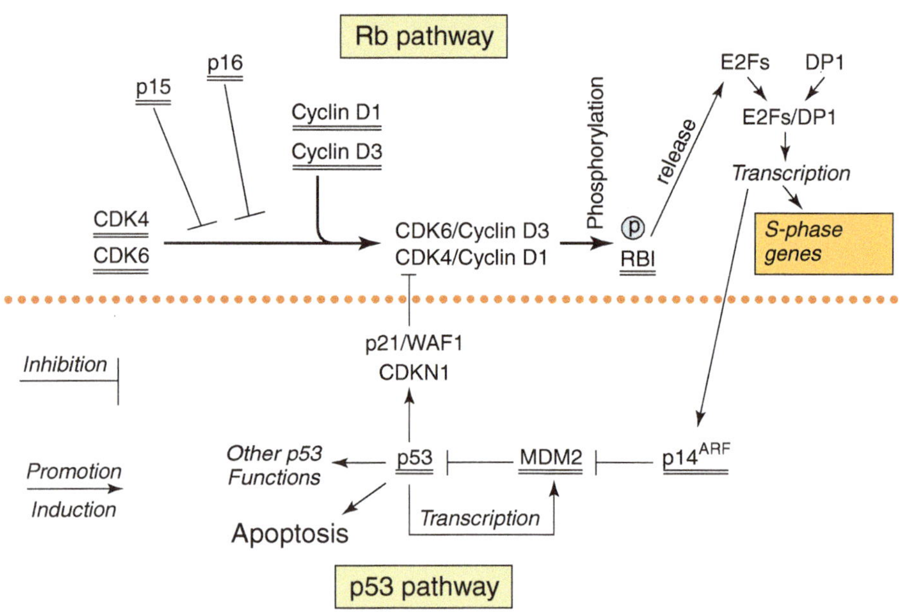

Figure 1-6 Simplified diagram outlining the interactions between the proteins of the Rb1 pathway (above) and the p53 pathway (below). The genes coding for p16 and p15 proteins are *CDKN2A* and *CDKN2B* respectively. The genes for all of the proteins underlined have been shown to be abnormal in the astrocytic and some other gliomas as well as in many other human tumor types. In the vast majority of cases, where a pathway is disrupted in a tumor it is due to only *one* of the genes coding for a protein in that pathway being abnormal (loss of both wild-type copies in the case of most tumor suppressor genes, or mutation, amplification and overexpression in the case of proto-oncogenes). Thus, the *pathways* targeted in oncogenesis and progression can be disrupted in many ways.

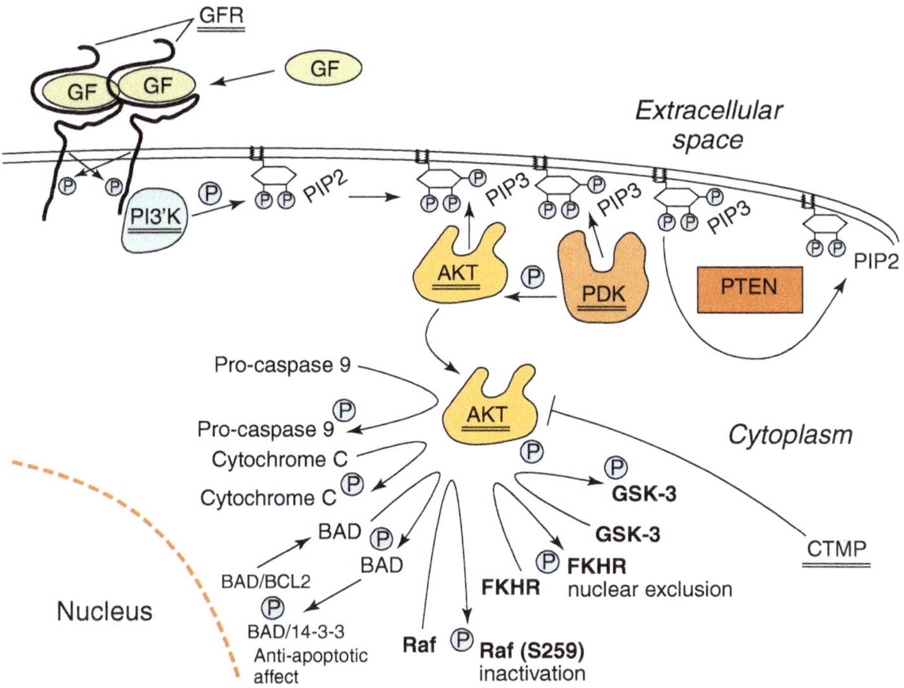

Figure 1-7 Simple diagram of signal transduction from cell surface growth factor receptors (GFR) via the PI3K/AKT pathway. Note that the well-known RAS/RAF/MAP kinase pathway is omitted. GF=growth factor; GFR = growth factor receptor. The genes for all the proteins underlined have been found to be mutated in human glioblastomas (see text for details).

diffuse astrocytomas (WHO grade II), as they are less common.[15,124,125] Over 60% of these tumors have loss of alleles on 17p including the *TP53* locus, and the retained *TP53* allele is mutated in the majority of cases.[60,126,127] The absence of wild-type p53 is therefore the commonest abnormal finding,[60,128] resulting in a nonfunctional p53 pathway. A small percentage of tumors have mutations of one allele but retain one wild-type allele. As the p53 protein is believed to function as a tetramer, and as tetramers with one abnormal p53 protein may not function normally, the finding of single mutated alleles together with a wild-type allele may be significant. Other genes coding for components of the p53 pathway (see Fig. 1-6), *MDM2* and *p14(ARF)* have been studied in small numbers of tumors and no abnormalities have been reported. Studies of the *TP53* related gene, *P73*, have not identified any mutations.[129] Loss of alleles from 6q, 13q, and 22q occur in some diffuse astrocytomas (WHO grade II). In tumors with LOH at 13q14.2 that encompass one copy of the *RB1* gene, there is no evidence of mutation of the single retained gene copy.[130] The same is true for the losses from 22q encompassing one *NF2* tumor suppressor gene.[131,132] Deletion mapping of chromosome 6 shows losses on 6q in a significant number of diffuse astrocytomas WHO grade II.[133] The potential tumor suppressor genes in all of these regions remain unknown. There are no consistently reported amplified genes or amplified regions of the genome in these astrocytomas.[130,134–137]

High-level expression of the PDGF ligands and receptors has been observed in all grades of astrocytic tumor, suggesting the presence of autocrine/paracrine loops.[138–141] Intracranial injection of a retrovirus containing *PDGF*-B induced glioblastomas in mice, suggesting involvement of the PDGF system in the pathogenesis of astrocytic tumors.[142] Overexpression is not associated with amplification except in the case of the PDGFA receptor gene (*PDGFAR*), which has been reported to be amplified and overexpressed in small subset of glioblastomas.[143–145]

Epigenetic changes such as hypermethylation of tumor suppressor gene promoters have only recently received attention. There is some evidence that some tumor suppressors are methylated in diffuse astrocytomas WHO grade II (e.g., the *PTEN* gene).[146] However, there are likely to be many other genes affected by aberrant methylation in the case of the astrocytomas WHO grade II.[147,148] The changes found in the astrocytomas WHO grade II form the baseline for studies of the genetic abnormalities associated with progression in the adult diffuse astrocytic tumors.

The genetic data on the anaplastic astrocytomas (WHO grade III) is also limited. Loss of one copy and mutation of the retained copy of *TP53* occur at approximately the same frequency as in the diffuse astrocytomas (WHO grade II).[60] Thus, the p53 pathway is nonfunctional in the majority of cases (more than 60%). Cytogenetics, comparative genomic hybridization, and molecular genetic techniques all show that losses of genetic material from 6q, 13q, 17p, and 22q, as seen in the WHO grade II astrocytomas, occur at similar or higher frequencies in anaplastic astrocytomas. With the sole exception of copy number abnormalities of 19q probably representing extra copies (targeted gene[s] unknown), there are no conclusively demonstrated abnormalities specific to this WHO grade. Around 20% of anaplastic astrocytomas show similar genetic abnormalities to those found in glioblastomas, involving other components of the p53 pathway (i.e., *MDM2* and *p14(ARF)*) and leading to disruption of the Rb1 pathway (Fig. 1-6); these are discussed in the glioblastoma section.[60]

The majority of glioblastomas arise de novo; this has ensured their study in considerable numbers.[12] Secondary glioblastomas are less frequent and have only been studied in comparatively small numbers.[149,150] Such patients will generally have been treated by irradiation and/or chemotherapy. Glioblastomas show the greatest numbers of genetic abnormalities among the astrocytic tumors, and clear patterns of genetic aberrations are emerging. The *TP53* gene is only mutated in about 37% of glioblastomas.[60] However, the p53 pathway is targeted by mutations of other genes coding for proteins that control cellular p53 levels. The two genes whose products are involved in controlling p53 levels are *p14(ARF)* and *MDM2*. *p14(ARF)* controls the activity of *MDM2*,[151] which in its turn controls the breakdown of p53.[152] Loss of both copies of the *p14(ARF)* gene or amplification and overexpression of *MDM2* will lead to the rapid breakdown of wild-type p53 protein, resulting in a cell with little or no wild-type p53 (see Fig. 1-6). The vast majority of glioblastomas (over 70%) have either no wild-type p53 *or* no p14(ARF) *or* have amplification and overexpression of MDM2 as mutually exclusive genetic abnormalities.[60] Methylation of the p14(ARF) promoter with decreased or no expression are further mechanisms that have been shown to be involved in some tumors.[153]

Similarly, one or another of the genes coding for proteins involved in the control of entry into the S-phase of the cell cycle (the retinoblastoma pathway) is mutated in glioblastomas (see Fig. 1-6). At the beginning of the G_1 phase of the cell cycle, RB1 is unphosphorylated. Unphosphorylated RB1 normally sequesters the E2F transcription factors.[154] Entry into S-phase is initiated by the release of the E2F transcription factors by the newly phosphorylated Rb1 at the restriction point in G_1. Loss of both wild-type copies of the *RB1* gene, resulting in nonfunctional or absent RB1 proteins or inappropriately phosphorylated RB1, will result in any expressed E2F being free to initiate transcription of the genes necessary for entry into S-phase. Inappropriate phosphorylation may be achieved in glioblastomas with wild-type RB1 by either loss of wild-type p16 expression or overexpression of CDK4 (secondary to amplification of its gene). Both of the latter events would make inappropriate phosphorylation of wild-type RB1 more likely with the release of the E2Fs. p16 normally binds CDK4 and inhibits the formation of the CDK4/cyclin D1 heterodimer that phosphorylates RB1.[155] In the absence of p16, all expressed CDK4 is available for heterodimer formation. When *CDK4* is amplified and overexpressed in the presence of normal levels of p16, there will be excess CDK4 available for heterodimer formation. One or the other of these genetic abnormalities is present in over 70% of glioblastomas; they are, with very few exceptions, mutually exclusive.[60] In addition, loss of *RB1* expression due to promoter methylation has been described in glioblastomas.[156] While disruption of both the p53 and Rb1 pathways seems essential for glioblastomas, the ways in which the pathways are rendered dysfunctional may confer slightly different biological characteristics on the individual tumors.

In addition to disruption of the p53 and Rb1 pathways, normal growth factor receptor signaling and signal transduction is also frequently disrupted in the glioblastomas. Starting at the surface of the cell, we will describe the abnormalities found (Fig. 1-7). About 35% of glioblastomas have amplification of the epidermal growth factor receptor *(EGFR)* gene (7p11–12). When amplified, this gene is always overexpressed, but it may also be overexpressed in the absence of amplification. Rearrangements of the amplified gene occur in almost half of the tumors with amplification. The most common rearrangement results in a transcript that is aberrantly spliced, but remains in frame[157–159] and codes for a mutated EGFR that has lost 267 amino acids of its extracellular domain and does not bind ligand.[160–161] This mutated EGFR is constitutively activated, and attempts are ongoing to target therapy to this aberrant cell surface molecule.[162,163] Other rearrangements of the amplified *EGFR* gene occur less frequently. These may result in abnormalities of the cytoplasmic domain, but also lead to increased signaling by the aberrant receptors.[164]

Signal transduction from the activated EGFR is through the RAS-RAF-MAP kinase pathway and through the activation of the PI3K (phosphoinositide 3-kinase)/AKT pathway. Aberrations of the RAS-RAF-MAP kinase pathway are uncommon in glioblastomas. However, signaling through the PI3K/AKT pathway is frequently aberrant. Normally, activated growth factor receptors' cytoplasmic domains activate the heterodimeric PI3K, which then phosphorylates local PIP2 (phosphatidylinositol-3,4-diphosphate) to PIP3 (phosphatidylinositol-3,4,5-triphosphate) (Fig. 1-7), resulting in the recruitment of AKT and PDK1 (3′-phosphoinositide-dependent kinase-1) to the inside of the membrane, due to their binding to PIP3 through PH domains. Here AKT comes into contact with

PDK1, which phosphorylates and activates AKT. Deregulation of this process occurs in a number of ways. Activating mutations of the *PIK3CA* (phosphotidylinositol 3-kinase, catalytic alpha) gene that codes for the catalytic component of the heterodimeric lipid kinase PI3K, resulting in constitutive activation, have been reported in WHO grade III and IV astrocytic tumors, some medulloblastomas and anaplastic oligodendrogliomas.[165–167] This would result in inappropriate levels of PIP3. The levels of PIP3 are negatively controlled by the presence of the dual-specificity phosphatase PTEN protein.[168–169] One of its major substrates is PIP3, which it dephosphorylates to PIP2.[170] The *PTEN* gene is located on 10q, and almost 90% of glioblastomas lose the region containing one *PTEN* gene at 10q23–24.[171–173] The retained copy of *PTEN* is mutated in over 40% of glioblastomas; thus, these tumors lack wild-type PTEN and cannot dephosphorylate PIP3 to PIP2[174] permitting stable high levels of PIP3 and activation of the Akt pathway (Fig. 1-7). This results in, among other things, decreased likelihood of apoptosis and the facilitation of HIF-1 (hypoxia inducible factor -1) activity.[175] Amplification and overexpression of *AKT* have also been described in at least one glioblastoma[176] and methylation and transcriptional downregulation of the *CTMP* gene (a negative regulator of AKT) have also been documented,[177] further events that would activate the AKT pathway. This is supported by reports on the affect of Akt activation in animal models of astrocytoma.[178] There is also data to suggest wild-type PTEN may contribute to growth arrest independently of the AKT pathway.[179] A more detailed discussion of the pathways targeted in gliomas has recently been published.[180]

There have been some attempts to correlate the genetic findings to patient outcome following conventional therapy (debulking surgery followed by 50 + 60 Gy irradiation). Amplification of the EGFR gene has not been shown to uniformly result in a better or worse outcome.[114,181–187] Combining the abnormalities has suggested that glioblastoma patients whose tumors have a disrupted RB1 pathway, disrupted p53 pathway, and no wild-type PTEN have the worst prognosis.[188] Similar findings have been reported for anaplastic astrocytomas WHO grade III.[189] While we still have no really well-documented genetic biomarkers for the astrocytic tumors that are diagnostic, predictive, prognostic, or therapeutic-response indicators (with the exception of methylation of the MGMT gene—see following discussion[190]), these insights into the genetic abnormalities of astrocytic tumors provide us with many potential therapeutic targets as well as an understanding of the complexity of the problem we are dealing with.

It is tempting to try to sort the genetic findings into a series of events explaining how de novo and secondary glioblastomas might develop. Both have disrupted p53 and Rb1 pathways—but these have occurred in different ways. In de novo tumors, amplification of the 12q14 region encompassing the *CDK4* and *MDM2* genes and resulting in their overexpression is found. This will disrupt both pathways by a single genetic event. Homozygous deletion of the region on 9p encompassing the genes coding for p16 (CDKN2A), p15 (CDKN2B) and p14(ARF) (*p14(ARF)*) requires two genetic events (deletion of both alleles), and is also mainly found in de novo glioblastomas.[116,191] Occasionally, de novo glioblastomas may also show greater numbers and more complex patterns of mutations with loss of one allele of each of *TP53* and *RB1* and mutation of the retained alleles, requiring 4 genetic mutational events. However, this is the rule in the secondary glioblastomas.[116,191] The data from the diffuse astrocytomas WHO grade II and the anaplastic astrocytomas WHO grade III indicate that they have, in over 60% of cases, no wild-type *TP53* gene through loss of one allele and mutation of the other.[60] Glioblastomas derived from these tumors would be expected to have a similar pattern of *TP53* mutations and this is what is found. The secondary glioblastomas also lose their functional Rb1 pathway but most often by a further two genetic events—loss of one allele and mutation of the retained *RB1*. In addition, losses on 10q, encompassing the *PTEN* gene, occur in the majority of secondary glioblastomas, while *EGFR* amplification is uncommon.[114] There are no data on the incidence of mutation of the retained allele of *PTEN* in secondary glioblastomas.

Methylation of tumor suppressor gene and DNA repair gene promoters has not received the same degree of attention as deletions and mutations, for practical methodological reasons. While some studies had shown methylation of known tumor suppressor genes, the association of *MGMT* (O(6)-methylguanine-DNA methyltransferase) methylation with improved survival in glioblastomas treated with alkylating agents made the field very relevant clinically.[192] This was subsequently confirmed in a clinical trial of combined radiation and temozolomide treatment.[123,190] The findings indicated that patients with methylation of the *MGMT* gene, and thus no expression or very limited expression of the protein, had a significant survival benefit—even with radiotherapy alone.[190] The cytotoxic and mutagenic actions of temozolomide have been attributed to its ability to form DNA adducts by methylation at the O^6 position of the purine base guanine to form O^6methylguanine.[193] Repair of these adducts is mediated by MGMT, which removes them from DNA in a single step mechanism, without cofactors but with the consumption of one MGMT molecule per adduct.[194] Thus constant expression of the MGMT protein is necessary for maintenance of the repair process.

Besides the well-characterized genes described above, astrocytic tumor genome analysis has shown many relatively consistent copy number alterations in additional chromosomal regions. At least some of these regions are likely to harbor novel oncogenes or TSGs, or their break points may be involved in the formation of fusion oncogenes. Some of the recurrent chromosomal imbalances include loss of 1p36, 6q23–27, 9p21–24, 10, 13p11–13, 13q14–34, and 22, and gain of 7.[120,195–197] The losses at 1p36 will be discussed in relation to the total 1p deletions seen in oligodendrogliomas in the next section. The consequences and genes targeted by many of these changes have yet to be identified.

OLIGODENDROGLIOMAS AND OLIGOASTROCYTOMAS

Oligodendrogliomas are divided into oligodendrogliomas WHO grade II and anaplastic oligodendrogliomas WHO grade III. They occur mainly in the cerebral hemispheres of adults. Classical oligodendrogliomas WHO grade II consist of moderately cellular, monomorphic tumors (Fig. 1-8) with round nuclei, often artifactually swollen cytoplasm on paraffin section, few or no mitoses, and a characteristic "chicken wire" pattern of normal-looking capillaries (no multilayered endothelial cells/microvascular proliferation permitted). There is no necrosis. They do not consistently express any known antigen characteristic of normal oligodendrocytes and may express GFAP. Oligodendrogliomas WHO grade II are relatively indolent, although they usually recur at the primary site and may display a tendency for subependymal spread with a 5% incidence of CSF seeding.

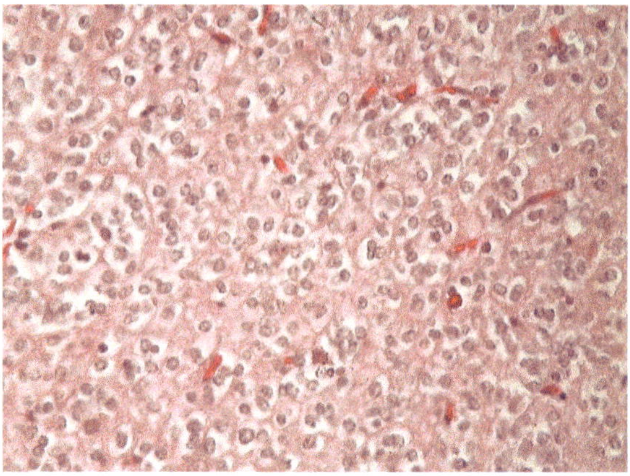

Figure 1-8 Oligodendroglioma WHO grade II with the typical tumor cell morphology: round nuclei and swollen empty cytoplasm. (H&E)

Anaplastic oligodendrogliomas WHO grade III are less common, more cellular, show nuclear atypia, pleomorphism, and mitotic activity. Microvascular proliferation and necrosis may be present. Both oligodendrogliomas and anaplastic oligodendrogliomas also invade diffusely into normal brain to varying degrees unique to each tumor.

Oligoastrocytomas consist of tumor cells with either astrocytic or oligodendroglial morphological characteristics, either diffusely mixed or combined as discrete areas in an individual tumor. Oligoastrocytomas are also divided into WHO grade II or III tumors; the latter are called anaplastic oligoastrocytomas and are more cellular with nuclear atypia, pleomorphism, microvascular proliferation, and mitotic activity. The current edition of the WHO classification recommends that if necrosis is present in an anaplastic oligoastrocytoma, it should be classified as glioblastoma with an oligodendroglial component and graded as WHO grade IV. Current data suggest that anaplastic oligoastrocytomas (but not anaplastic oligodendrogliomas) with necrosis do significantly worse than anaplastic oligoastrocytomas without necrosis.[198] However, they do better than conventional glioblastomas that lack an oligodendroglial component. Since 1990, when combination chemotherapy (procarbazine, CCNU (lomustine), and vincristine; PCV) was demonstrated to result in dramatic tumor responses,[199] the identification of all forms of glioma with oligodendroglial components has become clinically important. The morphological borderlines between astrocytomas, oligoastrocytomas, and oligodendrogliomas are still, however, ill-defined and controversial issues and this is particularly true of the anaplastic variants. Urgent agreement on definitions based on morphological or genetic characteristics, or a combination of both, is needed.

The majority of oligodendrogliomas show relatively specific genetic abnormalities that separate them from the other gliomas. Loss of all of 1 p and 19 q was demonstrated in a genomic wide analysis in 1994,[200] and this was later linked to a good response to PCV treatment providing the first molecular therapy response indicator for brain tumors.[201–203] The losses of 1 p and 19 q are most common among the grade II oligodendrogliomas (reports of up to 90%) and are present in over 50% of anaplastic oligodendrogliomas (WHO grade III). The explanation for this frequent co-deletion of two whole chromosomal arms was an unbalanced translocation t(1;19)(q10;p10).[204] It must be stressed that it is the *total* loss of one copy of 1p and 19q that is associated with oligodendrogliomas, and that losses involving the 1p36 region are a common event in astrocytic tumors, especially in glioblastomas.[196,205] Even homozygous deletions of the 1p36 region are not unusual in glioblastomas.[196] These findings in the astrocytic tumors makes it very important that the methods used can differentiate between partial and total 1p deletion if the results are to be used clinically. Oligodendrogliomas (WHO grade II) may show methylation of *p14(ARF)*with consequent loss of expression, as well as overexpression of EGFR and both the ligands and receptors of the PDGF system. In addition, MGMT hypermethylation with low or absent expression has been reported to be common in oligodendroglial tumors and likely contributes to the chemosensitivity of these tumors.[201]

Malignant progression is associated with additional genetic abnormalities similar to those described above for the astrocytic tumors, i.e., disruption of the Rb1 pathway due to homozygous deletions or, in some cases, hypermethylation of the *CDKN2A/p14(ARF)* locus or the *RB1* locus, or *CDK4* amplification and overexpression as is also seen in the progression of the diffuse astrocytic tumors.[206,207] Some anaplastic oligodendrogliomas have no wild-type PTEN, although this is usually seen only in tumors without 1p and 19q loss.[208,209] As is the case with the astrocytic tumors, there are many other chromosomal regions showing copy number abnormalities, particularly in the anaplastic oligodendrogliomas. These include chromosomes 4, 6, 7, 11, 13, 15, 18, and 22.[39,202,210] Oligoastrocytomas and anaplastic oligoastrocytomas tend to have aberrant genetic patterns similar to either the oligodendroglial tumors or the diffuse astrocytic tumors. As yet, there are no specific abnormalities associated with these mixed glial tumors.

MENINGIOMAS

Symptomatic meningiomas represent 13% to 26% of primary intracranial tumors, are most common in middle-aged and elderly patients, and show a marked female predominance. Small asymptomatic meningiomas are found incidentally in 1.4% of autopsies[211] or are identified during neuroimaging for other reasons.[212] Symptomatic meningiomas are usually solitary lobulated tumors, attached to the dura; they usually displace but do not invade adjacent brain. However, they may locally invade mesenchymal elements such as bone and subcutaneous tissue. This has no significance for WHO grading. Invasion of the skull may elicit an osteoblastic reaction. Brain invasion, although uncommon, can occur in meningiomas of all WHO malignancy grades and indicates a greater likelihood of recurrence. Brain invasion by a meningioma that otherwise morphologically fulfills the criteria for WHO grade I increases the grade to WHO grade II. Brain invasion in atypical or anaplastic meningiomas does not increase the WHO grade.

Meningiomas are thought to develop from meningothelial (arachnoidal) cells. Patients with NF2 as well as members of some other non-NF2 familial syndromes, where the genes involved are unknown, may develop multiple meningiomas, often early in life. Exposure to ionizing radiation is a well-recognized predisposing factor. The cellular morphology, the growth pattern, and the presence of extracellular material permit the differentiation of many histological subtypes (Fig. 1-9). Meningiomas are graded as WHO grade I, atypical meningiomas as WHO grade II, and anaplastic meningiomas as WHO grade III.[1]

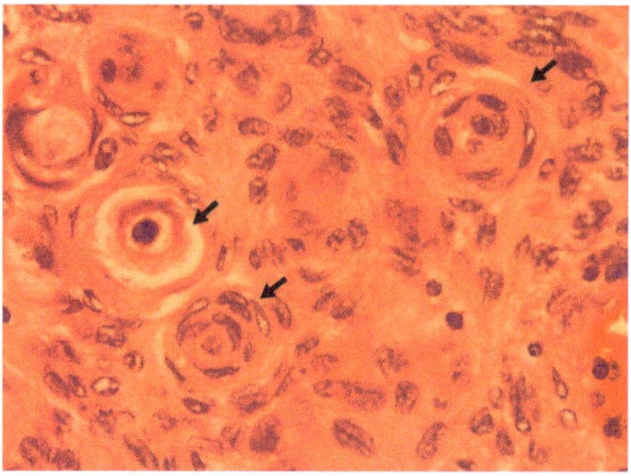

Figure 1-9 Typical meningioma specimen WHO grade I, showing an example of the common transitional meningioma with multiple whorls (arrows). (H&E)

Meningeal sarcomas are graded as WHO grade IV. Over 80% of meningiomas are WHO grade I. The current WHO classification recognizes 9 histological subtypes. Some histological subtypes are known to be associated with a less favorable outcome; these include the chordoid and clear cell meningiomas graded as WHO grade II, and the papillary and rhabdoid meningiomas graded as WHO grade III.[1] Atypical (WHO grade II) and anaplastic (WHO grade III) meningiomas can be of any of the recognized WHO grade I histological subtypes. The criteria for increasing the grade are strictly defined.[1] Most of the more aggressive meningioma variants are very rare, but atypical variants constitute 15% to 20%, with the anaplastic variants making up less than 2%. Both atypical and anaplastic meningiomas are more common in men. Meningiomas may progress, and therefore should be thoroughly sampled in order to identify areas with a histology associated with more aggressive behavior. The histological criteria indicating a less favorable outcome include frequent mitoses, regions of hypercellularity, uninterrupted or sheet-like growth, high nuclear-cytoplasmic ratio, prominent nucleoli and spontaneous necrosis.[1] Brain invasion should also be carefully excluded as this, if present, indicates a greater likelihood of recurrence and increases the WHO grade of otherwise grade I meningiomas to WHO grade II. The vast majority express epithelial membrane antigen (EMA) and vimentin and generally are negative for S-100 protein. The higher incidence of meningiomas in women, the apparently frequent manifestation of tumors during pregnancy, and the association of meningiomas with breast and genital cancer have suggested estrogen and progesterone dependency of the tumors. Meningiomas WHO grade I generally express progesterone receptors, and in some cases also express estrogen receptors. Expression of progesterone receptors is frequently lost in the atypical and anaplastic variants.

The consistent loss of one copy of chromosome 22 in meningiomas was one of the first genetic abnormalities reported in a human solid tumor.[213] The fact that the second most common tumor in neurofibromatosis type 2 patients was meningioma pointed to the *NF2* gene as the target on chromosome 22. Loss of both wild-type copies of *NF2* is found, overall, in about half of sporadic meningiomas and in the majority of NF2-associated meningiomas,[214,215] and the frequency varies with histological subtype—fibroblastic, transitional,and meningothelial meningiomas showing this trait in decreasing frequency. In the sporadic cases, this is usually by the loss of one copy (monosomy 22) and mutation of the retained copy,[214] while in the NF2 patients the single wild copy is lost, leaving the tumor cells with only the inherited mutated copy. It is important to note that at least 30% of all meningiomas and the majority of meningothelial meningiomas do not lose alleles on 22q nor do they have mutations or aberrant methylation of the *NF2* gene.[215] The genes involved in the oncogenesis of these meningiomas remain uncertain.

The NF2 tumor suppressor gene is made up of 17 exons and covers a genomic region of 95kb. It encodes transcripts with at least eight well-documented alternatively-spliced open reading frames. The full-length splice variants encode a deduced protein with approximately 47% identity to several members of the 4.1/ERM family of proteins, believed to be involved in linking cytoskeletal components to cell membrane proteins and including moesin, ezrin, and radixin—thus the name merlin.[216] The full-length splice variants have been shown to be involved in control of cell growth and motility in culture.[217,218] Genetically engineered mice with only one wild-type allele have been shown to develop many tumor forms,[219] while tissue-specific inactivation in Schwann cells or leptomeningeal cells results in schwannoma or meningioma formation respectively.[220,221]

Meningiomas may progress from grade I tumors to tumors of higher malignancy grade. This is associated with losses on chromosomal arms 1p, 6q, 9p, 10p and q, 14q, and 18q, as well as gains and some amplifications on many other chromosomes.[222–230] The genes targeted by these abnormalities are mostly unknown, but the losses on 9p are associated with loss of both wild-type copies of *CDKN2A*, *p14ARF*, and *CDKN2B*, as is commonly seen in the de novo glioblastomas and anaplastic oligodendrogliomas.[230] A candidate target for the losses on 14q has been identified and is the *NDRG2* gene, where hypermethylation of the retained copy has been shown together with loss of expression.[231]

LYMPHOMAS

Primary CNS lymphoma (PCNSL) is an uncommon form of extranodal non-Hodgkin lymphoma. Its incidence has increased worldwide over the last 30 years but appears to have stabilized or decreased in recent years, probably due to the introduction of highly active antiretroviral therapy to treat HIV infections in the western world. PCNSL is the most frequent brain tumor in patients with acquired or congenital immunodeficiency, but it also occurs in immunocompetent patients, with a peak incidence in the sixth and seventh decades. PCNSL is thought to represent about 3% of all brain tumors and 2% to 3% of all non-Hodgkin lymphomas.[1,232,233] Characteristic imaging features on contrast-enhanced MRI should lead to a suspicion of the diagnosis and the avoidance of corticosteroids (if at all possible) before early stereotactic biopsy. Diagnostic evaluation should include assessment of the brain, cerebrospinal fluid, and eyes, as all these regions may be involved.[234] Occult systemic disease is uncommon. Histopathologically, the lymphoma diffusely infiltrates the brain, initially spreading by characteristic angiocentric infiltration with concentric perivascular reticulin deposits, followed by invasion of the neural parenchyma. There may be multifocal growth and/or meningeal spread, and CSF cytology may be useful in some cases. The brain infiltration produces a variable reactive astrocytosis and microglial response and this, together with residual concentric perivascular reticulin, may be the only finding in a patient who has received steroids prior to biopsy. The vast majority are classified as diffuse large B-cell lymphomas (DLBCL). All morphological variants of DLBCL such as centroblastic, immunoblastic T-cell/histiocyte-rich, and anaplastic may occur. The tumor cells are immunoreactive for pan B-cell markers (CD19, CD20, and CD79a), and most tumor cell populations will express BCL-6 and MUM-1 as well as BCL-2. A reactive T-cell presence is almost always found. Other lymphoma types that occur, albeit infrequently, include low-grade B-cell lymphoma, marginal zone B-cell lymphoma, angiotrophic or intravascular B-cell lymphoma, T-cell lymphoma, anaplastic large-cell lymphoma NK/T-cell lymphoma, and, very rarely, Hodgkin disease. Diagnosis of all these lymphoma types requires immunophenotyping of the tumor cells, and the reader is referred to the WHO classification of tumors of hematopoetic and lymphoid tissues for the details of the antibodies and patterns of immunoreactivity characteristic for each of these lymphoma forms.[235] Also see the chapter on primary CNS lymphoma for further information about chromosomal deletions.

As resection is contraindicated and most diagnoses made on the basis of stereotactic biopsies, the amount of tumor tissue available for molecular studies is very limited. Most information has been derived from extraneural DLBCL and then confirmed to also be true in primary DLBCL of the CNS. Both have clonal rearrangement and somatic hypermutation of immunoglobulin genes.[236,237] Expression profiling indicates the existence of similar subtypes including germinal center B-cell type, activated B-cell type, and "type3" large B-cell type.[238,239] Aberrant somatic hypermutation targeting regions other than the immunoglobulin V-regions is also reported in both systemic and CNS forms.[240,241] Disruption of cell cycle control by abnormalities of the RB1 pathway have also been reported.[242] There are also many copy number abnormalities on various chromosomes reported, where the targeted genes are still unknown.[243]

METASTASES

Intracranial metastases are the commonest tumors in the brain in adults, occurring more than five times more frequently than primary tumors.[244] Autopsy studies show that up to a quarter of cancer patients develop brain metastases and around 5%, intraspinal metastases.[245] In adults the most common primary tumors responsible for brain metastases are lung cancer, breast cancer, cancers with an unknown primary, malignant melanoma, and colon cancer. The reader is referred to the specialist literature for information on the molecular genetics and biology of these many different tumor forms.

Conclusions

Histopathology has provided a morphological diagnosis on which therapy has been empirically based for at least 100 years. However, molecular data is more and more often being requested in addition to the histopathological findings. As yet, the most common requests are for the methylation status of the *MGMT* gene and the 1p/19q status of the glioma cells. In many other areas of oncology, molecular data are the norm (e.g., lymphoma, breast cancer, and sarcoma diagnosis). As new forms of molecular targeted therapy are introduced and found to be effective, the analysis of tumor specimens will have to be extended to provide clinically relevant data, and medical professionals must be able to both provide this information and interpret the findings. The ultimate aim is to provide tailored molecular targeted therapies that are specific to a patient's tumor cells, leaving their brain and other organs unharmed.

Since this chapter was completed, increasing evidence indicates that mutation at codon 132 of *IDH1* (or rarely mutation of codon 172 of *IDH2*) combined with either *TP53* mutation or total 1p/19q loss is a frequent and early change in the majority of oligodendroglial tumors, diffuse astrocytomas, anaplastic astrocytomas, and secondary glioblastomas but not in primary glioblastomas.[256,257] Patients with tumors with such mutations appear to have a better outcome than those with wild type *IDH* genes.

REFERENCES

1. Louis DN, Ohgaki H, Wiestler OD, Cavenee WK, editors. WHO Classification of Tumours of the Central Nervous System. Lyon: IARC; 2007.
2. Bailey P, Cushing H. A classification of tumours of the glioma group on a histogenetic basis with a correlated study of prognosis. Philadelphia, PA: J. B. Lippincott; 1926.
3. Davis RL, Onda K, Shubuya M, Lamborn K, Hoshino T. Proliferation markers in gliomas: a comparison of BUDR, KI-67, and MIB- 1. J Neurooncol 1995;24(1):9–12.
4. Williams GH, Romanowski P, Morris L, Madine M, Mills AD, Stoeber K, et al. Improved cervical smear assessment using antibodies against proteins that regulate DNA replication. Proc Natl Acad Sci U S A 1998;95(25):14932–7.
5. Galli R, Binda E, Orfanelli U, Cipelletti B, Gritti A, De Vitis S, et al. Isolation and characterization of tumorigenic, stem-like neural precursors from human glioblastoma. Cancer Res 2004;64(19):7011–21.
6. Hemmati HD, Nakano I, Lazareff JA, Masterman-Smith M, Geschwind DH, Bronner-Fraser M, et al. Cancerous stem cells can arise from pediatric brain tumors. Proc Natl Acad Sci U S A 2003;100(25):15178–83.
7. Singh SK, Clarke ID, Terasaki M, Bonn VE, Hawkins C, Squire J, et al. Identification of a cancer stem cell in human brain tumors. Cancer Res 2003;63(18):5821–8.
8. Singh SK, Hawkins C, Clarke ID, Squire JA, Bayani J, Hide T, et al. Identification of human brain tumour initiating cells. Nature 2004;432(7015):396–401.
9. Yuan X, Curtin J, Xiong Y, Liu G, Waschsmann-Hogiu S, Farkas DL, et al. Isolation of cancer stem cells from adult glioblastoma multiforme. Oncogene 2004;23(58):9392–400.
10. Dirks PB. Brain tumour stem cells: the undercurrents of human brain cancer and their relationship to neural stem cells. Philos Trans R Soc Lond B Biol Sci 2008;363(1489):139–52.
11. Fan X, Eberhart CG. Medulloblastoma stem cells. J Clin Oncol 2008;26(17):2821–7.
12. Ohgaki H, Kleihues P. Population-based studies on incidence, survival rates, and genetic alterations in astrocytic and oligodendroglial gliomas. J Neuropathol Exp Neurol 2005; 64(6):479–89.
13. Alshail E, Rutka JT, Becker LE, Hoffman HJ. Optic chiasmatic-hypothalamic glioma. Brain Pathol 1997;7(2):799–806.
14. Listernick R, Charrow J, Gutmann DH. Intracranial gliomas in neurofibromatosis type 1. Am J Med Genet 1999;89(1):38–44.
15. Jenkins RB, Kimmel DW, Moertel CA, Schultz CG, Scheithauer BW, Kelly PJ, et al. A cytogenetic study of 53 human gliomas. Cancer Genet Cytogenet 1989;39(2):253–79.
16. Bigner SH, McLendon RE, Fuchs H, McKeever PE, Friedman HS. Chromosomal characteristics of childhood brain tumors. Cancer Genet Cytogenet 1997;97(2):125–34.
17. Zattara-Cannoni H, Gambarelli D, Lena G, Dufour H, Choux M, Grisoli F, et al. Are juvenile pilocytic astrocytomas benign tumors? A cytogenetic study in 24 cases. Cancer Genet Cytogenet 1998;104(2):157–60.
18. Sanoudou D, Tingby O, Ferguson-Smith MA, Collins VP, Coleman N. Analysis of pilocytic astrocytoma by comparative genomic hybridization. Br J Cancer 2000;82(6):1218–22.

19. Jones DT, Ichimura K, Liu L, Pearson DM, Plant K, Collins VP. Genomic analysis of pilocytic astrocytomas at 0.97 Mb resolution shows an increasing tendency toward chromosomal copy number change with age. J Neuropathol Exp Neurol 2006;65(11):1049–58.
20. James CD, He J, Carlbom E, Mikkelsen T, Ridderheim PA, Cavenee WK, et al. Loss of genetic information in central nervous system tumors common to children and young adults. Genes Chromosom Cancer 1990;2(2):94–102.
21. Gutmann DH, Donahoe J, Brown T, James CD, Perry A. Loss of neurofibromatosis 1 (NF1) gene expression in NF1-associated pilocytic astrocytomas. Neuropathol Appl Neurobiol 2000;26(4):361–7.
22. Kluwe L, Hagel C, Tatagiba M, Thomas S, Stavrou D, Ostertag H, et al. Loss of NF1 alleles distinguish sporadic from NF1-associated pilocytic astrocytomas. J Neuropathol Exp Neurol 2001;60(9):917–20.
23. Patt S, Gries H, Giraldo M, Cervos-Navarro J, Martin H, Janisch W, et al. p53 gene mutations in human astrocytic brain tumors including pilocytic astrocytomas. Hum Pathol 1996;27(6):586–9.
24. Phelan CM, Liu L, Ruttledge MH, Muntzning K, Ridderheim PA, Collins VP. Chromosome 17 abnormalities and lack of TP53 mutations in paediatric central nervous system tumours. Hum Genet 1995;96(6):684–90.
25. Uhlmann K, Rohde K, Zeller C, Szymas J, Vogel S, Marczinek K, et al. Distinct methylation profiles of glioma subtypes. Int J Cancer 2003;106(1):52–9.
26. Gonzalez-Gomez P, Bello MJ, Lomas J, Arjona D, Alonso ME, Aminoso C, et al. Epigenetic changes in pilocytic astrocytomas and medulloblastomas. Int J Mol Med 2003;11(5):655–60.
27. Ebinger M, Senf L, Wachowski O, Scheurlen W. No aberrant methylation of neurofibromatosis 1 gene (NF1) promoter in pilocytic astrocytoma in childhood. Pediatr Hematol Oncol 2005;22(1):83–7.
28. Deshmukh H, Yeh TH, Yu J, Sharma MK, Perry A, Leonard JR, et al. High-resolution, dual-platform aCGH analysis reveals frequent HIPK2 amplification and increased expression in pilocytic astrocytomas. Oncogene 2008;.
29. Jones DTW, Kacialkowski S, Liu L, Pearson DM, Backlund LM, Ichimura K, et al. Tandem duplication producing a novel oncogenic BRAF fusion gene defines the majority of pilocytic astrocytomas. Cancer Res 2008; In Press.
30. Pfister S, Janzarik WG, Remke M, Ernst A, Werft W, Becker N, et al. BRAF gene duplication constitutes a mechanism of MAPK pathway activation in low-grade astrocytomas. J Clin Invest 2008;118(5):1739–49.
31. Hamilton RL, Pollack IF. The molecular biology of ependymomas. Brain Pathol 1997; 7(2):807–22.
32. Korshunov A, Golanov A, Timirgaz V. Immunohistochemical markers for intracranial ependymoma recurrence. An analysis of 88 cases. J Neurol Sci 2000;177(1):72–82.
33. Korshunov A, Sycheva R, Timirgaz V, Golanov A. Prognostic value of immunoexpression of the chemoresistance-related proteins in ependymomas: an analysis of 76 cases. J Neurooncol 1999;45(3):219–27.
34. Tabori U, Ma J, Carter M, Zielenska M, Rutka J, Bouffet E, et al. Human telomere reverse transcriptase expression predicts progression and survival in pediatric intracranial ependymoma. J Clin Oncol 2006;24(10):1522–8.
35. Taylor MD, Poppleton H, Fuller C, Su X, Liu Y, Jensen P, et al. Radial glia cells are candidate stem cells of ependymoma. Cancer Cell 2005;8(4):323–35.
36. Bijlsma EK, Voesten AM, Bijleveld EH, Troost D, Westerveld A, Merel P, et al. Molecular analysis of genetic changes in ependymomas. Genes Chromosomes Cancer 1995;13(4):272–7.
37. Ebert C, von Haken M, Meyer-Puttlitz B, Wiestler OD, Reifenberger G, Pietsch T, et al. Molecular genetic analysis of ependymal tumors. NF2 mutations and chromosome 22 q loss occur preferentially in intramedullary spinal ependymomas. Am J Pathol 1999;155(2):627–32.
38. Carter M, Nicholson J, Ross F, Crolla J, Allibone R, Balaji V, et al. Genetic abnormalities detected in ependymomas by comparative genomic hybridisation. Br J Cancer 2002;86(6):929–39.
39. Koschny R, Koschny T, Froster UG, Krupp W, Zuber MA. Comparative genomic hybridization in glioma: a meta-analysis of 509 cases. Cancer Genet Cytogenet 2002;135(2):147–59.
40. Huang B, Starostik P, Schraut H, Krauss J, Sorensen N, Roggendorf W. Human ependymomas reveal frequent deletions on chromosomes 6 and 9. Acta Neuropathol (Berl) 2003;106(4):357–62.
41. Mahler-Araujo MB, Sanoudou D, Tingby O, Liu L, Coleman N, Ichimura K, et al. Structural genomic abnormalities of chromosomes 9 and 18 in myxopapillary ependymomas. J Neuropathol Exp Neurol 2003;62(9):927–35.

42. Mendrzyk F, Korshunov A, Benner A, Toedt G, Pfister S, Radlwimmer B, et al. Identification of gains on 1q and epidermal growth factor receptor overexpression as independent prognostic markers in intracranial ependymoma. Clin Cancer Res 2006;12(7 Pt 1):2070–9.
43. Modena P, Lualdi E, Facchinetti F, Veltman J, Reid JF, Minardi S, et al. Identification of tumor-specific molecular signatures in intracranial ependymoma and association with clinical characteristics. J Clin Oncol 2006;24(33):5223–33.
44. Rickert CH, Korshunov A, Paulus W. Chromosomal imbalances in clear cell ependymomas. Mod Pathol 2006;19(7):958–62.
45. Rousseau E, Palm T, Scaravilli F, Ruchoux MM, Figarella-Branger D, Salmon I, et al. Trisomy 19 ependymoma, a newly recognized genetico-histological association, including clear cell ependymoma. Mol Cancer 2007;6:47.
46. Kurian KM, Jones DT, Marsden F, Openshaw SW, Pearson DM, Ichimura K, et al. Genome-Wide Analysis of Subependymomas Shows Underlying Chromosomal Copy Number Changes Involving Chromosomes 6, 7, 8 and 14 in a Proportion of Cases. Brain Pathol 2008;.
47. Pezzolo A, Capra V, Raso A, Morandi F, Parodi F, Gambini C, et al. Identification of novel chromosomal abnormalities and prognostic cytogenetics markers in intracranial pediatric ependymoma. Cancer Lett 2008;261(2):235–43.
48. von Haken MS, White EC, Daneshvar-Shyesther L, Sih S, Choi E, Kalra R, et al. Molecular genetic analysis of chromosome arm 17p and chromosome arm 22q DNA sequences in sporadic pediatric ependymomas. Genes Chromosomes Cancer 1996;17(1):37–44.
49. Alonso ME, Bello MJ, Arjona D, Gonzalez-Gomez P, Lomas J, de Campos JM, et al. Analysis of the NF2 gene in oligodendrogliomas and ependymomas. Cancer Genet Cytogenet 2002;134(1):1–5.
50. Lamszus K, Lachenmayer L, Heinemann U, Kluwe L, Finckh U, Hoppner W, et al. Molecular genetic alterations on chromosomes 11 and 22 in ependymomas. Int J Cancer 2001;91(6):803–8.
51. Begnami MD, Palau M, Rushing EJ, Santi M, Quezado M. Evaluation of NF2 gene deletion in sporadic schwannomas, meningiomas, and ependymomas by chromogenic in situ hybridization. Hum Pathol 2007;38(9):1345–50.
52. Kraus JA, de Millas W, Sorensen N, Herbold C, Schichor C, Tonn JC, et al. Indications for a tumor suppressor gene at 22q11 involved in the pathogenesis of ependymal tumors and distinct from hSNF5/INI1. Acta Neuropathol (Berl) 2001;102(1):69–74.
53. Rubio MP, Correa KM, Ramesh V, MacCollin MM, Jacoby LB, von Deimling A, et al. Analysis of the neurofibromatosis 2 gene in human ependymomas and astrocytomas. Cancer Res 1994;54(1):45–7.
54. Dyer S, Prebble E, Davison V, Davies P, Ramani P, Ellison D, et al. Genomic imbalances in pediatric intracranial ependymomas define clinically relevant groups. Am J Pathol 2002;161(6):2133–41.
55. Ward S, Harding B, Wilkins P, Harkness W, Hayward R, Darling JL, et al. Gain of 1q and loss of 22 are the most common changes detected by comparative genomic hybridisation in paediatric ependymoma. Genes Chromosomes Cancer 2001;32(1):59–66.
56. Urioste M, Martinez-Ramirez A, Cigudosa JC, Colmenero I, Madero L, Robledo M, et al. Complex cytogenetic abnormalities including telomeric associations and MEN1 mutation in a pediatric ependymoma. Cancer Genet Cytogenet 2002;138(2):107–10.
57. Gaspar N, Grill J, Geoerger B, Lellouch-Tubiana A, Michalowski MB, Vassal G. p53 Pathway dysfunction in primary childhood ependymomas. Pediatr Blood Cancer 2006;46(5):604–13.
58. Nozaki M, Tada M, Matsumoto R, Sawamura Y, Abe H, Iggo RD. Rare occurrence of inactivating p53 gene mutations in primary non-astrocytic tumors of the central nervous system: reappraisal by yeast functional assay. Acta Neuropathol (Berl) 1998;95(3):291–6.
59. Ohgaki H, Eibl RH, Wiestler OD, Yasargil MG, Newcomb EW, Kleihues P. p53 mutations in nonastrocytic human brain tumors. Cancer Res 1991;51(22):6202–5.
60. Ichimura K, Bolin MB, Goike HM, Schmidt EE, Moshref A, Collins VP. Deregulation of the p14ARF/MDM2/p53 pathway is a prerequisite for human astrocytic gliomas with G1-S transition control gene abnormalities. Cancer Res 2000;60(2):417–24.
61. Lukashova-v Zangen I, Kneitz S, Monoranu CM, Rutkowski S, Hinkes B, Vince GH, et al. Ependymoma gene expression profiles associated with histological subtype, proliferation, and patient survival. Acta Neuropathol 2007;113(3):325–37.
62. Suarez-Merino B, Hubank M, Revesz T, Harkness W, Hayward R, Thompson D, et al. Microarray analysis of pediatric ependymoma identifies a cluster of 112 candidate genes including four transcripts at 22q12.1–q13.3. Neuro Oncol 2005;7(1):20–31.

63. Burger PC, Yu IT, Tihan T, Friedman HS, Strother DR, Kepner JL, et al. Atypical teratoid/rhabdoid tumor of the central nervous system: a highly malignant tumor of infancy and childhood frequently mistaken for medulloblastoma: a Pediatric Oncology Group study. Am J Surg Pathol 1998;22(9):1083–92.
64. Biegel JA, Rorke LB, Emanuel BS. Monosomy 22 in rhabdoid or atypical teratoid tumors of the brain. N Engl J Med 1989;321(13):906.
65. Chen ML, McComb JG, Krieger MD. Atypical teratoid/rhabdoid tumors of the central nervous system: management and outcomes. Neurosurg Focus 2005;18(6A):E8.
66. Hilden JM, Meerbaum S, Burger P, Finlay J, Janss A, Scheithauer BW, et al. Central nervous system atypical teratoid/rhabdoid tumor: results of therapy in children enrolled in a registry. J Clin Oncol 2004;22(14):2877–84.
67. Tekautz TM, Fuller CE, Blaney S, Fouladi M, Broniscer A, Merchant TE, et al. Atypical teratoid/rhabdoid tumors (ATRT): improved survival in children 3 years of age and older with radiation therapy and high-dose alkylator-based chemotherapy. J Clin Oncol 2005;23(7):1491–9.
68. Biegel JA, Zhou JY, Rorke LB, Stenstrom C, Wainwright LM, Fogelgren B. Germ-line and acquired mutations of INI1 in atypical teratoid and rhabdoid tumors. Cancer Res 1999;59(1):74–9.
69. Verstegen MJ, Leenstra DT, Ijlst-Keizers H, Bosch DA. Proliferation- and apoptosis-related proteins in intracranial ependymomas: an immunohistochemical analysis. J Neurooncol 2002;56(1):21–8.
70. Adesina AM, Dunn ST, Moore WE, Nalbantoglu J. Expression of p27kip1 and p53 in medulloblastoma: relationship with cell proliferation and survival. Pathol Res Pract 2000;196(4):243–50.
71. Jaros E, Lunec J, Perry RH, Kelly PJ, Pearson AD. p53 protein overexpression identifies a group of central primitive neuroectodermal tumours with poor prognosis. Br J Cancer 1993;68(4):801–7.
72. Woodburn RT, Azzarelli B, Montebello JF, Goss IE. Intense p53 staining is a valuable prognostic indicator for poor prognosis in medulloblastoma/central nervous system primitive neuroectodermal tumors. J Neurooncol 2001;52(1):57–62.
73. Gajjar A, Hernan R, Kocak M, Fuller C, Lee Y, McKinnon PJ, et al. Clinical, histopathologic, and molecular markers of prognosis: toward a new disease risk stratification system for medulloblastoma. J Clin Oncol 2004;22(6):984–93.
74. Gilbertson R, Hernan R, Pietsch T, Pinto L, Scotting P, Allibone R, et al. Novel ERBB4 juxtamembrane splice variants are frequently expressed in childhood medulloblastoma. Genes Chromosomes Cancer 2001;31(3):288–94.
75. Gilbertson RJ, Clifford SC, MacMeekin W, Meekin W, Wright C, Perry RH, et al. Expression of the ErbB-neuregulin signaling network during human cerebellar development: implications for the biology of medulloblastoma. Cancer Res 1998;58(17):3932–41.
76. Gilbertson RJ, Pearson AD, Perry RH, Jaros E, Kelly PJ. Prognostic significance of the c-erbB-2 oncogene product in childhood medulloblastoma. Br J Cancer 1995;71(3):473–7.
77. Herms JW, Behnke J, Bergmann M, Christen HJ, Kolb R, Wilkening M, et al. Potential prognostic value of C-erbB-2 expression in medulloblastomas in very young children. J Pediatr Hematol Oncol 1997;19(6):510–5.
78. Grotzer MA, Janss AJ, Phillips PC, Trojanowski JQ. Neurotrophin receptor TrkC predicts good clinical outcome in medulloblastoma and other primitive neuroectodermal brain tumors. Klin Padiatr 2000;212(4):196–9.
79. Kim JY, Sutton ME, Lu DJ, Cho TA, Goumnerova LC, Goritchenko L, et al. Activation of neurotrophin-3 receptor TrkC induces apoptosis in medulloblastomas. Cancer Res 1999;59(3):711–9.
80. Fernandez-Teijeiro A, Betensky RA, Sturla LM, Kim JY, Tamayo P, Pomeroy SL. Combining gene expression profiles and clinical parameters for risk stratification in medulloblastomas. J Clin Oncol 2004;22(6):994–8.
81. Pomeroy SL, Tamayo P, Gaasenbeek M, Sturla LM, Angelo M, McLaughlin ME, et al. Prediction of central nervous system embryonal tumour outcome based on gene expression. Nature 2002;415(6870):436–42.
82. McCabe MG, Ichimura K, Liu L, Plant K, Backlund LM, Pearson DM, et al. High-resolution array-based comparative genomic hybridization of medulloblastomas and supratentorial primitive neuroectodermal tumors. J Neuropathol Exp Neurol 2006;65(6):549–61.

83. Scheurlen WG, Schwabe GC, Seranski P, Joos S, Harbott J, Metzke S, et al. Mapping of the breakpoints on the short arm of chromosome 17 in neoplasms with an i(17q). Genes Chromosomes Cancer 1999;25(3):230–40.
84. Bayani J, Zielenska M, Marrano P, Kwan Ng Y, Taylor MD, Jay V, et al. Molecular cytogenetic analysis of medulloblastomas and supratentorial primitive neuroectodermal tumors by using conventional banding, comparative genomic hybridization, and spectral karyotyping. J Neurosurg 2000;93(3):437–48.
85. Fruhwald MC, O'Dorisio MS, Rush LJ, Reiter JL, Smiraglia DJ, Wenger G, et al. Gene amplification in PNETs/medulloblastomas: mapping of a novel amplified gene within the MYCN amplicon. J Med Genet 2000;37(7):501–9.
86. Michiels EM, Weiss MM, Hoovers JM, Baak JP, Voute PA, Baas F, et al. Genetic alterations in childhood medulloblastoma analyzed by comparative genomic hybridization. J Pediatr Hematol Oncol 2002;24(3):205–10.
87. Raffel C, Gilles FE, Weinberg KI. Reduction to homozygosity and gene amplification in central nervous system primitive neuroectodermal tumors of childhood. Cancer Res 1990;50(3):587–91.
88. Reardon DA, Michalkiewicz E, Boyett JM, Sublett JE, Entrekin RE, Ragsdale ST, et al. Extensive genomic abnormalities in childhood medulloblastoma by comparative genomic hybridization. Cancer Res 1997;57(18):4042–7.
89. Shlomit R, Ayala AG, Michal D, Ninett A, Frida S, Boleslaw G, et al. Gains and losses of DNA sequences in childhood brain tumors analyzed by comparative genomic hybridization. Cancer Genet Cytogenet 2000;121(1):67–72.
90. Herms J, Neidt I, Luscher B, Sommer A, Schurmann P, Schroder T, et al. C-MYC expression in medulloblastoma and its prognostic value. Int J Cancer 2000;89(5):395–402.
91. Grotzer MA, Hogarty MD, Janss AJ, Liu X, Zhao H, Eggert A, et al. MYC messenger RNA expression predicts survival outcome in childhood primitive neuroectodermal tumor/medulloblastoma. Clin Cancer Res 2001;7(8):2425–33.
92. Boon K, Eberhart CG, Riggins GJ. Genomic amplification of orthodenticle homologue 2 in medulloblastomas. Cancer Res 2005;65(3):703–7.
93. Di C, Liao S, Adamson DC, Parrett TJ, Broderick DK, Shi Q, et al. Identification of OTX2 as a medulloblastoma oncogene whose product can be targeted by all-trans retinoic acid. Cancer Res 2005;65(3):919–24.
94. Hartmann W, Digon-Sontgerath B, Koch A, Waha A, Endl E, Dani I, et al. Phosphatidylinositol 3′-kinase/AKT signaling is activated in medulloblastoma cell proliferation and is associated with reduced expression of PTEN. Clin Cancer Res 2006;12(10):3019–27.
95. Koch A, Waha A, Hartmann W, Milde U, Goodyer CG, Sorensen N, et al. No evidence for mutations or altered expression of the Suppressor of Fused gene (SUFU) in primitive neuroectodermal tumours. Neuropathol Appl Neurobiol 2004;30(5):532–9.
96. Pang JC, Dong Z, Zhang R, Liu Y, Zhou LF, Chan BW, et al. Mutation analysis of DMBT1 in glioblastoma, medulloblastoma and oligodendroglial tumors. Int J Cancer 2003;105(1):76–81.
97. Rasheed BK, Stenzel TT, McLendon RE, Parsons R, Friedman AH, Friedman HS, et al. PTEN gene mutations are seen in high-grade but not in low-grade gliomas. Cancer Res 1997;57(19):4187–90.
98. Taylor MD, Liu L, Raffel C, Hui CC, Mainprize TG, Zhang X, et al. Mutations in SUFU predispose to medulloblastoma. Nat Genet 2002;31(3):306–10.
99. MacDonald TJ, Brown KM, LaFleur B, Peterson K, Lawlor C, Chen Y, et al. Expression profiling of medulloblastoma: PDGFRA and the RAS/MAPK pathway as therapeutic targets for metastatic disease. Nat Genet 2001;29(2):143–52.
100. Gilbertson RJ, Clifford SC. PDGFRB is overexpressed in metastatic medulloblastoma. Nat Genet 2003;35(3):197–8.
101. Vorechovsky I, Tingby O, Hartman M, Stromberg B, Nister M, Collins VP, et al. Somatic mutations in the human homologue of Drosophila patched in primitive neuroectodermal tumours. Oncogene 1997;15(3):361–6.
102. Pietsch T, Waha A, Koch A, Kraus J, Albrecht S, Tonn J, et al. Medulloblastomas of the desmoplastic variant carry mutations of the human homologue of Drosophila patched. Cancer Res 1997;57(11):2085–8.
103. Reifenberger J, Wolter M, Weber RG, Megahed M, Ruzicka T, Lichter P, et al. Missense mutations in SMOH in sporadic basal cell carcinomas of the skin and primitive neuroectodermal tumors of the central nervous system. Cancer Res 1998;58(9):1798–803.

104. Lam CW, Xie J, To KF, Ng HK, Lee KC, Yuen NW, et al. A frequent activated smoothened mutation in sporadic basal cell carcinomas. Oncogene 1999;18(3):833–6.
105. Zurawel RH, Allen C, Chiappa S, Cato W, Biegel J, Cogen P, et al. Analysis of PTCH/SMO/SHH pathway genes in medulloblastoma. Genes Chromosomes Cancer 2000;27(1):44–51.
106. Romer JT, Kimura H, Magdaleno S, Sasai K, Fuller C, Baines H, et al. Suppression of the Shh pathway using a small molecule inhibitor eliminates medulloblastoma in Ptc1(+/–)p53(–/–) mice. Cancer Cell 2004;6(3):229–40.
107. Bar EE, Stearns D. New developments in medulloblastoma treatment: the potential of a cyclopamine-lovastatin combination. Expert Opin Investig Drugs 2008;17(2):185–95.
108. Huang H, Mahler-Araujo BM, Sankila A, Chimelli L, Yonekawa Y, Kleihues P, et al. APC mutations in sporadic medulloblastomas. Am J Pathol 2000;156(2):433–7.
109. Zurawel RH, Chiappa SA, Allen C, Raffel C. Sporadic medulloblastomas contain oncogenic beta-catenin mutations. Cancer Res 1998;58(5):896–9.
110. Baeza N, Masuoka J, Kleihues P, Ohgaki H. AXIN1 mutations but not deletions in cerebellar medulloblastomas. Oncogene 2003;22(4):632–6.
111. Koch A, Waha A, Tonn JC, Sorensen N, Berthold F, Wolter M, et al. Somatic mutations of WNT/wingless signaling pathway components in primitive neuroectodermal tumors. Int J Cancer 2001;93(3):445–9.
112. Dahmen RP, Koch A, Denkhaus D, Tonn JC, Sorensen N, Berthold F, et al. Deletions of AXIN1, a component of the WNT/wingless pathway, in sporadic medulloblastomas. Cancer Res 2001;61(19):7039–43.
113. Kestler HA, Kuhl M. From individual Wnt pathways towards a Wnt signalling network. Philos Trans R Soc Lond B Biol Sci 2008;363(1495):1333–47.
114. Ohgaki H, Dessen P, Jourde B, Horstmann S, Nishikawa T, Di Patre PL, et al. Genetic pathways to glioblastoma: a population-based study. Cancer Res 2004;64(19):6892–9.
115. Sherer HJ. Cerebral astrocytomas and their derivatives. Am J Cancer 1940;40:159–98.
116. Biernat W, Tohma Y, Yonekawa Y, Kleihues P, Ohgaki H. Alterations of cell cycle regulatory genes in primary (de novo) and secondary glioblastomas. Acta Neuropathol (Berl) 1997;94(4):303–9.
117. von Deimling A, von Ammon K, Schoenfeld D, Wiestler OD, Seizinger BR, Louis DN. Subsets of glioblastoma multiforme defined by molecular genetic analysis. Brain Pathology 1993;3(1):19–26.
118. James CD, Carlbom E, Dumanski JP, Hansen M, Nordenskjold M, Collins VP, et al. Clonal genomic alterations in glioma malignancy stages. Cancer Res 1988;48(19):5546–51.
119. Reifenberger G, Ichimura K, Reifenberger J, Elkahloun AG, Meltzer PS, Collins VP. Refined mapping of 12q13-q15 amplicons in human malignant gliomas suggests CDK4/SAS and MDM2 as independent amplification targets. Cancer Res 1996;56(22):5141–5.
120. Ichimura K, Ohgaki H, Kleihues P, Collins VP. Molecular pathogenesis of astrocytic tumours. J Neurooncol 2004;70(2):137–60.
121. McCormack BM, Miller DC, Budzilovich GN, Voorhees GJ, Ransohoff J. Treatment and survival of low-grade astrocytoma in adults—1977–1988. Neurosurgery 1992;31(4):636–42 discussion 42.
122. Simpson JR, Horton J, Scott C, Curran WJ, Rubin P, Fischbach J, et al. Influence of location and extent of surgical resection on survival of patients with glioblastoma multiforme: results of three consecutive Radiation Therapy Oncology Group (RTOG) clinical trials. Int J Radiat Oncol Biol Phys 1993;26(2):239–44.
123. Stupp R, van den Bent MJ, Hegi ME. Optimal role of temozolomide in the treatment of malignant gliomas. Curr Neurol Neurosci Rep 2005;5(3):198–206.
124. Kimmel DW, O'Fallon JR, Scheithauer BW, Kelly PJ, Dewald GW, Jenkins RB. Prognostic value of cytogenetic analysis in human cerebral astrocytomas. Ann Neurol 1992;31(5):534–42.
125. Weber RG, Sabel M, Reifenberger J, Sommer C, Oberstrass J, Reifenberger G, et al. Characterization of genomic alterations associated with glioma progression by comparative genomic hybridization. Oncogene 1996;13(5):983–94.
126. Rasheed BK, McLendon RE, Herndon JE, Friedman HS, Friedman AH, Bigner DD, et al. Alterations of the TP53 gene in human gliomas. Cancer Res 1994;54(5):1324–30.
127. James CD, Carlbom E, Nordenskjold M, Collins VP, Cavenee WK. Mitotic recombination of chromosome 17 in astrocytomas. Proc Natl Acad Sci U S A 1989;86(8):2858–62.
128. Okamoto Y, Di Patre PL, Burkhard C, Horstmann S, Jourde B, Fahey M, et al. Population-based study on incidence, survival rates, and genetic alterations of low-grade diffuse astrocytomas and oligodendrogliomas. Acta Neuropathol 2004;108(1):49–56.

129. Alonso ME, Bello MJ, Lomas J, Gonzalez-Gomez P, Arjona D, De Campos JM, et al. Absence of mutation of the p73 gene in astrocytic neoplasms. Int J Oncol 2001;19(3):609–12.
130. Ichimura K, Schmidt EE, Goike HM, Collins VP. Human glioblastomas with no alterations of the CDKN2A (p16INK4A, MTS1) and CDK4 genes have frequent mutations of the retinoblastoma gene. Oncogene 1996;13(5):1065–72.
131. Hoang-Xuan K, Merel P, Vega F, Hugot JP, Cornu P, Delattre JY, et al. Analysis of the NF2 tumor-suppressor gene and of chromosome 22 deletions in gliomas. Int J Cancer 1995;60(4):478–81.
132. Ino Y, Silver JS, Blazejewski L, Nishikawa R, Matsutani M, von Deimling A, et al. Common regions of deletion on chromosome 22q12.3-q13.1 and 22q13.2 in human astrocytomas appear related to malignancy grade [In Process Citation.] J Neuropathol Exp Neurol 1999;58(8):881–5.
133. Miyakawa A, Ichimura K, Schmidt E, Varmeh-Ziaie S, Collins VP. Multiple deleted regions on the long arm of chromosome 6 in astrocytic tumours. Brit J Cancer 1999; In Press.
134. Reifenberger G, Liu L, Ichimura K, Schmidt EE, Collins VP. Amplification and overexpression of the MDM2 gene in a subset of human malignant gliomas without p53 mutations. Cancer Res 1993;53(12):2736–9.
135. Reifenberger G, Reifenberger J, Ichimura K, Meltzer PS, Collins VP. Amplification of multiple genes from chromosomal region 12q13–14 in human malignant gliomas: preliminary mapping of the amplicons shows preferential involvement of CDK4, SAS, and MDM2. Cancer Res 1994;54(16):4299–303.
136. Reifenberger G, Reifenberger J, Ichimura K, Collins VP. Amplification at 12q13–14 in human malignant gliomas is frequently accompanied by loss of heterozygosity at loci proximal and distal to the amplification site. Cancer Res 1995;55(4):731–4.
137. Ekstrand AJ, James CD, Cavenee WK, Seliger B, Pettersson RF, Collins VP. Genes for epidermal growth factor receptor, transforming growth factor alpha, and epidermal growth factor and their expression in human gliomas in vivo. Cancer Res 1991;51(8):2164–72.
138. Hermanson M, Funa K, Hartman M, Claesson-Welsh L, Heldin CH, Westermark B, et al. Platelet-derived growth factor and its receptors in human glioma tissue: expression of messenger RNA and protein suggests the presence of autocrine and paracrine loops. Cancer Res 1992;52(11):3213–9.
139. Lokker NA, Sullivan CM, Hollenbach SJ, Israel MA, Giese NA. Platelet-derived growth factor (PDGF) autocrine signaling regulates survival and mitogenic pathways in glioblastoma cells: evidence that the novel PDGF-C and PDGF-D ligands may play a role in the development of brain tumors. Cancer Res 2002;62(13):3729–35.
140. Huang H, Colella S, Kurrer M, Yonekawa Y, Kleihues P, Ohgaki H. Gene expression profiling of low-grade diffuse astrocytomas by cDNA arrays. Cancer Res 2000;60(24):6868–74.
141. Westermark B, Carlhendrik H, Nister M. Platelet-Derived Growth Factor In Human Glioma. Glia 1995;15(3):257–63.
142. Uhrbom L, Hesselager G, Nister M, Westermark B. Induction of brain tumors in mice using a recombinant platelet-derived growth factor B-chain retrovirus. Cancer Res 1998; 58(23):5275–9.
143. Fleming TP, Saxena A, Clark WC, Robertson JT, Oldfield EH, Aaronson SA, et al. Amplification and/or overexpression of platelet-derived growth factor receptors and epidermal growth factor receptor in human glial tumors. Cancer Res 1992;52(16):4550–3.
144. Kumabe T, Sohma Y, Kayama T, Yoshimoto T, Yamamoto T. Amplification of alpha-platelet-derived growth factor receptor gene lacking an exon coding for a portion of the extracellular region in a primary brain tumor of glial origin. Oncogene 1992;7(4):627–33.
145. Smith JS, Wang XY, Qian J, Hosek SM, Scheithauer BW, Jenkins RB, et al. Amplification of the platelet-derived growth factor receptor-A (PDGFRA) gene occurs in oligodendrogliomas with grade IV anaplastic features. J Neuropathol Exp Neurol 2000;59(6):495–503.
146. Wiencke JK, Zheng S, Jelluma N, Tihan T, Vandenberg S, Tamguney T, et al. Methylation of the PTEN promoter defines low-grade gliomas and secondary glioblastoma. Neuro Oncol 2007;9(3):271–9.
147. Costello JF, Plass C, Cavenee WK. Aberrant methylation of genes in low-grade astrocytomas. Brain Tumor Pathol 2000;17(2):49–56.
148. Yu J, Zhang H, Gu J, Lin S, Li J, Lu W, et al. Methylation profiles of thirty four promoter-CpG islands and concordant methylation behaviours of sixteen genes that may contribute to carcinogenesis of astrocytoma. BMC Cancer 2004;4(1):65.

149. Watanabe K, Sato K, Biernat W, Tachibana O, von Ammon K, Ogata N, et al. Incidence and timing of p53 mutations during astrocytoma progression in patients with multiple biopsies. Clin Cancer Res 1997;3(4):523–30.
150. Reifenberger J, Ring GU, Gies U, Cobbers L, Oberstrass J, An HX, et al. Analysis of p53 mutation and epidermal growth factor receptor amplification in recurrent gliomas with malignant progression. J Neuropathol Exp Neurol 1996;55(7):822–31.
151. Lowe SW, Sherr CJ. Tumor suppression by Ink4a-Arf: progress and puzzles. Curr Opin Genet Dev 2003;13(1):77–83.
152. Roth J, Dobbelstein M, Freedman DA, Shenk T, Levine AJ. Nucleo-cytoplasmic shuttling of the hdm2 oncoprotein regulates the levels of the p53 protein via a pathway used by the human immunodeficiency virus rev protein. Embo J 1998;17(2):554–64.
153. Nakamura M, Watanabe T, Klangby U, Asker C, Wiman K, Yonekawa Y, et al. p14ARF deletion and methylation in genetic pathways to glioblastomas. Brain Pathol 2001;11(2):159–68.
154. Wang JY, Knudsen ES, Welch PJ. The retinoblastoma tumor suppressor protein. Adv Cancer Res 1994;64:25–85.
155. Serrano M, Hannon GJ, Beach D. A new regulatory motif in cell-cycle control causing specific inhibition of cyclin D/CDK4: see comments. Nature 1993;366(6456):704–7.
156. Nakamura M, Yonekawa Y, Kleihues P, Ohgaki H. Promoter hypermethylation of the RB1 gene in glioblastomas. Lab Invest 2001;81(1):77–82.
157. Humphrey PA, Wong AJ, Vogelstein B, Zalutsky MR, Fuller GN, Archer GE, et al. Anti-synthetic peptide antibody reacting at the fusion junction of deletion-mutant epidermal growth factor receptors in human glioblastoma. Proc Natl Acad Sci U S A 1990;87(11):4207–11.
158. Wong AJ, Ruppert JM, Bigner SH, Grzeschik CH, Humphrey PA, Bigner DS, et al. Structural alterations of the epidermal growth factor receptor gene in human gliomas. Proc Natl Acad Sci U S A 1992;89(7):2965–9.
159. Sugawa N, Ekstrand AJ, James CD, Collins VP. Identical splicing of aberrant epidermal growth factor receptor transcripts from amplified rearranged genes in human glioblastomas. Proc Natl Acad Sci U S A 1990;87(21):8602–6.
160. Nishikawa R, Ji XD, Harmon RC, Lazar CS, Gill GN, Cavenee WK, et al. A mutant epidermal growth factor receptor common in human glioma confers enhanced tumorigenicity. Proc Natl Acad Sci U S A 1994;91(16):7727–31.
161. Ekstrand AJ, Longo N, Hamid ML, Olson JJ, Liu L, Collins VP, et al. Functional characterization of an EGF receptor with a truncated extracellular domain expressed in glioblastomas with EGFR gene amplification. Oncogene 1994;9(8):2313–20.
162. Jungbluth AA, Stockert E, Huang HJ, Collins VP, Coplan K, Iversen K, et al. A monoclonal antibody recognizing human cancers with amplification/overexpression of the human epidermal growth factor receptor. Proc Natl Acad Sci U S A 2003;100(2):639–44.
163. Mischel PS, Cloughesy TF. Targeted molecular therapy of GBM. Brain Pathol 2003; 13(1):52–61.
164. Ekstrand AJ, Sugawa N, James CD, Collins VP. Amplified and rearranged epidermal growth factor receptor genes in human glioblastomas reveal deletions of sequences encoding portions of the N- and/or C-terminal tails. Proc Natl Acad Sci U S A 1992;89(10):4309–13.
165. Samuels Y, Wang Z, Bardelli A, Silliman N, Ptak J, Szabo S, et al. High frequency of mutations of the PIK3CA gene in human cancers. Science 2004;304(5670):554.
166. Mueller W, Mizoguchi M, Silen E, D'Amore K, Nutt CL. Louis DN. Mutations of the PIK3CA gene are rare in human glioblastoma. Acta Neuropathol (Berl) 2005;109(6):654–5.
167. Broderick DK, Di C, Parrett TJ, Samuels YR, Cummins JM, McLendon RE, et al. Mutations of PIK3CA in anaplastic oligodendrogliomas, high-grade astrocytomas, and medulloblastomas. Cancer Res 2004;64(15):5048–50.
168. Furnari FB, Huang HJ, Cavenee WK. The phosphoinositol phosphatase activity of PTEN mediates a serum- sensitive G1 growth arrest in glioma cells. Cancer Res 1998;58(22): 5002–8.
169. Myers MP, Stolarov JP, Eng C, Li J, Wang SI, Wigler MH, et al. P-TEN, the tumor suppressor from human chromosome 10q23, is a dual-specificity phosphatase. Proc Natl Acad Sci U S A 1997;94(17):9052–7.
170. Myers MP, Pass I, Batty IH, Van der Kaay J, Stolarov JP, Hemmings BA, et al. The lipid phosphatase activity of PTEN is critical for its tumor supressor function. Proc Natl Acad Sci U S A 1998;95(23):13513–8.

171. Steck PA, Pershouse MA, Jasser SA, Yung WKA, Lin H, Ligon AH, et al. Identification of a candidate tumour suppressor gene, *MMAC1*, at chromosome 10q23.3 that is mutated in multiple advanced cancers. Nat Genet 1997;15(4):356–62.
172. Li J, Yen C, Liaw D, Podsypanina K, Bose S, Wang SI, et al. *PTEN*, a putative protein tyrosine phosphatase gene mutated in human brain, breast, and prostate cancer. Science 1997;275(5308):1943–7.
173. Ichimura K, Schmidt EE, Miyakawa A, Goike HM, Collins VP. Distinct patterns of deletion on 10p and 10q suggest involvement of multiple tumor suppressor genes in the development of astrocytic gliomas of different malignancy grades. Genes Chromosomes and Cancer 1998; In Press.
174. Schmidt E, Ichimura K, Goike HM, Moshref A, Liu L, Collins VP. Mutational profile of the PTEN/MMAC1 gene in primary human astrocytic tumors and xenografts. J Neuropathol Expt Neurol 1999; In Press.
175. Zundel W, Schindler C, Haas-Kogan D, Koong A, Kaper F, Chen E, et al. Loss of PTEN facilitates HIF-1-mediated gene expression. Genes Dev 2000;14(4):391–6.
176. Knobbe CB, Reifenberger G. Genetic alterations and aberrant expression of genes related to the phosphatidyl-inositol-3 -kinase/protein kinase B (Akt) signal transduction pathway in glioblastomas. Brain Pathol 2003;13(4):507–18.
177. Knobbe CB, Reifenberger J, Blaschke B, Reifenberger G. Hypermethylation and transcriptional downregulation of the carboxyl-terminal modulator protein gene in glioblastomas. J Natl Cancer Inst 2004;96(6):483–6.
178. Sonoda Y, Ozawa T, Hirose Y, Aldape KD, McMahon M, Berger MS, et al. Formation of intracranial tumors by genetically modified human astrocytes defines four pathways critical in the development of human anaplastic astrocytoma. Cancer Res 2001;61(13):4956–60.
179. Liu JL, Sheng X, Hortobagyi ZK, Mao Z, Gallick GE, Yung WK. Nuclear PTEN-Mediated Growth Suppression Is Independent of Akt Down-Regulation. Mol Cell Biol 2005;25(14):6211–24.
180. Collins VP. Mechanisms of disease: genetic predictors of response to treatment in brain tumors. Nat Clin Pract Oncol 2007;4(6):362–74.
181. Aldape KD, Ballman K, Furth A, Buckner JC, Giannini C, Burger PC, et al. Immunohistochemical detection of EGFRvIII in high malignancy grade astrocytomas and evaluation of prognostic significance. J Neuropathol Exp Neurol 2004;63(7):700–7.
182. Galanis E, Buckner J, Kimmel D, Jenkins R, Alderete B, O'Fallon J, et al. Gene amplification as a prognostic factor in primary and secondary high-grade malignant gliomas. Int J Oncol 1998;13(4):717–24.
183. Heimberger AB, Hlatky R, Suki D, Yang D, Weinberg J, Gilbert M, et al. Prognostic effect of epidermal growth factor receptor and EGFRvIII in glioblastoma multiforme patients. Clin Cancer Res 2005;11(4):1462–6.
184. Huncharek M, Kupelnick B. Epidermal growth factor receptor gene amplification as a prognostic marker in glioblastoma multiforme: results of a meta-analysis. Oncol Res 2000;12(2):107–12.
185. Olson JJ, Barnett D, Yang J, Assietti R, Cotsonis G, James CD. Gene amplification as a prognostic factor in primary brain tumors. Clin Cancer Res 1998;4(1):215–22.
186. Shinojima N, Tada K, Shiraishi S, Kamiryo T, Kochi M, Nakamura H, et al. Prognostic value of epidermal growth factor receptor in patients with glioblastoma multiforme. Cancer Res 2003;63(20):6962–70.
187. Smith JS, Tachibana I, Passe SM, Huntley BK, Borell TJ, Iturria N, et al. PTEN mutation, EGFR amplification, and outcome in patients with anaplastic astrocytoma and glioblastoma multiforme. J Natl Cancer Inst 2001;93(16):1246–56.
188. Backlund LM, Nilsson BR, Goike HM, Schmidt EE, Liu L, Ichimura K, et al. Short postoperative survival for glioblastoma patients with a dysfunctional Rb1 pathway in combination with no wild-type PTEN. Clin Cancer Res 2003;9(11):4151–8.
189. Backlund LM, Nilsson BR, Liu L, Ichimura K, Collins VP. Mutations in Rb1 pathway-related genes are associated with poor prognosis in Anaplastic Astrocytomas. Br J Cancer 2005;93(1):124–30.
190. Hegi ME, Diserens AC, Gorlia T, Hamou MF, de Tribolet N, Weller M, et al. MGMT gene silencing and benefit from temozolomide in glioblastoma. N Engl J Med 2005;352(10):997–1003.
191. Kleihues P, Ohgaki H. Primary and secondary glioblastomas: from concept to clinical diagnosis. Neuro-oncol 1999;1(1):44–51.
192. Esteller M, Garcia-Foncillas J, Andion E, Goodman SN, Hidalgo OF, Vanaclocha V, et al. Inactivation of the DNA-repair gene MGMT and the clinical response of gliomas to alkylating agents. N Engl J Med 2000;343(19):1350–4.

193. Lee SM, Thatcher N, Crowther D, Margison GP. Inactivation of O6-alkylguanine-DNA alkyltransferase in human peripheral blood mononuclear cells by temozolomide. Br J Cancer 1994;69(3):452–6.
194. Gander M, Leyvraz S, Decosterd L, Bonfanti M, Marzolini C, Shen F, et al. Sequential administration of temozolomide and fotemustine: depletion of O6-alkyl guanine-DNA transferase in blood lymphocytes and in tumours. Ann Oncol 1999;10(7):831–8.
195. Ichimura K, Mungall AJ, Fiegler H, Pearson DM, Dunham I, Carter NP, et al. Small regions of overlapping deletions on 6q26 in human astrocytic tumours identified using chromosome 6 tile path array-CGH. Oncogene 2006;25(8):1261–71.
196. Ichimura K, Vogazianou AP, Liu L, Pearson DM, Backlund LM, Plant K, et al. 1p36 is a preferential target of chromosome 1 deletions in astrocytic tumours and homozygously deleted in a subset of glioblastomas. Oncogene 2008;27(14):2097–108.
197. Seng TJ, Ichimura K, Liu L, Tingby O, Pearson DM, Collins VP. Complex chromosome 22 rearrangements in astrocytic tumors identified using microsatellite and chromosome 22 tile path array analysis. Genes Chromosomes Cancer 2005;43(2):181–93.
198. Miller CR, Dunham CP, Scheithauer BW, Perry A. Significance of necrosis in grading of oligodendroglial neoplasms: a clinicopathologic and genetic study of newly diagnosed high-grade gliomas. J Clin Oncol 2006;24(34):5419–26.
199. Macdonald DR, Gaspar LE, Cairncross JG. Successful chemotherapy for newly diagnosed aggressive oligodendroglioma. Ann Neurol 1990;27(5):573–4.
200. Reifenberger J, Reifenberger G, Liu L, James CD, Wechsler W, Collins VP. Molecular genetic analysis of oligodendroglial tumors shows preferential allelic deletions on 19 q and 1 p. Am J Pathol 1994;145(5):1175–90.
201. Mollemann M, Wolter M, Felsberg J, Collins VP, Reifenberger G. Frequent promoter hypermethylation and low expression of the MGMT gene in oligodendroglial tumors. Int J Cancer 2005;113(3):379–85.
202. Reifenberger G, Louis DN. Oligodendroglioma: toward molecular definitions in diagnostic neuro-oncology. J Neuropathol Exp Neurol 2003;62(2):111–26.
203. Cairncross JG, Ueki K, Zlatescu MC, Lisle DK, Finkelstein DM, Hammond RR, et al. Specific genetic predictors of chemotherapeutic response and survival in patients with anaplastic oligodendrogliomas. J Natl Cancer Inst 1998;90(19):1473–9.
204. Jenkins RB, Blair H, Ballman KV, Giannini C, Arusell RM, Law M, et al. A t(1;19)(q10;p10) mediates the combined deletions of 1 p and 19 q and predicts a better prognosis of patients with oligodendroglioma. Cancer Res 2006;66(20):9852–61.
205. Idbaih A, Marie Y, Pierron G, Brennetot C, Hoang-Xuan K, Kujas M, et al. Two types of chromosome 1 p losses with opposite significance in gliomas. Ann Neurol 2005;58(3):483–7.
206. Ueki K, Nishikawa R, Nakazato Y, Hirose T, Hirato J, Funada N, et al. Correlation of histology and molecular genetic analysis of 1 p, 19 q, 10 q, TP53, EGFR, CDK4, and CDKN2A in 91 astrocytic and oligodendroglial tumors. Clin Cancer Res 2002;8(1):196–201.
207. Wolter M, Reifenberger J, Blaschke B, Ichimura K, Schmidt EE, Collins VP, et al. Oligodendroglial tumors frequently demonstrate hypermethylation of the CDKN2A (MTS1, p16INK4a), p14ARF, and CDKN2B (MTS2, p15INK4b) tumor suppressor genes. J Neuropathol Exp Neurol 2001;60(12):1170–80.
208. Jeuken JW, Nelen MR, Vermeer H, van Staveren WC, Kremer H, van Overbeeke JJ, et al. PTEN mutation analysis in two genetic subtypes of high-grade oligodendroglial tumors. PTEN is only occasionally mutated in one of the two genetic subtypes. Cancer Genet Cytogenet 2000;119(1):42–7.
209. Sasaki H, Zlatescu MC, Betensky RA, Ino Y, Cairncross JG, Louis DN. PTEN is a target of chromosome 10 q loss in anaplastic oligodendrogliomas and PTEN alterations are associated with poor prognosis. Am J Pathol 2001;159(1):359–67.
210. Idbaih A, Marie Y, Lucchesi C, Pierron G, Manie E, Raynal V, et al. BAC array CGH distinguishes mutually exclusive alterations that define clinicogenetic subtypes of gliomas. Int J Cancer 2008;122(8):1778–86.
211. Rausing A, Ybo W, Stenflo J. Intracranial meningioma—a population study of ten years. Acta Neurol Scand 1970;46(1):102–10.
212. Vernooij MW, Ikram MA, Tanghe HL, Vincent AJ, Hofman A, Krestin GP, et al. Incidental findings on brain MRI in the general population. N Engl J Med 2007;357(18):1821–8.
213. Mark J, Levan G, Mitelman F. Identification by fluorescence of the G chromosome lost in human meningomas. Hereditas 1972;71(1):163–8.

214. Ruttledge MH, Sarrazin J, Rangaratnam S, Phelan CM, Twist E, Merel P, et al. Evidence for the complete inactivation of the NF2 gene in the majority of sporadic meningiomas. Nat Genet 1994;6(2):180–4.
215. Hansson CM, Buckley PG, Grigelioniene G, Piotrowski A, Hellstrom AR, Mantripragada K, et al. Comprehensive genetic and epigenetic analysis of sporadic meningioma for macro-mutations on 22 q and micro-mutations within the NF2 locus. BMC Genomics 2007;8:16.
216. Trofatter JA, MacCollin MM, Rutter JL, Murrell JR, Duyao MP, Parry DM, et al. A novel moesin-, ezrin-, radixin-like gene is a candidate for the neurofibromatosis 2 tumor suppressor. Cell 1993;72(5):791–800.
217. Shaw RJ, Paez JG, Curto M, Yaktine A, Pruitt WM, Saotome I, et al. The Nf2 tumor suppressor, merlin, functions in Rac-dependent signaling. Dev Cell 2001;1(1):63–72.
218. Lallemand D, Curto M, Saotome I, Giovannini M, McClatchey AI. NF2 deficiency promotes tumorigenesis and metastasis by destabilizing adherens junctions. Genes Dev 2003;17(9):1090–100.
219. McClatchey AI, Saotome I, Mercer K, Crowley D, Gusella JF, Bronson RT, et al. Mice heterozygous for a mutation at the Nf2 tumor suppressor locus develop a range of highly metastatic tumors. Genes Dev 1998;12(8):1121–33.
220. Kalamarides M, Niwa-Kawakita M, Leblois H, Abramowski V, Perricaudet M, Janin A, et al. Nf2 gene inactivation in arachnoidal cells is rate-limiting for meningioma development in the mouse. Genes Dev 2002;16(9):1060–5.
221. Giovannini M, Robanus-Maandag E, van der Valk M, Niwa-Kawakita M, Abramowski V, Goutebroze L, et al. Conditional biallelic Nf2 mutation in the mouse promotes manifestations of human neurofibromatosis type 2. Genes Dev 2000;14(13):1617–30.
222. Weber RG, Bostrom J, Wolter M, Baudis M, Collins VP, Reifenberger G, et al. Analysis of genomic alterations in benign, atypical, and anaplastic meningiomas: toward a genetic model of meningioma progression. Proc Natl Acad Sci U S A 1997;94(26):14719–24.
223. Ozaki S, Nishizaki T, Ito H, Sasaki K. Comparative genomic hybridization analysis of genetic alterations associated with malignant progression of meningioma. J Neurooncol 1999;41(2):167–74.
224. Lamszus K, Kluwe L, Matschke J, Meissner H, Laas R, Westphal M. *Allelic* losses at 1 p, 9 q, 10 q, 14 q, and 22 q in the progression of aggressive meningiomas and undifferentiated meningeal sarcomas. Cancer Genet Cytogenet 1999;110(2):103–10.
225. Cai DX, James CD, Scheithauer BW, Couch FJ, Perry A. PS6K amplification characterizes a small subset of anaplastic meningiomas. Am J Clin Pathol 2001;115(2):213–8.
226. Cai DX, Banerjee R, Scheithauer BW, Lohse CM, Kleinschmidt-Demasters BK, Perry A. Chromosome 1 p and 14 q FISH analysis in clinicopathologic subsets of meningioma: diagnostic and prognostic implications. J Neuropathol Exp Neurol 2001;60(6):628–36.
227. Lindblom A, Ruttledge M, Collins VP, Nordenskjold M, Dumanski JP. Chromosomal deletions in anaplastic meningiomas suggest multiple regions outside chromosome 22 as important in tumor progression. Int J Cancer 1994;56(3):354–7.
228. Buschges R, Ichimura K, Weber RG, Reifenberger G, Collins VP. Allelic gain and amplification on the long arm of chromosome 17 in anaplastic meningiomas. Brain Pathol 2002;12(2):145–53.
229. Perry A, Banerjee R, Lohse CM, Kleinschmidt-DeMasters BK, Scheithauer BW. A role for chromosome 9p21 deletions in the malignant progression of meningiomas and the prognosis of anaplastic meningiomas. Brain Pathol 2002;12(2):183–90.
230. Bostrom J, Meyer-Puttlitz B, Wolter M, Blaschke B, Weber RG, Lichter P, et al. Alterations of the tumor suppressor genes CDKN2A (p16(INK4a)), p14(ARF), CDKN2B (p15(INK4b)), and CDKN2C (p18(INK4c)) in atypical and anaplastic meningiomas. Am J Pathol 2001;159(2):661–9.
231. Lusis EA, Watson MA, Chicoine MR, Lyman M, Roerig P, Reifenberger G, et al. Integrative genomic analysis identifies NDRG2 as a candidate tumor suppressor gene frequently inactivated in clinically aggressive meningioma. Cancer Res 2005;65(16):7121–6.
232. Hochberg FH, Baehring JM, Hochberg EP. Primary CNS lymphoma. Nat Clin Pract Neurol 2007;3(1):24–35.
233. Gerstner E, Batchelor T. Primary CNS lymphoma. Expert Rev Anticancer Ther 2007;7(5): 689–700.
234. Abrey LE, Batchelor TT, Ferreri AJ, Gospodarowicz M, Pulczynski EJ, Zucca E, et al. Report of an international workshop to standardize baseline evaluation and response criteria for primary CNS lymphoma. J Clin Oncol 2005;23(22):5034–43.
235. Jaffe ES, Harris NL, Stein H, Vardiman JW, editors. Tumours of haematopoietic and lymphoid tissues. Lyon: IARC Press; 2001.

236. Larocca LM, Capello D, Rinelli A, Nori S, Antinori A, Gloghini A, et al. The molecular and phenotypic profile of primary central nervous system lymphoma identifies distinct categories of the disease and is consistent with histogenetic derivation from germinal center-related B cells. Blood 1998;92(3):1011–9.
237. Thompsett AR, Ellison DW, Stevenson FK, Zhu D. V(H) gene sequences from primary central nervous system lymphomas indicate derivation from highly mutated germinal center B cells with ongoing mutational activity. Blood 1999;94(5):1738–46.
238. Rubenstein JL, Fridlyand J, Shen A, Aldape K, Ginzinger D, Batchelor T, et al. Gene expression and angiotropism in primary CNS lymphoma. Blood 2006;107(9):3716–23.
239. Montesinos-Rongen M, Brunn A, Bentink S, Basso K, Lim WK, Klapper W, et al. Gene expression profiling suggests primary central nervous system lymphomas to be derived from a late germinal center B cell. Leukemia 2008;22(2):400–5.
240. Pasqualucci L, Neumeister P, Goossens T, Nanjangud G, Chaganti RS, Kuppers R, et al. Hypermutation of multiple proto-oncogenes in B-cell diffuse large-cell lymphomas. Nature 2001;412(6844):341–6.
241. Montesinos-Rongen M, Van Roost D, Schaller C, Wiestler OD, Deckert M. Primary diffuse large B-cell lymphomas of the central nervous system are targeted by aberrant somatic hypermutation. Blood 2004;103(5):1869–75.
242. Cobbers JM, Wolter M, Reifenberger J, Ring GU, Jessen F, An HX, et al. Frequent inactivation of CDKN2A and rare mutation of TP53 in PCNSL. Brain Pathol 1998;8(2):263–76.
243. Weber T, Weber RG, Kaulich K, Actor B, Meyer-Puttlitz B, Lampel S, et al. Characteristic chromosomal imbalances in primary central nervous system lymphomas of the diffuse large B-cell type. Brain Pathol 2000;10(1):73–84.
244. Wen PY, Loeffler JS. Management of brain metastases. Oncology (Williston Park) 1999;13(7): 941–54 57–61; discussion 61–2, 9.
245. Posner JB, Chernik NL. Intracranial metastases from systemic cancer. Adv Neurol 1978; 19:579–92.
246. Ward BA, Gutmann DH. Neurofibromatosis 1: from lab bench to clinic. Pediatr Neurol 2005; 32(4):221–8.
247. Uppal S, Coatesworth AP. Neurofibromatosis type 2. Int J Clin Pract 2003;57(8):698–703.
248. Raffel C. Medulloblastoma: molecular genetics and animal models. Neoplasia 2004;6(4): 310–22.
249. Lucci-Cordisco E, Zito I, Gensini F, Genuardi M. Hereditary nonpolyposis colorectal cancer and related conditions. Am J Med Genet A 2003;122(4):325–34.
250. Eng C, Parsons R. Cowden Syndrome. In: Vogelstein B, Kinzler KW, editors. The genetic basis of Cancer. New York, London: McGraw-Hill, Health Professions Division; 1998. p. 519–26.
251. Al-Saleem T, Wessner LL, Scheithauer BW, Patterson K, Roach ES, Dreyer SJ, et al. Malignant tumors of the kidney, brain, and soft tissues in children and young adults with the tuberous sclerosis complex. Cancer 1998;83(10):2208–16.
252. Flamme I, Krieg M, Plate KH. Up-regulation of vascular endothelial growth factor in stromal cells of hemangioblastomas is correlated with up-regulation of the transcription factor HRF/HIF-2alpha. Am J Pathol 1998;153(1):25–9.
253. Li YJ, Sanson M, Hoang-Xuan K, Delattre JY, Poisson M, Thomas G, et al. Incidence of germ-line p53 mutations in patients with gliomas. Int J Cancer 1995;64(6):383–7.
254. Malkin D. Li-Fraumeni Syndrome. In: Vogelstein B, Kinzler KW, editors. The genetic basis of Cancer. New York, London: McGraw-Hill, Health Professions Division; 1998. p. 393–422.
255. Kaufman DK, Kimmel DW, Parisi JE, Michels VV. A familial syndrome with cutaneous malignant melanoma and cerebral astrocytoma. Neurology 1993;43(9):1728–31.
256. Yan H, Parsons W, Genglin J, McLendon R, Rasheed A, Yuan W, et al. IDH1 and IDH2 mutations in gliomas. N Engl J Med 2009;360:765–73.
257. Ichimura K, Pearson DM, Kocialkowski S, Backlund LM, Chan R, Jones DT, Collins VP. IDH1 mutations are present in the majority of common adult gliomas but rare in primary glioblastomas. J. Neurooncol 2009;11:341–7.

2 Recent Advances in Epidemiology of Brain Tumors

JAMES L. FISHER • JUDITH SCHWARTZBAUM • MARGARET R. WRENSCH

In this chapter, we describe recent advances and challenges in the study of the epidemiology of brain tumors. We highlight the following: refinements in the histological categorization of brain tumors; progress in our understanding of the descriptive epidemiology of brain tumors; and advances in identifying both prognostic and causal factors associated with brain tumors. We focus on developments made in the past decade; however, where relevant or compelling, we briefly summarize literature preceding this period. Because approximately 75% of all primary brain tumors are classified as glioma or meningioma, we primarily discuss these more common brain tumors and further restrict our attention to research on adult brain tumors.

Refinements in Histological Categorization of Brain Tumors and Associated Developments

The International Classification of Diseases for Oncology, Third Edition (ICD-O-3) is the standard classification system for the registration of cancers in the United States (and most areas of the world) and contains widely-accepted histologic categories of brain tumors. Brain tumors are classified into the following major histologic groupings: tumors of neuroepithelial tissue (hereafter referred to as glioma, including astrocytoma [grade II], anaplastic astrocytoma [grade III], glioblastoma [grade IV], oligodendroglioma, and ependymoma), tumors of meninges (including meningioma and hemangioblastoma), germ cell tumors, and tumors of the sellar region (including pituitary tumors and craniopharyngioma). Glioma is the most common histological category, followed by meningioma, the category that includes the highest proportion of benign brain tumors (approximately 96% of meningiomas are considered benign).[1] Criteria for classifying brain tumors have varied substantially across time and geographic region. Prior to the past decade, most epidemiologic studies presented results for crude categories such as "all central nervous system (CNS) tumors" or "brain tumors." It is now well established that both the descriptive and analytic epidemiology of brain tumors varies considerably according to histologic grouping. A meaningful contribution of the Central Brain Tumor Registry of the United States (CBTRUS), which collects information on brain tumors occurring among residents of 19 U.S. states, has been the presentation of descriptive statistics according to categories detailed in the ICD-O-3.[1]

Progress in Understanding the Descriptive Epidemiology of Brain Tumors

Glioma incidence rates increased during the 1970s and 1980s (probably reflecting the use of new diagnostic imaging technologies[2]) and have remained relatively stable since the 1980s. Incidence rates for high grade gliomas among older age groups have increased over time from the late 1970s to the early 1990s, as have those for oligodendroglioma and mixed tumor histologies at the expense of less specific histologies.[2] A similar description of American meningioma incidence rates over time is not possible, because benign brain tumors were only recently required to be reported to American central cancer registries. However, Klaeboe et al.[3] report an increase in European meningioma incidence rates, which is also probably explained by new imaging technology introduced in the 1970s.

For all brain and CNS tumors combined, benign and malignant (brain tumors accounting for approximately 88%), the age-adjusted average annual (2000 to 2004) incidence rate for females (17.2 per 100,000 females) is greater than that for males (15.8 per 100,000 males).[1] Table 2-1 shows age-adjusted average annual (2000 to 2004) incidence rates and median ages at diagnosis for the major histologic groupings and their selected common histologic subtypes of brain tumors.[1] As shown in Table 2-1, men have higher incidence rates of gliomas, germ cell tumors and cysts, while women have a higher incidence rate of meningiomas.

TABLE 2-1 **Number of Cases, Median Ages at Diagnosis and Age-Adjusted Average Annual (2000-2004) Incidence Rates[a] of Primary Brain Tumors (Major Histologic Groupings and Selected Histologic Subtypes), According to Sex. Central Brain Tumor Registry of the United States (CBTRUS), reported in: CBTRUS Statistical Report: Primary Brain Tumors in the United States, 2000-2004.[1]**

Histologic Group	Median Age (Years)	Rate[a]	Male Rate[a]	Female Rate[a]
Tumors of Neuroepithelial Tissue/Glioma	53	6.45	7.70	5.39
Pilocytic Astrocytoma	12	0.34	0.34	0.34
Protoplasmic and Fibrillary Astrocytoma	45	0.09	0.10	0.08
Anaplastic Astrocytoma	51	0.44	0.53	0.37
Glioblastoma	64	3.09	3.94	2.38
Oligodendroglioma	41	0.32	0.35	0.30
Anaplastic Oligodendroglioma	49	0.17	0.19	0.15
Ependymoma/Anaplastic Ependymoma	41	0.26	0.29	0.24
Mixed Glioma	42	0.18	0.21	0.15
Malignant Glioma, NOS	41	0.41	0.44	0.39
Benign and Malignant Neuronal/Glial, Neuronal and Mixed	24	0.22	0.25	0.20
Embryonal/Primitive/Medulloblastoma	9	0.23	0.29	0.18
Tumors of Meninges	63	5.55	3.38	7.38
Meningioma	64	5.35	3.17	7.19
Germ Cell Tumors and Cysts	16	0.08	0.11	0.05
Tumors of Sellar Region	49	1.49	1.49	1.53
Pituitary	49	1.37	1.37	1.42
Craniopharyngioma	35	0.12	0.12	0.11

[a]Rates are per 100,000 persons, age-adjusted to the 2000 US (19 age groups) standard.

As described in a following section, results from analytic studies concerning reproductive and hormonal factors have suggested compelling possible explanations for the sex difference in glioma and meningioma risks.

Newly diagnosed glioma is approximately two times more common among whites than among blacks, as are germ cell tumors. In contrast, meningioma incidence rates are similar between whites and blacks.[1] Although there is no well-accepted mechanism for the race differences in glioma risk, differences in the distribution of human leukocyte antigens (HLA) among races, described later in the chapter, may explain it. In the United States, for diagnoses made between 2000 and 2004, the median age at diagnosis of a primary brain tumor was 57 years.[1] For all major histologic groups except germ cell tumors and cysts, incidence rates increase with advancing age.[1] Rates of cancers of nearly every anatomic site increase with advancing age; still, the reason for this increase is not known.

Brain tumor incidence rates vary moderately by geographic region in the United States and throughout the world.[1,4] However, differences in diagnostic practices, completeness of reporting, access to and quality of health care, make geographic and especially international comparisons difficult to interpret.[5,6]

Brain tumor survival time varies greatly by histologic type and age at diagnosis. In every adult age group, the lowest relative 2-year survival is found for patients with glioblastoma multiforme (GBM), ranging from 30.4% among those aged 20 to 44 years to 1.3% among those aged 75 years and older.[1] In general, within histologic types, survival time decreases with advancing age. The mechanisms for the strong and consistent inverse association between age and survival are poorly understood and deserve further exploration. Among adult (ages 20 years and older) patients diagnosed with primary malignant brain tumors between 2000 and 2005, only 32.5% and 23.7% survived 2 and 5 years, respectively, from the time of diagnosis.[4] Although there has been little change in the poor survival rates for patients diagnosed with GBM, for adult (ages 20 years and older) patients diagnosed with all malignant brain tumors combined, 2-year survival has increased from 21.7% in 1975 to 31.9% in 2004.[4] Among patients diagnosed with glioma, the largest improvements in survival occurred among patients with earlier stage glioma and those who were younger than 65 years of age. Population-based data from Norway and Finland suggest that survival for patients diagnosed with meningioma also improved between the 1950s and 1990s.[7,8] McCarthy et al.[9] estimate 5-year survival of 69% for meningioma, with those younger at diagnosis and those with benign meningioma having a more favorable prognosis.[9] It is likely that improvements in imaging technology, which allow the earlier identification of tumors, explain the progress for both glioma and meningioma. GBM probably has only a brief preclinical period; therefore, there may be little opportunity for technology-associated improvement in GBM survival. In the past decade, there has been very little improvement in 2-year survival among adults diagnosed with a primary malignant brain tumor (1.4% difference between the 2-year survival among patients diagnosed in 1994 and those diagnosed in 2004). The only relatively important difference in length of survival following GBM diagnosis, in the past decade, has resulted from concomitant addition of, and maintenance with, the chemotherapeutic agent, Temodar, which has improved median survival time for GBM patients by only 2.5 months.[10]

Advances in Identifying Prognostic Factors for Brain Tumors

Previous research has shown that GBM prognosis is associated with the following factors: age, marital status, tumor size, Karnofsky Performance Scale (KPS) score, patient condition before radiation therapy, degree of necrosis, enhancement on preoperative magnetic resonance imaging studies, therapeutic approach including extent of resection and capacity for complete resection, volume of residual disease, location of tumor, patient deterioration, presurgical serum albumin level, and persistent hyperglycemia 1 to 3 months following surgical resection.[11–16]

Most recent advances in the search for prognostic factors related to GBM and other high-grade gliomas have focused on molecular or serologic factors or on inherited genetic variation. Loss of heterozygosity (LOH) on chromosome 10q has been associated with shorter duration of survival from GBM,[17,18] and the combined LOH on 1p and 19q may afford a more favorable prognosis to GBM patients.[18] For oligodendroglioma, it is now well established that the combined tumor loss of 1p and 19q confers a more favorable prognosis.[19] Results submitted by Yang et al. showed that two genotypes associated with the 19q deletion region, GLTSCR1-exon-1 and ARCC2-exon-22, are independent predictors of glioma survival.[20] Results reported in the past decade provide evidence for the following as prognostic indicators for GBM and other glioma subtypes: p53 mutation and expression,[18,21–29] overexpression or amplification of epidermal growth factor receptor (EGFR),[22,24,25,27–29] CDKN2A alterations and deletions,[22,24,27] and MDM2 amplifications.[21,24,27,29,30] For example, EGFR expression is associated with nearly three-fold poorer survival among anaplastic astrocytoma patients.[29] In addition, Wrensch et al.[29] reported that glutathione-S-transferase (GST) theta (T)1 deletion afforded a less favorable prognosis for glioma patients, while higher survival is afforded to glioma patients with the ERCC1 (a DNA excision repair gene) C8092A polymorphism.

Recently, we have learned that p53 protein expression probably decreases with advancing age,[22,31] and investigators have reported interactions between age and molecular prognostic factors. For example, Simmons et al.[31] showed that there was a shorter survival time among younger patients whose tumors overexpressed EFGR but had normal p53 immunohistochemistry.[31] Age-dependent associations between GBM survival and 1p and CDKN2A have also been identified.[22]

GBM survival time varies with change in the MNS16A human telomerase polymorphism. Median survival time is 24.7 months for the SS-genotype, compared to 14.0 months and 13.1 months for the SL- and LL-genotypes respectively.[32] These results suggest that MNS16A may be used as a biomarker of treatment success.

In order to develop and progress, brain tumors must evade anti-tumor immunity. Recently, several immunological factors have been implicated in glioma prognosis. GBM patients with elevated immunoglobulin (Ig) E live an average of 9 months longer than do patients with lower or normal IgE levels.[29] Furthermore, amplification of interleukin (IL)-6, a cytokine which stimulates immune response, is significantly associated with decreased GBM survival time.[33]

Prognostic factors for meningioma patients have not been as thoroughly evaluated as those for glioma, perhaps because meningioma patients have more favorable prognoses. The recent requirement of central cancer registries to report benign brain tumors may increase our knowledge of demographic and geographic factors related to meningioma prognosis. Generally, younger meningioma patients survive longer than do older patients. A large study revealed that age, tumor size, and surgical and radiation treatments were associated with benign meningioma survival; however, only age and surgical and radiation treatments were associated with malignant meningioma survival.[9] Loss of tumor suppressor in lung cancer-1 (TSLC1) protein and abnormalities of chromosome 14 have been associated with meningioma prognosis.[34,35] We know little about the molecular and genetic factors that determine meningioma prognosis, but studies of such characteristics are being conducted at the present time.

Advances in Identifying Causal Factors for Brain Tumors

Only a few causal factors have been identified for brain tumors. Diseases or syndromes associated with rare mutations in highly penetrant genes (including neurofibromatosis types 1 and 2, tuberous sclerosis, retinoblastoma, Li-Fraumeni cancer family syndrome, and Turcot syndrome) and ionizing radiation are known to increase both glioma and meningioma risks. Analytic studies conducted over the past decade have sought to refine these established risk factors or to identify new factors.

Established Environmental Causal Factors for Brain Tumors

There are consistent and strong results from prospective studies of people exposed to ionizing radiation, providing unquestionable evidence of a linear dose-response association between ionizing radiation exposure and glioma risk.[36] Exposure to ionizing radiation comes from therapeutic and diagnostic medical procedures, occupation, atmospheric testing of nuclear weapons, natural sources, industrial accidents, and atomic bomb explosions. Therapeutic doses of ionizing radiation probably contribute to the development of only a small proportion of brain tumors, as exposure to therapeutic levels of ionizing radiation is rare.[37] Atomic bomb survivors have higher incidence rates of glioma and meningioma, as well as of schwannoma and pituitary tumors,[38] and meningioma risk increases with estimated radiation dose to the brain.[39] Ionizing radiation used to treat conditions such as tinea capitis in infants and children is associated with elevated relative risks for both glioma and meningioma, along with nerve sheath tumors and pituitary adenoma.[38,40,41] There are mixed results pertaining to diagnostic and therapeutic x-rays of the head and neck.[42–45] Second primary brain tumors occur more frequently than expected among patients previously treated for brain tumors with radiation therapy[46]; however, these results are confounded by the fact that people with higher grade tumors are more likely both to receive radiation and to have a recurrence. Future studies should consider the potential for underreporting of ionizing radiation exposure and imprecise estimates of age at first exposure.[36] There may be interaction between ionizing radiation and both age at exposure and genetic variation that may mediate exposure; future studies should consider these possible interactions.

In addition to rare mutations in penetrant genes and ionizing radiation, exogenous hormone use among women is now an established risk factor for meningioma. In part because females have a greater meningioma risk than do males, investigators have examined factors associated with estrogen (menopausal status, ages at menarche and menopause, parity, and uses of oral contraceptives and hormone replacement therapy [HRT]). The ratio of the female-to-male meningioma incidence rate has increased in European countries over time with the increased use of hormone replacement therapy by perimenopausal and postmenopausal women.[3] Several results suggest that meningioma risk is greatest among women during their reproductive years[7,47,48]; however, SEER statistics reveal that ratios of female-to-male meningioma incidence rates are greatest (greater than 2.5) during the ages 30 to 54 years.[4] There is no consistent or convincing evidence that parity and oral contraceptive use are associated with meningioma risk.[47–50] However, results from a population-based case-control study conducted by Wigertz et al.[48] revealed elevated meningioma risks among women who had used long-acting hormonal contraceptives (odds ratio [OR] for at least 10 years of use = 2.7; 95% CI: 0.9-7.5) and postmenopausal women who had ever used HRT (OR = 1.7; 95% CI: 1.0-2.8). While exogenous female hormones probably play a role in the development of some meningiomas, our understanding of mechanisms governing their role is limited, perhaps in part because the menstrual and reproductive factors that have been examined are insufficient to accurately characterize lifetime estrogen or other hormonal exposure.

Probable Causal Factors for Brain Tumors

Previous repeated null findings have allowed the dismissal of some risk factors (such as head injury/trauma and residential exposure to low-level electromagnetic fields), and more focused lines of inquiry have emerged to elucidate the complex roles of family history and allergic conditions and associated immunological factors, including varicella-zoster virus (VZV) infection and associated IgG levels. Over the past decade, the most compelling results from analytic epidemiologic studies have been those concerning immunological factors.

FAMILY HISTORY

The progressive accumulation of genetic and/or epigenetic alterations, permitting cells to evade normal regulatory mechanisms and/or escape destruction by the immune system, is thought to govern the development of glioma and meningioma, although these mechanisms have not yet been fully defined.[51–53] Evidence for the presence of genetic involvement in the causal pathways of glioma and meningioma is demonstrated most simply by studies which have shown an increased risk of brain tumors in close relatives of brain tumor patients, especially those with gliomas. Although brain tumors clearly aggregate in families, it can be difficult to distinguish shared environmental exposures from inherited characteristics. In fact, Grossman et al.[54] showed that brain tumors occur commonly in families with no known predisposing hereditary disease, and that the pattern of occurrence in many families suggests environmental, rather than genetic, causes.

However, important results presented by Malmer et al.[55] suggest that first-degree relatives, but not spouses, have a significantly increased brain tumor risk.

ALLERGIC AND ASSOCIATED IMMUNOLOGICAL CONDITIONS AND GLIOMA

There is consistent evidence for an association between allergy-related immune responses and glioma risk. Over the past two decades, results from ten case-control[56–65] and one of two cohort studies[66] show that self-reported allergies are inversely related to glioma risk. Linos et al.[67] conducted a formal meta-analysis of a subset of these studies and found that self-reported allergies are related to a 40% reduction in the risk of glioma (OR = 0.61; 95% CI: 0.55-0.67). Further evidence for this inverse association was contributed by Wiemels et al.[68] who found that total IgE levels were lower in glioma cases than in controls. Although mechanisms governing potential protection have not been identified, they may arise from the anti-inflammatory effects of IL- 4 and IL-13 cytokines involved in allergic and autoimmune disease[69] or from increased tumor immunosurveillance among those with allergies and autoimmune disease.[70] It is also possible that the inverse association results from immune suppression by a preclinical tumor.[71]

In addition to their role in allergic conditions, IL-4 and IL-13 cytokines also inhibit growth of glioma cell lines. IL-4 is strongly expressed during brain injury,[72] where invading T cells may be a source of this cytokine,[73] and IL-4 increases the number of T-cell precursors in GBM patients.[74] Barna et al.[73] found that three normal astrocytic, two low-grade astrocytoma, and three out of four GBM cell lines they evaluated expressed IL-4R alpha receptors. However, IL-4 suppressed DNA synthesis and cell proliferation only in the normal astrocytic and low-grade astrocytoma cell lines, not in the GBM cell lines. IL-4 could play a role in the inhibition of GBMs that arise from astrocytomas, but it may not be involved in de novo GBMs.[75] In view of a possible role for IL-4 and IL-13 in both allergic conditions and glioma, Schwartzbaum et al.[63] identified polymorphisms of the IL-4R alpha and IL-13 genes that increase allergic condition risk. Although these germline genetic variants are not sensitive indicators of the presence of allergic conditions, they do provide a measure of risk of these conditions free of recall bias. The working hypothesis was that individuals with IL-4R alpha or IL-13 polymorphisms that increase allergic condition risk would have a decreased risk of GBM. Using data from a small case-control study (111 GBM cases, 422 controls), the authors found results consistent with their hypothesis; each of the two IL-4R alpha and IL-13 single nucleotide polymorphisms (SNPs) associated with increased allergic condition risk were also related to decreased GBM risk. Wiemels et al.[76] confirmed their finding for one of the IL-13 SNPs in a larger case-control study of glioma (456 glioma cases, 541 controls). Furthermore, they reported that this IL-13 SNP was inversely associated with IgE levels among controls ($p = 0.04$). However, they did not find associations between the IL-4R alpha SNPs and glioma as had Schwartzbaum et al. They did note a borderline association between an IL-4R alpha haplotype (OR = 1.5; 95% CI: 1.0-2.3) and glioma. They also saw that a rare IL-4 haplotype was associated with decreased glioma risk (OR = 0.23; 95% CI: 0.07-0.83).

A larger study of the original four IL-4R alpha and IL-13 genetic variants by Schwartzbaum et al.[77] did not provide strong support for their original observations. Nonetheless, they found an IL-4R alpha haplotype associated with GBM

(OR = 2.26; 95% CI: 1.13-4.52) and inversely related to self-report of hay fever or asthma among controls (OR= 0.39; 95% CI: 0.16-0.98). Although Wiemels et al. also found suggestive evidence for an association of between an IL-4R alpha haplotype and glioma, when they restricted their haplotype to the same IL-4R alpha SNPs that Schwartzbaum et al. examined, they observed no evidence for an association with glioma (OR = 1.13; 95% CI: 0.83-1.53).

Immunosuppressive regulatory T-cells and their associated cytokines TGF-beta and IL-10 repress effective anti-glioma reactions and may provide a conceptual and mechanistic framework to explain an indirect relationship between allergies and anti-glioma immune reactions. The unique architecture of the brain does not exclude glioma from immune system interaction, although immune responses may be attenuated compared to those found in other organs. In addition, there is now evidence for infiltration of T and B cells into the brains of brain tumor patients; the enhancement of such responses is likely to form the basis of future effective glioma therapies. In recent in vitro studies of glioma, human glioma cell lines were found to secrete immunosuppressive cytokines that can selectively recruit regulatory T cells into the tumor microenvironment.[78] In addition, Chahlavi et al.[79] demonstrated that glioma cell lines mediate immunosuppression by promoting T cell death through tumor-associated antigens and gangliosides. Two of the major immunosuppressive cytokines that are present in both the glioma microenvironment and the peripheral blood of glioma patients, IL-10 and TGF-beta, induce immune tolerance, thereby inhibiting allergy and asthma.[80] Elevated IgE concentrations may therefore indicate low levels of immunosuppression and the resulting ability to conduct anti-tumor immunosurveillance against incipient glioma. Alternatively, the relative absence of allergies in glioma patients may merely show that these tumor-induced cytokines have suppressed the immune system.

Results pertaining to HLA—cell surface molecules that mediate interactions of tumor cells with the host immune response, in part by presenting antigenic peptides to T-lymphocytes—also suggest the importance of immunological responses in glioma development. Facoetti et al.[81] found that HLA class I antigen loss was significantly ($P<0.025$) correlated with tumor grade: HLA class I antigens were lost in approximately half of GBM tumors, but only in 20% of grade II astrocytoma tumors; selective HLA-A2 antigen loss was observed in approximately 80% of GBM lesions and half of the grade II astrocytoma tumors. GBM is positively associated with the HLA genotype B*13 and the HLA haplotype B*07-Cw*07 ($P=0.01$ and $P<0.001$, respectively), and is inversely associated with the genotype Cw*01.[82] Interestingly, these results could partially explain the increased GBM incidence among whites, because B*07 and B*07-Cw*07 are more common among whites than among nonwhites.

VARICELLA-ZOSTER VIRUS INFECTION AND ASSOCIATED IMMUNOGLOBULIN G AND GLIOMA

A reported history of varicella-zoster virus (VZV) infection and positive IgG to VZV is also associated with a reduced risk of glioma.[83–85] Results from case-control studies suggest that past clinical disease associated with VZV infection and anti-VZV IgG levels may be inversely associated with adult glioma risk.[83–85] It may be the specific nature of immune system response to antigens, and not exposure to the antigen per se, that is responsible for this inverse association with glioma.[68,86] Associations of glioma risk with VZV and IgG, along with other potentially important viral or bacterial infections, should be validated in studies in which serologic measurement of viral or bacterial exposure is ascertained before the development of brain tumors (to prevent the possibility of the tumor affecting the serologic assessment) and in which there is serologic or symptom-based confirmation of infection.

Possible Causal Factors for Brain Tumors Requiring Additional Study

CELLULAR TELEPHONE USE

In general, with the exception of analog cellular telephone use (which has largely been replaced by digital cell phone use), meningioma risk does not appear to increase as the result of cell phone use.[87–89,90,91] Mixed results have been reported for associations between cell phone use and acoustic neuroma risk[90–95]; however, relative risks from studies of more than one histologic type of brain tumor have been greater for acoustic neuroma, as compared to meningioma and glioma, especially when cell phone use is on the same side of the head as the tumor (ipsilateral).[93] Further study of cell phone use and acoustic neuroma risk is warranted. A relatively large number of epidemiologic studies of cell phone use and glioma risk have suggested that short-term cell phone use is probably not associated with glioma risk.[87–89,91,96–104] There are limited data and inconsistent results pertaining to long-term use and glioma risk,[87–89,91,97–99,102,104,105] with the most compelling results suggesting evidence of increased glioma risk as the result of ipsilateral cell phone use.[89,91,97,99,102] However, these results have likely been affected by small sample sizes, and selection and recall biases.[87,106] Some of the increased risk resulting from ipsilateral cell phone use may be attributable to recall bias because contralateral cell phone use appears to reduce risk; in the absence of recall bias, one would not expect cell phone use to decrease risk. The largest population-based case-control study reported to date (1522 glioma cases and 3301 controls) conducted in five Nordic countries and the United Kingdom[102] found no consistent evidence overall for increased risk of glioma related to use of cell phones; nor did they find increased glioma risk among the most highly-exposed group. However, if the latency period is at least 5 years long, then earlier studies lacked sufficient numbers of long-term cell phone users to adequately evaluate the relationship. The association of glioma risk with long-term cell phone use has not yet been convincingly demonstrated but will continue to be examined in the context of more refined studies, which will have greater statistical power because of the increasing numbers of the population who are long-term cell phone users and the potential release of individual records by cellular telephone companies for better exposure assessments.

POLYMORPHIC VARIATION IN DETOXIFICATION, DNA STABILITY AND REPAIR, AND CELL CYCLE REGULATION AND GLIOMA

Results from studies of polymorphic variation in detoxification, DNA stability and repair, and cell cycle regulation genes have produced suggestive but not definitive evidence for an association of these genes with glioma risk. Cytochrome p450s (CYP) and GST are involved in metabolizing many electrophilic compounds, including carcinogens, mutagens, cytotoxic drugs, metabolites, and products of reactive oxidation. For brain tumors, studies of CPY and GST have produced mixed results. Results from a recent meta-analysis of eight studies suggest that, although the T1 null genotype is significantly associated with a nearly twofold risk of meningioma, there are no associations between any of the GSTP1 105 and GSTP1 114 SNPs and glioma risk. Wrensch et al.[107] found little evidence for a general association of GST polymorphisms with glioma, but did show an association of GSTT1 deletion for glioma with p53 mutations. In a large Nordic and British population-based case-control study, Schwartzbaum et al.[108] reported no associations between the GSTM3, GSTP1 NQ01, CYP1A1, GSTM1, or GSTT1 polymorphisms and adult brain tumor risk; however, they found a weak association between the G-C (Val-Ala) GSTP1 105/114 haplotype and glioma.

Because DNA repair is important in maintaining DNA integrity, inherited variation in components of DNA repair pathways has been examined as potentially being related to glioma risk. Associations with glioma have been reported for variants in ERCC1,[109,110] ERCC2,[20,109,111] the nearby gene glioma tumor suppressor candidate of unknown function (GLTSCR1),[20] PRKDC (also known as XRCC7—a gene involved in nonhomologous end joining double-strand break repair),[112] and O^6–methylguanine-DNA methyltransferase (MGMT, which encodes a DNA repair protein that removes alkyl groups from an important DNA site—O^6),[113,114] but there are too few studies to assess consistency. Bethke et al.[115] recently reported that 16 SNPs (among over 1500 haplotype-tagging and putative functional SNPs selected to capture most common variation in the known 136 DNA repair genes) were significantly associated with glioma risk. Because DNA repair is complex (involving at least 136 known genes), studies focusing on constellations of variants involved in DNA repair pathways, as well as their interactions, might elucidate the roles of variants in gliomagenesis and progression.

Dysregulation of the cell cycle (control of proliferation and apoptosis) is a hallmark feature of most gliomas.[116] Results from large series of glioma cases and controls suggest that inherited variation in CASP8, a regulator of apoptosis, may be important in glioma development; risk for glioma was elevated among those with carrier status for the rare allele of D302H in CASP8 (OR = 1.7; 95% CI: 1.10-1.70).[117] In addition, MDM2, a key molecule in maintaining the fidelity of proliferation and apoptosis, appears to negatively regulate TP53 expression.[118,119] Findings from a recent study suggest that SNP309, in the promoter region of MDM2 and associated with MDM2 protein expression level, is not associated with histologic grade of glioma, age at onset, or p53 mutation rate or gliomagenesis.[120] In a study of glioma patients with Li-Fraumeni syndrome,[121] the G variant of SNP309 in the MDM2 promoter led to higher expression of MDM2 with concomitant reduced expression of TP53, and was significantly associated with earlier age of tumor development and multiple tumor sites. Associations between MDM2 and TP53 remain poorly understood and should be examined in studies with large sample sizes because of the potential need for smaller subgroup analyses.

HUMAN CYTOMEGALOVIRUS AND GLIOMA

Although several case-control studies found no evidence suggesting that human cytomegalovirus (HCMV) plays a role in the development of glioma,[85,122] HCMV nucleic acids and proteins have been observed in glioblastoma tissue and HCMV DNA has been found in the peripheral blood of glioblastoma patients.[123] Scheurer et al.[124] found

HCMV infection in 21 glioblastoma tumors that they evaluated. However, the presence of HCMV gene products in blood or tumor tissue may result from reactivation of infection caused by tumor-induced immunosuppression or from infected tumor cells shedding viral DNA[123] rather than from any role of HCMV in glioma development.

GENETIC FACTORS (OTHER THAN FAMILY HISTORY AND RARE MUTATIONS) AND MENINGIOMA

Mutations in the NF2 gene (probably accounting for more than half of meningiomas[125]) and loss of chromosome 22q are the most common genetic alterations associated with the initiation of meningiomas.[125,126] However, we do not understand the mechanisms governing the factors that allow meningioma to develop. Genetic results that may shape future studies of meningioma include the following findings: genetic changes of the APC gene play a role in meningioma formation;[127] a candidate common LOH region on 1p36.11 may harbor tumor suppressor genes related to malignant progression of meningioma;[128] the genotype combination of CC-CG-CC formed by three polymorphisms in p53 increases meningioma risk, but only among those with a family history of cancer;[129] SNPs in the Ki-ras and ERCC2 genes may be involved in meningioma formation; and SNPs in cyclin D1 and p16 may mark genes that have an inverse effect on risk of developing both radiation-associated and sporadic meningioma. One of the most intriguing findings concerning genetic factors related to meningioma resulted from a recent analysis of 136 DNA repair genes.[130] Bethke et al. found that the SNP rs4968451, which maps to the gene that encodes breast cancer susceptibility gene 1–interacting protein 1 (BRIP1), was consistently associated, across five studies, with an increased risk of developing meningioma.[130] This is compelling because: (1) greater than one fourth of the European population are carriers of at-risk genotypes for rs4968451; therefore, the variant is likely to contribute to 16% of meningiomas; and (2) BRIP1 encodes a helicase which interacts with BRCA1 and has BRCA1-dependent DNA repair and checkpoint functions, and this provides a possible explanation for the fact that both breast cancer and meningioma most commonly occur among women ages 50 to 70 years and that women with breast cancer have approximately 50% greater risk of meningioma and vice versa.[130]

Summary

Few causal factors (ionizing radiation, hereditary diseases/syndromes, and, for meningioma, exogenous female hormones) have been identified for brain tumors. There is a well-established association between the combined tumor loss of 1p and 19q and more favorable oligodendroglioma prognosis, and recent results have suggested that abnormal expression in several genes predicts GBM survival time. The mechanisms for the strong, consistent inverse association between age and survival are poorly understood and deserve further exploration. Focused hypotheses which consider recent developments and are examined within large, collaborative groups of investigators may shed light on unanswered questions concerning the complex relationship between immune response, gliomagenesis, and prognosis.

However, this year (2009) two published genome wide association studies for glioma, based on five sets of genome wide genotyping in glioma cases (University of California at san Francisco, Mayo Clinic, MD Anderson Cancer Center, UK and

The Cancer Genome Atlas) and several control groups discovered and confirmed the following five regions for glioma risk: chromosome 5p15.33 (TERT), 9p21.3 (CDKN2B), 8q24, 11q23 (PHLDB1), and, 20q13.3 (RTEL1).[131,132] These new discoveries open up tremendous opportunities for discovering mechanisms of glioma risk.

REFERENCES

1. CBTRUS. Statistical Report: Primary Brain Tumors in the United States 2000–2004. 2008.
2. McCarthy BJ. Descriptive Epidemiology of Glioma. Principles and Practices of Neuro-Oncology: A Multidisciplinary Approach. (In Press). 2008.
3. Klaeboe L, Stefan L, Scheie D, et al. Incidence of intracranial meningioma in Denmark, Finland, Norway and Sweden, 1968–1997. Int J Cancer 2005;117(6):996–1001.
4. SEER. Surveillance, Epidemiology, and End Results (SEER) Program (www.seer.cancer.gov) SEER*Stat Database, National Cancer Institute, DCCPS, Surveillance Research Program, Cancer Statistics Branch, released April 2008, based on the November 2007 submission. 2008.
5. Inskip PD, Linet MS, Heineman EF. Etiology of brain tumors in adults. Epidemiol Rev 1995;17(2):382–414.
6. Wrensch M, Minn Y, Chew T, Bondy M, Berger MS. Epidemiology of primary brain tumors: current concepts and review of the literature. Neuro-oncol 2002;4(4):278–99.
7. Helseth A. Incidence and survival of intracranial meningioma patients in Norway 1963–1992. Neuroepidemiology 1997;16(2):53–9.
8. Sankila R, Kallio M, Jaaskelainen J, Hakulinen T. Long-term survival of 1986 patients with intracranial meningioma diagnosed from 1953 to 1984 in Finland. Comparison of the observed and expected survival rates in a population-based series. Cancer 1992;70(6):1568–76.
9. McCarthy BJ, Davis FG, Freels S, et al. Factors associated with survival in patients with meningioma. J Neurosurg 1998;88(5):831–9.
10. Cohen MH, Johnson JR, Pazdur R. Food and Drug Administration Drug approval summary: temozolomide plus radiation therapy for the treatment of newly diagnosed glioblastoma multiforme. Clin Cancer Res 2005;11(19 Pt 1):6767–71.
11. Lacroix M, Abi-Said D, Fourney DR, et al. A multivariate analysis of 416 patients with glioblastoma multiforme: prognosis, extent of resection, and survival. J Neurosurg 2001; 95(2):190–8.
12. Lutterbach J, Sauerbrei W, Guttenberger R. Multivariate analysis of prognostic factors in patients with glioblastoma. Strahlentherapie und Onkologie 2003;179(1):8–15.
13. Jeremic B, Milicic B, Grujicic D, Dagovic A, Aleksandrovic J. Multivariate analysis of clinical prognostic factors in patients with glioblastoma multiforme treated with a combined modality approach. J Cancer Research Clinical Oncol 2003;129(8):477–84.
14. Schwartzbaum J, Lal P, Evanoff W, et al. Presurgical serum albumin levels predict survival time from glioblastoma multiforme. J Neuro-oncol 1999;43:35–41.
15. Chang S, Barker 2nd FG. Marital status, treatment, and survival in patients with glioblastoma multiforme. Cancer 2008;104(9):1975–84.
16. McGirt MJ, Chaichana KL, Gathinji M, et al. Persistent outpatient hyperglycemia is independently associated with decreased survival after primary resection of malignant brain astrocytomas. Neurosurg 2008;63(2):286–91.
17. Ohgaki H, Dessen P, Jourde B, et al. Genetic pathways to glioblastoma: a population-based study. Cancer Res 2004;64(19):6892–9.
18. Schmidt MC, Antweiler S, Urban N, et al. Impact of genotype and morphology on the prognosis of glioblastoma. J Neuropathol Exp Neurol 2002;61(4):321–8.
19. Aldape K, Burger PC, Perry A. Clinicopathologic aspects of 1p/19q loss and the diagnosis of oligodendroglioma. Arch Pathol Lab Med 2007;131(2):242–51.
20. Yang P, Kollmeyer TM, Buckner K, Bamlet W, Ballman KV, Jenkins RB. Polymorphisms in GLTSCR1 and ERCC2 are associated with the development of oligodendrogliomas. Cancer 2005;1(103):2363–72.
21. Ushio Y, Tada K, Shiraishi S, et al. Correlation of molecular genetic analysis of p53, MDM2, p16, PTEN, and EGFR and survival of patients with anaplastic astrocytoma and glioblastoma. Front Biosci 2003;8:e281–8.
22. Batchelor TT, Betensky RA, Esposito JM, et al. Age-dependent prognostic effects of genetic alterations in glioblastoma. Clin Cancer Res 2004;10(1 Pt 1):228–33.
23. Stander M, Peraud A, Leroch B, Kreth FW. Prognostic impact of TP53 mutation status for adult patients with supratentorial World Health Organization Grade II astrocytoma or oligoastrocytoma: a long-term analysis. Cancer 2004;101(5):1028–35.

24. Backlund LM, Nilsson BR, Liu L, Ichimura K, Collins VP. Mutations in Rb1 pathway-related genes are associated with poor prognosis in anaplastic astrocytomas. Brit J Cancer 2005;93(1):124–30.
25. Deb P, Sharma MC, Mahapatra AK, Agarwal D, Sarkar C. Glioblastoma multiforme with long term survival. Neurol India 2005;53(3):329–32.
26. McLendon RE, Herndon 2nd JE, West B, et al. Survival analysis of presumptive prognostic markers among oligodendrogliomas. Cancer 2005;104(8):1693–9.
27. Houillier C, Lejeune J, Benouaich-Amiel A, et al. Prognostic impact of molecular markers in a series of 220 primary glioblastomas. Cancer 2006;106(10):2218–23.
28. Layfield LJ, Willmore C, Tripp S, Jones C, Jensen RL. Epidermal growth factor receptor gene amplification and protein expression in glioblastoma multiforme: prognostic significance and relationship to other prognostic factors. Appl Immunohistochem Mol Morphol 2006;14(1):91–6.
29. Wrensch M, Wiencke JK, Wiemels J, et al. Serum IgE, tumor epidermal growth factor receptor expression, and inherited polymorphisms associated with glioma survival. Cancer Res 2006;66(8):4531–41.
30. Ranuncolo SM, Varela M, Morandi A, et al. Prognostic value of Mdm2, p53 and p16 in patients with astrocytomas. J Neuro-oncol 2004;68(2):113–21.
31. Simmons ML, Lamborn KR, Takahashi M, et al. Analysis of complex relationships between age, p53, epidermal growth factor receptor, and survival in glioblastoma patients. Cancer Res 2001;61(3):1122–8.
32. Wang L, Wang LE, El-Zein R, et al. Human telomerase genetic variation predicts survival of patients with glioblastoma multiforme (Abstract number 2823). Proc Amer Assoc Cancer Res 2005;46.
33. Tchirkov A, Khalil T, Chautard E, et al. Interleukin-6 gene amplification and shortened survival in glioblastoma patients. Brit J Cancer 2007;96(3):474–6.
34. Surace EI, Lusis E, Murakami Y, Scheithauer BW, Perry A, Gutmann DH. Loss of tumor suppressor in lung cancer-1 (TSLC1) expression in meningioma correlates with increased malignancy grade and reduced patient survival. J Neuropathol Exp Neurol 2004;63(10):1015–27.
35. Maillo A, Orfao A, Sayagues JM, et al. New classification scheme for the prognostic stratification of meningioma on the basis of chromosome 14 abnormalities, patient age, and tumor histopathology. J Clin Oncol 2003;21(17):3285–95.
36. Sadetzki S. Exposure to Ionizing Radiation and Glioma Risk. Principles and Practices of Neuro-Oncology: A Multidisciplinary Approach. (In Press).
37. Blettner M, Schlehofer B, Samkange-Zeeb F, Berg G, Schlaefer K, Schuz J. Medical exposure to ionising radiation and the risk of brain tumours: Interphone study group, Germany. Eur J Cancer 2007;43(13):1990–8.
38. Preston-Martin S. Epidemiology of primary CNS neoplasms. Neurol Clin 1996;14(2):273–90.
39. Shintani T, Hayakawa N, Hoshi M, et al. High incidence of meningioma among Hiroshima atomic bomb survivors. J Rad Res 1999;40(1):49–57.
40. Wrensch M, Minn Y, Chew T, Bondy M, Berger MS. Epidemiology of primary brain tumors: current concepts and review of the literature. Neuro-oncol 2002;4(4):278–99.
41. Juven Y, Sadetzki S. A possible association between ionizing radiation and pituitary adenoma: a descriptive study. Cancer 2002;95(2):397–403.
42. Wrensch M, Miike R, Lee M, Neuhaus J. Are prior head injuries or diagnostic X-rays associated with glioma in adults? The effects of control selection bias. Neuroepidemiology 2000;19(5):234–44.
43. Hardell L, Mild KH, Pahlson A, Hallquist A. Ionizing radiation, cellular telephones and the risk for brain tumours. Eur J Cancer Prev 2001;10(6):523–9.
44. Longstreth WTJ, Phillips LE, Drangsholt M, et al. Dental X-rays and the risk of intracranial meningioma: a population-based case-control study. Cancer 2004;100(5):1026–34.
45. Preston-Martin S, Yu MC, Henderson BE, Roberts C. Risk factors for meningiomas in men in Los Angeles County. J Natl Cancer Inst 1983;70(5):863–6.
46. Salminen E, Pukkala E, Teppo L. Second cancers in patients with brain tumours impact of treatment. Eur J Cancer 1999;35(1):102–5.
47. Schlehofer B, Blettner M, Wahrendorf J. Association between brain tumors and menopausal status. J Natl Cancer Inst 1992;84(17):1346–9.
48. Wigertz A, Lonn S, Mathiesen T, et al. Risk of brain tumors associated with exposure to exogenous female sex hormones. Am J Epidemiol 2006;164(7):629–36.
49. Jhawar BS, Fuchs CS, Colditz GA, Stampfer MJ. Sex steroid hormone exposures and risk for meningioma. J Neurosurg 2003;99(5):848–53.
50. Hatch EE, Linet MS, Zhang J, et al. Reproductive and hormonal factors and risk of brain tumors in adult females. Intl J Cancer 2005;114(5):797–805.

51. Fisher JL, Schwartzbaum J, Wrensch M, Wiemels JL. Epidemiology of Brain Tumors. Neurologic clinics. Brain Tumors in Adults 2007;25(4):867–90.
52. Schwartzbaum JA, Fisher JL, Aldape KD, Wrensch M. Epidemiology and molecular pathology of glioma. Nat Clin Pract Neurol 2006;2(9):494–503.
53. Wrensch M, Fisher JL, Schwartzbaum JA, Bondy M, Berger M, Aldape KD. The molecular epidemiology of gliomas in adults. Neurosurg Focus 2005;19(5):E5.
54. Grossman SA, Osman M, Hruban R, Piantadosi S. Central nervous system cancers in first-degree relatives and spouses. Cancer Invest 1999;17(5):299–308.
55. Malmer B, Henriksson R, Gronberg H. Familial brain tumours-genetics or environment? A nationwide cohort study of cancer risk in spouses and first-degree relatives of brain tumour patients. Int J Cancer 2003;106(2):260–3.
56. Brenner AV, Linet MS, Fine HA, et al. History of allergies and autoimmune diseases and risk of brain tumors in adults. Int J Cancer 2002;99(2):252–9.
57. Cicuttini FM, Hurley SF, Forbes A. Association of adult glioma with medical conditions, family, and reproductive history. Int J Cancer 1997;71(203–7).
58. Hochberg F, Toniolo P, Cole P, Salcman M. Nonoccupational risk indicators of glioblastoma in adults. J Neurooncol 1990;8(1):55–60.
59. Ryan P, Lee MW, North B, McMichael AJ. Risk factors for tumors of the brain and meninges: results from the Adelaide Adult Brain Tumor Study. Int J Cancer 1992;51(1):20–7.
60. Schlehofer B, Blettner M, Becker N, Martinsohn C, Wahrendorf J. Medical risk factors and the development of brain tumors. Cancer 1992;69:2541–7.
61. Schlehofer B, Blettner M, Preston-Martin S, et al. Role of medical history in brain tumour development. Results from the international adult brain tumour study. Int J Cancer 1999; 82(2):155–60.
62. Schoemaker MJ, Swerdlow AJ, Hepworth SJ, McKinney PA, van Tongeren M, Muir KR. History of allergies and risk of glioma in adults. Int J Cancer 2006.
63. Schwartzbaum J, Ahlbom A, Malmer B, et al. Polymorphisms associated with asthma are inversely related to glioblastoma multiforme. Cancer Res 2005;65(14):6459–65.
64. Wigertz A, Lonn S, Schwartzbaum J, et al. Allergic Conditions and Brain Tumor Risk. Am J Epidemiol 2007.
65. Wiemels JL, Wiencke JK, Sison JD, Miike R, McMillan A, Wrensch M. History of allergies among adults with glioma and controls. Int J Cancer 2002;98(4):609–15.
66. Schwartzbaum J, Jonsson F, Ahlbom A, et al. Cohort studies of association between self-reported allergic conditions, immune-related diagnoses and glioma and meningioma risk. Int J Cancer 2003;106(3):423–8.
67. Linos E, Raine T, Alonso A, Michaud D. Atopy and risk of brain tumors: a meta-analysis. J Natl Cancer Inst 2007;99(20):1544–50.
68. Wiemels JL, Wiencke JK, Patoka J, et al. Reduced immunoglobulin E and allergy among adults with glioma compared with controls. Cancer Res 2004;64(22):8468–73.
69. Dinarello CA. Setting the cytokine trap for autoimmunity. Nat Med 2003;9(1):20–2.
70. Dunn GP, Bruce AT, Ikeda H, Old LJ, Schreiber RD. Cancer immunoediting: from immunosurveillance to tumor escape. Nat Immunol 2002;3(11):991–8.
71. Schoemaker MJ, Swerdlow AJ, Hepworth SJ, McKinney PA, van Tongeren M, Muir KR. History of allergies and risk of glioma in adults. Int J Cancer 2006;119(9):2165–72.
72. Liu H, Prayson RA, Estes ML, et al. In vivo expression of the interleukin 4 receptor alpha by astrocytes in epilepsy cerebral cortex. Cytokine 2000;12(11):1656–61.
73. Barna BP, Estes ML, Pettay J, Iwasaki K, Zhou P, Barnett GH. Human astrocyte growth regulation: interleukin-4 sensitivity and receptor expression. J Neuroimmunol 1995;60(1–2):75–81.
74. Faber C, Terao E, Morga E, Heuschling P. Interleukin-4 enhances the in vitro precursor cell recruitment for tumor-specific T lymphocytes in patients with glioblastoma. J Immunother 2000;23(1):11–6.
75. Louis DN. A molecular genetic model of astrocytoma histopathology. Brain Pathol 1997; 7(2):755–64.
76. Wiemels JL, Wiencke JK, Kelsey KT, et al. Allergy-related polymorphisms influence glioma status and serum IgE levels. Cancer Epidemiol Biomarkers Prev 2007.
77. Schwartzbaum J, Ahlbom A, Lönn S, et al. An international case-control study of IL-4Ralpha, IL-13 and cyclooxygenase-2 polymorphisms and glioblastoma risk. Cancer Epidemiol Biomarkers Prev 2007;16(11):2448–54.
78. Jordan JT, Sun W, Hussain SF, DeAngulo G, Prabhu SS, Heimberger AB. Preferential migration of regulatory T cells mediated by glioma-secreted chemokines can be blocked with chemotherapy. Cancer Immunol Immunother 2008;57(1):123–31.

79. Chahlavi A, Rayman P, Richmond AL, et al. Glioblastomas induce T-lymphocyte death by two distinct pathways involving gangliosides and CD70. Cancer Res 2005;65(12):5428–38.
80. Umetsu DT, DeKruyff RH. The regulation of allergy and asthma. Immunol Rev 2006;212:238–55.
81. Facoetti A, Nano R, Zelini P, et al. Human leukocyte antigen and antigen processing machinery component defects in astrocytic tumors. Clin. Cancer Res 2005;11(23):8304–11.
82. Tang J, Shao W, Dorak MT, et al. Positive and negative associations of human leukocyte antigen variants with the onset and prognosis of adult glioblastoma multiforme. Cancer Epidemiol Biomarkers Prev 2005;14(8):2040–4.
83. Wrensch M, Weinberg A, Wiencke J, et al. Does prior infection with varicella-zoster virus influence risk of adult glioma?. Am J Epidemiol 1997;145(7):594–7.
84. Wrensch M, Weinberg A, Wiencke J, Miike R, Barger G, Kelsey K. Prevalence of antibodies to four herpesviruses among adults with glioma and controls. Am J Epidemiol 2001;154(2):161–5.
85. Wrensch M, Weinberg A, Wiencke J, et al. History of Chickenpox and Shingles and Prevalence of Antibodies to Varicella-Zoster Virus and Three Other Herpesviruses among Adults with Glioma and Controls. Am J Epidemiol 2005;161(10):929–38.
86. Wiemels JL, Wiencke JK, Sison JD, Miike R, McMillan A, Wrensch M. History of allergies among adults with glioma and controls. Intl J Cancer 2002;98(4):609–15.
87. Schuz J, Bohler E, Berg G, et al. Cellular phones, cordless phones, and the risks of glioma and meningioma (Interphone Study Group, Germany). Am J Epidemiol 2006;163(6):512–20.
88. Christensen HC, Schuz J, Kosteljanetz M, et al. Cellular telephones and risk for brain tumors: a population-based, incident case-control study. Neurology 2005;64(7):1189–95.
89. Lonn S, Ahlbom A, Hall P, Feychting M, Feychting M. Long-term mobile phone use and brain tumor risk. Am J Epidemiol 2005;161(6):526–35.
90. Hardell L, Carlberg M, Hansson Mild K. Pooled analysis of two case-control studies on the use of cellular and cordless telephones and the risk of benign brain tumours diagnosed during 1997–2003. Intl J Oncol 2006;28(2):509–18.
91. Hardell L, Carlberg M, Hansson Mild K. Case-control study on cellular and cordless telephones and the risk for acoustic neuroma or meningioma in patients diagnosed 2000–2003. Neuroepidemiology 2005;25(3):120–8.
92. Takebayashi T, Akiba S, Kikuchi Y, et al. Mobile phone use and acoustic neuroma risk in Japan. Occup Environ Med 2006;63(12):802–7.
93. Schoemaker MJ, Swerdlow AJ, Ahlbom A, et al. Mobile phone use and risk of acoustic neuroma: results of the Interphone case-control study in five North European countries. Brit J Cancer 2005;93(7):842–8.
94. Kundi M, Mild K, Hardell L, Mattsson M-O. Mobile telephones and cancer—a review of epidemiological evidence. J Toxicol Environ Health 2004;7(5):351–84.
95. Christensen HC, Schuz J, Kosteljanetz M, Poulsen HS, Thomsen J, Johansen C. Cellular telephone use and risk of acoustic neuroma. Am J Epidemiol 2004;159(3):277–83.
96. Auvinen A, Hietanen M, Luukkonen R, Koskela R-S. Brain tumors and salivary gland cancers among cellular telephone users. Epidemiology 2002;13(3):356–9.
97. Hardell L, Mild KH, Carlberg M. Case-control study on the use of cellular and cordless phones and the risk for malignant brain tumours. Intl J Rad Biol 2002;78(10):931–6.
98. Hardell L, Nasman A, Pahlson A, Hallquist A, Hansson Mild K. Use of cellular telephones and the risk for brain tumours: A case-control study. Intl J Oncol 1999;15(1):113–6.
99. Hepworth SJ, Schoemaker MJ, Muir KR, Swerdlow AJ, van Tongeren MJA, McKinney PA. Mobile phone use and risk of glioma in adults: case-control study. BMJ 2006;332(7546):883–7.
100. Inskip PD, Tarone RE, Hatch EE, et al. Cellular-telephone use and brain tumors. N Eng J Med 2001;344(2):79–86.
101. Johansen C, Boice JJ, McLaughlin J, Olsen J. Cellular telephones and cancer—a nationwide cohort study in Denmark. J Natl Cancer Inst 2001;93(3):203–7.
102. Lahkola A, Auvinen A, Raitanen J, et al. Mobile phone use and risk of glioma in 5 North European countries. Intl J Cancer 2007;120(8):1769–75.
103. Muscat JE, Malkin MG, Thompson S, et al. Handheld cellular telephone use and risk of brain cancer. JAMA 2000;284(23):3001–7.
104. Feychting M, Anders A. Radiofrequency fields and glioma. Principles and Practices of Neuro-Oncology: A Multidisciplinary Approach. (In Press).
105. Ahlbom A, Green A, Kheifets L, Savitz D, Swerdlow A, Swerdlow A. Epidemiology of health effects of radiofrequency exposure. Environ Health Perspect 2004;112(17):1741–54.
106. Hardell L, Carlberg M, Hansson Mild K. Pooled analysis of two case-control studies on use of cellular and cordless telephones and the risk for malignant brain tumours diagnosed in 1997–2003. Intl Arch Occup Environ Health 2006;79(8):630–9.

107. Wrensch M, Kelsey KT, Liu M, et al. Glutathione-S-transferase and adult glioma. Cancer Epidemiol Biomarkers Prev 2004;13(3):461–7.
108. Schwartzbaum JA, Ahlbom A, Lonn S, et al. An international case-control study of glutathione transferase and functionally related polymorphisms and risk of primary adult brain tumors. Cancer Epidemiol Biomarkers Prev 2007;16(3):559–96.
109. Wrensch M, Kelsey KT, Liu M, et al. ERCC1 and ERCC2 polymorphisms and adult glioma. Neuro-oncol 2005;7(4):495–507.
110. Chen P, Wiencke J, Aldape K, et al. Association of an ERCC1 polymorphism with adult-onset glioma. Cancer Epidemiol Biomarkers Prev 2000;9(8):843–7.
111. Caggana M, Kilgallen J, Conroy JM, et al. Associations between ERCC2 polymorphisms and gliomas. Cancer Epidemiol Biomarkers Prev 2001;10(4):355–60.
112. Wang L-E, Bondy ML, Shen H, et al. Polymorphisms of DNA repair genes and risk of glioma. Cancer Res 2004;64(16):5560–3.
113. Wiencke JK, Aldape K, McMillan A, et al. Molecular features of adult glioma associated with patient race/ethnicity, age, and a polymorphism in O6-methylguanine-DNA-methyltransferase. Cancer Epidemiol Biomarkers Prev 2005;14(7):1774–83.
114. Inoue R, Isono M, Abe M, Abe T, Kobayashi H. A genotype of the polymorphic DNA repair gene MGMT is associated with de novo glioblastoma. Neurol Res 2003;25(8):875–9.
115. Bethke L, Webb E, Murray A, et al. Comprehensive analysis of the role of DNA repair gene polymorphisms on risk of glioma. Hum Mol Genet 2007;17(6):800–5.
116. Ichimura K, Ohgaki H, Kleihues P, Collins VP. Molecular pathogenesis of astrocytic tumours. J Neuro-oncol 2004;70(2):137–60.
117. Bethke L, Sullivan K, Webb E, et al. The common D02H variant of CASP8 is associated with risk of glioma. Cancer Epidemiol Biomarkers Prev 2008;17(4):987–9.
118. Bond GL, Hu W, Levine AJ. MDM2 is a central node in the p53 pathway: 12 years and counting. Curr Cancer Drug Targets 2005;5(1):3–8.
119. Halatsch ME, Schmidt U, Unterberg A, Vougioukas VI. Uniform MDM2 overexpression in a panel of glioblastoma multiforme cell lines with divergent EGFR and p53 expression status. Anticancer Res 2006;26(6B):4191–4.
120. Tsuiki H, Nishi T, Takeshima H, et al. Single nucleotide polymorphism 309 affects murin-double-minute 2 protein expression but not glioma tumorigenesis. Neurol Med Chir (Tokyo) 2007;47(5):203–8; discussion 8–9.
121. Bond GL, Hu W, Bond EE, et al. A single nucleotide polymorphism in the MDM2 promoter attenuates the p53 tumor suppressor pathway and accelerates tumor formation in humans. Cell 2004;119(5):591–602.
122. Poltermann S, Schlehofer B, Steindorf K, Schnitzler P, Geletneky K, Schlehofer JR. Lack of association of herpesviruses with brain tumors. J Neurovirol 2006;12:90–9.
123. Mitchell DA, Xie W, Schmittling R, et al. Sensitive detection of human cytomegalovirus in tumors and peripheral blood of patients diagnosed with glioblastoma. Neuro-oncol 2008;10(1).
124. Scheurer ME, Bondy M, Aldape K, Albrecht T, El-Zein R. Detection of human cytomegalovirus in different histological types of gliomas. Acta Neuropathol 2008;116:79–86.
125. Simon M, Bostrom JP, Hartmann C. Molecular genetics of meningiomas: from basic research to potential clinical applications. Neurosurgery 2007;60(5):787–98; discussion -98.
126. Riemenschneider MJ, Perry A, Reifenberger G. Histological classification and molecular genetics of meningiomas. Lancet neurol 2006;5(12):1045–54.
127. Pecina-Slaus N, Nikuseva Martic T, Tomas D, Beros V, Zeljko M, Cupic H. Meningiomas exhibit loss of heterozygosity of the APC gene. J Neuro-oncol 2008;87(1):63–70.
128. Guan Y, Hata N, Kuga D, et al. Narrowing of the regions of allelic losses of chromosome 1p36 in meningioma tissues by an improved SSCP analysis. Intl J Cancer 2008;122(8):1820–6.
129. Malmer B, Feychting M, Lonn S, Ahlbom A, Henriksson R. p53 Genotypes and risk of glioma and meningioma. Cancer Epidemiol Biomarkers Prev 2005;14(9):2220–3.
130. Bethke L, Murray A, Webb E, et al. Comprehensive analysis of DNA repair gene variants and risk of meningioma. J Natl Cancer Inst 2008;100(4):270–6.
131. Sanjay S, Hosking FJ, Robertson LB, et al. Genome-wide association study identifies five susceptibility loci for glioma. Nature Genetics 2009;41(8):899–904.
132. Wrensch M, Jenkins RB, Chang JS, et al. Variants in the CDKN2B and RTEL1 regions are associated with high-grade glioma susceptibility. Nature Genetics [published online ahead of print July 5, 2009];41(8):905–8.

3 Clinical Features of Brain Tumors

LAKSHMI NAYAK • LISA M. DEANGELIS

Introduction

The symptoms and signs of a brain tumor resemble those seen in other focal neurological diseases, but they can also be generalized and nonspecific. If the clinician is not wary, brain tumors, especially slow-growing tumors, may be missed. Imaging is very important in the diagnosis of brain tumors, but clinical history and examination provide critical information to the diagnosis. Onset, duration, and progression of symptoms and signs can provide strong evidence for an intracranial mass and can often predict whether the lesion is slow or rapidly growing.

Pathophysiology of Symptoms and Signs

Symptoms and signs are caused by a variety of mechanisms, many of which may be active in a given patient. It is the combination of these mechanisms that produce the clinical syndromes observed in patients.[1,2]

DIRECT EFFECT OF TUMOR

Tumor can destroy normal neural tissue or displace and distort it by compression, leading to focal symptoms and signs. Direct invasion typically occurs in infiltrating gliomas and lymphomas, whereas meningiomas and metastases usually displace and distort brain tissue. The extent to which tissue is destroyed, as opposed to compressed, determines how reversible a patient's symptoms or signs may be following treatment of the tumor.

SECONDARY EFFECT OF EDEMA

Tumor, by disrupting the blood-brain barrier, leads to vasogenic edema, one of the most important causes of clinical impairment. White matter is particularly vulnerable to vasogenic edema, which tends to extend along neighboring white matter tracks. Edema leads to increasing mass effect and thus further compression of the surrounding brain. In some circumstances, local compression from increasing interstitial pressure in surrounding tissues may lead to local ischemia.

HYDROCEPHALUS AND CSF OBSTRUCTION

Tumors in the third or fourth ventricles, such as colloid cysts, ependymomas, choroid plexus papillomas, and meningiomas, can obstruct CSF outflow, resulting in hydrocephalus. In these situations, hydrocephalus may be the presenting feature. Tumor in the leptomeninges can lead to communicating hydrocephalus. Hydrocephalus and raised intracranial pressure may occur as a delayed complication of hemispheric tumors such as glioblastoma and metastases.

HERNIATION SYNDROMES

Brain tumors cause shift or herniation of brain tissue from one compartment to another. The most important clinical consequence of a shift is a depressed level of consciousness. False localizing signs may be seen, most commonly in patients with a herniation syndrome and raised intracranial pressure. A herniation syndrome is a rare presentation of an undiagnosed brain tumor. It is much more likely to be seen in a patient known to have an intracranial mass that has progressed despite treatment, usually late in the course of a brain tumor.

There are five common herniation syndromes.

Subfalcine herniation: The cingulate gyrus is pushed under the falx cerebri, leading to compression of both anterior frontal lobes or occlusion of an anterior cerebral artery with subsequent frontal lobe infarction.

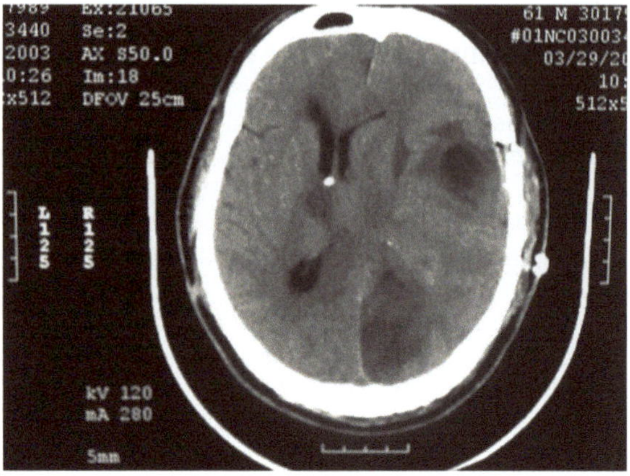

Figure 3-1 Non-contrast enhancing head CT scan demonstrating a left occipital infarct after herniation from a large left frontal malignant glioma. Note the significant persistent left-to-right shift.

Uncal herniation occurs when a mass lesion causes the uncus of the temporal lobe to herniate through the tentorium cerebelli. The key clinical sign of uncal herniation is ipsilateral oculomotor nerve palsy with a fixed and dilated pupil due to compression by the medial temporal lobe. Typically, a contralateral hemiparesis is also seen, but a false localizing sign of uncal herniation is an ipsilateral hemiparesis due to displacement of the brainstem to the opposite side causing compression of the contralateral cerebral peduncle against the tentorium (Kernohan notch). Additionally, unilateral or bilateral posterior cerebral artery occlusion can occur at the tentorial notch, leading to a homonymous hemianopsia or cortical blindness (Fig. 3-1).

Central herniation is due to pressure from a mass in the diencephalon and may lead to coma. Rostrocaudal shifts compress the brainstem, compromising its vascular supply and leading to Duret hemorrhages.

Tonsillar herniation occurs when the cerebellar tonsils herniate through the foramen magnum; this may cause obstruction of the fourth ventricular outflow, and compression of the medulla with sudden death.

Upward brainstem herniation is seen in patients with posterior fossa tumors, where the superior surface of the vermis and midbrain are pushed upward, compressing the dorsal mesencephalon and cerebral aqueduct. Dorsal midbrain compression leads to impairment of vertical eye movements and a reduced level of consciousness.[2,3]

Factors Determining Symptoms and Signs

There are several biological factors intrinsic to the tumor itself that affect the clinical manifestations of the disease (Table 3-1). The general location of the tumor, supratentorial vs. infratentorial, or cortical vs. subcortical, will affect the presentation. If the tumor is extraaxial, it will compress the underlying brain tissue instead

TABLE 3-1 Factors Determining the Signs and Symptoms of Brain Tumors

Location	
	Supratentorial vs. infratentorial
	Cortical vs. subcortical
	Intraparenchymal vs. extraparenchymal
Growth/Histology	
	Rapid vs. slow
	Infiltrative vs. discrete
Size	
	Large vs. small
Secretions	
	Pituitary hormones
	Melatonin
	Angiogenic factors
	Neuropeptides

of destroying it as a parenchymal tumor might. The rapidity of growth will determine how soon a tumor will manifest; slow-growing tumors are insidious. Discrete tumors usually present with focal localizing symptoms as compared to diffusely infiltrative ones. The size of the tumor can affect symptoms in that even large tumors in relatively silent areas of the brain may be asymptomatic, whereas small tumors in other areas, for instance the brainstem, will present early. Some tumors can cause non-neurological symptoms, such as pituitary tumors via secretions.

Neurologic Symptoms and Signs

Regardless of tumor location, patients can have generalized and/or lateralizing symptoms. Generalized symptoms are non-localizing and can include headache, seizures, nausea, vomiting, dizziness, mental status changes, and visual obscurations. Focal symptoms reflect the intracranial location of the tumor and include seizures, hemiparesis, diplopia, aphasia, vertigo, incoordination, sensory abnormalities, and dysphagia (Table 3-2). Finally, there are false localizing signs, which are caused by raised intracranial pressure and which may include diplopia, tinnitus, and hearing or visual loss. These signs may suggest focal neurologic dysfunction, but actually reflect a generalized increase in intracranial pressure.

GENERALIZED SYMPTOMS AND SIGNS

Headache

Headache is a very common symptom leading to neurologic referral, and when associated with a normal neurologic examination, is rarely due to a brain tumor. Intracranial neoplasms account for a small percentage (less than 10%) of patients with headache, but headache occurs in about 50% of patients with brain tumors,[4,5]

TABLE 3-2 Focal Signs and Symptoms of Brain Tumors (adapted from DeAngelis[50])

Location	Signs and symptoms
Frontal lobe	Contralateral hemiparesis Seizures: focal motor (contralateral) and generalized Aphasia (dominant side) Gait apraxia, incontinence, dementia (bilateral involvement) Behavioral changes Alien limb syndrome (supplementary motor cortex)
Parietal lobe	Contralateral sensory loss Seizures, typically sensory Agnosias Aphasias
Temporal lobe	Seizures: complex partial, generalized, olfactory Behavioral changes Memory problems Psychiatric manifestations Aphasia (dominant side) Visual field defect
Occipital lobe	Visual field defect Visual disturbances
Corpus callosum	Behavioral changes Memory loss (posterior) Dementia
Thalamus	Contralateral sensory loss Aphasia Behavioral changes
Basal ganglia	Contralateral hemiparesis Movement disorders
Pituitary, Sella, Optic nerve	Endocrine disturbances Visual defects, bitemporal hemianopsia (optic chiasm) Ophthalmoplegia (cavernous sinus)
Midbrain, Pineal gland	Pupillary abnormalities Paresis of vertical eye movements
Pons, Medulla	Hemiparesis Sensory loss Ataxia Cranial nerve abnormalities
Cerebellum	Ataxia Nystagmus Vertigo

and in some studies the prevalence has been shown to be as high as 60% to 70%.[6,7] However, most of these patients have accompanying neurologic signs. Headache is the sole presenting complaint in only 8% of patients with brain tumors.[6,8] A new-onset headache of sufficient severity that the patient seeks medical assistance, in an adult without a prior history of headache, requires a full investigation including neuroimaging.

Headache related to brain tumor is a result of raised intracranial pressure causing stimulation of pain-sensitive structures in the cranial vault (Table 3-3).[9,10] The pain-sensitive intracranial structures include the pachymeninges and all vascular structures in the brain; the brain parenchyma itself is insensitive to pain. Headaches occur due to involvement of the meninges and vessels by direct tumor invasion, inflammation or edema resulting from the tumor, or traction or pressure on the pain-sensitive structures by the tumor. Headache in brain tumor patients can be nonspecific, or may resemble tension-type headache, migraine, or a "classic tumor headache," which occurs in the morning and improves spontaneously over the course of the day. Tumor headache may get progressively severe over time; this is often related to an increase in the surrounding edema rather than the actual size of the tumor.[4,5]

The most common headache in brain tumor patients is similar to tension-type headache, and is characterized as a dull ache or pressure-like pain.[4,6] These headaches are usually bifrontal and are often worse on the side ipsilateral to the tumor. Nausea or vomiting may be associated, and usually indicate generalized elevation of intracranial pressure. However, headaches that mimic classical migraine can also occur in patients with brain tumors. They are seen predominantly in patients with a history of migraine who then develop a brain tumor. These headaches may be associated with nausea and vomiting which, in these cases, do not necessarily indicate raised intracranial pressure.[4] In some patients, a brain tumor can present as the worst headache of their life; this may be associated with intratumoral hemorrhage which is accompanied by neck stiffness, vomiting, mental status changes, and focal signs such as hemiparesis. More often, however, these severe headaches are not due to a bleed. In other cases, compression of the ophthalmic division of the trigeminal nerve or involvement of the nerve by tumor results in the typical pain of trigeminal neuralgia. Also, Gasserian ganglion involvement may cause neuralgia-type pain in the V2-3 distribution. Rarely, occipital neuralgia has been reported.[11,12] Some authors have demonstrated that there is a tendency for pulsatile pain with meningioma.[6] This may be related to the increased vasculature of meningiomas and innervation of the blood vessels by the trigeminal nerve.

The most common headache site in brain tumor patients is frontal, and is usually bilateral.[4] This is seen commonly with supratentorial tumors or with diffuse

TABLE 3-3 Factors Contributing to Headache in Patients with Brain Tumor

1. Raised ICP
2. Location of tumor
3. Size of tumor and surrounding edema
4. Midline shift
5. Prior history of headache

elevation of intracranial pressure. Occipital headaches, with or without neck pain, are seen in infratentorial tumors or when there is base of skull involvement by tumor, but tumors in these locations may also give rise to frontal pain. Thus, headache has poor localizing value. However, lateralization of the tumor can be reliable when the patient complains of headache on one side of the head or the other.

Headache caused by raised intracranial pressure is distinctive in its severity, its association with nausea and vomiting, and its resistance to common analgesics.[4] There may be associated papilledema, which is usually seen in children or young adults with raised intracranial pressure. Paroxysmal headaches can be seen in association with tumors of the third ventricle or pedunculated tumors intermittently obstructing CSF flow; occasionally, they are precipitated by changes in position. Rarely, Brunn syndrome can develop, which is characterized by attacks of sudden and severe headache, vomiting, and vertigo, triggered by head movement.[13] Episodic headaches may also be indicative of *plateau waves*. These occur in patients with elevation of baseline intracranial pressure (which may be asymptomatic) and episodic symptoms, including headaches, that are triggered by a change in body position. The act of assuming the upright posture triggers a marked increase in intracranial pressure due to loss of autoregulation. The brisk rise in intracranial pressure usually resolves on its own; however, it causes transient symptoms while the pressure is elevated, typically to a level exceeding systolic blood pressure. Generally, these symptoms last five to ten minutes and resolve spontaneously. In addition to headache, common symptoms that occur with plateau waves include visual loss or obscurations, lightheadedness, loss of tone in the legs and even loss of consciousness. These symptoms are often confused with seizures, but a careful history makes the diagnosis clear. Exacerbation of headache may also occur with changes in intracranial pressure, such as with coughing, sneezing, performing Valsalva maneuver, exertion, or sexual activity; however, these exacerbations are uncommon in brain tumor patients.[14]

Headaches occur more commonly with infratentorial than supratentorial tumors.[5,7,8] Dural-based tumors may present with headache. Subdural hematoma from dural metastases can also give rise to headache. Often, patients with supratentorial tumors without raised intracranial pressure do not have headaches despite large tumor size, and if they do have headaches, the pain is likely to be intermittent and less severe than with infratentorial tumors.[4] Young patients are also more likely to suffer from headaches than older patients, possibly because age-related atrophy allows better compensation for the growing mass.

Patients with a preexisting history of headache are predisposed to develop secondary headaches in the presence of brain tumors.[4,6] They are likely to suffer from headaches even when controlled for raised intracranial pressure. A change in quality, severity, and location of a pre-existing headache should be considered ominous and always warrants an evaluation.

Nausea and Vomiting

Nausea and vomiting occur when the chemotactic trigger zone in the area postrema, located on the floor of the fourth ventricle, is stimulated. Vomiting usually indicates raised intracranial pressure, but it can also occur because of direct compression of the vomiting center by posterior fossa tumors such as medulloblastoma or ependymomas of the fourth ventricle. It can also occur in the absence of elevated intracranial pressure in brainstem tumors involving the nucleus solitarius. Acute headache followed by an episode of vomiting suggests increased intracranial pressure. Projectile vomiting, usually seen in posterior fossa tumors in children, is uncommon in adults. Ictus emeticus or vomiting as an ictal phenomenon can, rarely, be a manifestation of epilepsy in tumors involving the insula and mesialtemporal lobe. It has been reported with temporal lobe astrocytoma[15] and mesial temporal glioma.[16]

Papilledema

Papilledema is an indicator of increased intracranial pressure; it is now rarely seen in patients at the time of presentation of a brain tumor. This is due to the widespread availability of modern neuroimaging, which is almost always performed before the tumor progresses far enough to cause papilledema. In its mildest form, or in acute cases, it may not lead to a change in visual acuity; enlargement of the blind spot may be the only finding on examination. Like headache, papilledema is seen more often in children and young adults; this is probably because older adults have more room for tumor expansion due to brain atrophy, or because, in older adults, optic nerve sheath fibrosis does not allow the pressure to be transmitted to the disc. Papilledema due to raised intracranial pressure is usually bilateral, although it may not be symmetrical. Certain chronic conditions, such as a frontal lobe tumor or olfactory groove meningioma, may, rarely, lead to the Foster Kennedy syndrome, in which there is optic atrophy on the side of the tumor due to chronic local compression, and papilledema on the contralateral side due to increased intracranial pressure.

Vertigo and Dizziness

Vertigo occurs commonly in cerebellopontine angle tumors; these include meningioma, schwannoma, and metastases. Occasionally, tumors such as astrocytoma, ependymoma, choroid plexus papilloma, or medulloblastoma arising from the pons or fourth ventricle may present with symptoms identical to those seen in cerebellopontine angle tumors. Vertigo may result from tumors invading the vestibular portion of cranial nerve VIII, the cerebellum, or the brainstem. Tumors in the cerebellum and brainstem cause vertigo in association with other signs and symptoms, such as dysmetria, appendicular and gait ataxia, and other cranial nerve signs. Some patients who have supratentorial tumors without involvement of the posterior fossa structures complain of dizziness or lightheadedness. These symptoms are usually nonspecific, but may indicate increased intracranial pressure.

Mental Status Changes

Mental and cognitive abnormalities may be specific or nonspecific.

Specific findings include aphasia, agnosia, abulia, alexia, or apraxia. These symptoms have localizing value but are often mistaken for global cognitive impairment. For example, a patient with a fluent Wernicke's type aphasia may be perceived as being confused rather than as having a language problem.

Nonspecific mental changes are among the most common symptoms and are often subtle, particularly early in the disease course. Irritability, change in personality, emotional lability, forgetfulness, lack of enthusiasm or spontaneity, and slowed response, progressing gradually to apathy and lethargy are seen in about 16% to 34% of patients.[17] These symptoms do not reflect tumor in a specific area of the brain, but, when present, are suggestive of tumors in deep structures affecting thalamocortical fibers, corpus callosum, reticular formation, and occasionally, the frontal lobes. Variations in behavior can be seen according to which area of the frontal lobe is involved; for example, apathy and abulia are seen in tumors involving the dorsolateral frontal lobe, whereas orbitofrontal tumors lead to disinhibition and impulsive behavior. Sometimes withdrawal and apathy are confused with depression, even when the patient denies feeling sad or depressed. Aggressive and impulsive behavior can be seen with lesions involving the amygdala. Occasionally, temporal lobe seizures present with behavioral disturbances. Malamud et al. have described outbursts of rage in patients with temporal lobe gliomas. Peduncular hallucinosis can occur with midbrain tumors, and has also been described in posterior fossa tumors compressing the brainstem.[18,19] Behavior and personality changes predominate as the presenting complaints, particularly in primary CNS lymphoma. This is due to its predilection for the frontal lobes and a 40% incidence of multiple lesions at diagnosis. Raised intracranial pressure can present with confusion, disorientation, lethargy, and coma.

Memory Problems

Tumors of the hippocampal formation of the medial temporal lobe and diencephalon can cause amnestic syndromes. An anterograde amnesia syndrome has been reported with tumors of the corpus callosum, particularly when the splenium is involved.[20,21] Korsakoff syndrome has been reported in primary CNS lymphoma involving the third ventricle.[22] Astrocytomas involving both temporal lobes can cause memory deficits.[23] Rarely, gliomas have been found in patients who present with transient global amnesia.[24]

Seizures

Many patients with brain tumors develop seizures, either as the presenting symptom or later in the course of their disease, usually due to tumor progression. The incidence varies depending on the patient's age and the type of tumor. Epilepsy occurs more commonly in primary tumors (30% to 90%) than metastases (35%). Among the primary tumors, slow-growing, low-grade tumors cause seizures more often (85% of patients) than high-grade neoplasms, such as glioblastoma (49%).[25–27] About 38% of patients with meningiomas develop seizures,[28] typically with convexity lesions; skull base meningiomas rarely cause seizures.

All seizures from brain tumors have a focal origin. Generalized seizures in a brain tumor patient always have a focal onset, but the discharge may proceed to secondary generalization so quickly that the focal signature may not be detected by the patient or an observer. If a lateralizing sign is detected in the postictal state, such as aphasia or a hemiparesis, this may also indicate that a focal lesion was responsible for the generalized convulsion. In addition, general postictal findings of confusion or lethargy are common.

The clinical manifestations of partial seizures depend on the location of the tumor; simple or complex partial seizures are more common in parietal, temporal, or frontal lobe lesions.[29] Aphasia in the absence of any other focal signs (such as hemiparesis or facial palsy) should alert the clinician to consider seizures; an EEG may be confirmatory. Mood or behavioral changes and hallucinations may be suggestive of seizures, particularly from temporal foci; in the undiagnosed patient, these may be confused with psychiatric disorders. Nonconvulsive status epilepticus should be considered in a patient presenting with lethargy or fluctuating mental status changes. Epilepsia partialis continua of Kozhevnikov, or focal motor status epilepticus, can be problematic, and is often refractory to a single and sometimes even to multiple antiepileptic agents. Laughter as an ictal event, known as gelastic seizures, has been seen with hypothalamic hamartomas[30] and has also been reported in a case of a low-grade hypothalamic astrocytoma.[31]

LATERALIZING SYMPTOMS AND SIGNS

Visual Problems

Visual obscurations and decreased visual acuity can occur in patients with elevated intracranial pressure. Orbital or retro-orbital tumors can lead to scotomas. Loss of vision can develop from tumors of the optic nerve.

Lesions of the chiasm lead to bitemporal hemianopsia; the most common causes are pituitary adenoma, craniopharyngioma, meningioma, hypothalamic glioma, ectopic pinealoma or dysgerminoma, and metastases. Homonymous hemianopsia is the result of a tumor in the contralateral occipital cortex or optic tract. Tumors in the parietal lobe and adjacent temporal lobe can give rise to visual neglect on the contralateral side. Compression of a posterior cerebral artery directly by tumor or from herniation can result in cortical blindness. When a patient is unaware of his blindness, the condition is known as Anton syndrome. Other causes of altitudinal field defect include compression of the optic nerve by frontal tumor[32] and increased pressure from a posterior fossa tumor compressing the chiasm by upward herniation.[33]

Direct involvement of the third, fourth, or sixth cranial nerves can give rise to diplopia. This is commonly due to invasion of the cavernous sinus, or because of orbital tumors compressing the nerves or, occasionally, the extraocular muscles. However, diplopia can result from raised intracranial pressure causing dysfunction of the abducens nerve as a false localizing sign. Ipsilateral pupillary dilatation followed by diplopia suggesting oculomotor nerve impairment is an ominous sign; such a patient should be evaluated for uncal herniation.

Prosopagnosia, or the inability to recognize faces, occurs in lesions of the right or bilateral occipitotemporal cortex. It has been documented in a case of leptomeningeal involvement of the brain.[34] Posterior parietal lesions give rise to simultanagnosia which is the inability to perceive different parts of a visual scene as a whole. Balint syndrome, a triad of optic ataxia, ocular apraxia, and simultanagnosia can occasionally be seen.

Hemiparesis

Contralateral hemiparesis develops in tumors located in the motor cortex, basal ganglia, internal capsule, or brainstem. Hemiparesis from tumors usually begins as mild loss of fine motor control and gradually progresses. Often patients are unaware of minor deficits that may be identified by the clinician on neurological examination. The onset of symptoms is unlike a stroke, unless there is hemorrhage into the tumor causing acute symptoms. In rare circumstances, infarcts may develop from compression of blood vessels by the tumor mass, venous sinus thrombosis leading to venous infarcts, or, rarely, in patients with intravascular lymphoma, where the tumor fills a blood vessel in the brain.

Aphasia

Language deficit or aphasia results from tumor invasion of the language areas located in the dominant hemisphere, including subcortical structures such as the basal ganglia and thalamus. Aphasia due to large brain tumors is usually associated with other focal signs such as a hemiparesis; however, a seizure can present as an isolated transient aphasia that may be mistaken for a transient ischemic attack in the undiagnosed patient. The language disturbance of many patients with brain tumors may not fit into the classical categories of aphasia as outlined in Table 3-4. This is due to the highly infiltrative nature of tumors such as gliomas and lymphomas, where there can be extensive involvement throughout the language pathways. Furthermore, tumors can occur anywhere and their growth is not defined by vascular territories. This is important to remember, as most aphasia syndromes were classified in patients with stroke. Therefore, while patients may have features suggestive of a typical Wernicke or Broca aphasia, many have a mixed picture that defies simple classification.

Ataxia

Gait abnormalities can present as a hemiparetic gait, cerebellar ataxia, or frontal ataxia. A tumor in a hemisphere will cause circumduction of the contralateral leg which may be evident only on examination of gait. Tumors in the cerebellar hemisphere give rise to ipsilateral limb ataxia; the anterior portion of the anterior lobe

TABLE 3-4 Types of Aphasia with Localization

Type of aphasia	Characteristics	Localization
Broca	Nonfluent, normal comprehension, impaired repetition	Inferior frontal gyrus
Wernicke	Fluent, impaired comprehension & repetition	Superior temporal gyrus
Global	Nonfluent, impaired comprehension & repetition	Perisylvian (frontal and temporal)
Conduction	Fluent, normal comprehension, impaired repetition	Insula
Transcortical motor	Nonfluent, normal comprehension and repetition	Anterior to Broca's area
Transcortical sensory	Fluent, impaired comprehension, preserved repetition	Around Wernicke's area

affects the legs, whereas the posterior portion of the anterior lobe affects the arms. The patient may veer to one side; this helps localize the lesion to the ipsilateral hemisphere. Truncal ataxia results from tumors in the cerebellar vermis. Frontal lobe tumors and hydrocephalus can cause gait disturbances or apraxia.[35] Lesions in the vestibular system can lead to vertigo and gait imbalance.

Primary Intra-axial Tumors

Astrocytomas are graded by the World Health Organization (WHO) classification scheme. In order of increasing malignancy, they are classified as pilocytic (WHO grade I), fibrillary (WHO grade II), anaplastic astrocytomas (WHO grade III) and glioblastoma multiforme (WHO grade IV). Low grade tumors usually present with seizures. High-grade tumors are more likely to present with focal symptoms and deficits (Table 3-5). Patients with grade III astrocytomas and glioblastomas present with headaches (53% to 57%), seizures (57% of patients with grade III, 24% of patients with GBM), hemiparesis (25% to 36%), aphasia (23% to 36%), and visual problems (21%).[17] Memory loss and cognitive changes are more frequent in GBM (39%), as compared to grade III tumors (23%).[17] Low-grade tumors almost always present with a seizure (75% to 85%). Typically, this occurs in a young adult, and the neurologic examination is otherwise normal, even if the lesion is found to be quite large on neuroimaging. Preservation of neurologic function can be attributed to the infiltrative nature of these lesions and the lack of tissue destruction. Other presenting symptoms for pilocytic astrocytomas are headaches (27%) and visual complaints (12%).[36]

Oligodendrogliomas are slower growing than astrocytomas. They are found only as either grade II or grade III lesions. The low-grade tumors typically present with seizures alone, and these patients can go for over a decade before other neurologic symptoms develop. In 72% of patients, a seizure is the initial presenting complaint[37,38]; seizures occur in 90% of patients at some point during the disease course.[38] Headaches are the initial symptom in 10% of patients, whereas hemiparesis and aphasia occur only in 3% of patients at diagnosis.[38] In patients who have oligodendrogliomas with a combined loss of 1p and 19q, 93% present with low-grade tumors and seizures of long standing duration.[39] The high-grade oligodendrogliomas present similarly to the high-grade astrocytomas.

TABLE 3-5 Signs and Symptoms over the Duration of the Disease by Tumor Type[2,5,17,26,27,28,36,43,48]

Tumor type	Headache	Seizure	Hemiparesis
Low-grade glioma	10%	75–85%	16%
Glioblastomas	57%	24–49%	36%
Meningiomas	36–59%	29–60%	30–50%
Brain metastases	49–77%	18–35%	39–59%

Gliomatosis cerebri is seen when astrocytomas and, rarely, oligodendrogliomas widely infiltrate the brain in a diffuse fashion. Symptoms may be generalized (such as headaches, papilledema, behavioral changes) or focal.

Optic gliomas involve the optic nerve or optic chiasm. They may be associated with neurofibromatosis type 1. The clinical course is characterized by progressive or stepwise visual loss.

Brainstem gliomas present with cranial nerve palsies (91%),[40] followed by the subsequent development of long-tract signs. Headaches with nausea are seen in 57% of patients.[40] Brainstem gliomas may be associated with neurofibromatosis type 1.

Medulloblastomas are seen usually in children and young adults. Obstructive hydrocephalus is common at presentation. Clinically, patients of all ages present with headache, nausea, and vomiting. In adults, papilledema is seen in about 75% of patients, cerebellar symptoms in 45%, and nystagmus in 50%.[41]

Primary CNS lymphomas often present with behavioral and cognitive changes (43%). Headaches, nausea, and vomiting suggestive of raised intracranial pressure (33%) and focal deficits (70%) are seen, although seizures are less common (14%), as these tumors typically involve the deep structures of brain.[42] Ocular involvement leads to visual complaints.

Primary Extra-axial Tumors

Meningiomas are usually benign and very slow-growing; they are often very large by the time they are symptomatic. They typically involve the cortical convexity or skull base. The symptoms depend on the location of the tumor, but headaches (36% to 59%), seizures (29% to 60%), and personality changes (22%) may develop due to compression of the underlying brain tissue (Table 3-5). Hemiparesis is more frequently seen with malignant meningiomas (50%) than benign (30%).[5,27,43]

Vestibular schwannomas present with hearing loss (75%), tinnitus (18%), unsteadiness of gait (20%), vertigo (16%), and/or ipsilateral facial numbness or weakness.[44] Bilateral vestibular schwannomas are pathognomonic for neurofibromatosis type 2.

Pineal tumors usually compress the aqueduct and result in hydrocephalus. Compression of the colliculi leads to development of Parinaud syndrome with impaired upgaze, convergence, retraction nystagmus, eyelid retraction (Collier sign), and pupillary light-near dissociation. Other symptoms are headache, nausea, vomiting, vertigo, ataxia, cognitive changes, and, rarely, insomnia.

Pituitary tumors may be adenomas, carcinomas, or metastases. Adenomas are the most common and are usually benign. When the tumors are of microadenoma size (<1 cm), patients often present with hormone hypersecretion (e.g., ACTH, growth hormone, prolactin). Alternatively, macroadenomas (>1 cm) usually present with

TABLE 3-6 Endocrine Disturbances Associated with Pituitary Tumors

Hormone	Endocrine abnormality
Hypersecretion	
Prolactin	Amenorrhea, galactorrhea (in women) Impotence (in men)
Growth hormone	Acromegaly
TSH	Hyperthyroidism
ACTH	Cushing syndrome, Nelson syndrome
FSH, LH	Hypogonadism, asymptomatic
Hyposecretion	
FSH, LH	Impotence, loss of libido, osteoporosis
Growth hormone	Central obesity, reduced muscle mass Premature atherosclerosis Psychiatric manifestations
TSH	Hypothyroidism
ACTH	Addison disease
Vasopressin	Polydipsia, polyuria, nocturia

TSH: Thyroid stimulating hormone
ACTH: Adrenocorticotropic hormone
FSH: Follicle-stimulating hormone
LH: Luteinizing hormone

hormone hyposecretion and compression of neighboring structures, particularly the optic chiasm, causing visual field defects (68%) including bitemporal hemianopia (16%).[45] Table 3-6 outlines endocrine disturbances associated with pituitary tumors.

Other signs may include unilateral visual loss with optic atrophy, and ptosis, diplopia, or facial numbness from cavernous sinus involvement. Rarely, pituitary apoplexy occurs, leading to the sudden onset of severe headache, visual loss, and loss of consciousness. This can occur from hemorrhage into or infarction of the adenoma.

Brain Metastases

Cancer can spread to any part of the central nervous system. Often, patients with no known cancer present with symptoms from brain metastases.[2] Certain cancers, such as lung, breast, and melanoma, have a predilection to metastasize to the nervous system. Autopsy studies have shown that 24% to 29% of patients dying from systemic cancer have intracranial metastases; 15% are intraparenchymal, 9% are dural, and 8% are leptomeningeal metastases.[46,47]

The site and nature of the CNS metastasis depends on the primary cancer; for example, lung cancer commonly leads to brain metastases, whereas prostate cancer is most likely to produce skull lesions and dural metastases. Lymphoma and leukemia usually cause leptomeningeal metastases.[47]

Brain Metastases

The most common cancers associated with metastases to the brain are lung, breast, and melanoma.[46,47] Common symptoms and signs are headache (49% to 77%), hemiparesis (39% to 59%), cognitive changes (22% to 58%), seizures (18% to 35%), aphasia (10% to 18%), and gait ataxia (19%) (Table 3-5).[2,5,27,48]

Dural Metastases

Intracranial dural metastases result from extension of skull lesions or hematogenous spread. Prostate and breast cancer are the most common offenders.[46,47] Symptoms are usually based on the tumor site; however, other presentations of dural involvement include venous sinus invasion or compression leading to venous infarcts, hemorrhage and hydrocephalus, malignant subdural effusions, and ophthalmoplegia from cranial nerve involvement in the cavernous sinus. Common symptoms and signs are headaches (39%), cranial neuropathies (30%), visual problems (16%), mental status changes (16%), and seizures (11%).[49]

Leptomeningeal Metastases

Lymphoma, leukemia, breast and lung cancer, and melanoma frequently metastasize to the leptomeninges.[46,47] Cranial nerve involvement leading to diplopia (20%), peripheral facial weakness (26%), sensorineural hearing loss (20%), and bulbar weakness (4%) are common manifestations. Metastases to the leptomeninges over the cerebral cortex can give rise to seizures (15%).[2] Hydrocephalus and symptoms of raised intracranial pressure can result from leptomeningeal infiltration at the base of the brain or by infiltration of the arachnoid villi obstructing CSF flow and reabsorption.

CONCLUSIONS

Symptoms and signs of brain tumors vary based on the tumors' site of origin, histologic features, growth potential, extent of invasiveness, tendency for progression, and recurrence. Tumors in the brain can lead to focal deficits or generalized symptoms. Focal deficits are usually of localizing value, but occasionally false localizing signs and symptoms can mislead the clinician. When the history and neurological examination suggests a brain tumor, an MRI with gadolinium contrast is required for definitive diagnosis.

REFERENCES

1. DeAngelis LM, Gutin PH, Leibel SA, Posner JB. In: Intracranial Tumors: Diagnosis and Treatment. London: Martin Dunitz; 2002. p. 65–96.
2. DeAngelis LM, Posner JB, editors. Neurologic Complications of Cancer. New York: Oxford University Press; 2008. p. 141–281.
3. Posner JB, Saper CB, Schiff ND, Plum F, editors. Plum and Posner's Diagnosis of Stupor and Coma. 4th ed New York: Oxford University Press; 2007. p. 88–118.
4. Forsyth PA, Posner JB. Headaches in patients with brain tumors: a study of 111 patients. Neurology 1993;43:1678–83.

5. Pfund Z, Szapary L, Jaszberenyi O, Nagy F, Czopf J. Headache in intracranial tumors. Cephalalgia 1999;19:787–90.
6. Schankin CJ, Ferrari U, Reinisch VM, Birnbaum T, Goldbrunner R, Straube A. Characteristics of brain tumour-associated headache. Cephalalgia 2007;27:904–11.
7. Suwanwela N, Phanthumchinda K, Kaoropthum S. Headache in brain tumor: a cross-sectional study. Headache 1994;34:435–8.
8. Vazquez-Barquero A, Ibanez FJ, Herrera S, Izquierdo JM, Berciano J, Pascual J. Isolated headache as the presenting clinical manifestation of intracranial tumors: a prospective study. Cephalalgia 1994;14:270–2.
9. Cutrer FM. Pain-sensitive cranial structures:chemical anatomy. In: Silberstein SD, Lipton RB, Dalessio DJ, editors. Wolff's Headache and other head pain. New York: Oxford University Press; 2001. p. 50–6.
10. Fricke B, Andres KH, Von During M. Nerve fibers innervating the cranial and spinal meninges: morphology of nerve fiber terminals and their structural integration. Microsc Res Tech 2001;53:96–105.
11. Garza I. Craniocervical junction schwannoma mimicking occipital neuralgia. Headache 2007;47:1204–5.
12. Piovesan EJ, Werneck LC, Teive HA, Navarro F, Kowacs PA. Neurophysiology of pain in tentorial irritation: description of a case secondary to medulloblastoma. Arq Neuropsiquiatr 1998;56:677–82.
13. Krasnianski M, Muller T, Stock K, Zierz S. Bruns syndrome caused by intraventricular tumor. Eur J Med Res 2007;12:582–4.
14. Pascual J, Iglesias F, Oterino A, Vazquez-Barquero A, Berciano J. Cough, exertional, and sexual headaches: an analysis of 72 benign and symptomatic cases. Neurology 1996;46:1520–4.
15. Chen C, Yen DJ, Yiu CH, Shih YH, Yu HY, Su MS. Ictal vomiting in partial seizures of temporal lobe origin. Eur Neurol 1999;42:235–9.
16. Schauble B, Britton JW, Mullan BP, Watson J, Sharbrough FW, Marsh WR. Ictal vomiting in association with left temporal lobe seizures in a left hemisphere language-dominant patient. Epilepsia 2002;43:1432–5.
17. Chang SM, Parney IF, Huang W, et al. Patterns of care for adults with newly diagnosed malignant glioma. JAMA 2005;293:557–64.
18. Leiva-Santana C, Jerez-Garcia PT, del Real-Francia MA, Sanchez RM. Peduncular hallucinosis associated with a space occupying lesion of the brain stem. Rev Neurol 1999;28:1174–6.
19. Nadvi SS, van Dellen JR. Transient peduncular hallucinations secondary to brain stem compression by a medulloblastoma. Surg Neurol 1994;41:250–2.
20. Bustamante J, Lopera F. Tumour of the corpus callosum: the association between interhemispheric disconnection and an anterograde amnesia syndrome. Rev Neurol 2006;43:207–12.
21. Rudge P, Warrington EK. Selective impairment of memory and visual perception in splenial tumours. Brain 1991;114(Pt 1B):349–60.
22. Toth C, Voll C, Macaulay R. Primary CNS lymphoma as a cause of Korsakoff syndrome. Surg Neurol 2002;57:41–5.
23. Gillespie JS, Craig JJ, McKinstry CS. Bilateral astrocytoma involving the limbic system precipitating disabling amnesia and seizures. Seizure 2000;9:301–3.
24. Shuping JR, Toole JF, Alexander Jr E. Transient global amnesia due to glioma in the dominant hemisphere. Neurology 1980;30:88–90.
25. Herman ST. Epilepsy after brain insult: targeting epileptogenesis. Neurology 2002;59:S21–6.
26. Lote K, Stenwig AE, Skullerud K, Hirschberg H. Prevalence and prognostic significance of epilepsy in patients with gliomas. Eur J Cancer 1998;34:98–102.
27. van Breemen MS, Wilms EB, Vecht CJ. Epilepsy in patients with brain tumours: epidemiology, mechanisms, and management. Lancet Neurol 2007;6:421–30.
28. Liigant A, Haldre S, Oun A, et al. Seizure disorders in patients with brain tumors. Eur Neurol 2001;45:46–51.
29. Lynam LM, Lyons MK, Drazkowski JF, et al. Frequency of seizures in patients with newly diagnosed brain tumors: a retrospective review. Clin Neurol Neurosurg 2007;109:634–8.
30. Cascino GD, Andermann F, Berkovic SF, et al. Gelastic seizures and hypothalamic hamartomas: evaluation of patients undergoing chronic intracranial EEG monitoring and outcome of surgical treatment. Neurology 1993;43:747–50.
31. Coppola G, Spagnoli D, Sciscio N, Russo F, Villani RM. Gelastic seizures and low-grade hypothalamic astrocytoma: a case report. Brain and Development 2002;24:183–6.
32. Newsom RS, Simcock P, Zambarakji H. Cerebral metastasis presenting with altitudinal field defect. J Neuroophthalmol 1999;19:10–1.

33. Fierro B, Castiglione MG, Turrisi G, Savettieri G. Inferior altitudinal hemianopia associated with a tumor in the posterior fossa: report of a case. Ital J Neurol Sci 1984;5:89–91.
34. Miura M, Iijima N, Hayashida K, Kitazawa K, Ishii K, Ohara S. [Case of leptomeningeal carcinomatosis effectively treated with intrathecal chemotherapy using ventriculoperitoneal shunt]. Rinsho Shinkeigaku 2006;46:404–9.
35. Terry JB, Rosenberg RN. Frontal lobe ataxia. Surg Neurol 1995;44:583–8.
36. Forsyth PA, Shaw EG, Scheithauer BW, O'Fallon JR, Layton Jr DD, Katzmann JA. Supratentorial pilocytic astrocytomas. A clinicopathologic, prognostic, and flow cytometric study of 51 patients. Cancer 1993;72:1335–42.
37. Lebrun C, Fontaine D, Ramaioli A, et al. Long-term outcome of oligodendrogliomas. Neurology 2004;62:1783–7.
38. Olson JD, Riedel E, DeAngelis LM. Long-term outcome of low-grade oligodendroglioma and mixed glioma. Neurology 2000;54:1442–8.
39. van den Bent MJ, Looijenga LH, Langenberg K, et al. Chromosomal anomalies in oligodendroglial tumors are correlated with clinical features. Cancer 2003;97:1276–84.
40. Nishio S, Fukui M, Tateishi J. Brain stem gliomas: a clinicopathological analysis of 23 histologically proven cases. J Neurooncol 1988;6:245–50.
41. Maleci A, Cervoni L, Delfini R. Medulloblastoma in children and in adults: a comparative study. Acta Neurochir (Wien) 1992;119:62–7.
42. Bataille B, Delwail V, Menet E, et al. Primary intracerebral malignant lymphoma: report of 248 cases. J Neurosurg 2000;92:261–6.
43. Rohringer M, Sutherland GR, Louw DF, Sima AA. Incidence and clinicopathological features of meningioma. J Neurosurg 1989;71:665–72.
44. Rosenberg SI. Natural history of acoustic neuromas. Laryngoscope 2000;110:497–508.
45. Halle AA, Drewry RD, Robertson JT. Ocular manifestations of pituitary adenomas. South Med J 1983;76:732–5.
46. Hojo S, Hirano A. Pathology of Metastases Affecting the Central Nervous System. In: Takakura K, Sano K, Hojo S, Hirano A, editors. Metastatic tumors of the central nervous system. Tokyo-New York: Igaku-Shoin; 1982.
47. Posner JB, Chernik NL. Intracranial metastases from systemic cancer. Adv Neurol 1978;19:579–92.
48. Takakura K, Sano K. Clinical features of intracranial metastatic tumors. In: Takakura K, Sano K, Hojo S, Hirano A, editors. Metastatic tumors of the central nervous system. Tokyo-New York: Igaku-Shoin; 1982. p. 112–37.
49. Nayak L, Iwamoto FM, Abrey LE. Intracranial Dural Metastases. Neurology 2008;70(Suppl. 1): A160.
50. DeAngelis LM. Tumors of the central nervous system and intracranial hypertension and hypotension. In: Goldman L, Ausiello D, editors. Cecil Textbook of Medicine. 23rd ed Philadelphia: Saunders; 2008. p. 1437–49.

4

Advanced Imaging of Adult Brain Tumors with MRI and PET

GEOFFREY S. YOUNG • JAN STAUSS •
SRINIVASAN MUKUNDAN

Abstract

We briefly review the major advanced MRI techniques used in clinical brain tumor imaging: diffusion-weighted imaging (DWI), perfusion-weighted imaging (DSC PWI), dynamic contrast-enhanced T1 permeability imaging (DCE T1P), diffusion-tensor imaging (DTI), and MR spectroscopy and spectroscopic imaging (MRS and MRSI, respectively). These techniques provide information about tumor cellularity (DWI), white matter invasion (DTI), metabolic derangement including hypoxia and necrosis (MRS), neovascular capillary blood volume (DSC PWI), and permeability (DCE T1P). These techniques, when combined with conventional anatomical imaging (T2WI, FLAIR T2WI and delayed gadolinium [Gd] enhanced T1WI MRI) may improve diagnostic yield by providing insight into the underlying physiology described in previous chapters. Application of these techniques in clinical primary brain tumor diagnosis, grading, therapeutic planning, and monitoring of therapy are introduced, concentrating on high-grade malignant infiltrative glioma (HGG).

Introduction

As with conventional sequences, image contrast in the advanced MRI techniques is also derived from fundamental properties, such as spin density, T1, T2, T2,* and contrast enhancement of the underlying tissues. Thus, advanced techniques are also affected by the same artifacts as conventional pulse sequences; moreover, additional artifacts specific to the advanced acquisition and data processing are also seen. By subjecting the tissues to additional magnetic gradients and or radiofrequency pulses beyond what is typical for the fundamental pulse sequences, the signal emitted by the tissue is modulated, resulting in images with advanced tissue contrasts that are more reflective of relevant functional characteristics such as blood volume, permeability, hypercellularity, etc. Unfortunately, the price paid for this additional information is reduced signal-to-noise ratio and spatial resolution in comparison to the conventional anatomical images. For these reasons, it is critical that the neuroimager interpret information from advanced MRI sequences in the context of high-resolution conventional MR examination. Frequently, in fact, advanced sequences are co-registered to high-resolution conventional Gd enhanced T1WI with 1 mm or smaller voxel size to facilitate better interpretation.

Knowledge of the conventional morphological MRI and CT appearance of brain tumor forms an essential foundation for the interpretation of advanced imaging. Although it is beyond the scope of this chapter, it seems reasonable to bring to the reader's attention one recent morphologic imaging report that, pending prospective validation, suggests that in anaplastic astrocytoma an expansile growth pattern and lack of enhancement may predict longer survival.[1] In addition, this clinical introduction will not review the more than half-century-long literature on MR physics, engineering, and basic tissue physiology that has preceded the recent clinical application of these techniques. This background understanding is not essential for the neurologist, oncologist, or surgeon caring for brain tumor patients, but is critical for the neuroimaging researcher and practitioner. Numerous other advanced MRI techniques are excluded from this review because they have not yet achieved widespread clinical application. Finally, the reader is cautioned that the rapid progress of commercial MRI hardware, software, and clinical literature necessitates frequent reevaluation of the conclusions of this review.

Increasingly widespread research use of advanced brain imaging techniques in humans and animal models is making a great contribution to scientific understanding of brain tumor pathophysiology, to evaluation of new therapies, and in discovery of predictive markers that promise to assist in HGG phenotyping for personalization of therapy. These vital and exciting efforts, should not be confused with the clinical goals of advanced brain tumor imaging, which primarily focus on four issues that present significant challenges for conventional MRI:[2] (1) differentiation of primary infiltrative glioma from other primary brain tumors, metastatic tumors, strokes, infection, and tumefactive demyelination; (2) preoperative grading of primary glioma; (3) planning of biopsy, resection, and radiation therapy, including detection of tumor margin; (4) sensitive early detection of recurrence or progression in HGG, with distinction from radiation necrosis. In particular, in the last few years, the problem of detecting recurrence has become far more difficult because of the widespread use of temozolomide. This has increased both the incidence of postradiation enhancement mimicking progression (pseudoprogression) in approximately 20% of treated patients[3] and that of angiogenesis inhibitors. The latter appear to alter the pattern of recurrence and progression by decreasing enhancement without definitely prolonging survival.[4,5] Advanced MRI aims to address these challenges by characterizing and monitoring the four most important independent pathophysiologic attributes of each individual patient's brain tumor: (1) hypercellularity, (2) high invasiveness, (3) hypermetabolism, (4) hypervascularity. These four attributes are known as the "4-Hs." The pathophysiologic heterogeneity of brain tumors makes assessment of all 4-Hs crucial to a modern multiparametric brain tumor characterization. All HGGs have a least one of these attributes, and a few will have all four. Thus assessment of all 4-Hs is essential, at least at baseline.

Diffusion Weighted Imaging (DWI) of Cellularity

DWI image contrast is based on random thermal diffusion (Brownian motion) of water molecules in each voxel of brain tissue. In bulk water, the movement (diffusion) of a given water molecule is not constrained by boundaries, and the average diffusivity (diffusion per unit time) is proportional to the temperature. At higher temperatures, molecules have greater Brownian motion and therefore have greater diffusivity. In brain, the temperature is constant, and the distance water diffuses during a fixed time is mainly determined by physical constraints to water diffusion at the cellular and subcellular levels. Formally, diffusivity is determined by the fraction of tissue water in the intracellular compartment, where the tightly packed membranes of intracellular organelles hinders the free diffusion of water. In comparison, water in the extravascular extracellular space (EES) has a diffusivity (ADCe) that is an order of magnitude greater than the intracellular diffusivity (ADCi). Since the size of neurons is much smaller than the size of the DWI voxels, the average apparent diffusion coefficient (ADC) of each voxel is primarily influenced by the ratio of extracellular to intracellular water, referred to as the extracellular volume fraction (EVF) or local tissue "cellularity."[6,7] While

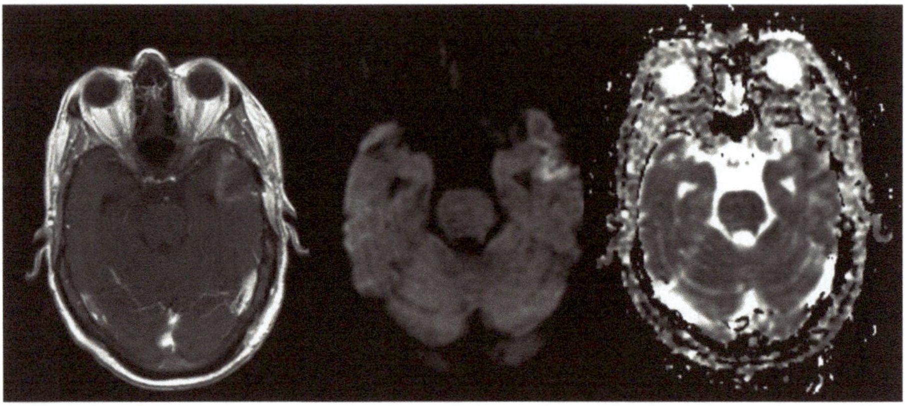

Figure 4-1 60-year-old man with treated gliosarcoma in the left temporal lobe. Hyperintensity in the left temporal lobe on the DWI (middle), confirmed by the ADC map (right) representing low diffusivity, suggests high cellular tumor, more marked than the degree of abnormal contrast enhancement (left).

this oversimplification of a very complex and technically heterogeneous literature may provoke controversy among imaging experts, it is generally accepted as a first approximation. See Figure 4-1.

CELLULARITY IN DIFFERENTIAL DIAGNOSIS

DWI can be crucial in helping to distinguish brain tumor from tumefactive non-neoplastic disorders. The use of DWI in ischemia is well known. This can be of significance in rare cases where mass-like presentations of embolic and vasculitic ischemia are difficult to distinguish from brain tumor.[8] In addition, sensitivity and specificity of over 90% are routinely achieved using DWI to distinguish the low ADC of epidermoid (due to the presence of sloughed epithelial cells, cholesterol, and keratin) from the high ADC of pure CSF-containing arachnoid cyst. Similar accuracy is achieved in distinguishing the low ADC of abscess, filled with white blood cells, from the high diffusivity of CSF-filled necrotic tumor cavities. A rim of low diffusivity at the periphery of a lesion may also be helpful in suggesting tumefactive demyelination.[9–12]

DWI can also be useful in preoperative differential diagnosis of brain tumors. In intra-axial tumors, low ADC suggests that lymphoma, medulloblastoma, or metastasis should be considered; the high cellularity of these lesions typically results in a much lower ADC than for HGG.[13,14] Similarly, low diffusivity in extra-axial masses suggests highly cellular meningioma or dural metastasis. Nevertheless, glioblastoma and gliosarcoma cannot be completely excluded; a small number are very cellular and present with a high ADC that overlaps with that of the other tumor types.[13,15–17] This illustrates the most important biological insight and, at the same time, the most important caution critical to responsible clinical use of advanced imaging: *because HGG genetics, pathophysiology, and imaging phenotypes are so diverse, no single image data subtype can reliably be interpreted in isolation from the other advanced imaging data, conventional imaging data, and clinical history.*

CELLULARITY IN TUMOR GRADING AND THERAPEUTIC PLANNING

A number of studies support the correlation of low minimum ADC (ADC_{min}) with high cellularity in tumors, including low-grade glioma, high-grade glioma, medulloblastoma, lymphoma, meningioma, and metastasis.[13,18–22] Lower ADC correlates with atypical and malignant pathologic subtypes of meningioma, but the ADC overlap between low and high grade populations is too great to allow reliable prediction of tumor pathology or behavior in individual patients.[21] In part, this seems likely to reflect the importance of vasogenic edema produced by vascular endothelial growth factor (VEGF) secretion and tissue invasion in determining meningioma behavior. Several groups have reported that ADC_{min} less than 1.7 to 2.5×10^{-3} mm^2/s within the cellular portion of glioma correlates with high grade.[23,24] ADC varies significantly within each grade, especially among HGG.[14,23,25–27] In addition to variation in cellularity, variation in the degree of necrosis, hemorrhage, and calcification likely contribute to this finding, as does variation in vascular permeability, related to angiogenesis and secretion of VEGF and other vasoactive paracrine factors. Although this variation reduces the likelihood that DWI alone can reliably predict histopathology, it suggests that ADC or other metrics derived from DWI may help in prediction of response to radiation.[28]

DWI MONITORING OF THERAPEUTIC RESPONSE

Detection of low ADC at the surgical resection margin on immediate postoperative imaging should suggest marginal ischemic necrosis rather than residual tumor.[29,30] While persistently low or decreasing ADC within the cavity or extra-axial space should suggest the possibility of pyogenic infection, the temporal evolution of postoperative hematoma and necrotic debris often produces a complex DWI and ADC appearance, so careful correlation with changes over time in the imaging studies and clinical presentation is essential.[31]

Beyond detection of these postoperative complications, low ADC offers an independent parameter for predicting malignancy and aggressive behavior in gliomas. In patients whose preoperative MRI demonstrates an atypical MRI pattern, low ADC evidence of high cellularity predicts aggressive clinical behavior and may, in some cases, be a better predictor than histopathology.[32] Although published thresholds vary, it has been shown that patients with minimum intratumoral ADC (minADC) less than 1.0×10^{-3} mm^2/s have a much worse prognosis than those with higher-ADC tumors.[33] Because EPI DWI-derived ADC estimates vary greatly with instrument, precise acquisition parameters, and postprocessing, investigations of normalized ADC ratios would seem to be indicated and, indeed, are beginning to be published.

In tumors with high baseline cellularity, such as highly cellular GBM or medulloblastoma, ADC may aid in early detection of treatment response to chemoradiation, as cellularity decreases in response to cytotoxic chemoradiation.[19,20,34–37] Because of interscan variation in ADC estimates, normalized ADC ratios (nADC) may prove more robust than absolute ADC measurements in separating radiation necrosis and pseudoprogression from recurrence after XRT. These measures are attracting increasing interest, since ADC in brain tumor seems relatively less affected by steroid use and angiogenesis inhibition than are enhancement, tumor edema, and permeability.[38] As suppression of enhancement by angiogenesis inhibition makes follow-up with conventional enhanced imaging less reliable, ADC may offer an

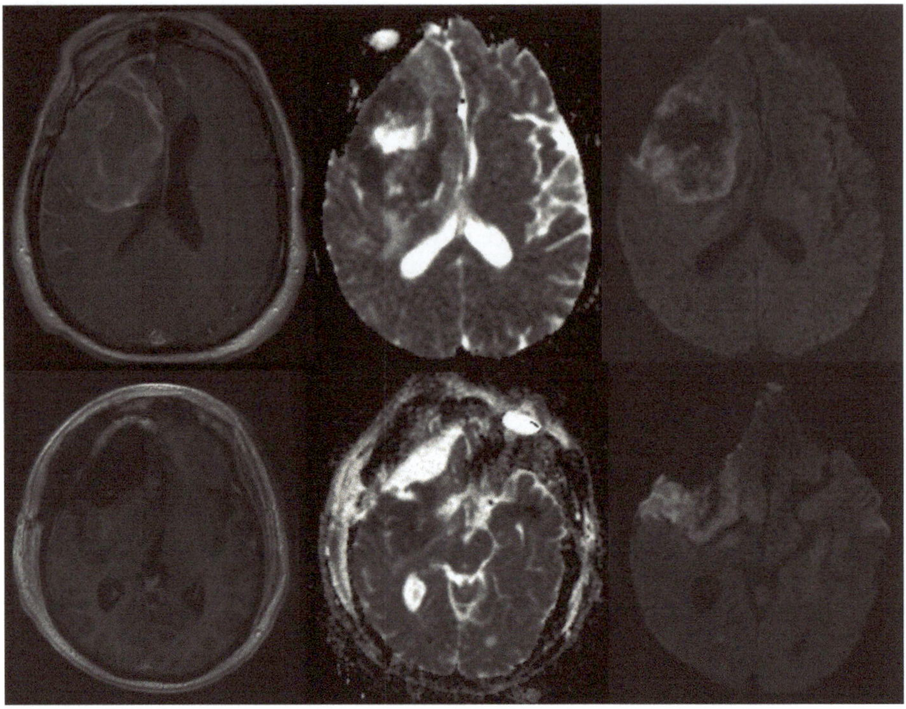

Figure 4-2 In a patient with GBM, the presurgery MRI (top row) shows very low diffusivity on ADC map (middle) and DWI (right), corresponding to abnormal gadolinium enhancement (left). While high doses of perioperative steroids decrease the permeability and eliminate contrast enhancement almost completely, they do not affect the cellularity, which is reflected by persistent reduced diffusivity as is seen on the postsurgical MRI (bottom row). This illustrates the utility of DWI in follow-up of patients on steroids and angiogenesis inhibitors, both of which strongly suppress permeability and enhancement.

important complement to blood volume imaging for longitudinal follow-up. This promise justifies ongoing development of higher b-value and multiple b-value echo-planar (EPI) sequences as well as non-EPI techniques to improve estimates of ADC, estimates of cell volume fraction. and longitudinal registration. "Functional diffusion mapping" is one investigational method of quantifying longitudinal change in ADC, among a number of such methods under study.[39,40] See Figure 4-2.

White Matter Invasion Assessment with Diffusion Tensor Imaging (DTI)

DWI, by imaging the motion of water in one to three spatial directions, acquires enough information to estimate the magnitude of random thermal diffusion. DTI acquires information in at least six directions, and completely defines a tensor (three-dimensional vector) describing both the magnitude and direction of water diffusion.[41,42] A large number of techniques that acquire many more diffusion directions to much more precisely define local water diffusion direction have been published under various names (q-ball imaging, diffusion spectrum imaging, etc.). Precise detection of the preferred direction of water diffusion is of interest in brain imaging because the myelinated axon bundles assist water diffusion along white matter tracts and prevent water diffusion across the tracts, a tissue property referred to as "anisotropy." The relative degree of white matter "diffusion anisotropy" in each voxel can be characterized by a number of derived scalar metrics comparing diffusivity in one direction with another, of which the most widely used is termed the fractional anisotropy (FA).

DTI TRACTOGRAPHY FOR SURGICAL GUIDANCE

Alternatively, the exact vector diffusion tensor can be depicted graphically in each voxel and the voxels connected to depict the mean fiber orientation in various major white matter tracts. A large number of algorithms for producing such "tractograms" have been published.

In conjunction with blood oxygen level dependent (BOLD) functional MRI (fMRI) depiction of sensorimotor, visual, and primary language cortical activation, DTI tractography have evolved into robust techniques for detecting the location of critical white matter tracts that are next to, displaced by, or invaded by tumor, allowing avoidance of operative injury to functional tracts and prediction of postoperative disability that may result from their transection.[43–47]

DTI Assessment of White Matter Invasion

Interest in imaging the white matter infiltrative component of HGG continues to increase because temozolomide chemoradiation and angiogenesis inhibition have been shown to alter the pattern of recurrence[4] by improving control of the enhancing solid component. FLAIR T2WI is very sensitive to the presence of vasogenic edema elicited by microscopic tumor invasion, but does not allow reliable distinction of direct tumor infiltration from peritumoral edema. A number of studies suggest that a decrease in FA or other DTI-derived measures of white matter anisotropy may be a marker for white matter disruption due to local glioma infiltration, as other causes of vasogenic edema would not be expected to actually disrupt white matter tracts. Observation of lower white matter anisotropy near to the high-grade tumor masses was encouraging; this remains an exciting research focus,[43] although one not yet ready for translation to clinical use. Reports of widely different results from groups employing different combinations of angular resolution, b-value, and signal-to-noise ratio (SNR) illustrate that acquisition and postprocessing techniques will need to mature before clinical trials demonstrating effective detection of the margins of WM invasion are likely to be successful.[27,48–54] Unfortunately, since no effective treatment for infiltrative tumor exists, biopsy of involved white matter is difficult to justify ethically. Many resections are performed with suction, which makes it difficult to track the origin of the tissue; also, no widespread robust method has been developed to correlate tissue with MRI on a millimeter scale. Therefore, human DTI translation research remains hampered by lack of a valid gold standard. A successful alternative strategy has been to use DTI to predict clinical outcome; classification of preoperative glioma margins as infiltrative or expansile by qualitative interpretation of DTI tractography correlates with survival.[55] See Figure 4-3.

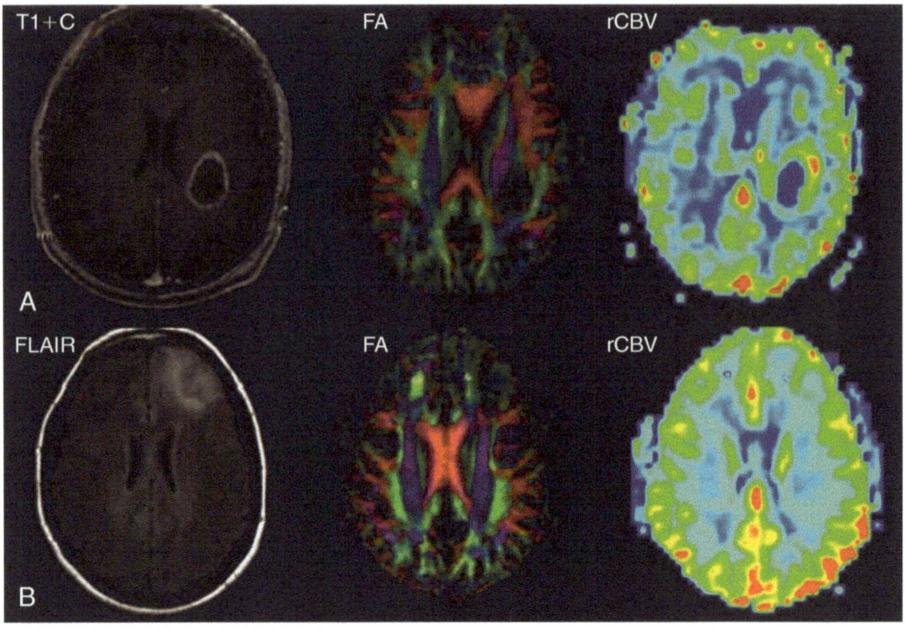

Figure 4-3 Post-Gd T1WI (top left) depicts a focal ring-enhancing glioma with peripheral high blood volume on the CBV map (top right). Although hypervascular, this glioma is expansile rather than infiltrative, as is seen on the tricolor FA map (top center). The infiltrative-appearing glioma on the FLAIR image (bottom left), in contrast, has low blood volume (bottom right), but while hypervascular, has an infiltrative pattern on the FA map (bottom center). (Figure courtesy Shuohui Yang, MD and X. Joe Zhou, PhD.)

Another strategy may be to try to demonstrate the efficacy of DTI-derived anisotropy, in combination with ADC, as an early indicator of response or potential survival in patients undergoing chemoradiation.[56] Such studies are ongoing using a large number of more sophisticated metrics of white matter coherence. These measures promise to achieve greater sensitivity and specificity by exploiting the tensor directional information from DTI and DSI more fully than simple FA.[48,51,57–59]

Spectroscopy of Tumor Metabolic Derangement

MR spectroscopy (MRS) and spectroscopic imaging (MRSI) essentially represent in vivo application of nuclear magnetic resonance (NMR). NMR revolutionized analytic chemistry in the 1940s by allowing chemists to nondestructively assay the chemical composition and bond structure of organic molecules. Differences in the spin density of the surrounding electron cloud produce a different degree of magnetic shielding at each chemically unique position in a molecule. This "chemical shift" alters the applied external magnetic field experienced by each proton in a molecule, causing it to precess at a slightly different frequency and emit a slightly different frequency of radio waves when excited. The radiofrequency is detected and plotted on a graph in which the x-axis displays the spectrum of frequencies emitted by the sample in parts per million (ppm) relative to a standard reference, and the y-axis displays the magnitude of each frequency in arbitrary units relative. The use of ppm rather than hertz (Hz) allows spectra acquired at different field strengths to be directly compared.[60,61] Different chemical compounds are identified in the spectrum ("assigned") by recognition of one or more peaks representing the resonance from distinct species of protons in that compound. The spectrum can be acquired from a single voxel (MRS), a two dimensional matrix of voxels from a single slice (2-D MRSI), or a rectangular three-dimensional matrix of voxels (3-D MRSI). MRSI data are sometimes displayed as color "metabolite maps" that give a qualitative impression of the anatomic distribution of the height, area, or ratio of height or area corresponding to important peaks or assigned compounds, but interpretation relies principally on inspection of the graphed spectra.

Although MRI and NMR are in principle the same, certain physical and practical limitations of clinical human MRS make it unlikely that human MRS will ever completely fulfill the high hopes that surrounded initial implementation over 20 years ago. These limitations include: much lower achievable field strength (3T vs. 20+T), much higher sample temperature (37° C vs. freezing in liquid nitrogen), much shorter tolerable scan times (less than 10 minutes vs. hours or days), rarity of MR detectable spin 1/2 nuclei other than protons ($^{1}H_{0}$) in human tissue, inability to perform heavy isotope labeling in vivo or centrifugally spin patients, and extremely complicated mixtures of metabolites in tissue. Nevertheless, progress has made MRS valuable for a number of important niche applications in clinical neuroimaging care and research.

The most important assigned peaks observed with 1.5 T to 3.0 T in vivo MRS of brain tumor patients are: branch chain amino acids produced by lysosomal catabolism in activated polymorphonuclear leukocytes (PMN) (AA: 0.9–1.0 ppm), lipid products of necrosis (Lip: 0.9–1.5 ppm), lactate from anaerobic glycolysis (Lac: 1.3 ppm), alanine (Ala: 1.5 ppm), n-acetyl aspartate associated with intact neuronal membranes (NAA: 2.0 ppm), choline released during cell membrane synthesis or degradation (Cho: 3.2 ppm), energy storage creatine compounds (Cr: 3.0 ppm and 3.9 ppm) and myoinositol (mI: 3.6 ppm). Lipid and lactate peaks represent a number of compounds with similar structures and so produce broad peaks, and creatine produces two easily detectable peaks corresponding to two chemically nonequivalent species of protons. AA and Lac can be differentiated from the overlapping broad Lip peak, when needed, by acquiring spectra at different TEs, since the protons forming these two peaks precess out of phase with the Lip, NAA, Cr, and Cho peaks. Analysis of these major assigned peaks in brain spectra can provide important information about pathophysiology but not etiology. Decreased NAA is seen with neuronal injury of any cause, and increased Cho with glial growth or injury of any cause; Lac appears with all causes of anaerobic glycolysis, and increased Lip and decreased Cr with all causes of necrosis.[62,63,64]

Spectroscopy in Differential Diagnosis

Elevated Cho and decreased NAA with variable occurrence of Lac and Lip represent the typical spectra seen in glioma, but identical abnormal spectra may be seen in ischemia, demyelination, infection, and other pathologies. For this reason, MRS is not generally useful in differential diagnosis of brain masses; however, it has been carefully studied in a number of niche applications, such as distinction of meningioma from dural metastasis and peripheral HGG. All three may have very high Cho, but because meningioma and metastases contain no neurons, the spectra demonstrate no detectable NAA. However, this signature is not definitive, since focal HGG may also contain no detectable NAA. The addition of Lac and Lip in this context favors HGG, but may also occur in metastasis. Similarly, the small ALA peak detected in 80% of meningioma spectra is found in roughly the same proportion of metastases and schwannomas.[65] Nevertheless, observation of very high ALA in the context of characteristic PWI, DWI, and basic imaging patterns may help to distinguish meningioma, peripheral GBM, gliosarcoma or other intra-axial tumors. Similarly, extensive clinical research has failed to support early hopes that MRS would help to distinguish tumor from tumefactive ischemia and demyelination.[66–69] As noted, the reason for this failure is that the principle peaks in MRS reflect pathophysiology rather than etiology: rapid breakdown of glial membranes in ischemia and demyelination releases as much choline as rapid membrane synthesis in HGG, neuronal injury reduces the NAA peak regardless of the cause, and Lac and Lip derived from anaerobic glycolysis and necrosis are common to many pathologies. Nevertheless, in adult neuroimaging there is one clinically useful application of MRS in differential diagnosis: distinction of bacterial, fungal, or parasitic abscesses from cystic necrosis due to tumor or radiation by detection of the AA peak specific for presence of activated PMNs.[10,70] See Figure 4-4.

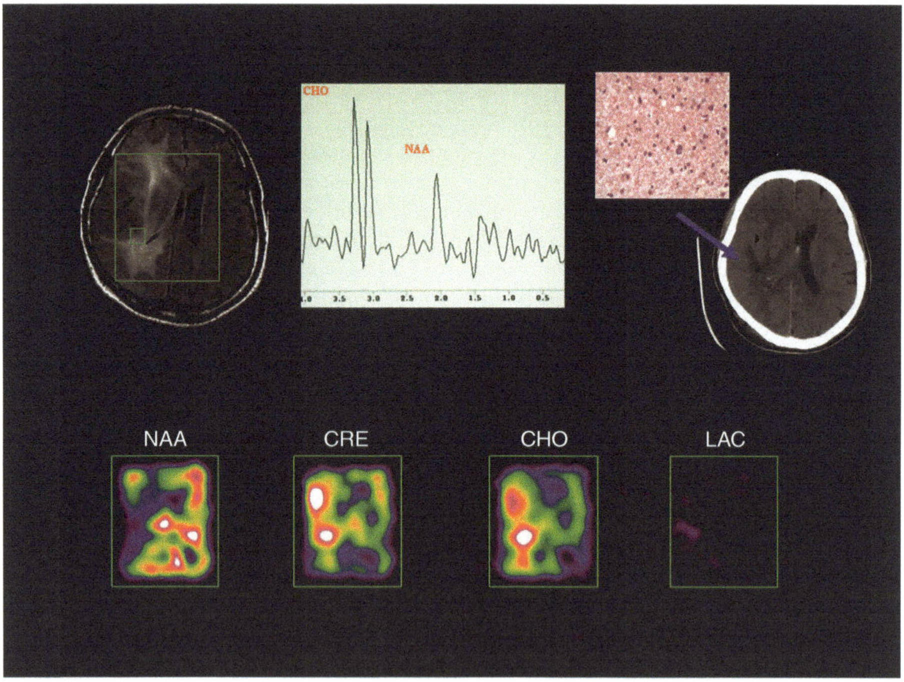

Figure 4-4 One voxel from a 2-D MRSI (top center) of infiltrative glioma seen on FLAIR image (top left) demonstrates an increased Cho/NAA ratio, suggesting increased membrane turnover and neuronal injury typical of low-grade glioma. The voxel displayed, selected based on the MRSI color maps of NAA, CR, Cho (bottom row), contains the highest Cho/NAA ratio and was selected as the target for biopsy (top right) in order to reduce the risk of undergrading.

Spectroscopy in Glioma Grading and Biopsy Guidance

In clinical practice, MRS can help to suggest the presence of high-grade tumor in areas where Cho/NAA peak height ratios (CNR) are greater than 1.5.[24,71,72–74] A number of derived semi-quantitative metrics, such as CNR R-values normalized to the contralateral white matter, can be helpful in accounting for anatomic and individual variation of these ratios. One important caution is that higher NAA/Cho ratios are more often found in grade III than in grade IV glioma. For this reason, detection of Lip and Lac evidence of necrosis and anaerobic metabolism in spectra of untreated glioma can add to suspicion of WHO grade IV tumor.[24,75] MRS is a particularly useful adjunct to PWI for preoperative grading of oligodendroglioma, since high blood volumes on PWI may be misleading.[76–79] Interpretation of MRS in the context of PWI and basic imaging characteristics is critical to avoiding this pitfall.

Targeting metabolically active tissue with high Cho/NAA ratios can decrease rates of "undergrading" and false negatives related to sampling error in biopsy of heterogeneous HGG.[80,81] These successes have motivated application of MRS to guide radiosurgery,[82–84] and suggest that wider utility may emerge as the automation, speed, resolution, and reproducibility of MRS gradually increases. Unfortunately, confirmation of the utility of MRS for guidance is hampered by the pathologic heterogeneity of HGG, the poor efficacy of current ablative therapies and the intractable problem of obtaining precise correlation with tissue samples.

More recent analyses have shown that whole brain ratios of NAA (WBNAA) may be decreased by up to 30%—far more than can be explained by focally detectable tumor.[85] This approach seems particularly timely since whole brain markers of infiltrative tumor burden are becoming a more significant contributor to patient mortality as control of focal recurrence improves. MRS assessment of CH_2/CH_3 ratios within the lipid spectrum of normal-appearing white matter may offer a complementary nonlocalized tumor burden assay.[86]

MRS in Posttreatment Monitoring

Differentiation of recurrent or progressive HGG from early radiation effect and chemoradiation necrosis remains difficult, especially because a mixture of both processes is present in many patients. Here again MRS may prove a valuable adjunct to PWI, although its efficacy remains unproven.[87] Since Lac and Lip are seen in both processes, observation of these peaks is not sufficient to exclude recurrence unless accompanied by absence of Cho and NAA peaks, or evidence of decreasing Cho over the course of MRSI follow-up. This is particularly convincing if corroborated by increasing ADC and decreasing CBV. Similarly, increasing Cho/NAA ratios over time are a sensitive sign for early tumor recurrence.[81,83,88–90] Interpreted in the context of other basic and advanced imaging data, technically meticulous serial MRSI has been shown to be valuable in early detection of tumor recurrence. Unfortunately, because voxel to voxel variation in Cho, NAA, Lac, and Lip at each time point is usually greater than the change in spectra over time, minute differences in technique can render longitudinal comparison invalid. Similarly, very significant errors in interpretation can result from slight errors in MRS or MRSI voxel positioning resulting in accidental inclusion of small amounts of fat from skull marrow; scalp; choroid plexus; dural ossification; magnetic susceptibility artifact from bone or metal; or CSF in ventricles.

For this reason, the groups that have been most successful in use of serial MRSI have found it essential to have a neuroimager expert in MRS supervise each acquisition, a requirement that, in combination with the long time required for MRS—typically 20-plus minutes per patient—and lack of insurance reimbursement, has made high-quality, reliable MRS unachievable in routine clinical care at many of the largest centers. Hopefully, progress in automation of MRSI acquisition may address these issues in future, but for the moment, MRSI remains the advanced imaging modality most subject to individual variation in resources and expertise.

Perfusion and Permeability Imaging of Tumor Microvessels

DSC PWI

Although rapid cell division, extensive white matter invasion, and disordered metabolism are important pathophysiologic attributes, the most important attributes of infiltrative glioma biology may be the cooption of existing brain capillaries and the development of neovascularization (and the biological switch between these two states). In particular, the genetic and humoral mechanisms by which HGG induces neovascularization are the target of intensive research and of imaging biomarker, molecular biomarker, and chemotherapeutic agent development.[91] Intermediate grade gliomas may produce varying degrees of upregulation of vascular growth factor/receptor signaling—including VEGF, PDGF, EGFR and IL-8 among others—and expression of AQP4 and other aquaporins that disrupt endothelial tight junctions. These factors act directly on existing brain capillaries to increase permeability of the blood-brain barrier (BBB), resulting in varying degrees of edema; they may produce mild contrast enhancement.[92] On the other hand, high density, morphologically abnormal, tortuous, high-density neocapillaries are seen nearly exclusively in HGG and often result in markedly elevated local cerebral capillary blood volume (CBV). Because the endothelia of these tumor vessels express very low levels of occludins and other normal cell surface proteins, lack normal pericyte and basal lamina support, and have disordered intercellular tight junctions and large gaps in the neovessel wall, their permeability both to small molecules and to the much larger Gd chelate contrast agents (Gd) is markedly increased.[93,94] This combination of abnormal blood volume and permeability is the basis of the oldest "advanced" tumor imaging method—delayed Gd-enhanced T1-weighted imaging. The degree of contrast enhancement reflects an admixture of CBV and permeability. In addition, it is strongly affected by contrast agent dose and imaging delay, making it a less reliable marker of tumor biology than semi-quantitative techniques for independently estimating CBV and permeability: dynamic susceptibility contrast (DSC) perfusion-weighted imaging (PWI) of CBV performed during the first pass of Gd, and DSC PWI dynamic contrast-enhanced (DCE) T1-weighted imaging of permeability (T1P) performed during the first 3 to 5 minutes of Gd recirculation.

First Pass Dynamic Susceptibility Contrast Perfusion Imaging (DSC PWI) of CBV

In DSC PWI a rapid intravenous power injection of Gd produces a concentrated bolus of paramagnetic Gd-infused blood that rapidly decreases tissue signal intensity during continuous fast susceptibility-weighted echoplanar (EPI) whole brain imaging. It should be understood that although Gd chelates are primarily described as T1 relaxation agents, at high concentration, such as during bolus administration, they are also very effective T2* agents. Thus, on first pass imaging in DSC PWI approaches, a time-intensity curve shows loss of signal during the wash-in phase, with recovery of signal demonstrated during wash-out. After estimation of Gd concentration from the dynamic time-intensity curve, the area under the Gd concentration curve during the bolus is computed. This area is proportional to the CBV and is thus referred to as relative CBV (rCBV); it is typically displayed as a color map in which the color of each pixel corresponds to the rCBV in arbitrary units (AU). Absolute quantitation is impractical because of the large number of variables that affect each image acquisition (injection rate, local contrast dose, contrast leakage, patient-MR coil coupling, radiofrequency preamplifier transmitter and receiver gain, etc.), so the measurements are typically normalized to the contralateral normal-appearing white matter (NAWM) producing a semi-quantitative normalized CBV (nCBV) ratio.[95,96] Clinical interpretation of CBV maps requires careful quality assurance of the dynamic data in each acquisition to ensure that patient motion, bolus concentration, bolus timing, signal-to-noise ratios, susceptibility artifacts, and partial volume averaging of vessels and cortex do not lead to false positive or false negative interpretation. This involves careful inspection of the source images and time-intensity curves (TIC), window-level adjustment, placement of regions of interest (ROI) for rCBV and nCBV calculation, and correlation with basic MRI images, as well as inspection of the color maps themselves. Visual inspection and correlation with prior anatomic knowledge and basic sequences are essential. Normal gray matter CBV is approximately 2.7 times higher than white matter; therefore, inclusion of gray matter in an ROI or nCBV calculation can result in false positive detection of hypervascular tumor.

DSC PWI Contribution to Differential Diagnosis

Like DWI and MRS, DSC PWI can aid in distinguishing necrotic hypervascular tumor from brain abscess by demonstrating high CBV in the tissue around the cystic cavity.[11] Because tumefactive demyelinating lesions, lymphoma, and many histologies of brain metastases have low blood volume on gradient-echo EPI (GE-EPI) DSC PWI, care must be taken to correlate with DWI and anatomical sequences.[97–99] In contrast, observation of nCBV > 1.8-2.0 can help confirm the presence of HGG, as high nCBV is not seen in lymphoma, tumefactive demyelination, or abscess (although some cases will fall into the intermediate range).[100] Further, although broad overlap between categories limits the clinical utility of these findings, nCBV is significantly higher in malignant than benign meningioma, and differs among histologic meningioma subtypes.[101,102] While high nCBV is detected relatively commonly in metastases when GE-EPI DSC PWI technique is used, SE-EPI technique can provide much greater specificity, probably because of its greater selectivity for microvascular blood volume.[103] Nevertheless, even GE-EPI PWI-derived nCBV has been shown to help differentiate dural metastasis from meningioma and parenchymal metastasis from HGG.[104]

In addition, attention to the shape of the upslope of the TIC in PWI can give a crude qualitative assessment of the degree of contrast leakage from the intravascular space across the BBB during first pass. Lesions with no BBB—generally those derived from nonglial precursors such as meningioma, metastasis, lymphoma, or choroid plexus papilloma/carcinoma—usually have a higher first-pass permeability than HGG, which generates microvessels with grossly impaired but not completely absent BBB. The TIC in an ROI placed inside one of these lesions will often show minimal or no recovery of signal intensity after the minimum point of the TIC, whereas normal brain shows nearly complete recovery of signal intensity to baseline, and HGG, an intermediate degree of recovery. This crude "first-pass permeability" estimate can provide a clue to the nature of some enhancing lesions.[14,105–107] When the differential diagnosis of a peripheral-enhancing tumor includes meningioma as well as HGG, or when the differential diagnosis of a periventricular tumor includes choroid plexus papillocarcinoma and GBM, attention to the TIC shape may help with differential diagnosis. See Figures 4-5 and 4-6.

Quantitative assessment of first pass leakage has also been investigated and a DSC PWI-based index of "relative recirculation" (rR) derived by estimating, with a gamma-variate curve, the shape of the curve that would be expected in a normal capillary bed with minimal recirculation and leakage, and subtracting this from the observed TIC. The hypothesis that rR in part reflects the degree of microvascular tortuosity in tumor microvessels is attractive but difficult to establish definitively, and so although rR has been demonstrated to correlate with tumor grade, it remains to be demonstrated that rR imaging provides significant hemodynamic or clinical information independent of better-established measures of CBV and permeability.[108,109]

Again, attention to DWI and conventional sequences can provide essential supportive evidence of high cellularity, location, and morphology. Likewise, when high nCBV is detected, attention to anatomical imaging morphology provides

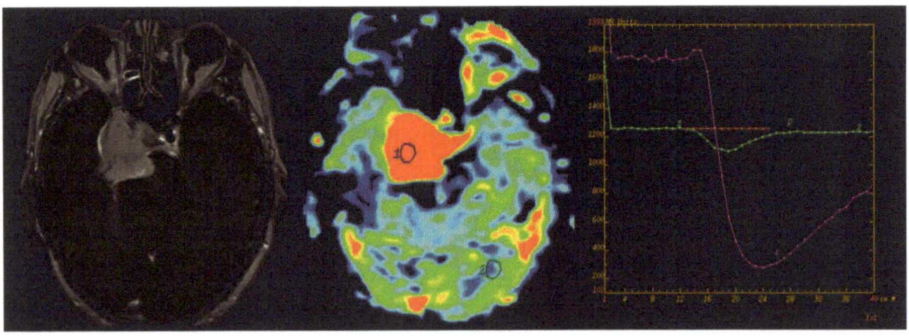

Figure 4-5 Large right suprasellar extra-axial lesion shows avid Gd enhancement (left). Relative cerebral blood volume map (middle) demonstrates very high CBV as compared to normal brain tissue. The purple time-intensity curve of the lesion (right) shows a characteristic low return to baseline, typical of meningioma because of the high first-pass permeability.

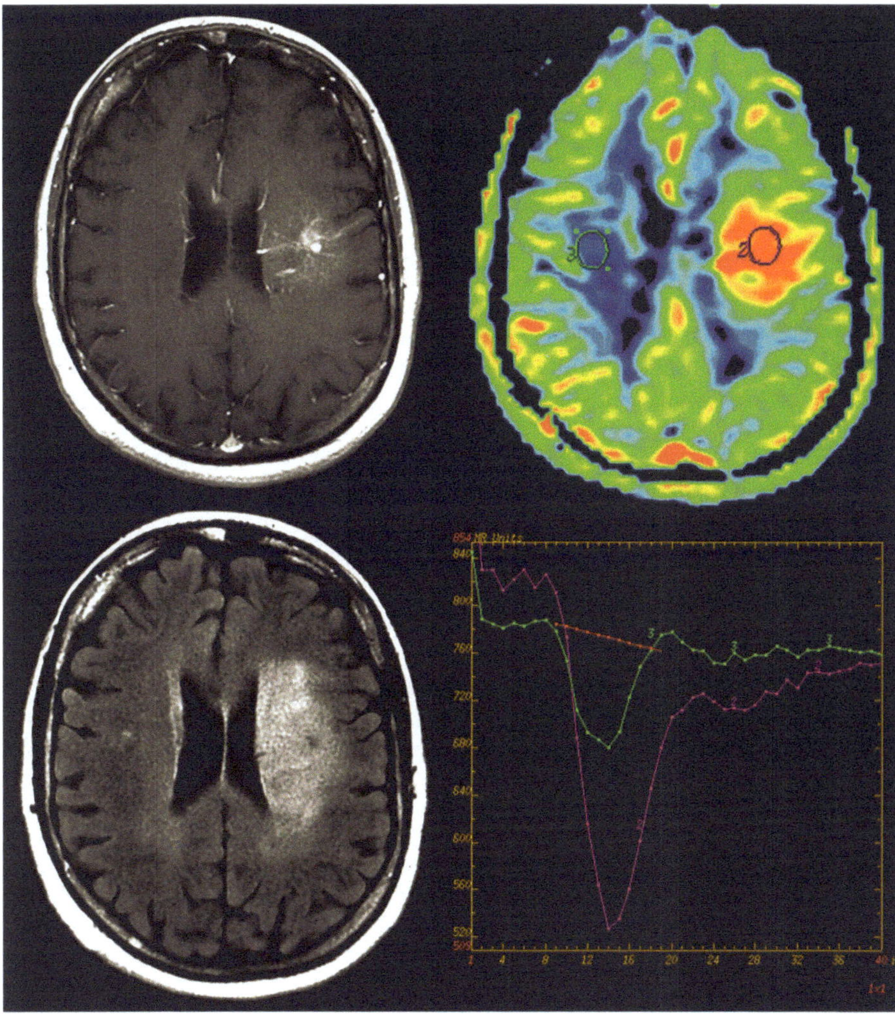

Figure 4-6 The large hyperintense lesion (FLAIR, bottom left), with multiple small central foci of enhancement (pGd T1WI, top left) in the left centrum semiovale, has very high relative blood volume (top right), strongly suggestive of a high-grade glioma. Purple time-intensity curve (bottom right) from an ROI selected in the tumor demonstrates more than 60% signal intensity recovery to baseline after the first pass, typical of a glial lesion with a BBB.

critical context for PWI interpretation. When a cortically based circumscribed tumor with little associated infiltration is detected, especially if it is coarsely calcified, oligodendroglioma and related low-grade primary brain tumors must be considered, as the "chicken-wire" neo-capillaries of oligodendroglioma have a much higher nCBV for a given grade than does infiltrative glioma.[76–79] For this reason, pending advances in clinical use of quantitative PWI, MRS remains important in grading of oligodendroglioma. Similarly, observation of high nCBV in a mural tumor nodule within a circumscribed cyst does not indicate high tumor grade, because histologically benign hemangioblastoma tumor nodules generally have nCBV greater than 6.0.[110] In contrast, as is expected for low-grade glioma, mural nodules in WHO grade I pilocytic astrocytoma have been reported to have nCBV less than 1.5.[111] Thus, DSC PWI promises to be able to differentiate between these lesions, despite the fact that both have high vascular permeability leading to indistinguishably avid Gd enhancement on conventional imaging and both show an enhancing mural nodule and tumor cyst morphology.[112]

DSC PWI in Infiltrative Astrocytoma: Preoperative Grading, Prognosis, Treatment Planning and Follow-up

Notwithstanding the caveat discussed above for tumors of other histologies, in astrocytoma, a maximum nCBV within the tumor (nCBVmax) is unequivocally and strongly correlated with histologic grade.[113–119] Areas of nCBVmax greater than 1.8 to 2.0 are strongly suggestive of foci of HGG and are an important target for biopsy, resection, or focal ablation.[119–121] Furthermore, nCBV has been shown to predict survival in HGG, with nCBV greater than 2.3 correlating with particularly poor outcome.[122]

In low-grade glioma, an nCBV threshold of 1.8 has been reported to be strongly predictive of survival.[123] The similarity of this threshold to published values for distinction of low and high grade tumor suggests the possibility that the effect could be due, at least in part, to identification of a subset of undergraded HGG. This is supported by the observation that increase in nCBV in LGG predicts high-grade transformation as much as a year before gadolinium enhancement.[124] Most recently, a retrospective analysis has extended this literature by suggesting that high nCBV with a similar threshold can be used to predict outcome independent of tumor grade.[125] Whether PWI nCBV is identifying a subset of LGG patients who are undergraded by standard histopathology because of surgical sampling error or revealing a limitation in the prognostic value of histopathology in LGG, there would seem to be an urgent need for formulation and validation of a combined histopathologic, molecular diagnostic, and advanced imaging-based prognostic sub-classification of glioma.

Use of DSC PWI during longitudinal follow-up to detect recurrence of HGG and distinguish it from chemoradiation effect is technically more challenging because of low spatial resolution, difficulties in longitudinal registration of EPI data, and susceptibility artifacts from blood products and metal that are often present in the postoperative setting. Nevertheless, increase in nCBV has been shown to predict recurrence in HGG following surgery and chemoradiation.[126] As might be expected, especially in the setting of high ADC, low nCBV appears to be a useful indicator that recurrent enhancement represents radiation effect rather than recurrent HGG.[36,127–129] Because nCBV correlates with angiogenesis, a decrease in nCBV during therapy may also offer a powerful marker of response to angiogenesis inhibition.[116,130] Because of the heterogeneity of HGG hypervascularity between and within patients, careful comparison of follow-up PWI to baseline pretherapy and posttherapy time points is critical.[120]

In addition, careful attention to DSC PWI technique and correlation with steroid and antiangiogenic agent dosing are critical for accurate interpretation. There is evidence from animal models that high-dose steroids decrease CBV as measured by GE-EPI DSC PWI by up to 30% to 50%, but either do *not* significantly affect, or at some doses may *increase* CBV as measured by SE-EPI DSC PWI.[38,131,132]

This difference reflects the greater selectivity of SE-EPI PWI technique for neocapillaries smaller than 10 microns in diameter as compared to GE-EPI PWI technique, which is sensitive both to neocapillaries and to small arterioles and venules larger than 25 microns in diameter. A variant of PWI that exploits this difference by using interleaved gradient echo (GE) and spin echo (SE) echoplanar (EPI) DSC PWI data to semi-quantitatively estimate the relative size and/or density of tumor neovessels has been shown to be clinically practical and to correlate with tumor grade, although at press time it is not yet available as FDA-approved software for clinical scanners.[133,134] Preliminary vessel-size imaging reports that both antiangiogenic and steroid therapy may decrease the average size of tumor microvessels, and preliminary reports from small-animal models suggesting equal or greater antiangiogenesis therapy change in nCBV estimated from SE-EPI DSC PWI nCBV suggest that vessel-size imaging and SE-EPI DSC nCBV may offer the most robust and promising surrogate markers for monitoring response to antiangiogenic therapy.[130] These issues are not yet fully resolved but merit discussion, as the unequivocal effect of increasingly widespread antiangiogenic therapy to suppress permeability makes traditional Gd-enhanced T1WI ever less reliable for tumor follow-up.[38,132,135] Intensive investigation of the effects of antiangiogenic therapy on the interdependent attributes of vessel size, CBV, and permeability in glioma in humans and animals will be required to clarify this critical issue.

Microvascular Permeability Imaging During Recirculation

Gliomas secrete angiogenic peptides and other factors that increase the permeability of the native brain capillary BBB to small molecules and electrolytes, resulting in vasogenic edema. GBM, in addition, induces formation of neovessels with large endothelial defects that allow virtually unimpeded passage of larger molecules including the "low molecular weight" Gd MR contrast agents. This leakage results in signal intensity enhancement on delayed T1-weighted images, which correlates roughly with increased permeability and imperfectly with tumor grade.[2] Increased permeability in neovessels is due to abnormal morphology with the presence of large fenestrations in neovascular walls. This mechanism is qualitatively different from that giving rise to increased permeability in co-opted native vessels, which is likely due to the secondary effects of VEGF, also known as vascular permeability factor (VPF). Thus, permeability is a rational marker for tumor grade. Dynamic contrast-enhanced (DCE) T1-weighted permeability (T1P) imaging represents the best-established method of assessing tumor vessel microstructure. T1-weighted images of the whole brain are acquired continuously for 3 to 5 minutes, starting just before arrival of the contrast bolus. In contrast to DSC PWI, in which a decrease in signal intensity on T2*WI due to the initial pass of concentrated intravascular Gd is used to assess MTT, CBF, and CBV, in T1P an increase in signal intensity on T1WI due to the leakage of Gd into the extravascular extracellular space during recirculation is used to assess the pharmacokinetics of BBB integrity. Although many metrics have been derived to characterize permeability, the most widely accepted is the intravascular to extravascular leakage transfer constant [K(trans)] calculated from the two-compartment modeling equation. This is derived from the slope of the T1P TIC, after exclusion of first pass effects and correction for T2* effects, flow, and venous concentration. Other methods and metrics that have been proposed in order to characterize Gd leakage during the first pass of the bolus, rather than the delayed phase, are beyond the scope of this discussion, as their physiologic significance and utility remains unclear. These include controversial estimates of Ktrans derived from DSC PWI data, and measures such as max dI/dt, rR, etc., derived from T1P data.[136–139]

Permeability for Tumor Grading and Follow-up

Increase in permeability metrics derived from careful application of established DCE T1P technique correlates well with higher tumor grade,[93,136,138–140] although not quite as well as Ncbv.[141,142] These two measures are independent[143] but strongly correlated,[144] probably due to the prominent contribution of high-volume highly leaky tumor neovessels to glioma biology. The optimal combination of T1P and PWI for HGG imaging remains to be determined, but inflammation, ischemia, corticosteroids, chemotherapeutic agents, and radiation seem to affect permeability more directly than blood volume. T1P has not achieved widespread clinical acceptance, despite good evidence of its utility in distinguishing necrosis from tumor recurrence,[137,140] because the technique requires longer acquisition time and more complicated postprocessing. As improvements in technique addresses both of these drawbacks, this may change in the years ahead.

Positron Emission Tomography in Brain Tumors

Positron emission tomography (PET) is based on the detection of annihilation photons (see Figure 4-7). An intravenously injected positron-emitting radiotracer

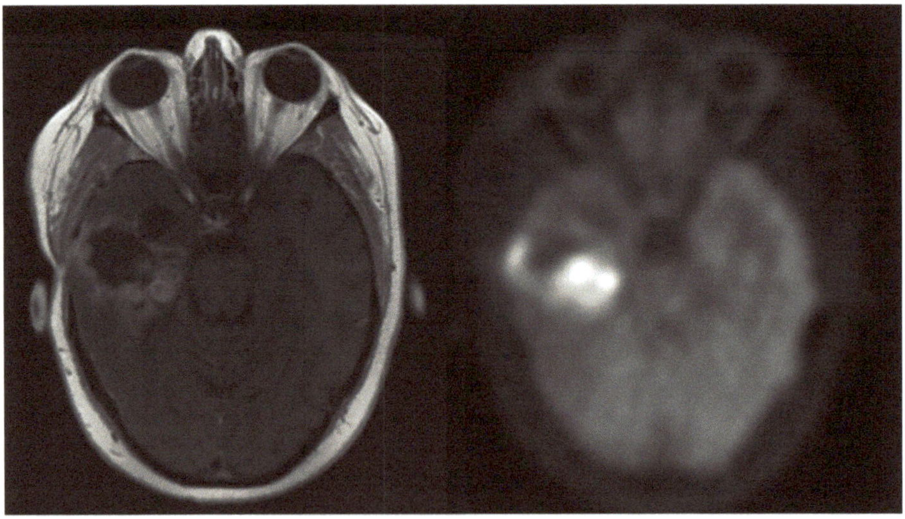

Figure 4-7 29-year-old woman with glioblastoma, status post surgery, radiation, and chemotherapy. PET demonstrates markedly increased FDG uptake (right figure) corresponding to nodular contrast enhancement on MR adjacent to the resection cavity (left figure). FDG uptake is much higher in intensity as compared to the background FDG uptake of normal gray matter, favoring recurrent disease over radiation necrosis.

distributes in the brain depending on its biochemical properties. The emitted positron combines with a negatively charged electron in tissue, resulting in two 511 keV annihilation photons. These two photons travel in opposite directions and are detected by two of multiple detector elements surrounding the patient. The origin of the annihilation event in the brain can be localized to the line between the two activated detectors, which allows the reconstruction of a three dimensional dataset reflecting the radionuclide concentration in individual brain voxels.

RADIOTRACERS

Several radiotracers have been investigated for brain tumor imaging, with the predominant focus being on glucose and amino acid tracers.

(18)F-fluorodeoxyglucose (FDG)

FDG is a glucose analogue that is actively transported across the blood-brain barrier (BBB) and phosphorylated within cells. FDG uptake reflects the tissue glucose metabolism and is usually high in high-grade tumors and relatively low in low-grade tumors. A significant drawback of FDG for brain tumor imaging is the high physiological FDG uptake of the brain (in particular of gray matter) resulting in a relatively low tumor-to-background ratio. FDG uptake of WHO II tumors is normally similar to that of white matter, while FDG uptake of WHO III and IV lesions is often less than or similar to that of gray matter.[145] FDG uptake is also seen in inflammatory processes, limiting the specificity of FDG for tumor imaging in certain cases.

Amino acid tracers

Amino acid tracers are an emerging alternative to FDG for brain tumor imaging. The more commonly used amino acid tracers for brain tumor imaging are ^{11}C-methionine (MET), ^{18}F-fluoroethyltyrosine (FET) and ^{18}F-fluorodihydroxyphenylalanine (DOPA). Cell uptake of amino acids occurs via carrier-mediated transport mechanisms, which are in general upregulated in malignant cells.[146,147] Background uptake of amino acids in normal brain tissue is generally low, resulting in better tumor-to-background contrast as compared to FDG.[148] MET has been more extensively investigated, but requires an on-site cyclotron because of the short half-life of ^{11}C (20 minutes). FET and DOPA are labeled with ^{18}F, which has a more favorable halftime of 110 minutes, and are likely to gain wider acceptance because of the lack of requirement for an on-site cyclotron.

Detection of recurrence

FDG is useful for detecting growing high-grade gliomas, but is insensitive for detection of low-grade tumor recurrence because of the often low tumor-to-background contrast.[149] Nevertheless, FDG can provide useful information when used in the surveillance of low-grade tumors, as a new finding of high FDG uptake in a known low-grade glioma that previously showed low FDG-avidity is strongly suggestive of anaplastic transformation and has prognostic value.[150]

Amino acid tracers are a promising means of detection of recurrent brain tumors, in particular for low-grade gliomas because of their higher uptake as compared to normal brain uptake. Amino acid tracer uptake of low-grade and high-grade glioma is generally very similar, and amino acid tracer cannot reliably differentiate low-grade from high-grade tumors. Chen and Silverman compared DOPA to FDG in 81 patients with various brain tumors and demonstrated the superiority of DOPA over FDG for imaging of low-grade tumors and recurrence evaluation, with sensitivity for DOPA of 98% and specificity of 86%.[151]

Differentiation of recurrence from treatment effects

A particularly challenging clinical question is the differentiation of tumor progression and/or recurrence from the benign changes that follow multi-modality treatment. PET has been considered a promising modality, overcoming the limited specificity of MRI for this distinction. The first study, including five patients, reported in 1982 that FDG PET was able to reliably distinguish between radiation necrosis and recurrent glioma.[152] Subsequent studies at first supported the accuracy of FDG.[153,154] More recent studies have been less favorable; the specificity of FDG was reported to be as low as 40% and comparable to the specificity of ^{201}Thallium-SPECT.[155] The low FDG specificity might be explained by FDG uptake in inflammatory cells in radiation necrosis. The importance of co-registering FDG images with MRI for more accurate interpretation has been emphasized.[156]

There has been hope that amino acid tracers might improve the specificity of PET in the differentiation of recurrence from treatment-related changes, based on the good tumor-to-background contrast and the assumption that amino acid tracer uptake is upregulated in neoplasm and to a much lesser degree in inflammatory processes. In a recent study, Terakawa et al. evaluated PET with MET in 77 patients with glioma or metastatic brain tumor and found a sensitivity and specificity of 75% for MET.[157] The false-positive cases showed high uptake of MET in necrotic tissue; previous reports have raised the concern that the value of MET is limited in cases of disrupted blood-brain barrier.[158]

Very promising results have been published for PET using FET in selected patients with MRI-based suspicion of glioma. A sensitivity of 92% and specificity of 100% have been reported, with that specificity being superior to conventional MRI.[159–161] A recently published prospective study that included 31 patients with glioma and suspicion for recurrence based on MRI and FET-PET found a positive predictive value of FET for recurrence of 84%.[162] The conclusion was made that the positive predictive value of FET-PET is high, but not quite high enough to replace stereotactic biopsy.

In short, FDG is particularly useful for imaging of high-grade glioma and detection of transformation of low-grade into high-grade glioma. Amino acid tracers appear more promising than FDG in the differentiation of tumor recurrence from treatment-related changes, at which task they may prove more specific than MRI. Amino acid tracers outperform FDG in the detection of low-grade tumors, but cannot reliably differentiate low-grade from high-grade glioma.

Summary

The past few years have seen an explosion in the ability of advanced MRI and PET techniques to directly image elements of brain tumor pathophysiology and genetics including the critical HGG attributes of hypercellularity, hypoxia, necrosis, white matter invasion, neoangiogenesis, and induced microvessel permeability. The pace of basic tumor imaging research continues to accelerate, and the advent of disease-altering chemotherapy is demanding clinical translation of advanced techniques. Even today, novel computer-assisted image analysis, data-reduction, and multiparametric classification systems are desperately needed to allow full exploitation of the imaging data explosion. The most important hindrance to widespread clinical translation and validation of these techniques is the fact that current advanced imaging sequences are EPI-based. EPI-based sequences suffer from susceptibility artifacts, low spatial resolution, and anatomic distortion that decrease reproducibility and require meticulous attention for valid reliable longitudinal and quantitative use. Furthermore, the most widely used and easily implemented method for quantitation—the hot spot method—is subject to well documented problems with reproducibility and bias. Nevertheless, as the use of these new techniques to differentiate between genetically-valid tumor subcategories and, especially, to predict prognosis and treatment response, is validated, a profound revision of the current brain tumor classification and treatment algorithms may be underway.[116,119,163,164] With careful correlation with basic imaging, multimodality physiologic brain tumor imaging can play an important complementary role to histopathology and molecular markers in guiding brain tumor diagnosis and therapy.

Acknowledgments

Shuohui Yang, MD and X. Joe Zhou, PhD for provision of figures, and Nicholas Young, BS for text editing.

REFERENCES

1. Moulding HD, Friedman DP, Curtis M, Kenyon L, Flanders AE, Paek SH, et al. Revisiting anaplastic astrocytomas I: an expansive growth pattern is associated with a better prognosis. J Magn Reson Imaging 2008;28(6):1311–21.
2. Ginsberg LE, Fuller GN, Hashmi M, et al. The significance of lack of MR contrast enhancement of supratentorial brain tumors in adults: histopathological evaluation of a series. Surg Neurol 1998;49(4):436–40.
3. Brandsma D, Stalpers L, Taal W, Sminia P, van den Bent MJ. Clinical features, mechanisms, and management of pseudoprogression in malignant gliomas. Lancet Oncol 2008;9(5):453–61. Review.
4. Norden AD, Young GS, Setayesh K, Muzikansky A, Klufas R, Ross GL, et al. Bevacizumab for recurrent malignant gliomas: efficacy, toxicity, and patterns of recurrence. Neurology 2008;70(10):779–87.
5. Dietrich J, Norden AD, Wen PY. Emerging antiangiogenic treatments for gliomas—efficacy and safety issues. Curr Opin Neurol 2008;21(6):736–44.
6. Provenzale J, Mukundan S, Barboriak DP. Diffusion-weighted and Perfusion MR Imaging for Brain Tumor Characterization and Assessment of Treatment Response. Radiology 2006; 239(3):632–49.

7. Mardor Y, Pfeffer R, Spiegelmann R, et al. Early detection of response to radiation therapy in patients with brain malignancies using conventional and high b-value diffusion-weighted magnetic resonance imaging. J Clin Oncol 2003;21:1094–100.
8. Molly ES, Calabrese LH. Tumor-like mass lesion (ML): an under-recognized presentation of primary angiitis of the central nervous system (PACNS). Arthritis Rheum 2006;54:486.
9. Reddy JS, Mishra AM, Behari S, et al. The role of diffusion-weighted imaging in the differential diagnosis of intracranial cystic mass lesions: a report of 147 lesions. Surg Neurol 2006;66(3):246–50.
10. Mishra AM, Gupta RK, Jaggi RS, et al. Role of diffusion-weighted imaging and in vivo proton magnetic resonance spectroscopy in the differential diagnosis of ring-enhancing intracranial cystic mass lesions. J Comput Assist Tomogr 2004;28(4):540–7.
11. Erdogan C, Hakyemez B, Yildirim N, et al. Brain abscess and cystic brain tumor: discrimination with dynamic susceptibility contrast perfusion-weighted MRI. J Comput Assist Tomogr 2005;29(5):663–7.
12. Tsui EY, Leung WH, Chan JH, et al. Tumefactive demyelinating lesions by combined perfusion-weighted and diffusion weighted imaging. Comput Med Imaging Graph 2002;26(5):343–6.
13. Guo AC, Cummings TJ, Dash RC, et al. Lymphomas and high-grade astrocytomas: comparison of water diffusibility and histologic characteristics. Radiology 2002;224:177–83.
14. Calli C, Kitis O, Yunten N, et al. Perfusion and diffusion MR imaging in enhancing malignant cerebral tumors. Eur J Radiol 2006;58(3):394–403.
15. Okamoto K, Ito J, Ishikawa K, et al. Diffusion-weighted echo-planar MR imaging in differential diagnosis of brain tumors and tumor-like conditions. Eur Radiol 2000;10:1342–50.
16. Toh CH, Chen YL, Hsieh TC, et al. Glioblastoma multiforme with diffusion-weighted magnetic resonance imaging characteristics mimicking primary lymphoma. Case report. J Neurosurg 2006;105:132–5.
17. Krabbe K, Gideon P, Wagn P, et al. MR diffusion imaging of human intracranial tumours. Neuroradiology 1997;39(7):483–9.
18. Kotsenas AL, Roth TC, Manness WK, et al. Abnormal diffusion-weighted MRI in medulloblastoma: does it reflect small cell histology? Pediatr Radiol 1999;29(7):524–6.
19. Chenevert TL, Stegman LD, Taylor JM, et al. Diffusion magnetic resonance imaging: an early surrogate marker of therapeutic efficacy in brain tumors. J Natl Cancer Inst 2000;92(24):2029–36.
20. Chenevert TL, McKeever PE, Ross BD. Monitoring early response of experimental brain tumors to therapy using diffusion magnetic resonance imaging. Clin Cancer Res 1997;3(9):1457–66.
21. Filippi CG, Edgar MA, Ulug AM, et al. Appearance of meningiomas on diffusion-weighted images: correlating diffusion constants with histopathologic findings. AJNR Am J Neuroradiol 2001;22(1):65–72.
22. Hayashida Y, Hirai T, Morishita S, et al. Diffusion-weighted imaging of metastatic brain tumors: comparison with histologic type and tumor cellularity. AJNR Am J Neuroradiol 2006;27(7):1419–25.
23. Sugahara T, Korogi Y, Kochi M, et al. Usefulness of diffusion-weighted MRI with echo-planar technique in the evaluation of cellularity in gliomas. J Magn Reson Imaging 1999;9:53–60.
24. Catalaa I, Henry R, Dillon WP, et al. Perfusion, diffusion and spectroscopy values in newly diagnosed cerebral gliomas. NMR Biomed 2006;19(4):463–75.
25. Yang D, Korogi Y, Sugahara T, et al. Cerebral gliomas: prospective comparison of multivoxel 2D chemical-shift imaging proton MR spectroscopy, echoplanar perfusion and diffusion-weighted MRI. Neuroradiology 2002;44:656–66.
26. Bulakbasi N, Kocaoglu M, Ors F, et al. Combination of single-voxel proton MR spectroscopy and apparent diffusion coefficient calculation in the evaluation of common brain tumors. *AJNR* Am J Neuroradiol 2003;24:225–33.
27. Castillo M, Smith JK, Kwock L, et al. Apparent diffusion coefficients in the evaluation of high-grade cerebral gliomas. AJNR Am J Neuroradiol 2001;22:60–4.
28. Mardor Y, Roth Y, Ochershvilli A, et al. Pretreatment prediction of brain tumors' response to radiation therapy using high b-value diffusion-weighted MRI. Neoplasia 2004;6(2):136–42.
29. Khan RB, Gutin PH, Rai SN, et al. Use of diffusion weighted magnetic resonance imaging in predicting early postoperative outcome of new neurological deficits after brain tumor resection. Neurosurgery 2006;59(1):60–6.
30. Smith JS, Cha S, Mayo MC, McDermott MW, Parsa AT, Chang SM, et al. Serial diffusion-weighted magnetic resonance imaging in cases of glioma: distinguishing tumor recurrence from postresection injury. J Neurosurg 2005;103(3):428–38.
31. Schaefer PW, Grant PE, Gonzalez RG. Diffusion-weighted MR imaging of the brain. Radiology 2000;217:331–45.

32. Baehring JM, Bi WL, Bannykh S, Piepmeier JM, Fulbright RK. Diffusion MRI in the early diagnosis of malignant glioma. J Neurooncol 2007;82(2):221–5.
33. Murakami R, Sugahara T, Nakamura H, Hirai T, Kitajima M, Hayashida Y, et al. Malignant supratentorial astrocytoma treated with postoperative radiation therapy: prognostic value of pretreatment quantitative diffusion-weighted MR imaging. Radiology 2007;243(2):493–9.
34. Hein PA, Eskey CJ, Dunn JF, et al. Diffusion-weighted imaging in the follow-up of treated high-grade gliomas: tumor recurrence versus radiation injury. AJNR Am J Neuroradiol 2004;25:201–9.
35. Chan YL, Yeung DK, Leung SF, et al. Diffusion-weighted magnetic resonance imaging in radiation-induced cerebral necrosis. Apparent diffusion coefficient in lesion components. J Comput Assist Tomogr 2003;27(5):674–80.
36. Tsui EY, Chan JH, Ramsey RG, et al. Late temporal lobe necrosis in patients with nasopharyngeal carcinoma: evaluation with combined multi-section diffusion weighted and perfusion weighted MR imaging. Eur J Radiol 2001;39(3):133–8.
37. Schubert MI, Wilke M, Müller-Weihrich S, Auer DP. Diffusion-weighted magnetic resonance imaging of treatment-associated changes in recurrent and residual medulloblastoma: preliminary observations in three children. Acta Radiol 2006;47(10):1100–4.
38. Bastin ME, Carpenter TK, Armitage PA, et al. Effects of dexamethasone on cerebral perfusion and water diffusion in patients with high-grade glioma. AJNR Am J Neuroradiol 2006;27(2):402–8.
39. Moffat BA, Chenevert TL, Lawrence TS, et al. Functional diffusion map: a noninvasive MRI biomarker for early stratification of clinical brain tumor response. Proc Natl Acad Sci U S A 2005;102(15):5524–9.
40. Hamstra DA, Chenevert TL, Moffat BA, et al. Evaluation of the functional diffusion map as an early biomarker of time-to-progression and overall survival in high-grade glioma. Proc Natl Acad Sci U S A 2005;102(46):16759–64.
41. Inoue T, Ogasawara K, Beppu T, et al. Diffusion tensor imaging for preoperative evaluation of tumor grade in gliomas. Clin Neurol Neurosurg 2005;107(3):174–80.
42. Field AS, Wu YC, Alexander AL. Principal diffusion direction in peritumoral fiber tracts: Color map patterns and directional statistics. Ann N Y Acad Sci 2005;1064:193–201.
43. Goebell E, Fiehler J, Ding XQ, et al. Disarrangement of fiber tracts and decline of neuronal density correlate in glioma patients—a combined diffusion tensor imaging and 1H-MR spectroscopy study. AJNR Am J Neuroradiol 2006;27(7):1426–31.
44. Yu CS, Li KC, Xuan Y, et al. Diffusion tensor tractography in patients with cerebral tumors: a helpful technique for neurosurgical planning and postoperative assessment. Eur J Radiol 2005;56(2):197–204.
45. Nimsky C, Grummich P, Sorensen AG, et al. Visualization of the pyramidal tract in glioma surgery by integrating diffusion tensor imaging in functional neuronavigation. Zentralbl Neurochir 2005;66(3):133–41.
46. Lazar M, Alexander AL, Thottakara PJ, et al. White matter reorganization after surgical resection of brain tumors and vascular malformations. AJNR Am J Neuroradiol 2006;27(6):1258–71.
47. Schonberg T, Pianka P, Hendler T, et al. Characterization of displaced white matter by brain tumors using combined DTI and fMRI. Neuroimage 2006;30(4):1100–11.
48. Provenzale JM, McGraw P, Mhatre P, et al. Peritumoral brain regions in gliomas and meningiomas: investigation with isotropic diffusion-weighted MR imaging and diffusion-tensor MR imaging. Radiology 2004;232(2):451–60.
49. Price SJ, Burnet NG, Donovan T, et al. Diffusion tensor imaging of brain tumours at 3 T: a potential tool for assessing white matter tract invasion? Clin Radiol 2003;58:455–62.
50. Lu S, Ahn D, Johnson G, et al. Peritumoral diffusion tensor imaging of highgrade gliomas and metastatic brain tumors. AJNR Am J Neuroradiol 2003;24:937–41.
51. Lu S, Ahn D, Johnson G, et al. Diffusion-tensor MR imaging of intracranial neoplasia and associated peritumoral edema: introduction of the tumor infiltration index. Radiology 2004;232(1):221–8.
52. Chiang IC, Kuo YT, Lu CY, et al. Distinction between high-grade gliomas and solitary metastases using peritumoral 3-T magnetic resonance spectroscopy, diffusion, and perfusion imagings. Neuroradiology 2004;46:619–27.
53. Kono K, Inoue Y, Nakayama K, et al. The role of diffusion-weighted imaging in patients with brain tumors. AJNR Am J Neuroradiol 2001;22:1081–8.
54. Stadnik TW, Chaskis C, Michotte A, et al. Diffusion-weighted MR imaging of intracerebral masses: comparison with conventional MR imaging and histologic findings. AJNR Am J Neuroradiol 2001;22:969–76.
55. Guan X, Lai S, Lackey J, Shi J, Techavipoo U, Moulding HD, et al. Revisiting anaplastic astrocytomas II: further characterization of an expansive growth pattern with visually enhanced diffusion tensor imaging. J Magn Reson Imaging 2008;28(6):1322–36.

56. Sundgren PC, Fan X, Weybright P, et al. Differentiation of recurrent brain tumor versus radiation injury using diffusion tensor imaging in patients with new contrast-enhancing lesions. Magn Reson Imaging 2006;24(9):1131–42.
57. Stieltjes B, Schluter M, Didinger B, et al. Diffusion tensor imaging in primary brain tumors: reproducible quantitative analysis of corpus callosum infiltration and contralateral involvement using a probabilistic mixture model. Neuroimage 2006;31(2):531–42.
58. Zhou XJ, Leeds NE, Kumar AJ, et al. Differentiation of Tumor Recurrence from Treatment-Induced Necrosis Using Quantitative Diffusion MRI. Proceedings ISMRM. 2001. p. 726.
59. van Westen D, Latt J, Englund E, et al. Tumor extension in high-grade gliomas assessed with diffusion magnetic resonance imaging: values and lesion-to-brain ratios of apparent diffusion coefficient and fractional anisotropy. Acta Radiol 2006;47(3):311–9.
60. Marshall I, Wardlaw J, Cannon J, et al. Reproducibility of metabolite peak areas in 1H MRS of brain. Magn Reson Imaging 1996;14(3):281–92.
61. Calvar JA. Accurate (1)H tumor spectra quantification from acquisitions without water suppression. Magn Reson Imaging 2006;24(9):1271–9.
62. Birken DL, Oldendorf WH. N-acetyl-L-aspartic acid: a literature review of a compound prominent in 1H-NMR spectroscopic studies of brain. Neurosci Biobehav Rev 1989;13(1):23–31.
63. Moffett JR, Ross B, Arun P, et al. N-Acetylaspartate in the CNS: From neurodiagnostics to neurobiology. Prog Neurobiol 2007;81(2):89–131.
64. Wyss M, Kaddurah-Daouk R. Creatine and creatinine metabolism. Physiol Rev 2000; 80(3):1107–213.
65. Cho YD, Choi GH, Lee SP, et al. (1)H-MRS metabolic patterns for distinguishing between meningiomas and other brain tumors. Magn Reson Imaging 2003;21(6):663–72.
66. Gajewicz W, Papierz W, Szymczak W, et al. The use of proton MRS in the differential diagnosis of brain tumors and tumor like processes. Med Sci Monit 2003;9(9):MT97–105.
67. Preul MC, Caramanos Z, Collins DL, et al. Accurate, noninvasive diagnosis of human brain tumors by using proton magnetic resonance spectroscopy. Nat Med 1996;2:323–5.
68. Del Sole A, Falini A, Ravasi L, et al. Anatomical and biochemical investigation of primary brain tumours review.. Eur J Nucl Med 2001;28(12):1851–72.
69. Delorme S, Weber MA. Applications of MRS in the evaluation of focal malignant brain lesions. Cancer Imaging 2006;22(6):95–9.
70. Lai PH, Ho JT, Chen WL, et al. Brain abscess and necrotic brain tumor: discrimination with proton MR spectroscopy and diffusion-weighted imaging. AJNR Am J Neuroradiol 2002;23(8):1369–77.
71. Devos A, Lukas L, Suykens JA, et al. Classification of brain tumours using short echo time 1H MR spectra. J Magn Reson 2004;170:164–75.
72. Law M, Yang S, Wang H, et al. Glioma grading: sensitivity, specificity, and predictive values of perfusion MR imaging and proton MR spectroscopic imaging compared with conventional MR imaging. AJNR Am J Neuroradiol 2003;24(10):1989–98.
73. Fayed N, Morales H, Modrego PJ, et al. Contrast/Noise ratio on conventional MRI and choline/creatine ratio on proton MRI spectroscopy accurately discriminate low-grade from high-grade cerebral gliomas. Acad Radiol 2006;13(6):728–37.
74. Chen J, Huang SL, Li T, et al. In vivo research in astrocytoma cell proliferation with 1H-magnetic resonance spectroscopy: correlation with histopathology and immunohistochemistry. Neuroradiology 2006;48(5):312–8.
75. Li X, Vigneron DB, Cha S, et al. Relationship of MR-derived lactate, mobile lipids, and relative blood volume for gliomas in vivo. AJNR Am J Neuroradiol 2005;26(4):760–9.
76. Jenkinson MD, Smith TS, Joyce K, et al. MRS of oligodendroglial tumors: correlation with histopathology and genetic subtypes. Neurology 2005;64(12):2085–9.
77. White ML, Zhang Y, Kirby P, Ryken TC. Can tumor contrast enhancement be used as a criterion for differentiating tumor grades of oligodendrogliomas? Am J Neuroradiol 2005;26:784–90.
78. Lev MH, Ozsunar Y, Henson JW, et al. Glial tumor grading and outcome prediction using dynamic spin-echo MR susceptibility mapping compared with conventional contrast-enhanced MR: confounding effect of elevated rCBV of oligodendrogliomoas [sic]. Am J Neuroradiol 2004;25:214–21.
79. Xu M, See SJ, Ng WH, et al. Comparison of magnetic resonance spectroscopy and perfusion-weighted imaging in presurgical grading of oligodendroglial tumors. Neurosurgery 2005;56:919–24.
80. Gajewicz W, Grzelak P, Gorska-Chrzastek M, et al. The usefulness of fused MRI and SPECT images for the voxel positioning in proton magnetic resonance spectroscopy and planning the biopsy of brain tumors: presentation of the method. Neurol Neurochir Pol 2006;40(4):284–90.

81. Hall WA, Martin A, Liu H, et al. Improving diagnostic yield in brain biopsy: coupling spectroscopic targeting with real-time needle placement. J Magn Reson Imaging 2001;13(1):12–5.
82. Payne GS, Leach MO. Applications of magnetic resonance spectroscopy in radiotherapy treatment planning. Br J Radiol 2006;79(Special Issue 1):S16–S26.
83. Graves EE, Nelson SJ, Vigneron DB, et al. A preliminary study of the prognostic value of 1H-spectroscopy in gamma knife radiosurgery of recurrent malignant gliomas. Neurosurgery (Baltimore) 2000;46:319–28.
84. Graves EE, Pirzkall A, Nelson SJ, et al. Registration of magnetic resonance spectroscopic imaging to computed tomography for radiotherapy treatment planning. Med Phys 2001; 28:2489–96.
85. Cohen BA, Knopp EA, Rusinek H, et al. Assessing global invasion of newly diagnosed glial tumors with whole-brain proton MR spectroscopy. AJNR Am J Neuroradiol 2005;26(9):2170–7.
86. Matulewicz L, Sokol M, Wydmanski J, et al. Could lipid CH2/CH3 analysis by in vivo 1H MRS help in differentiation of tumor recurrence and post-radiation effects? Folia Neuropathol 2006;44(2):116–24.
87. Chernov M, Hayashi M, Izawa M, et al. Differentiation of the radiation-induced necrosis and tumor recurrence after gamma knife radiosurgery for brain metastases: importance of multi-voxel proton MRS. Minim Invasive Neurosurg 2005;48(4):228–34.
88. Graves EE, Nelson SJ, Vigneron DB, et al. Serial proton MR spectroscopic imaging of recurrent malignant gliomas after gamma knife radiosurgery. AJNR 2001;2:613–24.
89. Plotkin M, Eisenacher J, Bruhn H, et al. 123I-IMT SPECT and 1H MR-spectroscopy at 3.0T in the differential diagnosis of recurrent or residual gliomas: a comparative study. J Neurooncol 2004;70(1):49–58.
90. Hollingworth W, Medina LS, Lenkinski RE, et al. A systematic literature review of magnetic resonance spectroscopy for the characterization of brain tumors. AJNR Am J Neuroradiol 2006;27(7):1404–11 Review.
91. Kaur B, Tan C, Brat DJ, et al. Genetic and hypoxic regulation of angiogenesis in gliomas. J Neurooncol 2004;70(2):229–43. Review.
92. Manoonkitiwongsa PS, Schultz RL, Whitter EF, et al. Contraindications of VEGF-based therapeutic angiogenesis: effects on macrophage density and histology of normal and ischemic brains. Vascul Pharmacol 2006;44(5):316–25.
93. Liebner S, Fischmann A, Rascher G, et al. Claudin-1 and claudin-5 expression and tight junction morphology are altered in blood vessels of human glioblastoma multiforme. Acta Neuropathol (Berl) 2000;100(3):323–31.
94. Davies DC. Blood-brain barrier breakdown in septic encephalopathy and brain tumours. J Anat 2002;200(6):639–46. Review.
95. Nakagawa T, Tanaka R, Takeuchi S, et al. Haemodynamic evaluation of cerebral gliomas using XeCT. Acta Neurochir (Wien) 1998;140(3):223–33.
96. Muizelaar JP, Fatouros PP, Schroder ML. A new method for quantitative regional cerebral blood volume measurements using computed tomography. Stroke 1997;28(10):1998–2005.
97. Essig M, Waschkies M, Wenz F, et al. Assessment of brain metastases with dynamic susceptibility-weighted contrast-enhanced MR imaging: initial results. Radiology 2003;228(1):193–9.
98. Kremer S, Grand S, Berger F, et al. Dynamic contrast-enhanced MRI: differentiating melanoma and renal carcinoma metastases from high-grade astrocytomas and other metastases. Neuroradiology 2003;45(1):44–9.
99. Kremer S, Grand S, Remy C, et al. Contribution of dynamic contrast MR imaging to the differentiation between dural metastasis and meningioma. Neuroradiology 2004;46(8):642–8.
100. Cha S, Pierce S, Knopp EA, Johnson G, Yang C, Ton A, et al. Dynamic contrast-enhanced T2*-weighted MR imaging of tumefactive demyelinating lesions. AJNR Am J Neuroradiol 2001;22(6):1109–16.
101. Zhang H, Rödiger LA, Shen T, Miao J, Oudkerk M. Perfusion MR imaging for differentiation of benign and malignant meningiomas. Neuroradiology 2008;50(6):525–30.
102. Zhang H, Rödiger LA, Shen T, Miao J, Oudkerk M. Preoperative subtyping of meningiomas by perfusion MR imaging. Neuroradiology 2008;50(10):835–40.
103. Young GS, Setayesh K. Spin-Echo Echo-Planar Perfusion MR Imaging in the Differential Diagnosis of Solitary Enhancing Brain Lesions: Distinguishing Solitary Metastases from Primary Glioma. AJNR Am J Neuroradiol 2008.
104. Kremer S, Grand S, Rémy C, Pasquier B, Benabid AL, Bracard S, et al. Contribution of dynamic contrast MR imaging to the differentiation between dural metastasis and meningioma. Neuroradiology 2004;46(8):642–8.

105. Yang S, Law M, Zagzag D. Dynamic contrast-enhanced perfusion MR imaging measurements of endothelial permeability: differentiation between atypical and typical meningiomas. AJNR Am J Neuroradiol 2003;24:1554–9.
106. Hartmann M, Heiland S, Harting I, et al. Distinguishing of primary cerebral lymphoma from high-grade gliomas with perfusion-weighted magnetic resonance imaging. Neurosci Lett 2003; 338:119–22.
107. Rollin N, Guyotat J, Streichenberger N, et al. Clinical relevance of diffusion and perfusion magnetic resonance imaging in assessing intra-axial brain tumors. Neuroradiology 2006;48(3):150–9.
108. Kassner A, Annesley DJ, Zhu XP, et al. Abnormalities of the contrast re-circulation phase in cerebral tumors demonstrated using dynamic susceptibility contrast-enhanced imaging: a possible marker of vascular tortuosity. J Magn Reson Imaging 2000;11:103–13.
109. Jackson A, Kassner A, Zhu XP, Li KL. Reproducibility of T2* blood volume and vascular tortuosity maps in cerebral gliomas. J Magn Reson Imaging 2001;14:510–6.
110. Neuroradiology 2007;49(7):5. Hakyemez B, Erdogan C, Bolca N, Yildirim N, Gokalp G, Parlak M. Evaluation of different cerebral mass lesions by perfusion-weighted MR imaging. *J Magn Reson Imaging* 2006 Oct;24(4):817–24
111. Grand SD, Kremer S, Tropres IM, Hoffmann DM, Chabardes SJ, Lefournier V, et al. Perfusion-sensitive MRI of pilocytic astrocytomas: initial results. Neuroradiology 2007;49(7):545–50.
112. Bing F, Kremer S, Lamalle L, Chabardes S, Ashraf A, Pasquier B, et al. Value of perfusion MRI in the study of pilocytic astrocytoma and hemangioblastoma: Preliminary findings. J Neuroradiol 2008; Oct 17—Abstract only (Article in French).
113. Hakyemez B, Erdogan C, Ercan I, et al. High-grade and low-grade gliomas: differentiation by using perfusion MR imaging. Clin Radiol 2005;60(4):493–502.
114. Knopp EA, Cha S, Johnson G, et al. Glial neoplasms: dynamic contrast-enhanced T2*-weighted MR imaging. Radiology 1999;211:791–8.
115. Sugahara T, Korogi Y, Kochi M, et al. Correlation of MR imaging-determined cerebral blood volume maps with histologic and angiographic determination of vascularity of gliomas. AJR Am J Roentgenol 1998;171:1479–86.
116. Maia AC, Malheiros SM, da Rocha AJ, et al. MR cerebral blood volume maps correlated with vascular endothelial growth factor expression and tumor grade in nonenhancing gliomas. AJNR Am J Neuroradiol 2005;26(4):777–83.
117. Shin JH, Lee HK, Kwun BD, et al. Using relative cerebral blood flow and volume to evaluate the histopathologic grade of cerebral gliomas: preliminary results. AJR Am J Roentgenol 2002;179(3):783–9.
118. Aronen HJ, Gazit IE, Louis DN, et al. Cerebral blood volume maps of gliomas: comparison with tumor grade and histologic findings. Radiology 1994;191(1):41–51.
119. Chaskis C, Stadnik T, Michotte A, et al. Prognostic value of perfusion-weighted imaging in brain glioma: a prospective study. Acta Neurochir (Wien) 2006;148(3):277–85; comment 285.
120. Lupo JM, Cha S, Chang SM, et al. Dynamic susceptibility-weighted perfusion imaging of high-grade gliomas: characterization of spatial heterogeneity. AJNR Am J Neuroradiol 2005;26(6):1446–54.
121. Maia AC, Malheiros SM, da Rocha AJ, et al. Stereotactic biopsy guidance in adults with supratentorial nonenhancing gliomas: role of perfusion-weighted magnetic resonance imaging. J Neurosurg 2004;101(6):970–6.
122. Hirai T, Murakami R, Nakamura H, Kitajima M, Fukuoka H, Sasao A, et al. Prognostic value of perfusion MR imaging of high-grade astrocytomas: long-term follow-up study. AJNR Am J Neuroradiol 2008;29(8):1505–10.
123. Law M, Oh S, Babb JS, Wang E, Inglese M, Zagzag D, et al. Low-grade gliomas: dynamic susceptibility-weighted contrast-enhanced perfusion MR imaging—prediction of patient clinical response. Radiology 2006;238(2):658–67.
124. Danchaivijitr N, Waldman AD, Tozer DJ, Benton CE, Brasil Caseiras G, Tofts PS, et al. Low-grade gliomas: do changes in rCBV measurements at longitudinal perfusion-weighted MR imaging predict malignant transformation? Radiology 2008;247(1):170–8.
125. Law M, Young RJ, Babb JS, Peccerelli N, Chheang S, Gruber ML, et al. Gliomas: predicting time to progression or survival with cerebral blood volume measurements at dynamic susceptibility-weighted contrast-enhanced perfusion MR imaging. Radiology 2008;247(2):490–8.
126. Cha S, Knopp EA, Johnson G, et al. Dynamic contrast-enhanced T2-weighted MR imaging of recurrent malignant gliomas treated with thalidomide and carboplatin. AJNR Am J Neuroradiol 2000;21:881–90.
127. Tsui EY, Chan JH, Leung TW, et al. Radionecrosis of the temporal lobe: dynamic susceptibility contrast MRI. Neuroradiology 2000;42(2):149–52.

128. Siegal T, Rubinstein R, Tzuk-Shina T, et al. Utility of relative cerebral blood volume mapping derived from perfusion magnetic resonance imaging in the routine follow up of brain tumors. J Neurosurg 1997;86(1):22–7.
129. Sugahara T, Korogi Y, Tomiguchi S, et al. Posttherapeutic intraaxial brain tumor: the value of perfusion-sensitive contrast-enhanced MR imaging for differentiating tumor recurrence from nonneoplastic contrast-enhancing tissue. AJNR Am J Neuroradiol 2000;21(5):901–9.
130. Quarles CC, Schmainda KM. Assessment of the morphological and functional effects of the anti-angiogenic agent SU11657 on 9 L gliosarcoma vasculature using dynamic susceptibility contrast MRI. Magn Reson Med 2007;57(4):680–7.
131. Badruddoja MA, Krouwer HG, Rand SD, Rebro KJ, Pathak AP. Schmainda KM. Antiangiogenic effects of dexamethasone in 9 L gliosarcoma assessed by MRI cerebral blood volume maps. Neuro Oncol 2003;5(4):235–43.
132. Wilkinson ID, Jellineck DA, Levy D, et al. Dexamethasone and enhancing solitary cerebral mass lesions: alterations in perfusion and blood-tumor barrier kinetics shown by magnetic resonance imaging. Neurosurgery 2006;58(4):640–6.
133. Schmainda KM, Rand SD, Joseph AM, Lund R, Ward BD, Pathak AP, et al. Characterization of a first-pass gradient-echo spin-echo method to predict brain tumor grade and angiogenesis. AJNR Am J Neuroradiol 2004;25(9):1524–32.
134. Kiselev VG, Strecker R, Ziyeh S, Speck O, Hennig J. Vessel size imaging in humans. Magn Reson Med 2005;53(3):553–63. .Jensen JH, Lu H, Inglese M. Microvessel density estimation in the human brain by means of dynamic contrast-enhanced echo-planar imaging. *J Magn Reson Med.* 2006 Nov;56(5):1145–50.
135. Ostergaard L, Hochberg FH, Rabinov JD, et al. Early changes measured by magnetic resonance imaging in cerebral blood flow, blood volume, and blood-brain barrier permeability following dexamethasone treatment in patients with brain tumors. J Neurosurg 1999;90(2):300–5.
136. Roberts HC, Roberts TP, Ley S, et al. Quantitative estimation of microvascular permeability in human brain tumors: correlation of dynamic Gd-DTPA-enhanced MR imaging with histopathologic grading. Acad Radiol 2002;9(1, Suppl 1):S151–5.
137. Hazle JD, Jackson EF, Schomer DF, et al. Dynamic imaging of intracranial lesions using fast spin-echo imaging: differentiation of brain tumors and treatment effects. J Magn Reson Imaging 1997;7(6):1084–93.
138. Uematsu H, Maeda M, Sadato N, et al. Vascular permeability: quantitative measurement with double-echo dynamic MR imaging-theory and clinical application. Radiology 2000;214:912–7.
139. Roberts HC, Roberts TPL, Brasch RC, et al. Quantitative measurement of microvascular permeability in human brain tumors achieved using dynamic contrast-enhanced MR imaging: correlation with histologic grade. AJNR Am J Neuroradiol 2000;21:891–9.
140. Provenzale JM, Wang GR, Brenner T, et al. Comparison of permeability in high-grade and low-grade brain tumors using dynamic susceptibility contrast MR imaging. AJR Am J Roentgenol 2002;178:711–6.
141. Law M, Yang S, Babb JS, et al. Comparison of cerebral blood volume and vascular permeability from dynamic susceptibility contrast enhanced perfusion MR imaging with glioma grade. AJNR Am J Neuroradiol 2003;25:746–55.
142. Law M, Young R, Babb J, et al. Comparing perfusion metrics obtained from a single compartment versus pharmacokinetic modeling methods using dynamic susceptibility contrast-enhanced perfusion MR imaging with glioma grade. AJNR Am J Neuroradiol 2006;27(9):1975–82.
143. Jackson A, Kassner A, Annesley-Williams D, et al. Abnormalities in the recirculation phase of contrast agent bolus passage in cerebral gliomas: comparison with relative blood volume and tumor grade. AJNR Am J Neuroradiol 2002;23(1):7–14.
144. Provenzale JM, York G, Moya MG, et al. Correlation of relative permeability and relative cerebral blood volume in high-grade cerebral neoplasms. AJR Am J Roentgenol 2006;187(4):1036–42.
145. Chen W, Silverman DH. Advances in Evaluation of Primary Brain Tumors. Semin Nucl Med 2008;38(4):240–50.
146. Isselbacher KJ. Sugar and amino acid transport by cells in culture: differences between normal and malignant cells. N Engl J Med 1972;286:929–33.
147. Busch H, Davis JR, Honig GR, Anderson DC, Nair PV, Nyhan WL. The uptake of a variety of amino acids into nuclear proteins of tumors and other tissues. Cancer Res 1959;19:1030–9.
148. Jager PL, Vaalburg W, Pruim J, de Vries EG, Langen KJ, Piers DA. Radiolabeled amino acids: basic aspects and clinical applications in oncology. J Nucl Med 2001;42(3):432–45.
149. Chen W, Silverman DH. Advances in Evaluation of Primary Brain Tumors. Semin Nucl Med 2008;38(4):240–50.

150. De Witte O, Levivier M, Violon P, et al. Prognostic value of positron emission tomography with 18F. Fluoro-2-D-glucose in the low-grade glioma. J Neurosurg 1996;39:470–7.
151. Chen W, Silverman DHS, Delaloye S, et al. 18F-FDOPA PET imaging of brain tumors: Comparison study with 18F-FDG PET and evaluation of diagnostic accuracy. J Nucl Med 2006;47:904–11.
152. Patronas NJ, Di Chiro G, Brooks RA, DeLaPaz RL, Kornblith PL, Smith BH, et al. Work in progress: [18F] fluorodeoxyglucose and positron emission tomography in the evaluation of radiation necrosis of the brain. Radiology 1982;144(4):885–9.
153. Kim EE, Chung SK, Haynie TP, Kim CG, Cho BJ, Podoloff DA, et al. Differentiation of residual or recurrent tumors from post-treatment changes with F-18 FDG PET. Radiographics 1992;12(2):269–79.
154. Di Chiro G, Oldfield E, Wright DC, De Michele D, Katz DA, Patronas NJ, et al. Cerebral necrosis after radiotherapy and/or intraarterial chemotherapy for brain tumors: PET and neuropathologic studies. AJR Am J Roentgenol 1988;150(1):189–97.
155. Kahn D, Follett KA, Bushnell DL, Nathan MA, Piper JG, Madsen M, et al. Diagnosis of recurrent brain tumor: value of 201Tl SPECT vs 18F-fluorodeoxyglucose PET. AJR Am J Roentgenol 1994;163(6):1459–65.
156. Chao ST, Suh JH, Raja S, Lee SY, Barnett G. The sensitivity and specificity of FDG PET in distinguishing recurrent brain tumor from radionecrosis in patients treated with stereotactic radiosurgery. Int J Cancer 2001;96(3):191–7.
157. Terakawa Y, Tsuyuguchi N, Iwai Y, Yamanaka K, Higashiyama S, Takami T, et al. Diagnostic accuracy of 11C-methionine PET for differentiation of recurrent brain tumors from radiation necrosis after radiotherapy. J Nucl Med 2008;49(5):694–9.
158. Roelcke U, Radü EW, von Ammon K, Hausmann O, Maguire RP, Leenders KL. Alteration of blood-brain barrier in human brain tumors: comparison of [18F] fluorodeoxyglucose, [11C] methionine and rubidium-82 using PET. J Neurol Sci 1995;132(1):20–7.
159. Pöpperl G, Gotz C, Rachinger W, et al. Value of O-(2-[18F] fluoroethyl)-L-tyrosine PET for the diagnosis of recurrent glioma. Eur J Nucl Med Mol Imaging 2004;31:1464–70.
160. Pöpperl G, Götz C, Rachinger W, Schnell O, Gildehaus FJ, Tonn JC, et al. Serial O-(2-[(18)F] fluoroethyl)-L-tyrosine PET for monitoring the effects of intracavitary radioimmunotherapy in patients with malignant glioma. Eur J Nucl Med Mol Imaging 2006;33(7):792–800.
161. Rachinger W, Goetz C, Popperl G, et al. Positron emission tomography with O-(2-[18F] fluoroethyl)-L-tyrosine versus magnetic resonance imaging in the diagnosis of recurrent gliomas. Neurosurgery 2005;57:505–11.
162. Mehrkens JH, Pöpperl G, Rachinger W, Herms J, Seelos K, Tatsch K, et al. The positive predictive value of O-(2-[18F] fluoroethyl)-L-tyrosine (FET) PET in the diagnosis of a glioma recurrence after multimodal treatment. J Neurooncol 2008;88(1):27–35.
163. Preusser M, Haberler C, Hainfellner JA. Malignant glioma: neuropathology and neurobiology. Wien Med Wochenschr 2006;156(11–12):332–7. Review.
164. Law M, Oh S, Babb JS, et al. Low-grade gliomas: dynamic susceptibility-weighted contrast-enhanced perfusion MR imaging—prediction of patient clinical response. Radiology 2006;238(2):658–67.

5 Malignant Gliomas in Adults

ANDREW D. NORDEN • JAN DRAPPATZ • PATRICK Y. WEN

Introduction

Malignant gliomas (MG) account for more than 75% of the approximately 20,500 newly diagnosed malignant primary brain tumors in the United States each year.[1] They represent the most common type of malignant primary brain tumor in adults. More than half of MGs are glioblastomas (GBM), the most aggressive subtype. The majority of the remainder include anaplastic astrocytomas (AA), anaplastic oligodendrogliomas (AO), and anaplastic oligoastrocytomas (AOA).[1,2] Other MG subtypes are rare. Glioblastoma is a disease of middle age, with a median age at diagnosis of 64 years. Anaplastic gliomas (AG) affect a younger adult population with a median age of 45 years.[1,3] Despite being relatively uncommon, MGs are incurable and are responsible for a disproportionate share of cancer-related morbidity and mortality.[4] With optimal treatment, median survival is only 12 to 15 months for GBM and 2 to 5 years for AG. Established adverse prognostic factors in MG include increasing age, GBM histology, poor performance status, and unresectable tumor.[5] Recently, there have been important advances in the molecular pathogenesis of MG, some of which may provide additional prognostic information that will help in therapeutic decision-making.[6–12] This chapter summarizes the pathology, pathogenesis, diagnosis, and management of adult MGs with a focus on therapy and recent therapeutic advances. This topic has been recently reviewed elsewhere.[4,13]

Epidemiology

The only established risk factors for MG are exposure to ionizing radiation and rare familial syndromes such as neurofibromatosis types 1 and 2, Li-Fraumeni syndrome, and Turcot syndrome.[3,14] Approximately 5% of patients with malignant gliomas have a family history of gliomas. The genetic basis for most of these tumors is unknown. An international consortium, GLIOGENE, has been established to study the genetic basis of familial gliomas.[15] Exposures to various carcinogens, infections such as cytomegalovirus, diet, elevated IgE, electromagnetic radiation, and cellular phones have not been conclusively linked to MG risk.[3] Malignant glioma epidemiology is reviewed in detail elsewhere in this volume.

Pathology

MGs are infiltrative tumors with a presumptive glial cell of origin. The World Health Organization (WHO) classification scheme defines four histologic grades for astrocytomas. These include grade I (pilocytic astrocytoma), grade II (diffuse astrocytoma), grade III (AA), and grade IV (GBM).[2] Grade I tumors occur primarily in children. Grade II tumors are considered low-grade gliomas, while grade III and IV tumors are MGs. Typical histologic features of AAs include hypercellularity, nuclear atypia, and mitoses. The presence of microvascular proliferation and/or necrosis often indicates progression to GBM. Oligodendrogliomas are classified as well-differentiated oligodendrogliomas (grade II) or AOs (grade III). Mixed tumors, or oligoastrocytomas, are also classified as well-differentiated (grade II) or AOA (grade III). Tumors with oligodendroglial components may have distinctive features such as perinuclear clearing, giving rise to a "fried-egg" appearance, and a reticular pattern of blood vessel growth.

Molecular Pathogenesis

Recent studies have begun to elucidate the molecular pathogenesis of MGs.[10–12,16] Such information may help to improve tumor classification and prognostication.[8,9,17–19] As has been observed for many cancers, increasing malignancy in glial tumors is associated with an accumulation of genetic abnormalities that results in impairment of cell cycle control, DNA repair, and signaling.[12,20] On the basis of differences in molecular pathogenesis and natural history, GBMs are often classified as primary or secondary tumors (Figure 5-1).[12,20] Primary GBMs arise de novo in older patients, and have a characteristic molecular genetic profile that includes epidermal growth factor receptor (*EGFR*) amplification and mutations, loss of heterozygosity (LOH) of chromosome 10q, phosphatase and tensin homolog deleted on chromosome 10 (*PTEN*) mutations, and p16 deletion. Secondary GBMs are much rarer, evolve from lower-grade gliomas, and typically occur in younger patients.

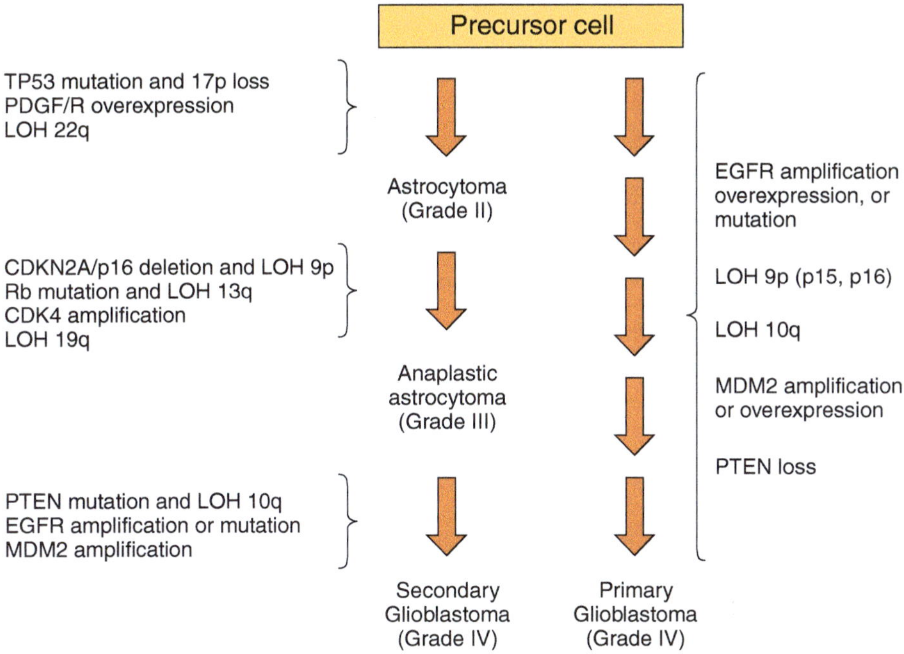

Figure 5-1 Molecular genetic changes associated with glioma progression. Abbreviations: *CDK,* cyclin-dependent kinase; *EGFR,* epidermal growth factor receptor; *LOH,* loss of heterozygosity; *MDM2,* murine double minute 2; *PDGF/R,* platelet-derived growth factor/receptor; *PTEN,* phosphate and tensin homolog deleted on chromosome 10; *Rb,* retinoblastoma. (Adapted from Wen PY, Kesari S, Drappatz J. Expert Rev Anticancer Ther 2006;6:733–54.)

Typical genetic abnormalities include *TP53* mutations,[21] platelet-derived growth factor (PDGFR) overexpression, abnormalities in the p16/retinoblastoma (Rb) pathway, and LOH 10q.[12,22] These tumors may also have mutations of the isocitrate dehydrogenase gene.[23] None of these features allow for definitive GBM classification. Primary and secondary GBMs cannot be distinguished histologically and have not been shown to respond differentially to treatment.

Abnormalities in EGFR signaling are common in MGs.[12] EGFR amplification and overexpression are observed in about 40% of primary GBMs. EGFRvIII is a constitutively active EGFR mutant that is expressed by approximately 30% of GBMs, and represents a potentially important therapeutic target because of its exclusive expression by tumor cells.[12,18] Activating mutations in the extracellular domain of the EGFR are also present in a subset of GBMs.[24] Activation of the PDGFR promotes tumor growth as well, and MGs frequently coexpress PDGF and PDGFR.[12] Signaling through these and other growth factor receptors activates fundamental signal transduction pathways such as the Ras/mitogen-activated protein kinase (MAP-kinase) pathway and the phosphoinositide 3′-kinase (PI3K)/Akt/mammalian target of rapamycin (mTOR) pathway, both of which promote cell proliferation.[12] PTEN is an endogenous inhibitor of PI3K signaling that is mutated or lost in up to 50% of GBMs.[12,25] Downstream targets of these growth factor signaling pathways activate transcriptional programs for cell survival, proliferation, and invasion. Additionally, many of these pathways serve to upregulate vascular endothelial growth factor (VEGF) and angiogenesis, which has an emerging pathogenic role in MGs that is discussed in greater detail below.[26,27]

For cancer in general and MG specifically, there is growing interest in "personalized medicine," which refers to the effort to individualize therapy based on a particular tumor's molecular genetic profile.[7,9] Examples of molecular predictors with probable therapeutic value are chromosomes 1p/19q, the loss of which may confer chemosensitivity in oligodendroglial tumors,[28–30] and *MGMT* promoter methylation, which may predict temozolomide sensitivity in GBM.[8,31] Advances in gene sequencing and expression profiling are helping to define molecular subtypes of MG that will allow for optimal selection of targeted therapeutics for individual patients.[32,33]

Cellular Origins

Despite recent advances, the cell of origin for MGs remains unknown. Emerging evidence suggests that neural stem cells, or related progenitor cells, may undergo malignant transformation and give rise to these tumors.[16,34–38] Additionally, glioma stem cells contribute to the treatment resistance of MGs[38,39]; a recent study found that expression of stem cell markers such as CD133 in MG specimens may predict resistance to both radiation and chemotherapy.[40] The radioresistance of stem cells is mediated by robust activation of DNA damage response pathways.[41] Mechanisms that contribute to stem cell chemoresistance are different and include increased production of O^6-methylguanine-DNA-methyltransferase (MGMT), overexpression of multi-drug resistance genes, and apoptosis inhibition.[42–44]

Diagnosis

Like other space-occupying lesions, MGs often present with a combination of generalized and focal symptoms. Generalized symptoms include headaches, mood changes, altered mental status, and psychomotor slowing. Focal symptoms reflect the location of the lesion in the brain and may include seizures, hemiparesis or hemisensory loss, and aphasia. Among the generalized symptoms, headaches are common and are frequently indistinguishable from tension headaches.[45] The classical pattern of headaches that are worse in the morning and with recumbency is only occasionally reported. In the face of suspicious neurological symptoms, the possibility of MG is often suggested by findings on contrast-enhanced magnetic resonance imaging (MRI) or computerized tomography (CT). A typical appearance of MG on either MRI or CT is an irregularly enhancing mass with associated edema and mass effect. Although GBMs often have a central necrotic cavity and more peritumoral edema than AGs,[46] pathological confirmation of the diagnosis is crucial, as radiographic features are currently inadequate to reliably determine histology and tumor grade.

Medical Management

Common medical and neurological problems in MG patients include seizures, peritumoral edema, venous thromboembolic disease, fatigue, mood disorders, and cognitive dysfunction.[47] Patients who experience seizures require treatment with antiepileptic drugs (AED). Many of the older AEDs (e.g., phenytoin, carbamazepine, and phenobarbital) are inducers of hepatic cytochrome P450, the same enzyme system that metabolizes many chemotherapeutic agents. For this reason, newer AEDs that neither induce nor inhibit the cytochrome P450 system (e.g., gabapentin, levetiracetam, and lamotrigine) are recommended. Although the American Academy of Neurology suggests that AEDs not be routinely prescribed to brain tumor patients who have not had seizures,[48] many practitioners continue to administer AED prophylaxis.[49]

Because many MG patients experience symptomatic peritumoral edema, corticosteroids such as dexamethasone are often required.[50] Adverse effects such as Cushing syndrome and steroid myopathy frequently develop due to prolonged corticosteroid administration. This treatment also increases the risk of *Pneumocystis jirovecii* pneumonia. Prophylactic antibiotics are generally prescribed for these patients,[47] although the value of this practice is unproven.[51] Late complications of corticosteroid use, such as osteoporosis with vertebral body compression fractures, are increasingly observed as new treatments prolong survival. Routine prophylaxis with calcium and vitamin D supplementation and bisphosphonates is an important consideration. Emerging antiangiogenic therapies such as bevacizumab (a humanized monoclonal antibody against VEGF) and VEGFR inhibitors effectively treat peritumoral edema and may permit reduction in corticosteroid doses.[47,50,52]

Venous thromboembolism from leg and pelvic veins is an important risk for MG patients, with a lifetime incidence of 20% to 30%.[47,53] Anticoagulation in MG patients with venous thromboembolism confers a low risk of intratumoral hemorrhage.[47,54] Therefore, in most circumstances, anticoagulation is appropriate treatment for venous thromboembolism in a MG patient. When a MG patient has recently had brain surgery or has intracerebral hemorrhage, inferior vena cava filters are a reasonable alternative, although they have high complication rates.[55] Results from a large randomized clinical trial performed in cancer patients with venous thromboembolism indicate that treatment with low molecular weight heparin confers a lower risk of recurrent thromboembolic disease than does treatment with warfarin (9% versus 17%), without a difference in bleeding rates or mortality.[56] On the basis of these data, which included 27 brain tumor patients, low molecular weight heparin is recommended by many physicians for treatment of venous thromboembolism in MG patients.

Fatigue is a common complaint among MG patients, and may respond to treatment with modafinil or methylphenidate.[57] Methylphenidate is also used to treat apathy or abulia. Limited evidence supports the use of donepezil[58] and memantine for memory impairment. Depression and anxiety respond to standard psychopharmacological interventions[59] and are likely underdiagnosed in this population.

Tumor-Directed Therapy (See Table 5-1)

SURGERY

Standard therapy for newly diagnosed MGs begins with a surgical procedure, as a definitive diagnosis cannot be made based on radiographic features alone. Although the infiltrative nature of gliomas precludes surgical cure, maximal surgical resection is recommended in all newly diagnosed patients. Benefits of surgical resection

TABLE 5-1 Summary of Therapeutic Options for Malignant Gliomas

Setting	Histology	Treatment Options
Newly Diagnosed Tumor*	Glioblastoma	• RT with concomitant and adjuvant TMZ • RT and carmustine wafers
	Anaplastic Astrocytoma**	• RT with concomitant and adjuvant TMZ • RT with adjuvant TMZ or PCV only
	Anaplastic Oligodendroglioma or Oligoastrocytoma**	• RT alone • RT with concomitant and adjuvant TMZ • RT with adjuvant TMZ or PCV only • Adjuvant TMZ or PCV alone
Recurrent Tumor**	Any	• Clinical trial enrollment*** • Surgical resection, SRS, or re-irradiation for selected candidates • Carmustine wafers • Chemotherapy (PCV, TMZ, carmustine, lomustine, carboplatin, etoposide, irinotecan, others) • Bevacizumab and irinotecan

Adapted from: Wen PY, Kesari S. Malignant gliomas in adults. N Engl J Med 2008;359:492–507.

*Treatment should always begin with maximal surgical resection.

**No standard of care has been defined.

***Clinical trial enrollment should be offered to recurrent malignant glioma patients whenever possible.

Abbreviations: *PCV*, procarbazine, lomustine (CCNU), and vincristine; *RT*, radiation therapy; *SRS*, stereotactic radiosurgery; *TMZ*, temozolomide.

include improvement of symptoms related to mass effect, reduction of tumor volume remaining to be treated with other modalities,[60] and removal of the necrotic tumor core which may be poorly accessible to circulating chemotherapy and resistant to radiation therapy (RT). Surgical resection also increases diagnostic accuracy, as biopsy provides a small specimen for pathological review that may not be representative of the entire lesion.[61] Mounting evidence of variable quality suggests that surgical resection confers a modest survival benefit as compared to biopsy.[62,63] Advances including MRI-guided neuro-navigation, intraoperative MRI, functional MRI, intraoperative mapping,[64] and fluorescent-guided surgery[65] have reduced surgical complication rates and allowed more complete tumor resections.[66] Patients with inoperable tumors located in eloquent areas require stereotactic biopsies for tissue diagnosis.

Surgery may also be considered in recurrent MG patients with good performance status when the tumor is accessible, symptomatic, and distant from eloquent areas. Surgical resection in the recurrent setting may improve quality of life and allow time for additional therapy.[67] The impact of resection on survival in recurrent MG patients is uncertain.

RADIATION THERAPY

Radiation therapy is generally considered to be the most important treatment modality for MGs. The addition of RT to surgery provides a robust survival benefit for GBM patients, increasing median survival from 3 to 4 months to 7 to 12 months.[68,69] Standard RT for MG is involved-field external beam irradiation to a total dose of 60 Gy, delivered in 1.8 Gy to 2.0 Gy fractions over approximately 6 weeks. The definition of the involved field varies, but it generally includes the area of T2 hyperintensity on MRI plus a 1 cm to 2 cm margin, often with a boost to the area of contrast enhancement. Conformal planning is used to reduce radiation exposure to surrounding brain. Although MG is an infiltrative disease, 90% of conventionally irradiated tumors recur locally at the original site.[70]

Many variations on standard RT have been investigated in an attempt to increase efficacy. Randomized studies with higher total radiation doses have confirmed the early impression that doses greater than 60 Gy yield no additional benefit.[71] A number of studies using altered fractionation schemes have failed to show any benefit over conventional fractionation.[72] Various radiosensitizing agents have been administered to patients with MGs, though none has demonstrated substantial efficacy. Strategies designed to provide additional radiation dose to the resection cavity, such as brachytherapy[73] and stereotactic radiosurgery (SRS),[74,75] have neither improved local control nor survival. Newer approaches including chemotherapy,[13] targeted molecular agents,[76] and antiangiogenic agents[77] may potentially work synergistically with RT and improve outcomes and are under investigation.

Patients over the age of 70 represent a challenging subgroup of MG patients with an extremely poor prognosis. In this population, the addition of RT to supportive care alone increases median survival from 16.9 weeks to only 29.1 weeks.[78] Furthermore, older patients are at increased risk for both acute and delayed radiation toxicity. Common manifestations include disabling fatigue that may last weeks to months,[79] nausea, and headache. Treatment options include an abbreviated course of RT (40 Gy in 15 fractions over 3 weeks)[80] or chemotherapy alone[81]; in elderly patients, both approaches produce similar outcomes to conventional RT regimens.

Additional involved-field RT is rarely offered to patients with recurrent MG, as doses higher than 60 Gy offer marginal benefit and increase the risk of radiation necrosis.[82] Small nonrandomized studies have demonstrated a survival benefit for MG patients treated with SRS at recurrence.[75] However, much of the data is subject to selection bias, and this approach is not routinely utilized. Fractionated stereotactic RT has also been evaluated for treatment of recurrent MG.[83] Fractionation allows for increased radiation doses to the tumor bed with less risk of injury to surrounding brain, but its efficacy is also unproven.

CHEMOTHERAPY

The importance of chemotherapy in MG treatment has grown in recent years. Early studies of adjuvant nitrosourea therapy for MGs were methodologically flawed and failed to demonstrate a significant survival advantage.[68,84] Subsequent meta-analyses confirmed that adjuvant chemotherapy produces a modest survival benefit (6% to 10% increase in 1-year survival).[85,86] In 2005, the European Organization for Research and Treatment of Cancer (EORTC) and the National

Cancer Institute of Canada (NCIC) reported the results of a large randomized phase III trial in newly diagnosed GBM, comparing RT alone (60 Gy over 6 weeks) with RT and concomitant daily temozolomide (Temodar®, Schering-Plough, Kenilworth, New Jersey; 75 $mg/m^2/d$), followed by adjuvant temozolomide therapy (150 to 200 $mg/m^2/day$ for 5 consecutive days out of every 28-day cycle, for 6 cycles).[69] Grade 3 or 4 toxicity in the chemotherapy group was modest and included fatigue (13%), nausea (2%), thrombocytopenia (12%), and neutropenia (7%). The addition of temozolomide to RT increased median survival compared to RT alone (14.6 mo vs. 12.1 mo; $p < 0.0001$). At two years, the proportion of surviving patients in the chemotherapy group was 26.5% as compared to 10.4% in the RT alone group. On the basis of these results, RT with concomitant and adjuvant temozolomide became the standard of care for newly diagnosed GBM (Figure 5-2). Recently, updated results from this study showed that the survival benefit with temozolomide was maintained even at 5 years (9.8% were alive at 5 years with temozolomide, versus 1.9% with radiotherapy alone (hazard ratio 0.6, 95% CI 0.5-0.7; $p<0.0001$).[87]

In a companion study, tumor specimens from the EORTC/NCIC study were evaluated for methylation status of the *MGMT* gene promoter.[8] MGMT is an endogenous DNA repair enzyme that removes alkyl groups from DNA and thus confers resistance to temozolomide and other alkylating agents. Methylation is an epigenetic modification that results in decreased gene transcription. Therefore, tumor cells with methylated *MGMT* promoters have less MGMT enzyme, resulting in less effective DNA repair and increased temozolomide sensitivity. As predicted, the benefit of temozolomide was more dramatic in patients with *MGMT* promoter methylation. Among GBM patients with *MGMT* promoter methylation who were treated with temozolomide, median survival was 21.7 months and 2-year survival, 46%. Temozolomide-treated patients with unmethylated *MGMT* promoters had a significantly shorter median survival of only 12.7 months, and a 2-year survival of 13.8%.[8] Because this study was conducted retrospectively in a relatively small sample of patients, temozolomide remains the standard of care for newly diagnosed GBM patients, regardless of *MGMT* promoter methylation status. A randomized phase III trial sponsored by the Radiation Therapy Oncology Group (RTOG 0525) will definitively evaluate the utility of *MGMT* promoter methylation in determining temozolomide sensitivity. In the future, patients whose tumors have unmethylated *MGMT* promoters may be offered alternatives to the standard temozolomide

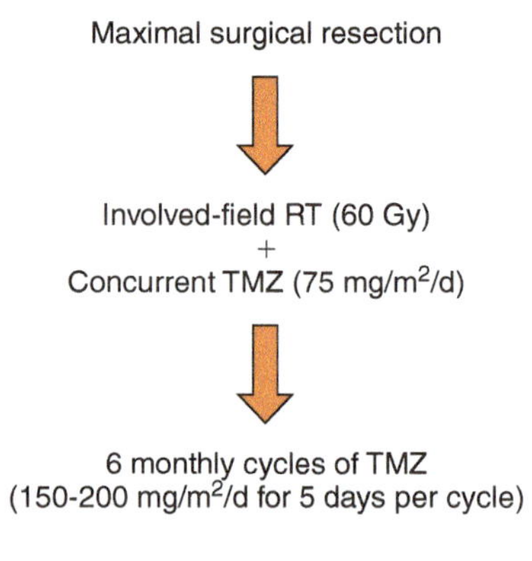

Figure 5-2 Standard treatment algorithm for newly-diagnosed glioblastoma. Abbreviations: *RT*, radiation therapy; *TMZ*, temozolomide

regimen. Investigational approaches to suppress MGMT activity include dose-intense temozolomide regimens (e.g., 21 days on/7 days off,[88] 7 days on/7days off,[89] or continuous dosing[90]), which may deplete the enzyme,[91] and combination therapy with O^6-benzylguanine or other MGMT inhibitors.[92–94] Inhibitors of other DNA repair enzymes such as poly-(ADP-ribose)-polymerase (PARP) may also improve the efficacy of temozolomide.[95]

An alternative to systemic chemotherapy involves the implantation of carmustine-containing biodegradable wafers (Gliadel® wafers, MGI Pharma, Bloomington, Minnesota) into the resection cavity following tumor debulking. These wafers gradually release carmustine over several weeks, allowing for a high local chemotherapy concentration with minimal systemic toxicity. In a double-blind, randomized, phase III trial of 240 newly diagnosed MG patients, patients received either conventional therapy (surgery followed by RT) with placement of a carmustine wafer or conventional therapy with placement of an identical placebo wafer. Carmustine wafer treatment increased median survival from 11.6 to 13.9 months ($P = 0.03$).[96] Carmustine wafers were FDA-approved for treatment of newly-diagnosed GBM on the basis of these data.

Although chemotherapy is often considered in treating recurrent MGs, the benefit of standard chemotherapy has been modest in this setting. Phase II trials of temozolomide for recurrent glioblastomas have demonstrated response rates of only 5%, with stable disease in 40% of patients and 6-month progression-free survival (PFS6) in the range of 21%.[97-99] Alternative temozolomide dosing regimens may be more effective. Other agents such as carmustine, carboplatin, etoposide, irinotecan, and PCV (procarbazine, lomustine [CCNU], and vincristine) combination therapy produce low response rates and no significant survival benefit.[100] In selected patients with recurrent glioblastomas who can undergo resection, carmustine-containing biodegradable wafers (Gliadel® wafers, MGI Pharma, Bloomington, Minnesota) produces a modest survival advantage of approximately 8 weeks.[101] In light of limited data, treatment decisions for patients with recurrent glioblastomas must be made on an individual basis. Factors to consider include tumor histology, prior therapy, time to relapse, and performance status. In general, patients with recurrent disease should be enrolled in clinical trials whenever feasible.

THERAPY FOR ANAPLASTIC GLIOMAS

Anaplastic astrocytomas are also treated with a dual-modality approach. Options include the same treatment regimen used for GBM, RT with concurrent and adjuvant temozolomide, or a somewhat less aggressive regimen of RT with adjuvant temozolomide only. Concurrent chemotherapy has not yet been tested in a clinical trial for AAs. Carmustine wafers are also used in some cases, as described above.

Tumors with oligodendroglial elements, AOs and AOAs, are less common than other subtypes of MG. However, they confer a better prognosis than do pure astrocytic tumors, and they have increased sensitivity to treatment.[102] The majority of AOs and 14% to 20% of AOAs have deletions of chromosomes 1 p and 19 q,[102] due to an unbalanced translocation of 19 p to 1 q.[103] Tumors with 1 p/19 q codeletion are particularly sensitive to PCV chemotherapy.[6,104] Codeletion of 1 p/19 q also may confer sensitivity to temozolomide, with an increase in response rate from 34% to 59% in one study.[28] The reason for the increased chemosensitivity conferred by 1p/19q codeletion is an area of ongoing investigation, but decreased levels of stathmin may be important.[105]

The value of chemotherapy for newly-diagnosed AO/AOA has recently been evaluated in two large phase III trials.[106,107] Although neither study showed an overall survival benefit (2.5 to 4.7 years), patients treated with both RT and PCV chemotherapy had 10 to 12 months of additional time to tumor progression as compared to RT alone. The lack of an overall survival benefit may relate to the fact that most patients who initially received RT alone were subsequently treated with chemotherapy at relapse. In both studies, 1p/19q codeletion was associated with marked survival prolongation. Because most published studies in AO/AOA were initiated prior to 2005, the majority of available data involve PCV chemotherapy. Although PCV and temozolomide have not yet been directly compared, temozolomide is likely to have similar activity and less toxicity.[102] Several large intergroup trials are underway evaluating the optimal combination of radiation therapy and temozolomide in patients with newly diagnosed AO/AOA.

Experimental Therapies

TARGETED MOLECULAR THERAPIES

As the molecular pathogenesis of MG is elucidated, there is growing interest in targeted molecular therapies against signaling pathways that regulate glioma cell growth, division, and other critical functions.[12,76,108,109] Targets of particular importance include receptor tyrosine kinases such as EGFR,[110] PDGFR,[111,112] and VEGFR.[52] Inhibitors of intracellular signaling molecules are also being developed against mTOR,[113,114] farnesyltransferase,[115] and PI3K, among many others (Figure 5-3).

The EGFR came to attention as a potential therapeutic target because the gene is amplified in more than 40% of primary GBMs.[116] Approximately one quarter to one third of GBMs have a constitutively active EGFR mutant known as EGFRvIII, and all of these EGFRvIII-expressing tumors also exhibit EGFR amplification or overexpression.[117] Unchecked EGFR pathway signaling promotes cell proliferation, tumor invasion, angiogenesis, and apoptosis inhibition. Several small-molecule inhibitors of the EGFR such as gefitinib (Iressa®, AstraZeneca, Wilmington, Delaware) and erlotinib (Tarceva®, OSI, Melville, New York) have been evaluated in MGs. Though these agents are generally well-tolerated, reported responses have been limited (0% to 25%) and short-lived. EGFR expression is not predictive of response, but patients with EGFRvIII mutations and intact PTEN may be more likely to benefit from therapy.[118]

PDGF pathway upregulation is another common feature of MGs that suggests a potential therapeutic target.[119] The first clinically useful small-molecule tyrosine kinase inhibitor was imatinib mesylate (Gleevec®, Novartis, East Hanover, New Jersey), an inhibitor of the Bcr-Abl, PDGF, and c-Kit receptor tyrosine kinases, which has activity against chronic myelogenous leukemia and gastrointestinal stromal tumors. Phase II trials of imatinib monotherapy in patients with recurrent MG showed minimal activity.[111,112] Preliminary studies of the combination of imatinib with hydroxyurea suggested possible activity in recurrent AG[120] and recurrent GBM.[121] However, a large multicenter phase III trial failed to confirm any benefit.[122]

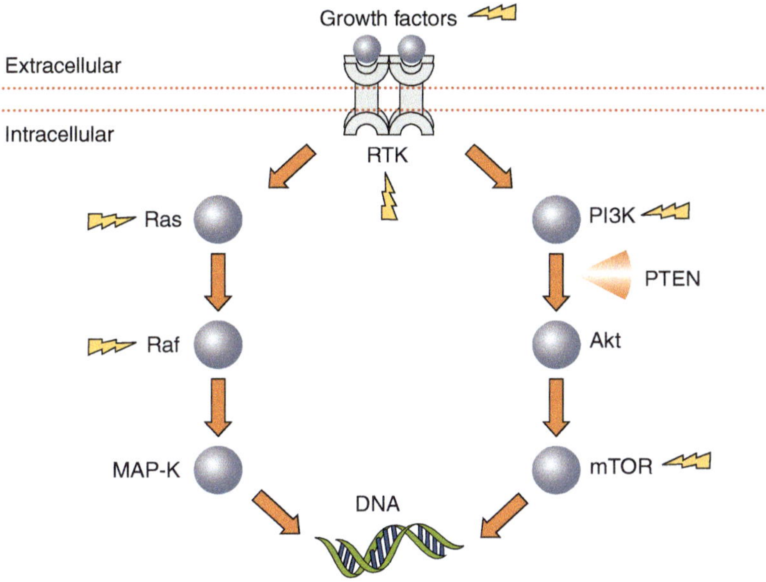

Figure 5-3 Selected signaling pathways in malignant gliomas. By transcriptional regulation, these pathways have important effects on cell growth, division, invasion, apoptosis, and angiogenesis. Lightning bolts indicate targets for which inhibitors are currently available. Some examples of receptor tyrosine kinase inhibitors include the epidermal growth factor receptor (EGFR) inhibitors erlotinib and gefitinib, the platelet-derived growth factor receptor (PDGFR) inhibitor imatinib, and the vascular endothelial growth factor receptor (VEGFR) inhibitor cediranib. An example of an inhibitor directed against a growth factor ligand is bevacizumab, the humanized monoclonal antibody against VEGF. Sorafenib is a multi-targeted tyrosine kinase inhibitor that blocks VEGF, PDGFR, and Raf. PI3K inhibitors such as XL765 (Exelixis, South San Francisco, California) and many others are now entering clinical trials for malignant glioma. A variety of mTOR inhibitors have been evaluated in malignant glioma including rapamycin (sirolimus, Rapamune®, Wyeth, Madison, New Jersey), temsirolimus (CCI-779, Torisel™, Wyeth, Madison, New Jersey), and everolimus (RAD001, Novartis, Basel, Switzerland). Abbreviations: *MAP-K*, mitogen-associated protein kinase; *mTOR*, mammalian target of rapamycin; *PI3K*, phosphoinositide 3′-kinase; *PTEN*, phosphatase and tensin homolog deleted on chromosome 10; *RTK*, receptor tyrosine kinase

Receptor tyrosine kinase signaling is mediated in part by the MAP-kinase and PI3K pathways. As such, components of these signaling pathways represent potential targets in MG therapy. An early step in activation of the MAP-kinase pathway is localization of Ras to the cell membrane, which depends upon Ras farnesylation by the enzyme farnesyltransferase. Farnesyltransferase inhibitors (FTI) such as tipifarnib[123] (R115777, Zarnestr™, Johnson and Johnson, New Brunswick, New Jersey) and lonafarnib (SCH66366, Sarasar®, Schering-Plough, Kenilworth, New Jersey) have shown modest activity as monotherapy in recurrent MG. The mammalian target of rapamycin is a downstream molecule in the PI3K pathway that is an attractive target for therapy.[124] The mTOR inhibitor and rapamycin analog temsirolimus (CCI-779, Torisel™, Wyeth, Madison, New Jersey) has been studied in recurrent MG with modest results thus far.[125,126] A pilot study of neoadjuvant rapamycin therapy for recurrent PTEN-deficient GBM demonstrated variable mTOR inhibition in tumor tissue and marked reduction in tumor cell proliferation in 7 of 14 (50%) patients, supporting in vitro evidence of increased sensitivity to mTOR inhibitors in this population.[127] Inhibitors of PI3K itself are currently in early clinical development for MG.

As these results imply, monotherapy with targeted molecular agents has shown modest activity, with disappointing response rates of 0% to 15% and no improvement in PFS6.[76,108,128] These results are not surprising when one considers that most MGs have coactivation of multiple tyrosine kinases[129] and highly redundant signaling pathways. In addition, many of the targeted molecular agents are hydrophilic and fail to penetrate tumor tissue sufficiently to inhibit critical targets. In light of these difficulties, efforts are under way to identify biomarkers that may enable prediction of responsiveness to targeted molecular drugs. For example, tumors with EGFRvIII and intact PTEN seem to be more sensitive to EGFR inhibitors in some studies,[130] although not in others.[131] Similarly, tumors with increased activity of the PI3K/Akt pathway are resistant to these same drugs.[132] Approaches that are now being evaluated in clinical trials involve the use of rational combinations of drugs that inhibit multiple targets, drugs that target multiple relevant targets at once, and combinations of drugs with radiotherapy and chemotherapy.[12,76,108,128,133] There is also growing interest in clinical trial designs that include posttreatment tissue specimens to verify appropriate target inhibition.[134]

ANTIANGIOGENIC THERAPIES

It is now well established that angiogenesis is required for the growth of most solid tumors, including MG.[27,135,136] The importance of angiogenesis in the pathogenesis of MG was long suspected, because GBMs are highly vascular tumors with abundant endothelial proliferation. Angiogenic factors produced by GBM cells include VEGF,[137] basic fibroblast growth factor (bFGF),[138] hepatocyte growth factor/scatter factor (HGF/SF).[139] The endothelial cells within MG tumor vasculature express VEGFR2 (KDR, Fkl-1), resulting in a paracrine loop in which VEGF secreted locally by the tumor promotes endothelial cell growth and division.[140] Higher levels of VEGF expression are observed in more malignant tumors; in one study, VEGF levels were increased more than ten-fold in high-grade gliomas as compared to their low-grade counterparts.[139] Other important angiogenic signaling pathways in MGs involve Tie2 and its ligands angiopoietin-1 and -2[141] and the Notch-Delta-like ligand (Dll) pathway.[142]

As described above, glioma stem cells may contribute to treatment resistance[41,143] and produce pro-angiogenic molecules such as VEGF.[144] Recent data shows that glioma stem cells are found in close proximity to tumor blood vessels,[145,146] suggesting that antiangiogenic treatment might preferentially target these treatment-resistant MG constituents. This may also suggest a mechanism by which antiangiogenic treatments and cytotoxic chemotherapy could achieve synergistic antitumor efficacy.[147]

For these reasons, MGs have become targets of interest for antiangiogenic drug therapy.[148] Early and relatively weak antiangiogenic agents such as thalidomide had modest activity,[149] but newer agents appear to be more promising (Figure 5-4). In initial studies for recurrent MG, combination therapy with bevacizumab and irinotecan resulted in radiographic response rates of 34% to 66%.[150-153] The regimen was well-tolerated with a low incidence of hemorrhage, an adverse effect of major concern for this class of drugs based on initial solid tumor data. Although it has been suggested that the impressive radiographic responses observed in patients

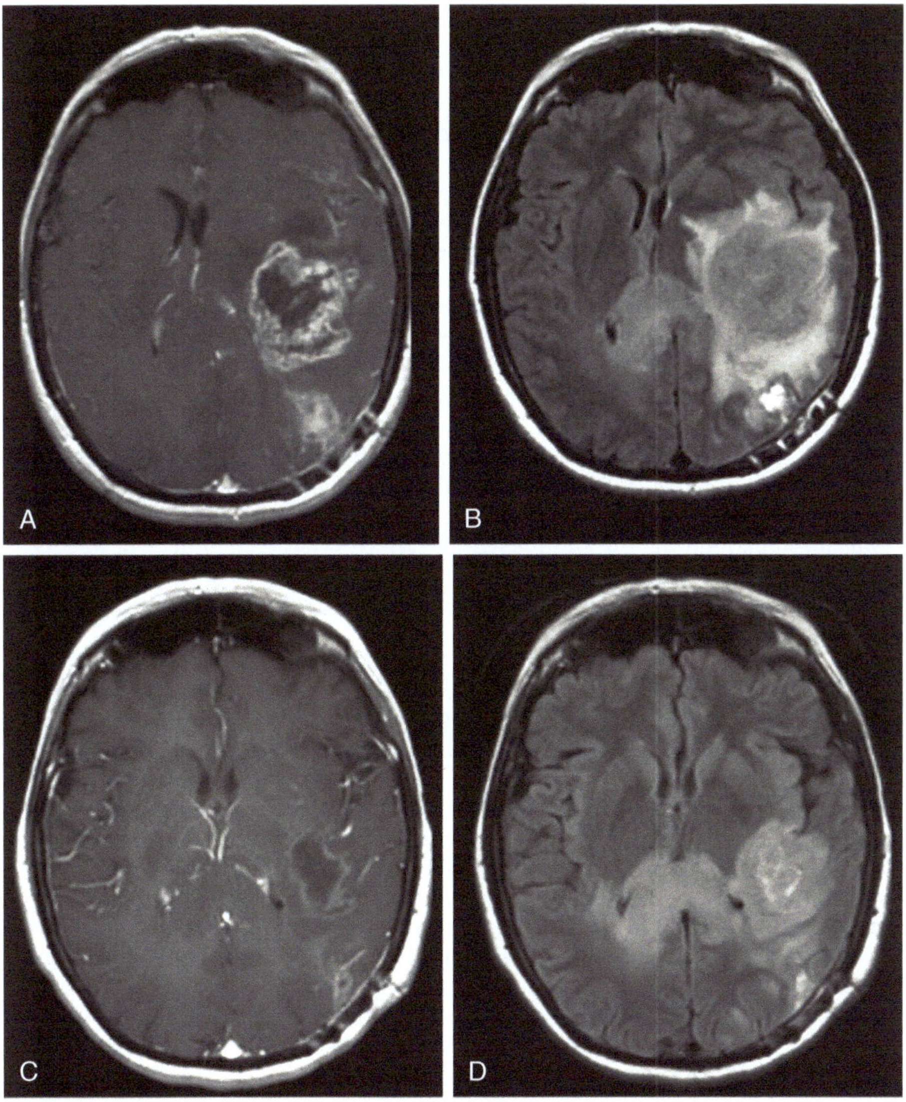

Figure 5-4 Radiographic response to antiangiogenic therapy. T1 post-gadolinium **(A)** and fluid-attenuated inversion recovery (FLAIR) **(B)** brain MRI from a patient with a recurrent left hemisphere glioblastoma following treatment with radiation therapy and temozolomide. After two doses of bevacizumab (10 mg/kg) and irinotecan (125 mg/m^2), there is marked reduction in gadolinium enhancement **(C)** and FLAIR hyperintensity **(D)**, consistent with a partial response. Responses of this magnitude are frequently observed in patients treated with this regimen. The marked reduction in edema often permits reduction in corticosteroid dosing.

treated with bevacizumab may be the result of decreased permeability of the vasculature rather than a true antitumor effect, subsequent clinical trial data have confirmed prolongation of PFS. In the first phase II trial, PFS6 was 43% for GBM patients and 59% for AG patients; these data are substantially better than the PFS6 of 21% reported in recurrent GBM patients treated with temozolomide.[99] The radiographic response rate was 57% for GBM patients and 61% for AG patients.[154] Treatment was well-tolerated with a single intracranial hemorrhage and four cases of venous thromboembolism, another adverse effect reported in previous solid tumor trials.[155,156] A subsequent phase II trial evaluated recurrent GBM patients in first or second relapse who were treated with bevacizumab with or without irinotecan.[157] In the monotherapy arm, PFS6 was 42.6% and radiographic response rate 28.2%. In the combination therapy arm, PFS6 was 50.3% and radiographic response rate 37.8%. Median overall survival was approximately 9 months in both groups. The study lacked statistical power to identify any benefit of adding irinotecan to bevacizumab. Most patients were able to reduce their corticosteroid doses by 50% or more. Again, treatment was well-tolerated with rare hemorrhagic complications. More recently, a phase II trial of bevacizumab in heavily pretreated patients with recurrent GBM produced similar results with a response rate of 35% and a PFS6 of 29%.[158]

There is emerging evidence that inhibitors of angiogenesis may work synergistically with RT.[77] Several trials are ongoing in which newly diagnosed GBM patients receive bevacizumab with RT and temozolomide. The regimen appears to be safe, despite a possible increase in wound-healing complications.[159] Bevacizumab is being combined in ongoing studies with a variety of targeted molecular agents as well.[160]

Aside from inhibitors of VEGF like bevacizumab, there are many small-molecule tyrosine kinase inhibitors directed against VEGFR. Cediranib (AZD2171, Recentin; AstraZeneca, London, UK), is an oral pan-VEGFR inhibitor that also has activity against PDGFR and c-Kit. Cediranib was tested in a phase II clinical trial in patients with recurrent GBM. The treatment achieved a promising response rate of 56% and PFS6 of 26%.[161,162] As had been noted in the bevacizumab studies, there was a striking steroid-sparing effect. All of the patients who required corticosteroids were able to reduce their doses or stop treatment entirely. Among the 31 patients enrolled, there were no intracranial hemorrhages, although adverse effects such as hypertension, diarrhea, and fatigue were common. The authors used advanced MRI techniques to show that cediranib produced reversible reductions in blood vessel size and permeability, lending support to the concept of vascular normalization, which asserts that antiangiogenic treatment may "normalize" structurally and functionally abnormal tumor blood vessels.[27] By virtue of vascular normalization, antiangiogenic therapies may facilitate delivery of chemotherapeutics into the tumor and reduce hypoxia, perhaps improving the efficacy of RT as well.[163]

Mechanisms of resistance to antiangiogenic therapy are beginning to be elucidated.[164,165] Failure of anti-VEGF/VEGFR therapy may correlate with upregulation of alternative pro-angiogenic factors such as bFGF,[162] stromal-derived factor-1α (SDF1α),[162] Tie2, and placental growth factor (PlGF),[166] or with mobilization of circulating endothelial cells or their bone marrow–derived precursor cells.[142,162] Some preclinical data suggest that blockade of VEGF-mediated angiogenesis may promote tumor infiltration by cooption of existing cerebral blood vessels.[141,167–171] In recurrent MG patients who are treated with bevacizumab, there is an increased risk of infiltrative tumor growth observed on MRI scans, which suggests that bevacizumab may promote tumor infiltration in patients.[150,172–174] These findings imply that anti-VEGF/VEGFR therapy may function optimally when combined with agents that target tumor invasion and non–VEGF-mediated angiogenesis.

OTHER THERAPIES

An array of other therapeutic modalities are being explored for MG. Examples include gene therapy,[175,176] stem cell targeting,[177] synthetic chlorotoxins (TM-601),[178] chemotherapeutic agents with enhanced ability to penetrate into tumor tissue, and convection-enhanced delivery of drugs and toxins.[179] Antitumor vaccines based on peptide antigens, dendritic cells, or whole tumor cells represent a major avenue of investigation. Among the many promising vaccines are CDX-110,[180] a peptide vaccine directed against EGFRvIII, and GVAX,[181] which involves administration of irradiated autologous tumor cells mixed with GM-CSF producing cells.

Conclusions

Despite progress in recent years, the prognosis for most patients with MG remains poor. The addition of temozolomide to the therapeutic arsenal was an important advance, and antiangiogenic therapy has now emerged as a critical component of treatment for recurrent tumors. Thus far, the potential of targeted molecular drug therapy has not been fully realized. Future approaches include the use of treatment regimens that inhibit complementary targets and combinations of targeted molecular drugs with RT, chemotherapy, and antiangiogenic therapies. Additionally, our understanding of glioma biology and treatment resistance is evolving at a rapid pace. Tactics for circumventing treatment resistance mediated by MGMT and PARP as well as the intrinsic resistance of glioma stem cells are beginning to materialize. These and other novel treatment approaches are much needed.

Acknowledgments

We gratefully acknowledge the support of the Melinda Wanatick Brain Tumor Research Fund.

REFERENCES

1. CBTRUS. Statistical Report: Primary Brain Tumors in the United States, 2000–2004. Published by the Central Brain Tumor Registry of the United States; 2008.
2. Louis DN, Ohgaki H, Wiestler OD, et al. The 2007 WHO classification of tumors of the central nervous system. Lyon, France: IARC Press; 2007.
3. Fisher JL, Schwartzbaum JA, Wrensch M, Wiemels JL. Epidemiology of brain tumors. Neurol Clin 2007;25:867–90.
4. Wen PY, Kesari S. Malignant gliomas in adults. N Engl J Med 2008;359:492–507.
5. Curran Jr WJ, Scott CB, Horton J, et al. Recursive partitioning analysis of prognostic factors in three Radiation Therapy Oncology Group malignant glioma trials. J Natl Cancer Inst 1993;85:704–10.
6. Ino Y, Betensky RA, Zlatescu MC, et al. Molecular subtypes of anaplastic oligodendroglioma: implications for patient management at diagnosis. Clin Cancer Res 2001;7:839–45.
7. Colman H, Aldape K. Molecular predictors in glioblastoma: toward personalized therapy. Arch Neurol 2008;65:877–83.
8. Hegi ME, Diserens AC, Gorlia T, et al. MGMT gene silencing and benefit from temozolomide in glioblastoma. N Engl J Med 2005;352:997–1003.

9. Phillips HS, Kharbanda S, Chen R, et al. Molecular subclasses of high-grade glioma predict prognosis, delineate a pattern of disease progression, and resemble stages in neurogenesis. Cancer Cell 2006;9:157–73.
10. McLendon R, Friedman A, Bigner D, et al. Comprehensive genomic characterization defines human glioblastoma genes and core pathways. Nature 2008.
11. Parsons DW, Jones S, Zhang X, et al. An integrated genomic analysis of human glioblastoma multiforme. Science 2008;321:1807–12.
12. Furnari FB, Fenton T, Bachoo RM, et al. Malignant astrocytic glioma: genetics, biology, and paths to treatment. Genes Dev 2007;21:2683–710.
13. Stupp R, Hegi ME, Gilbert MR, Chakravarti A. Chemoradiotherapy in malignant glioma: standard of care and future directions. J Clin Oncol 2007;25:4127–36.
14. Farrell CJ, Plotkin SR. Genetic causes of brain tumors: neurofibromatosis, tuberous sclerosis, von Hippel-Lindau, and other syndromes. Neurol Clin 2007;25:925–46.
15. Malmer B, Adatto P, Armstrong G, et al. GLIOGENE an International Consortium to Understand Familial Glioma. Cancer Epidemiol Biomarkers Prev 2007;16:1730–4.
16. Lee DY, Gutmann DH. Cancer stem cells and brain tumors: uprooting the bad seeds. Expert Rev Anticancer Ther 2007;7:1581–90.
17. Nutt CL, Mani DR, Betensky RA, et al. Gene expression-based classification of malignant gliomas correlates better with survival than histological classification. Cancer Res 2003;63:1602–7.
18. Pelloski CE, Ballman KV, Furth AF, et al. Epidermal growth factor receptor variant III status defines clinically distinct subtypes of glioblastoma. J Clin Oncol 2007;25:2288–94.
19. Collins VP. Mechanisms of disease: genetic predictors of response to treatment in brain tumors. Nat Clin Pract Oncol 2007;4:362–74.
20. Ohgaki H, Kleihues P. Genetic pathways to primary and secondary glioblastoma. Am J Pathol 2007;170:1445–53.
21. Watanabe K, Tachibana O, Sata K, Yonekawa Y, Kleihues P, Ohgaki H. Overexpression of the EGF receptor and p53 mutations are mutually exclusive in the evolution of primary and secondary glioblastomas. Brain Pathol 1996;6:217–23; discussion 23–4.
22. Ueki K, Ono Y, Henson JW, Efird JT, von Deimling A, Louis DN. CDKN2/p16 or RB alterations occur in the majority of glioblastomas and are inversely correlated. Cancer Res 1996;56:150–3.
23. Yan H, Parsons DW, Jin G, et al. IDH1 and IDH2 mutations in gliomas. N Engl J Med 2009;360:765–73.
24. Lee JC, Vivanco I, Beroukhim R, et al. Epidermal growth factor receptor activation in glioblastoma through novel missense mutations in the extracellular domain. PLoS Med 2006;3:e485.
25. Steck P, Perhouse MA, Jasser SA, et al. Identification of a candidate tumour suppressor gene, MMAC 1, at chromosome 10q23.3 that is mutated in multiple advanced cancers. Nature Genet 1997;15:356–62.
26. Guo P, Hu B, Gu W, et al. Platelet-derived growth factor-B enhances glioma angiogenesis by stimulating vascular endothelial growth factor expression in tumor endothelia and by promoting pericyte recruitment. Am J Pathol 2003;162:1083–93.
27. Jain RK, di Tomaso E, Duda DG, Loeffler JS, Sorensen AG, Batchelor TT. Angiogenesis in brain tumours. Nat Rev Neurosci 2007;8:610–22.
28. Brandes AA, Tosoni A, Cavallo G, et al. Correlations between O6-methylguanine DNA methyltransferase promoter methylation status, 1p and 19q deletions, and response to temozolomide in anaplastic and recurrent oligodendroglioma: a prospective GICNO study. J Clin Oncol 2006;24:4746–53.
29. Ino Y, Zlatescu MC, Sasaki H, et al. Long survival and therapeutic responses in patients with histologically disparate high-grade gliomas demonstrating chromosome 1p loss. J Neurosurg 2000;92:983–90.
30. Cairncross JG, Ueki K, Zlatescu MC, et al. Specific chromosomal losses predict chemotherapeutic response and survival in patients with anaplastic oligodendrogliomas. J Natl Cancer Inst 1998;90:1473–9.
31. Hegi ME, Liu L, Herman JG, et al. Correlation of O6-methylguanine methyltransferase (MGMT) promoter methylation with clinical outcomes in glioblastoma and clinical strategies to modulate MGMT activity. J Clin Oncol 2008;26:4189–99.
32. McLendon R, Friedman A, Bigner D, et al. Comprehensive genomic characterization defines human glioblastoma genes and core pathways. Nature 2008.
33. Parsons DW, Jones S, Zhang X, et al. An Integrated Genomic Analysis of Human Glioblastoma Multiforme. Science 2008.

34. Assanah M, Lochhead R, Ogden A, Bruce J, Goldman J, Canoll P. Glial progenitors in adult white matter are driven to form malignant gliomas by platelet-derived growth factor-expressing retroviruses. J Neurosci 2006;26:6781–90.
35. Sanai N, Alvarez-Buylla A, Berger MS. Neural stem cells and the origin of gliomas. N Engl J Med 2005;353:811–22.
36. Clarke MF, Fuller M. Stem cells and cancer: two faces of eve. Cell 2006;124:1111–5.
37. Singh SK, Hawkins C, Clarke ID, et al. Identification of human brain tumour initiating cells. Nature 2004;432:396–401.
38. Stiles CD, Rowitch DH. Glioma stem cells: a midterm exam. Neuron 2008;58:832–46.
39. Dirks PB. Brain tumor stem cells: bringing order to the chaos of brain cancer. J Clin Oncol 2008;26:2916–24.
40. Murat A, Migliavacca E, Gorlia T, et al. Stem cell-related "self-renewal" signature and high epidermal growth factor receptor expression associated with resistance to concomitant chemoradiotherapy in glioblastoma. J Clin Oncol 2008;26:3015–24.
41. Bao S, Wu Q, McLendon RE, et al. Glioma stem cells promote radioresistance by preferential activation of the DNA damage response. Nature 2006;444:756–60.
42. Liu G, Yuan X, Zeng Z, et al. Analysis of gene expression and chemoresistance of CD133 + cancer stem cells in glioblastoma. Mol Cancer 2006;5:67.
43. Salmaggi A, Boiardi A, Gelati M, et al. Glioblastoma-derived tumorospheres identify a population of tumor stem-like cells with angiogenic potential and enhanced multidrug resistance phenotype. Glia 2006;54:850–60.
44. Dean M, Fojo T, Bates S. Tumour stem cells and drug resistance. Nat Rev Cancer 2005;5:275–84.
45. Loghin M, Levin VA. Headache related to brain tumors. Curr Treat Options Neurol 2006;8:21–32.
46. Cha S. Update on brain tumor imaging: from anatomy to physiology. AJNR Am J Neuroradiol 2006;27:475–87.
47. Wen P, Schiff D, Kesari S, Drappatz J, Gigas D, Doherty L. Medical management of patients with brain tumors. J Neurooncol 2006;80:313–32.
48. Glantz MJ, Cole BF, Forsyth PA, et al. Practice parameter: anticonvulsant prophylaxis in patients with newly diagnosed brain tumors. Report of the Quality Standards Subcommittee of the American Academy of Neurology. Neurology 2000;54:1886–93.
49. Siomin V, Angelov L, Li L, Vogelbaum MA. Results of a survey of neurosurgical practice patterns regarding the prophylactic use of anti-epilepsy drugs in patients with brain tumors. J Neurooncol 2005;74:211–5.
50. Gerstner ER, Duda DG, di Tomaso E, et al. VEGF inhibitors in the treatment of cerebral edema in patients with brain cancer. Nat Rev Clin Oncol 2009;6:229–36.
51. Green H, Paul M, Vidal L, Leibovici L. Prophylaxis of Pneumocystis pneumonia in immunocompromised non-HIV-infected patients: systematic review and meta-analysis of randomized controlled trials. Mayo Clin Proc 2007;82:1052–9.
52. Batchelor T, Sorensen A, di Tomaso E, et al. AZD2171, a Pan-VEGF Receptor Tyrosine Kinase Inhibitor, Normalizes Tumor Vasculature and Alleviates Edema in Glioblastoma Patients. Cancer Cell 2007;11:83–95.
53. Gerber DE, Grossman SA, Streiff MB. Management of venous thromboembolism in patients with primary and metastatic brain tumors. J Clin Oncol 2006;24:1310–8.
54. Ruff RL, Posner JB. Incidence and treatment of peripheral venous thrombosis in patients with glioma. Ann Neurol 1983;13:334–6.
55. Levin JM, Schiff D, Loeffler JS, Fine HA, Black PM, Wen PY. Complications of therapy for venous thromboembolic disease in patients with brain tumors. Neurology 1993;43:1111–4.
56. Lee AY, Levine MN, Baker RI, et al. Low-molecular-weight heparin versus a coumarin for the prevention of recurrent venous thromboembolism in patients with cancer. N Engl J Med 2003;349:146–53.
57. Meyers CA, Weitzner MA, Valentine AD, Levin VA. Methylphenidate therapy improves cognition, mood, and function of brain tumor patients. J Clin Oncol 1998;16:2522–7.
58. Shaw EG, Rosdhal R, D'Agostino Jr RB, et al. Phase II study of donepezil in irradiated brain tumor patients: effect on cognitive function, mood, and quality of life. J Clin Oncol 2006;24:1415–20.
59. Litofsky NS, Farace E, Anderson Jr F, Meyers CA, Huang W, Laws Jr ER. Depression in patients with high-grade glioma: results of the Glioma Outcomes Project. Neurosurgery 2004;54:358–66; discussion 66–7.

60. Keles GE, Lamborn KR, Chang SM, Prados MD, Berger MS. Volume of residual disease as a predictor of outcome in adult patients with recurrent supratentorial glioblastomas multiforme who are undergoing chemotherapy. J Neurosurg 2004;100:41–6.
61. Jackson RJ, Fuller GN, Abi-Said D, et al. Limitations of stereotactic biopsy in the initial management of gliomas. Neuro-oncol 2001;3:193–200.
62. Sanai N, Berger MS. Glioma extent of resection and its impact on patient outcome. Neurosurgery 2008;62:753–64; discussion 264–6.
63. Stummer W, Reulen HJ, Meinel T, et al. Extent of resection and survival in glioblastoma multiforme: identification of and adjustment for bias. Neurosurgery 2008;62:564–76; discussion -76.
64. Asthagiri AR, Pouratian N, Sherman J, Ahmed G, Shaffrey ME. Advances in brain tumor surgery. Neurol Clin 2007;25:975–1003.
65. Stummer W, Pichlmeier U, Meinel T, Wiestler OD, Zanella F, Reulen HJ. Fluorescence-guided surgery with 5-aminolevulinic acid for resection of malignant glioma: a randomised controlled multicentre phase III trial. Lancet Oncol 2006;7:392–401.
66. Asthagiri AR, Pouratian N, Sherman J, Ahmed G, Shaffrey ME. Advances in brain tumor surgery. Neurol Clin 2007;25:975–1003; viii-ix.
67. Brown PD, Maurer MJ, Rummans TA, et al. A prospective study of quality of life in adults with newly diagnosed high-grade gliomas: the impact of the extent of resection on quality of life and survival. Neurosurgery 2005;57:495–504; discussion 495–504.
68. Walker MD, Alexander Jr E, Hunt WE, et al. Evaluation of BCNU and/or radiotherapy in the treatment of anaplastic gliomas. A cooperative clinical trial. J Neurosurg 1978;49:333–43.
69. Stupp R, Mason WP, van den Bent MJ, et al. Radiotherapy plus concomitant and adjuvant temozolomide for glioblastoma. N Engl J Med 2005;352:987–96.
70. Hochberg FH, Pruitt A. Assumptions in the radiotherapy of glioblastoma. Neurology 1980;30:907–11.
71. Lee SW, Fraass BA, Marsh LH, et al. Patterns of failure following high-dose 3-D conformal radiotherapy for high-grade astrocytomas: a quantitative dosimetric study. Int J Radiat Oncol Biol Phys 1999;43:79–88.
72. Fiveash JB, Spencer SA. Role of radiation therapy and radiosurgery in glioblastoma multiforme. Cancer J 2003;9:222–9.
73. Selker RG, Shapiro WR, Burger P, et al. The Brain Tumor Cooperative Group NIH Trial 87–01: a randomized comparison of surgery, external radiotherapy, and carmustine versus surgery, interstitial radiotherapy boost, external radiation therapy, and carmustine. Neurosurgery 2002;51: 343–55 discussion 55–7.
74. Souhami L, Seiferheld W, Brachman D, et al. Randomized comparison of stereotactic radiosurgery followed by conventional radiotherapy with carmustine to conventional radiotherapy with carmustine for patients with glioblastoma multiforme: report of Radiation Therapy Oncology Group 93–05 protocol. Int J Radiat Oncol Biol Phys 2004;60:853–60.
75. Tsao MN, Mehta MP, Whelan TJ, et al. The American Society for Therapeutic Radiology and Oncology (ASTRO) evidence-based review of the role of radiosurgery for malignant glioma. Int J Radiat Oncol Biol Phys 2005;63:47–55.
76. Chi A, Wen P. Inhibiting kinases in malignant gliomas. Expert Opin Ther Targets 2007; 11:473–96.
77. Duda DG, Jain RK, Willett CG. Antiangiogenics: the potential role of integrating this novel treatment modality with chemoradiation for solid cancers. J Clin Oncol 2007;25:4033–42.
78. Keime-Guibert F, Chinot O, Taillandier L, et al. Radiotherapy for glioblastoma in the elderly. N Engl J Med 2007;356:1527–35.
79. Davies E, Clarke C, Hopkins A. Malignant cerebral glioma—I: Survival, disability, and morbidity after radiotherapy. BMJ 1996;313:1507–12.
80. Roa W, Brasher PM, Bauman G, et al. Abbreviated course of radiation therapy in older patients with glioblastoma multiforme: a prospective randomized clinical trial. J Clin Oncol 2004;22:1583–8.
81. Glantz M, Chamberlain M, Liu Q, Litofsky NS, Recht LD. Temozolomide as an alternative to irradiation for elderly patients with newly diagnosed malignant gliomas. Cancer 2003;97:2262–6.
82. Stieber VW, Mehta MP. Advances in radiation therapy for brain tumors. Neurol Clin 2007;25: 1005–33; ix.
83. Combs SE, Thilmann C, Edler L, Debus J, Schulz-Ertner D. Efficacy of fractionated stereotactic reirradiation in recurrent gliomas: long-term results in 172 patients treated in a single institution. J Clin Oncol 2005;23:8863–9.
84. Randomized trial of procarbazine, lomustine, and vincristine in the adjuvant treatment of high-grade astrocytoma: a Medical Research Council trial. J Clin Oncol 2001;19:509–18.

85. Fine HA, Dear KB, Loeffler JS, Black PM, Canellos GP. Meta-analysis of radiation therapy with and without adjuvant chemotherapy for malignant gliomas in adults. Cancer 1993;71:2585–97.
86. Stewart LA. Chemotherapy in adult high-grade glioma: a systematic review and meta-analysis of individual patient data from 12 randomised trials. Lancet 2002;359:1011–8.
87. Stupp R, Hegi ME, Mason WP, et al. Effects of radiotherapy with concomitant and adjuvant temozolomide versus radiotherapy alone on survival in glioblastoma in a randomised phase III study: 5-year analysis of the EORTC-NCIC trial. Lancet Oncol 2009.
88. Brandes AA, Tosoni A, Cavallo G, et al. Temozolomide 3 weeks on and 1 week off as first-line therapy for recurrent glioblastoma: phase II study from gruppo italiano cooperativo di neuro-oncologia (GICNO). Br J Cancer 2006;95:1155–60.
89. Wick A, Felsberg J, Steinbach JP, et al. Efficacy and tolerability of temozolomide in an alternating weekly regimen in patients with recurrent glioma. J Clin Oncol 2007;25:3357–61.
90. Perry JR, Mason WP, Belanger K, et al. The temozolomide RESCUE study: A phase II trial of continuous (28/28) dose-intense temozolomide (TMZ) after progression on conventional 5/28 day TMZ in patients with recurrent malignant glioma. J Clin Oncol 2010;2008:26.
91. Tolcher AW, Gerson SL, Denis L, et al. Marked inactivation of O6-alkylguanine-DNA alkyltransferase activity with protracted temozolomide schedules. Br J Cancer 2003;88:1004–11.
92. Broniscer A, Gururangan S, MacDonald TJ, et al. Phase I trial of single-dose temozolomide and continuous administration of o6-benzylguanine in children with brain tumors: a pediatric brain tumor consortium report. Clin Cancer Res 2007;13:6712–8.
93. Quinn JA, Jiang SX, Reardon DA, et al. Phase 1 trial of temozolomide plus irinotecan plus O(6)-benzylguanine in adults with recurrent malignant glioma. Cancer 2009.
94. Quinn JA, Jiang SX, Reardon DA, et al. Phase II trial of temozolomide plus o6-benzylguanine in adults with recurrent, temozolomide-resistant malignant glioma. J Clin Oncol 2009;27:1262–7.
95. Zaremba T, Curtin NJ. PARP inhibitor development for systemic cancer targeting. Anticancer Agents Med Chem 2007;7:515–23.
96. Westphal M, Hilt D, Bortey E, et al. A phase 3 trial of local chemotherapy with biodegradable carmustine (BCNU) wafers (Gliadel wafers) in patients with primary malignant glioma. Neurooncol 2003;5:79–88.
97. Brada M, Hoang-Xuan K, Rampling R, et al. Multicenter phase II trial of temozolomide in patients with glioblastoma multiforme at first relapse. Ann Oncol 2001;12:259–66.
98. Brandes AA, Ermani M, Basso U, et al. Temozolomide as a second-line systemic regimen in recurrent high-grade glioma: a phase II study. Ann Oncol 2001;12:255–7.
99. Yung WK, Albright RE, Olson J, et al. A phase II study of temozolomide vs. Procarbazine in patients with glioblastoma multiforme at first relapse. Br J Cancer 2000;83:588–93.
100. Laterra J, Grossman S, Carson K, Lesser G, Hochberg F, Gilbert M. Suramin and radiotherapy in newly diagnosed glioblastoma: phase 2 NABTT CNS Consortium study. Neuro-oncol 2004;6:15–20.
101. Brem H, Piantadosi S, Burger PC, et al. Placebo-controlled trial of safety and efficacy of intraoperative controlled delivery by biodegradable polymers of chemotherapy for recurrent malignant gliomas: The Polymer-brain Tumor Treatment Group. Lancet 1999;345:1008–12.
102. van den Bent MJ. Anaplastic oligodendroglioma and oligoastrocytoma. Neurol Clin 2007;25: 1089–109.
103. Jenkins RB, Blair H, Ballman KV, et al. A t(1;19)(q10;p10) mediates the combined deletions of 1p and 19q and predicts a better prognosis of patients with oligodendroglioma. Cancer Res 2006;66:9852–61.
104. Cairncross JG, Ueki K, Zlatescu MC, et al. Specific genetic predictors of chemotherapeutic response and survival in patients with anaplastic oligodendrogliomas. J Natl Cancer Inst 1998;90:1473–9.
105. Ngo T, Peng T, Liang X, et al. The 1p-encoded protein stathmin and resistance of malignant gliomas to nitrosoureas. J Natl Cancer Inst 2007;99:639–52.
106. Cairncross G, Berkey B, Shaw E, et al. Phase III trial of chemotherapy plus radiotherapy compared with radiotherapy alone for pure and mixed anaplastic oligodendroglioma: Intergroup Radiation Therapy Oncology Group Trial 9402. J Clin Oncol 2006;24:2707–14.
107. van den Bent MJ, Carpentier AF, Brandes AA, et al. Adjuvant procarbazine, lomustine, and vincristine improves progression-free survival but not overall survival in newly diagnosed anaplastic oligodendrogliomas and oligoastrocytomas: a randomized European Organisation for Research and Treatment of Cancer phase III trial. J Clin Oncol 2006;24:2715–22.
108. Sathornsumetee S, Reardon DA, Desjardins A, Quinn JA, Vredenburgh JJ, Rich JN. Molecularly targeted therapy for malignant glioma. Cancer 2007;110:13–24.

109. Idbaih A, Ducray F, Sierra Del Rio M, Hoang-Xuan K, Delattre JY. Therapeutic application of noncytotoxic molecular targeted therapy in gliomas: growth factor receptors and angiogenesis inhibitors. Oncologist 2008;13:978–92.
110. Rich J, Reardon D, Peery T, et al. Phase II trial of gefitinib in recurrent glioblastoma. J Clin Oncol 2004;22:133–42.
111. Wen PY, Yung WK, Lamborn KR, et al. Phase I/II study of imatinib mesylate for recurrent malignant gliomas: North American Brain Tumor Consortium Study 99–08. Clin Cancer Res 2006;12:4899–907.
112. Raymond E, Brandes AA, Dittrich C, et al. Phase II study of imatinib in patients with recurrent gliomas of various histologies: a European Organisation for Research and Treatment of Cancer Brain Tumor Group Study. J Clin Oncol 2008;26:4659–65.
113. Galanis E, Buckner J, Maurer M, et al. Phase II trial of temsirolimus (CCI-779) in recurrent glioblastoma multiforme: a North Central Cancer Treatment Group Study. J Clin Oncol 2005;23:5294–304.
114. Chang S, Wen P, Cloughesy T, et al. Phase II study of CCI-779 in patients with recurrent glioblastoma multiforme. Invest New Drugs 2005;23:357–61.
115. Cloughesy T, Wen P, Robins H, et al. Phase II trial of tipifarnib in patients with recurrent malignant glioma either receiving or not receiving enzyme-inducing antiepileptic drugs: a North American Brain Tumor Consortium Study. J Clin Oncol 2006;24:3651–6.
116. Maher EA, Furnari FB, Bachoo RM, et al. Malignant glioma: genetics and biology of a grave matter. Genes Dev 2001;15:1311–33.
117. Aldape KD, Ballman K, Furth A, et al. Immunohistochemical detection of egfrviii in high malignancy grade astrocytomas and evaluation of prognostic significance. J Neuropathol Exp Neurol 2004;63:700–7.
118. Mellinghoff I, Wang M, Vivanco I, et al. Molecular determinants of the response of glioblastomas to EGFR kinase inhibitors. N Engl J Med 2005;353:2012–24.
119. Shih AH, Holland EC. Platelet-derived growth factor (PDGF) and glial tumorigenesis. Cancer Lett 2006;232:139–47.
120. Desjardins A, Quinn JA, Vredenburgh JJ, et al. Phase II study of imatinib mesylate and hydroxyurea for recurrent grade III malignant gliomas. J Neurooncol 2007;83:53–60.
121. Reardon DA, Egorin MJ, Quinn JA, et al. Phase II study of imatinib mesylate plus hydroxyurea in adults with recurrent glioblastoma multiforme. J Clin Oncol 2005;23:9359–68.
122. Dresemann G, Rosenthal M, Höffken K, et al. Imatinib plus hydroxyurea versus hydroxyurea monotherapy in progressive glioblastoma (GBM)–an international open label randomised phase III study. Neuro Oncol 2007;9:519.
123. Cloughesy TF, Wen PY, Robins HI, et al. Phase II trial of tipifarnib in patients with recurrent malignant glioma either receiving or not receiving enzyme-inducing antiepileptic drugs: a North American Brain Tumor Consortium Study. J Clin Oncol 2006;24:3651–6.
124. Chiang GG, Abraham RT. Targeting the mtor signaling network in cancer. Trends Mol Med 2007;13:433–42.
125. Chang SM, Wen P, Cloughesy T, et al. Phase II study of CCI-779 in patients with recurrent glioblastoma multiforme. Invest New Drugs 2005;23:357–61.
126. Galanis E, Buckner JC, Maurer MJ, et al. Phase II trial of temsirolimus (CCI-779) in recurrent glioblastoma multiforme: a North Central Cancer Treatment Group Study. J Clin Oncol 2005;23:5294–304.
127. Cloughesy TF, Yoshimoto K, Nghiemphu P, et al. Antitumor activity of rapamycin in a Phase I trial for patients with recurrent PTEN-deficient glioblastoma. PLoS Med 2008;5:e8.
128. Sathornsumetee S, Rich JN, Reardon DA. Diagnosis and Treatment of High-Grade Astrocytoma. Neurol Clin 2007;25:1111–39.
129. Stommel JM, Kimmelman AC, Ying H, et al. Coactivation of receptor tyrosine kinases affects the response of tumor cells to targeted therapies. Science 2007;318:287–90.
130. Mellinghoff IK, Wang MY, Vivanco I, et al. Molecular determinants of the response of glioblastomas to EGFR kinase inhibitors. N Engl J Med 2005;353:2012–24.
131. Brown PD, Krishnan S, Sarkaria JN, et al. Phase I/II trial of erlotinib and temozolomide with radiation therapy in the treatment of newly diagnosed glioblastoma multiforme: North Central Cancer Treatment Group Study N0177. J Clin Oncol 2008;26:5603–9.
132. Haas-Kogan D, Prados M, Lamborn K, Tihan T, Berger M, Stokoe D. Biomarkers to predict response to epidermal growth factor receptor inhibitors. Cell Cycle 2005;4:1369–72.
133. Wen PY. New developments in targeted molecular therapies for glioblastoma. Expert Rev Anticancer Ther 2009;9:7–10.

134. Chang SM, Lamborn KR, Kuhn JG, et al. Neurooncology clinical trial design for targeted therapies: lessons learned from the North American Brain Tumor Consortium. Neuro Oncol 2008;10:631–42.
135. Folkman J. Tumor angiogenesis: therapeutic implications. N Engl J Med 1971;285:1182–6.
136. Folkman J. Angiogenesis. Annu Rev Med 2006;57:1–18.
137. Plate K, Breier G, Weich H, Risau W. Vascular endothelial growth factor is a potential tumour angiogenesis factor in human gliomas in vivo. Nature 1992;359:845–8.
138. Stefanik DF, Rizkalla LR, Soi A, Goldblatt SA, Rizkalla WM. Acidic and basic fibroblast growth factors are present in glioblastoma multiforme. Cancer Res 1991;51:5760–5.
139. Schmidt NO, Westphal M, Hagel C, et al. Levels of vascular endothelial growth factor, hepatocyte growth factor/scatter factor and basic fibroblast growth factor in human gliomas and their relation to angiogenesis. Int J Cancer 1999;84:10–8.
140. Millauer B, Shawver LK, Plate KH, Risau W, Ullrich A. Glioblastoma growth inhibited in vivo by a dominant-negative Flk-1 mutant. Nature 1994;367:576–9.
141. Holash J, Maisonpierre PC, Compton D, et al. Vessel cooption, regression, and growth in tumors mediated by angiopoietins and VEGF. Science 1999;284:1994–8.
142. Kerbel RS. Tumor angiogenesis. N Engl J Med 2008;358:2039–49.
143. Rich JN. Cancer stem cells in radiation resistance. Cancer Res 2007;67:8980–4.
144. Bao S, Wu Q, Sathornsumetee S, et al. Stem cell-like glioma cells promote tumor angiogenesis through vascular endothelial growth factor. Cancer Res 2006;66:7843–8.
145. Calabrese C, Poppleton H, Kocak M, et al. A perivascular niche for brain tumor stem cells. Cancer Cell 2007;11:69–82.
146. Gilbertson RJ, Rich JN. Making a tumour's bed: glioblastoma stem cells and the vascular niche. Nat Rev Cancer 2007;7:733–6.
147. Folkins C, Man S, Xu P, Shaked Y, Hicklin DJ, Kerbel RS. Anticancer therapies combining antiangiogenic and tumor cell cytotoxic effects reduce the tumor stem-like cell fraction in glioma xenograft tumors. Cancer Res 2007;67:3560–4.
148. Norden AD, Drappatz J, Wen PY. Novel anti-angiogenic therapies for malignant gliomas. Lancet Neurol 2008;7:1152–60.
149. Fine HA, Wen PY, Maher EA, et al. Phase II trial of thalidomide and carmustine for patients with recurrent high-grade gliomas. J Clin Oncol 2003;21:2299–304.
150. Norden AD, Young GS, Setayesh K, et al. Bevacizumab for recurrent malignant gliomas: efficacy, toxicity, and patterns of recurrence. Neurology 2008;70:779–87.
151. Pope WB, Lai A, Nghiemphu P, Mischel P, Cloughesy TF. MRI in patients with high-grade gliomas treated with bevacizumab and chemotherapy. Neurology 2006;66:1258–60.
152. Stark Vance V. Bevacizumab (Avastin®) and CPT-11 (Camptosar®) in the Treatment of Relapsed Malignant Glioma [abstract]. Neuro-oncol 2005;7:369.
153. Nghiemphu PL, Liu W, Lee Y, et al. Bevacizumab and chemotherapy for recurrent glioblastoma: a single-institution experience. Neurology 2009;72:1217–22.
154. Wagner SA, Desjardins A, Reardon DA, et al. Update on survival from the original phase II trial of bevacizumab and irinotecan in recurrent malignant gliomas [abstract]. J Clin Oncol 2008;26:2021.
155. Vredenburgh JJ, Desjardins A, Herndon 2nd JE, et al. Phase II trial of bevacizumab and irinotecan in recurrent malignant glioma. Clin Cancer Res 2007;13:1253–9.
156. Vredenburgh JJ, Desjardins A, Herndon 2nd JE, et al. Bevacizumab plus irinotecan in recurrent glioblastoma multiforme. J Clin Oncol 2007;25:4722–9.
157. Cloughesy TF, Prados MD, Mikkelsen T, et al. A phase II, randomized, non-comparative clinical trial of the effect of bevacizumab (BV) alone or in combination with irinotecan (CPT) on 6-month progression free survival (PFS6) in recurrent, treatment-refractory glioblastoma (GBM) [abstract]. J Clin Oncol 2008;26:2010b.
158. Kreisl TN, Kim L, Moore K, et al. Phase II trial of single-agent bevacizumab followed by bevacizumab plus irinotecan at tumor progression in recurrent glioblastoma. J Clin Oncol 2009;27:740–5.
159. Lai A, Filka E, McGibbon B, et al. Phase II Pilot Study of Bevacizumab in Combination With Temozolomide and Regional Radiation Therapy for Up-Front Treatment of Patients With Newly Diagnosed Glioblastoma Multiforme: Interim Analysis of Safety and Tolerability. Int J Radiat Oncol Biol Phys 2008.
160. Norden AD, Drappatz J, Wen PY. Antiangiogenic therapy in malignant gliomas. Curr Opin Oncol 2008;20:652–61.
161. Batchelor T, Sorensen AG, Ancukiewicz M, et al. A phase II trial of AZD2171 (cediranib), an oral pan-VEGF receptor tyrosine kinase inhibitor, in patients with recurrent glioblastoma [abstract]. J Clin Oncol 2007;25:2001.

162. Batchelor TT, Sorensen AG, di Tomaso E, et al. AZD2171, a pan-VEGF receptor tyrosine kinase inhibitor, normalizes tumor vasculature and alleviates edema in glioblastoma patients. Cancer Cell 2007;11:83–95.
163. Jain RK. Normalization of tumor vasculature: an emerging concept in antiangiogenic therapy. Science 2005;307:58–62.
164. Bergers G, Hanahan D. Modes of resistance to anti-angiogenic therapy. Nat Rev Cancer 2008;8:592–603.
165. Ellis LM, Hicklin DJ. Pathways mediating resistance to vascular endothelial growth factor-targeted therapy. Clin Cancer Res 2008;14:6371–5.
166. Willett CG, Boucher Y, Duda DG, et al. Surrogate markers for antiangiogenic therapy and dose-limiting toxicities for bevacizumab with radiation and chemotherapy: continued experience of a phase I trial in rectal cancer patients. J Clin Oncol 2005;23:8136–9.
167. Chi A, Norden AD, Wen PY. Inhibition of angiogenesis and invasion in malignant gliomas. Expert Rev Anticancer Ther 2007;7:1537–60.
168. Kunkel P, Ulbricht U, Bohlen P, et al. Inhibition of glioma angiogenesis and growth in vivo by systemic treatment with a monoclonal antibody against vascular endothelial growth factor receptor-2. Cancer Res 2001;61:6624–8.
169. Lamszus K, Kunkel P, Westphal M. Invasion as limitation to anti-angiogenic glioma therapy. Acta Neurochir Suppl 2003;88:169–77.
170. Rubenstein JL, Kim J, Ozawa T, et al. Anti-VEGF antibody treatment of glioblastoma prolongs survival but results in increased vascular cooption. Neoplasia 2000;2:306–14.
171. Paez-Ribes M, Allen E, Hudock J, et al. Antiangiogenic therapy elicits malignant progression of tumors to increased local invasion and distant metastasis. Cancer Cell 2009;15:220–31.
172. Lassman AB, Iwamoto FM, Gutin PH, Abrey LE. Patterns of relapse and prognosis after bevacizumab (BEV) failure in recurrent glioblastoma (GBM) [abstract]. J Clin Oncol 2008;26:2028.
173. Zuniga RM, Torcuator R, Doyle T, et al. Retrospective analysis of patterns of recurrence seen on MRI in patients with recurrent glioblastoma multiforme treated with bevacizumab plus irinotecan [abstract]. J Clin Oncol 2008;26:13013.
174. Narayana A, Raza S, Golfinos JG, et al. Bevacizumab therapy in recurrent high grade glioma: Impact on local control and survival [abstract]. J Clin Oncol 2008;26:13000.
175. Fulci G, Chiocca EA. The status of gene therapy for brain tumors. Expert Opin Biol Ther 2007;7:197–208.
176. Aghi M, Rabkin S, Martuza RL. Effect of chemotherapy-induced DNA repair on oncolytic herpes simplex viral replication. J Natl Cancer Inst 2006;98:38–50.
177. Nakamizo A, Marini F, Amano T, et al. Human bone marrow-derived mesenchymal stem cells in the treatment of gliomas. Cancer Res 2005;65:3307–18.
178. Mamelak A, Rosenfeld S, Bucholz R, et al. Phase I single-dose study of intracavitary-administered iodine-131-TM-601 in adults with recurrent high-grade glioma. J Clin Oncol 2006;24:3644–50.
179. Ferguson S, Lesniak MS. Convection enhanced drug delivery of novel therapeutic agents to malignant brain tumors. Curr Drug Deliv 2007;4:169–80.
180. Sampson JH, Archer GE, Bigner DD, et al. Effect of egfrviii-targeted vaccine (CDX-110) on immune response and TTP when given with simultaneous standard and continuous temozolomide in patients with GBM. J Clin Oncol 2008;26:2011.
181. Nemunaitis J, Jahan T, Ross H, et al. Phase 1/2 trial of autologous tumor mixed with an allogeneic GVAX vaccine in advanced-stage non-small-cell lung cancer. Cancer Gene Ther 2006;13:555–62.

6 Low Grade Astrocytomas

LAWRENCE D. RECHT • HANNES VOGEL • GRIFFITH R. HARSH

Introduction

In the 1970s, 80% of nonglioblastoma gliomas were considered to be diffuse astrocytomas. The percentages of oligodendrogliomas and oligoastrocytomas have risen progressively subsequently; these tumors now account for 65% of grade II primary glioma diagnoses in the SEER database from 1994 to 2001.[1] This increase reflects not a biological change, but, instead, an evolution in pathological interpretation prompted by the identification of a favorable-risk chemosensitive oligodendroglioma; this has created an "incentive" to find oligodendroglial elements and to determine whether there are deletions in 1p and 19q.

Each revision of the WHO classification schema, most recently published in 2007, alters the relative incidences of astrocytomas; with each version, new types are added and old ones modified. The term "low-grade glioma" should be avoided since it lumps together almost two dozen WHO grade I and grade II glial neoplasms, many of which have significantly different biological properties, prognoses, and optimal therapies. The most common entities are WHO grade I pilocytic astrocytomas (PA) and gangliogliomas, WHO grade II diffuse astrocytomas, and the favorable-risk 1p/19q deleted oligodendrogliomas.

In this chapter, we will focus primarily on WHO grade I pilocytic astrocytomas and WHO grade II diffuse astrocytomas, and emphasize that they represent very distinct clinical entities. The oligodendrogliomas are covered in another chapter in this monograph.

Diffuse Astrocytoma, WHO Grade II

PATHOLOGICAL AND MOLECULAR ASPECTS

Diffuse astrocytoma is the most common astrocytoma. Because its cells produce neuroglial fibrils, this tumor is firm and rubbery. Its epicenter is typically in white matter. Cytologically, the more common *fibrillary* subtype is composed of atypical fibrillary astrocytes with hyperchromatic, elongated nuclei that appear "naked" within a fibrillary background or display discernable eosinophilic cytoplasmic processes. Fine and coarse neuroglial fibrils occupy the matrix and lie in random orientation among the cells from which they are derived (Figure 6-1). Mitotic activity is, by definition, absent in small biopsies and rare even in large resection specimens. Vasculature is inconspicuous, and necrosis is characteristically absent. Two pathological variants of the diffuse astrocytoma are the *protoplasmic* and the *gemistocytic*. The former is composed of cells resembling protoplasmic astrocytes. Protoplasmic tumors generally involve the cerebral cortex. *Gemistocytic* astrocytomas, by contrast, have cells with prominent eosinophilic cytoplasm that imparts a distended or globoid appearance and strong glial fibrillary acidic protein (GFAP) immunopositivity.

Unlike oligodendrogliomas, which frequently demonstrate losses of 1p and 19q and rarely have p53 mutations, many WHO grade II diffuse astrocytomas demonstrate loss of chromosome 17p, and roughly half harbor p53 mutations.[2,3] The prognostic value of a p53 mutation is debated.[2,4,5]

Many WHO grade II diffuse astrocytomas harbor an alteration of a component of either the RB1 or the TP53 pathway, but few have alterations in both pathways. One study of 46 patients found a defect in the TP53 pathway in 70% and in the Rb pathway in 13%.[6] The authors concluded that disruption of either the TP53 or the p14ARF pathway is frequent in low-grade astrocytomas and correlates with an unfavorable clinical course.

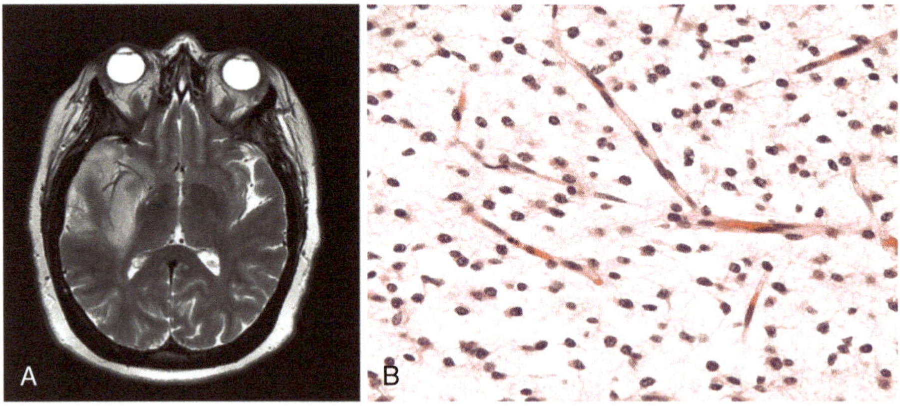

Figure 6-1 Diffuse Fibrillary Astrocytoma. A, Characteristic MR imaging appearance of Grade II fibrillary astrocytoma, demonstrating T2 hyperintensity with minimal mass effect. The infiltrating nature of these neoplasms makes complete resection difficult. **B,** Photomicrograph of a WHO grade II diffuse fibrillary astrocytoma, characterized by slight nuclear atypia, delicate vasculature in a fibrillar background, without mitotic activity or necrosis.

Even more common in WHO grade II diffuse astrocytomas is abnormal p53 protein immunoreactivity, which can occur even when mutations are not present.[2] PDGFr-alpha overexpression is also common[7] in these tumors.

A recent study comparing WHO grade II diffuse astrocytomas with primary and secondary GBMs using cDNA array analysis noted that WHO grade II diffuse astrocytomas had highly specific and homogenous expression profiles compared with the less specific and heterogenous profiles of primary GBMs; those of secondary GBM were intermediate.[8] The distinguishing factor for primary GBMs was the upregulation of genes involved in angiogenesis. Such genes were not upregulated in WHO grade II diffuse astrocytomas, suggesting that angiogenesis is intimately linked with aggressive behavior.

CLINICAL ASPECTS

WHO grade II diffuse astrocytomas are generally slowly growing, locally infiltrative tumors in young or middle-aged adults.[9,10] They rarely metastasize within[11] or outside[12] the CNS. They usually present as nonenhancing lesions on MRI (Figure 6-1). They are best viewed as "diffuse"; in other words, they are infiltrative, ill-defined tumors that can spread for many centimeters throughout the cortex and along white matter tracts, perivascular spaces, and periventricular ependyma in the form of secondary structures of Scherer, namely in perivascular and perineuronal locations. Regional heterogeneities in morphology, proliferative activity, ploidy and genetic aberrations are common.[13] Although some patients survive for decades,[14,15] these tumors have a propensity to evolve gradually into more aggressive anaplastic gliomas or GBMs,[16,17] especially in older patients.[16]

Patients with supratentorial WHO grade II diffuse astrocytomas have a much higher incidence of seizures as a presenting symptom than do those with higher grade gliomas. Epilepsy is by far the most common and important symptom in WHO grade II diffuse astrocytomas. Seizures occur as a presenting symptom in approximately 50% of cases, and have a prevalence greater than 80%.[18] Furthermore, patients with WHO grade II diffuse astrocytomas often suffer from neuropsychological and psychological problems that are aggravated by epilepsy and its treatment.[19]

The seizures originate not from the mass lesion but from adjacent brain tissue.[20,21] Nevertheless, both radiation therapy[22] and lesionectomy[21,23,24] may significantly reduce or even eliminate medically refractory seizures.

Anticonvulsants, even multiple agents in combination, fail to control seizures in up to 50% of patients.[19,25] They may also impair cognitive functioning.[19] Since differences in efficacy are small, clinicians should choose an anticonvulsant with few side effects. Due to their effects on cytochrome P450 metabolism, the potential for interaction between anticonvulsants and other drugs (e.g., chemotherapeutics) can make it difficult to maintain adequate drug levels. Newer nonenzyme-inducing antiepileptic drugs such as levetiracetam and lamotrigine have equal efficacy, fewer side effects, and less frequent drug interactions than the more conventional agents, and are thus preferable to phenytoin and phenobarbital.

In a recent review of patients with intractable epilepsy and supratentorial tumors, including many with WHO grade II diffuse astrocytomas, improved seizure outcome was associated with a short duration of epilepsy before surgery, a single EEG focus, and the absence of hippocampal sclerosis or cortical dysplasia.[26]

The authors concluded that tumor resection was indicated for seizure control and prevention of malignant progression.

PROGNOSTIC FEATURES

Before CT scanning became readily available, reported median survival times for patients with WHO grade II diffuse astrocytomas were 5 years or less.[27–30] More recent studies, however, show much longer median survival times, usually between 7 and 9 years, and 5- and 10-year survival rates range from 25% to 97% and 10% to 63% respectively.[14,17,31–37] Two explanations have been offered for this longer reported survival: either patients are being diagnosed earlier or they are being more effectively treated. One recent study[38] noted that use of newer imaging methods added no more than 6 months to the duration of survival following imaging diagnosis. Because radiation therapy has not been shown to improve survival, the authors speculated that longer survival resulted from more effective surgery, although they did note that macroscopically complete resections did not significantly improve survival duration as compared to less complete resections.

The outcome for patients with low-grade glioma (LGG) is intimately linked to anaplastic transformation. Pathologic progression of a diffuse astrocytoma to GBM produces an abrupt change in clinical behavior. The incidence of malignant transformation has been reported in various clinical studies to range from 13% to 86%.[28,39–43] Because many of these series included previously treated patients, the natural history of this transformation is difficult to determine. A recent study reviewed 40 patients with progressive tumors who had undergone surgery but no further therapy for at least 3 months after the diagnosis of diffuse astrocytoma was made.[44] Half had grade III or IV tumors when a second biopsy or operation was performed. Patients with progression had longer median times to reoperation (47 months vs. 22.5 months). The authors noted that complete resection delayed the time to reoperation but did not affect whether progression occurred.

The prognosis of adult patients with diffuse astrocytomas is largely determined by the inherent biology of the tumor[27,32,37,43,45] and patient age.[14,32,37,39,46,47] Adverse prognostic factors include poor performance status, tumor contrast enhancement, cognitive dysfunction, focal neurological deficits, and steroid dependency.[14,27,32,37,39,43,46,48] In one study of several hundred patients accrued to two EORTC studies, multivariate analysis identified age greater than 40 years, astrocytoma histology subtype, largest diameter of tumor greater than 6 cm, tumor crossing the midline, and neurologic deficit present prior to surgery as the most important poor prognostic factors.[49]

TREATMENT ISSUES

Treatment options include surgical resection, radiation, and chemotherapy. That acceptable practice patterns range from observation to radical resection plus radiochemotherapy exemplifies the controversial aspects of this tumor type.

Surgery provides tissue for histopathological analysis and can be helpful in relieving mass effect. However, because of the infiltrative nature of this tumor, gross total resection is often not possible. Nevertheless, most neurosurgeons favor attempting maximal resection at the time of surgery.[49–52] However, it must be emphasized that these observations are difficult to interpret because of a bias in comparing these patients to those for whom it was not possible to do a maximal resection; therefore, the data should not be considered definitive and less extensive surgeries or even observation can still be justified.

Radiation therapy is also frequently advocated for diffuse astrocytomas, but the data supporting this approach are weak. An important study from the EORTC examined the effect of either immediate or delayed RT (54 Gy in 6 weeks) in a randomized study that included over 300 patients.[53,54] Although immediate RT prolonged progression-free survival and seemed to result in better seizure control, no difference in survival was noted. The absence of a survival benefit suggested that although RT seemed to slow progression, it did not avert transformation into more aggressive GBMs. In addition, escalating the RT dose does not improve survival for these patients.[46,50]

Thus, there are no firm recommendations concerning RT in diffuse astrocytoma. Generally, clinicians use prognostic factors to choose patients who might benefit from immediate RT. These include persistence of significant disease-associated neurological dysfunction (including seizures), recurrent or progressive disease, age over 40, tumor size greater than 6 cm or crossing midline, and MIB proliferation index greater than 3%.[49,50,55]

There is no evidence that administration of *chemotherapy* prolongs survival in patients with diffuse astrocytoma.[56] However, a recent report from the RTOG suggested some improvement in progression-free survival when RT was combined with procarbazine, CCNU, and vincristine (PCV), although 5-year survival was not significantly altered.[57]

Pilocytic Astrocytoma

PATHOLOGICAL ASPECTS

Pilocytic astrocytomas (PA) differ microscopically from fibrillary astrocytomas in that there is a tendency for biphasic morphology, alternating between compact perivascular and microcystic regions. The hallmark, although quite nonspecific, is the piloid or hairlike neoplastic astrocyte, appearing as a slender unipolar cell. Tumor cells remote from blood vessels have a rarefied and sparsely cellular appearance and tend to undergo microcystic degeneration. Rosenthal fibers and eosinophilic granular bodies are commonly seen and are useful pathological hallmarks in differentiating these tumors from other astrocytomas (Figure 6-2).

CLINICAL ASPECTS

PAs are well-circumscribed tumors that occur mostly in children. They occur most frequently in the cerebellum (Figure 6-2), but also arise in supratentorial regions, chiefly the optic-hypothalamic region, as well as dorsally exophytic brainstem lesions.

PAs are frequently cystic and well-demarcated radiographically and almost always enhance on MRI[58] due to the paradoxical prominence of microvasculature, an important histological feature distinguishing the PA from a WHO grade II glioma.

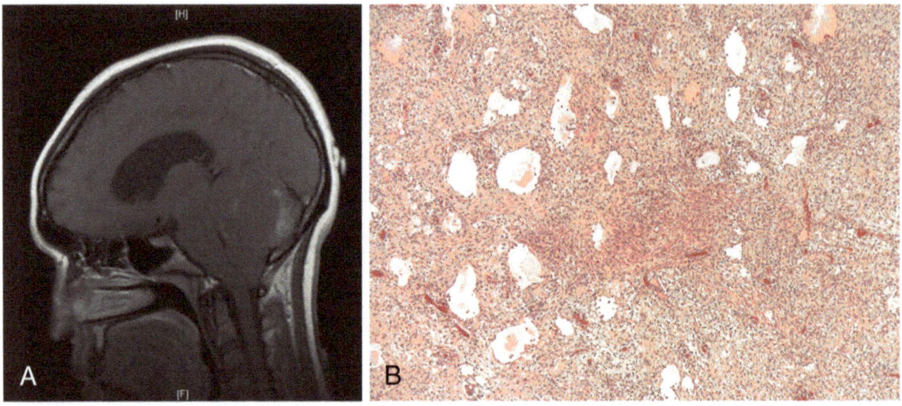

Figure 6-2 Pilocytic astrocytoma. A, Characteristic imaging appearance of cystic mass surrounded by eccentric enhancement. This is counterintuitive because contrast enhancement is usually considered a hallmark of aggressive glioma behavior; however, PAs typically enhance avidly. This is because enhancement is due to prominent microvasculature that would not be seen in a WHO grade II astrocytoma. **B,** Low-power photomicrograph of a pilocytic astrocytoma exhibiting the typical biphasic morphology, with dense eosinophilic regions alternating with microcystic or looser areas.

PROGNOSTIC ASPECTS

PAs are distinguished from WHO grade II through IV gliomas by their excellent prognosis; over 95% of patients survive 10 years or more.[59] Furthermore, they are much less likely to transform into GBM, although there are several reports of such an occurrence many years after diagnosis. Multicentric spread has also been reported, especially with hypothalamic tumors.[60]

TREATMENT ISSUES

Surgery is the primary treatment. Since prognosis is excellent, even after partial resection, irradiation minimally impacts survival or the risk of tumor progression.[59] Additionally, since RT may be associated with eventual malignant transformation of PAs,[61] RT should be reserved for symptomatic patients with extensive residual disease.

Chemotherapy has been used to treat young patients with PAs at inaccessible sites such as the optic pathways,[62] but evidence supporting a routine role for this modality in PAs is lacking.

Other Astrocytoma Subtypes

PLEOMORPHIC XANTHOASTROCYTOMA (PXA) WHO GRADE II

Once termed *giant cell glioblastoma* or *monstrocellular sarcoma*, PXAs were officially recognized as a distinct entity in the 1993 WHO classification. They account for less than 1% of astrocytic neoplasms. Although their histological features include marked cellular pleomorphism, nuclear atypia and the presence of bizarre, multinucleate giant cells (Figure 6-3), they behave in a comparatively benign fashion. Long-term survival is common following complete resection,

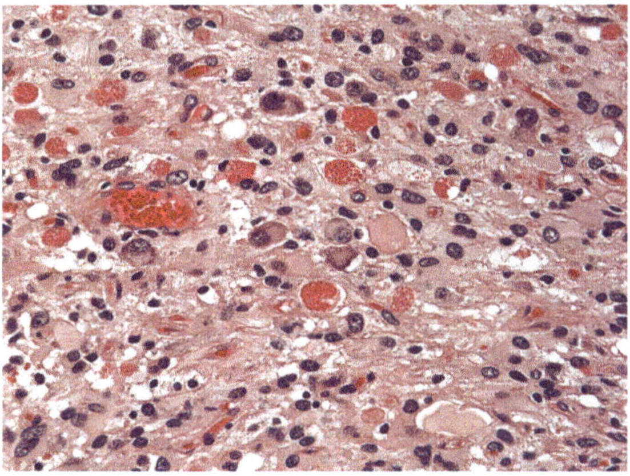

Figure 6-3 **Pleomorphic xanthoastrocytoma (PXA), WHO grade II.** Prominent cytological pleomorphism with a focal abundance of eosinophilic granular bodies (EGBs).

which is generally possible due to their superficial location, relative circumscription, and cyst/mural architecture.[63–65] Nonetheless, although the 10-year survival rate for patients is greater than 70%, PXAs are distinguished from the truly benign astrocytomas, such as PAs, by their tendency to recur and to transform into more anaplastic forms (as often as 20% of the time). They are thus assigned a WHO grade of II. Pathological correlates of this more malignant behavior include less pleomorphism and a higher mitotic rate (more than 5 mitoses/HPF).[65]

SUBEPENDYMAL GIANT CELL ASTROCYTOMAS (SEGA) WHO GRADE I

SEGAs occur in approximately 5% to 10% of patients with tuberous sclerosis, an autosomal dominant, multisystem, neurocutaneous syndrome characterized by a triad of seizures, adenoma sebaceum, and mental retardation. They are presumed to arise from the distinctive cortical tubers that are characteristics of these tumors. Although the characteristic giant cells are of mixed glioneuronal lineage,[66] SEGAs are still grouped with the astrocytomas. They are histologically benign (Figure 6-4), although their location in the lateral ventricles at the level of the foramen of Munro can often result in hydrocephalus. Surgery provides for a better outcome when performed before, rather than after, obstructive hydrocephalus occurs.[67,68]

Although most studies have addressed the SEGAs in the context of tuberous sclerosis, at least half of SEGAs occur sporadically.[69] It is not clear whether spontaneously occurring SEGAs are as benign, as several cases have been reported wherein spontaneous SEGAs behaved aggressively.

NEW ASTROCYTOMA VARIANTS

The fourth edition of the WHO classification of CNS tumors identifies two new subtypes of astrocytoma.[70] The *angiocentric glioma* is a WHO grade I neoplasm that occurs in children and young adults. It presents as a hemispheric mass in a patient with epilepsy. It does not enhance on neuroimaging. Pathologically, tumors are composed of bipolar cells intimately associated with blood vessels, often oriented perpendicular to the vascular lumen. They are probably curable by surgery.[71,72]

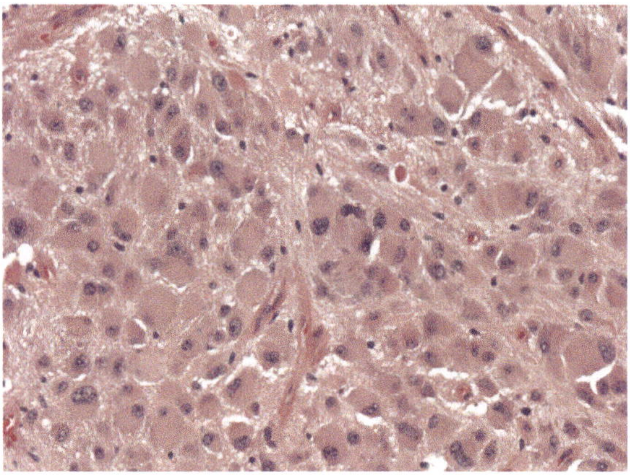

Figure 6-4 Subependymal giant cell astrocytoma (SEGA) WHO grade I. The dominant feature of SEGAs is the presence of large cells with hybrid features between gemistocytic astrocytes, with eccentric eosinophilic cytoplasm and neurons with large, round nuclei bearing prominent nucleoli.

The *pilomyxoid astrocytoma* is a variant of the PA that often arises in the hypothalamus.[73] Pilomyxoid astrocytomas are well circumscribed on MRI and typically enhance. Histologically, this tumor is dominated by a hypercellular monomorphous population of piloid cells without Rosenthal fibers and eosinophilic granular bodies (EGBs).

Despite their being a PA variant, these tumors are often aggressive; in the new classification schema, they are therefore classified as WHO grade II neoplasms.[74–76]

ASTROCYTOMAS IN NF1 PATIENTS

Neurofibromatosis type 1 is the most common inherited neurocutaneous syndrome, whose manifestations usually include CNS and peripheral neural tumors. The most common site of CNS tumor origin is the optic pathways, and most optic tumors are PAs. However, NFI patients may also develop diffuse astrocytomas in later life.[77,78]

PAs in NF1 have a distinctive predilection to involve the optic nerve, optic chiasm, and hypothalamus. In young patients with NF1,15% to 20% have an optic PA.[79] Tumors arising in these areas, even those with high mitotic activity, are often indolent, suggesting that this location affects clinical behavior.

Patients with NF1 also develop tumors, in other locations, with indeterminate features. They are low grade but lack typical PA features and can be diffusely infiltrative; they tend to behave similarly to the PA.[77] Diffusely infiltrating astrocytomas are rare, but their frequency rises with age.[78] They can resemble a GBM. While RT is discouraged for PAs, it appears necessary for these more aggressive infiltrative astrocytomas, especially those with malignant histology.

REFERENCES

1. Claus EB, Black PM. Survival rates and patterns of care for patients diagnosed with supratentorial low-grade gliomas: data from the SEER program, 1973–2001. Cancer 2006;106:1358–63.
2. Watanabe K, Sato K, Biernat W, et al. Incidence and timing of p53 mutations during astrocytoma progression in patients with multiple biopsies. Clin Cancer Res 1997;3:523–30.

3. Reifenberger J, Ring GU, Gies U, et al. Analysis of p53 mutation and epidermal growth factor receptor amplification in recurrent gliomas with malignant progression. J Neuropathol Exp Neurol 1996;55:822–31.
4. Peraud A, Kreth FW, Wiestler OD, et al. Prognostic impact of TP53 mutations and p53 protein overexpression in surpratentorial WHO grade II astrocytomas and oligoastrocytoma. Clin Cancer Res 2002;8:1117–24.
5. Ishii N, Tada M, Hamou M-F, et al. Cells with TP53 mutations in low grade astrocytic tumors evolve clonally to malignancy and are an unfavorable prognostic factor. Oncogene 1999;18:5870–8.
6. Watanabe T, Katayama Y, Yoshino A, et al. Deregulation of the TP53/p14(ARF) tumor suppressor pathway in low-grade diffuse astrocytomas and its influence on clinical course. Clin Cancer Res 2003;9:4884–90.
7. Hermanson M, Funa K, Koopmann J, et al. Association of loss of heterozygosity on chromosome 17p with high platelet-derived growth factor a expression in human malignant gliomas. Cancer Res 1996;56:164–71.
8. Godard S, Getz G, Delorenzi M, et al. Classification of human astrocytic gliomas on the basis of gene expression: A correlated group of genes with angiogenic activity emerges as a strong predictor of subtypes. Cancer Res 2003;63:6613–25.
9. McLendon RE, Enterline DS, Tien RD, et al. Tumors of central neuroepithelial origin. In: Bigner DD, McLendon RE, Bruner JM, editors. Russel and Rubinstein's Pathology of Tumors of the Nervous System. 6th ed. New York: Arnold; 1998. p. 307–572.
10. Kleihues P, Davis RL, Ohgaki H, et al. Diffuse astrocytoma. In: Kleihues P, Cavenee WK, editors. Pathology and Genetics of Tumours of the Nervous System. Lyon: IARC Press; 2000. p. 22–6.
11. Laerum OD, Mork SJ. Mechanisms of altered growth control: invasion and metastasis. In: Bigner DD, McLendon RE, Bruner JM, editors. Russell and Rubinstein's Pathology of Tumors of the Nervous System, vol. 1. 6th ed New York: Arnold; 1998. p. 117–40.
12. Hoffman HJ, Duffner PK. Extraneural metastases of central nervous system tumors. Cancer 1985;56:1778–82.
13. Perry A. Pathology of low-grade gliomas: An update of emerging concepts. Neuro-Oncology 2003;5:168–78.
14. Bauman G, Lote K, Larson D, et al. Pretreatment factors predict overall survival for patients with low-grade glioma: A recursive partitioning analysis. Int J Rad Oncol Biol Phys 1999;45:923–9.
15. Davis FG, Freels S, Grutsch J, et al. Survival rates in patients with primary malignant brain tumors stratified by patient age and tumor histologic type: an analysis based on Surveillance, Epidemiology, and End Results (SEER) data, 1973-1991. J Neurosurg 1998;88:1–10.
16. Shafqat S, Hedley-Whyte ET, Henson JW. Age-dependent rate of anaplastic transformation in low-grade astrocytoma. Neurology 1999;52:867–9.
17. Vertosick FT, Selker RG, Arena VC. Survival of patients with well-differentiated astrocytomas diagnosed in the era of computed tomography. Neurosurgery 1991;28:496–501.
18. Lote K, Stenwig AE, Skullerud K, Hirschberg H. Prevalence and prognostic significance of epilepsy in patients with gliomas. Eur J Cancer 1998;34:98–102.
19. Klein M, Engelberts NHJ, van der Ploeg HM, et al. Epilepsy in low-grade gliomas: The impact on cognitive function and quality of life. Ann Neurol 2003;54:514–20.
20. Haglund MM, Berger MS, Kunkel DD, et al. Changes in gamma-aminobutyric acid and somatostatin in epileptic cortex associated with low-grade gliomas. J Neurosurg 1992;77:209–16.
21. Berger MS, Ghatan S, Haglund MM, et al. Low-grade gliomas associated with intractable epilepsy: seizure outcome utilizing electrocorticography during tumor resection. J Neurosurg 1993;79:62–9.
22. Rogers LR, Morris HH, Lupica K. Effect of cranial irradiation on seizure frequency in adults with low-grade astrocytoma and medically intractable epilepsy. Neurology 1993;43:1599–601.
23. Zentner J, Hufnagel A, Wolf HK, et al. Surgical treatment of neoplasms associated with medically intractable epilepsy. Neurosurgery 1997;41:378–86.
24. Hennessy MJ, Elwes RD, Honavar M, et al. Predictors of outcome and pathological considerations in the surgical treatment of intractable epilepsy associated with temporal lobe lesions. J Neurol Neurosurg Psychiatr 2001;70:450–8.
25. Semah F, Picot MC, Adam C, et al. Is the underlying cause of epilepsy a major prognostic factor for recurrence. Neurology 1998;51:1256–62.
26. Luyken C, Blumcke H, Fimmers R, et al. The spectrum of long-term epilepsy-associated tumors: Long-term seizure and tumor outcome and neurosurgical aspects. Epilepsia 2003;44:822–30.
27. Soffietti R, Chio A, Giordana MT, et al. Prognostic factors in well-differentiated cerebral astrocytomas in the adult. Neurosurgery 1989;24:686–92.

28. Laws ER, Taylor WF, Clifton MB, Okazaki H. Neurosurgical management of low-grade astrocytoma of the cerebral hemispheres. J Neurosurg 1984;61:665–73.
29. Fazekas JT. Treatment of grades I and II brain astrocytomas. The role of radiotherapy. Intl J Rad Oncol Biol Phys 1977;2:661–6.
30. Silverman C, Marks JE. Prognostic significance of contrast enhancement in low-grade astrocytomas of the adult cerebrum. Radiology 1981;139:211–3.
31. Leighton C, Fisher B, Bauman G, et al. Supratentorial low-grade glioma in adults: An analysis of prognostic factors and timing of radiation. J Clin Oncol 1997;15:1294–301.
32. Lote K, Egeland T, Hager B, et al. Survival, prognostic factors, and therapeutic efficacy in low-grade glioma: A retrospective study in 379 patients. J Clin Oncol 1997;15:3129–40.
33. McCormack BM, Miller DC, Budzilovich GN, et al. Treatment and survival of low-grade astrocytoma in adults—1977–1988. Neurosurgery 1992;31:636–42.
34. Medbery CA, Straus KL, Steinberg SM, et al. Low-grade astrocytomas: Treatment results and prognostic variables. Intl J Rad Oncol Biol Phys 1988;15:837–41.
35. Scerrati M, Roselli R, Iacoangeli M, et al. Prognostic factors in low grade (WHO grade II) gliomas of the cerebral hemispheres: the role of surgery. J Neurol Neurosurg Psychiatr 1996;61:291–6.
36. Shaw EG, Scheithauer BW, Gilbertson DT, et al. Postoperative radiotherapy of supratentorial low-grade gliomas. Intl J Rad Oncol Biol Phys 1989;16:663–8.
37. van Veelen MLC, Avezaat CJJ, Kros JM, et al. Supratentorial low grade astrocytoma: prognostic factors, dedifferentiation, and the issue of early versus late surgery. J Neurol Neurosurg Psychiatr 1998;64:581–7.
38. Johannesen TB, Langmark F, Lote K. Progress in long-term survival in adult patients with supratentorial low-grade tumors: a population-based study of 993 patients in whom tumors were diagnosed between 1970 and 1993. J Neurosurg 2003;99:854–62.
39. Piepmeier JM. Observations on the current treatment of low-grade astrocytic tumors of the cerebral hemispheres. J Neurosurg 1987;67:177–81.
40. Afra D, Muller W, Benoist G, et al. Supratentorial recurrences of gliomas. Results of reoperations on astrocytomas and oligodendrogliomas. Acta Neurochir 1978;43:217–27.
41. Muller W, Afra D, Schroder R. Supratentorial recurrences of gliomas. Morphological studies in relation to time intervals with astrocytomas. Acta Neurochir 1977;37:75–91.
42. Muller W, Afra D, Schroder R. Supratentorial recurrences of gliomas. Morphological studies in relation to time intervals with oligodendrogliomas. Acta Neurochir 1977;39:15–25.
43. Philippon JH, Clemenceau SH, Fauchon FH, Foncin JF. Supratentorial low-grade astrocytomas in adults. Neurosurgery 1993;32:554–9.
44. Schmidt M, Berger MS, Lamborn K, et al. Repeated operations for infiltrative low-grade gliomas without intervening therapy. J Neurosurg 2003;98:1165–9.
45. Shaw EG, Scheithauer BW, O'Fallon J. Supratentorial gliomas: a comparative study by grade and histologic type. J Neuro-Oncol 1997;31:273–8.
46. Karim AB, Maat B, Hatlevoll R, et al. A randomized trial on dose-response in radiation therapy of low-grade cerebral glioma: European Organization for Research and Treatment of Cancer (EORTC) study 22844. Intl J Rad Oncol Biol Phys 1996;36:549–56.
47. Vecht CJ. The influence of age on treatment decisions in low grade glioma. J Neurol Neurosurg Psychiatr 1993;56:1259–64.
48. Lote K, Egeland T, Hager B, et al. Prognostic significance of CT contrast enhancement within histological subgroups of intracranial glioma. J Neuro-Oncol 1998;40:161.
49. Pignatti F, van den Bent M, Curran D, et al. Prognostic factors for survival in adult patients with cerebral low-grade glioma. J Clin Oncol 2002;20:2076–84.
50. Shaw E, Arusell R, Scheithauer B, et al. Prospective randomized trial of low- versus high-dose radiation therapy in adults with supratentorial low-grade glioma: Initial report of a North Central Cancer Treatment Group/Radiation Therapy Oncology Group/Eastern Cooperative Oncology Group study. J Clin Oncol 2002;20:2267–76.
51. Keles GE, Lamborn KR, Berger MS. Low-grade hemispheric gliomas in adults: a critical review of extent of resection as a factor influencing outcome. J Neurosurg 2001;95:735–45.
52. Smith JS, Chang EF, Lamborn KR, et al. Role of extent of resection in the long-term outcome of low-grade hemispheric gliomas. J Clin Oncol 2008;26:1338–45.
53. Karim AB, Afra D, Cornu P, et al. Randomized trial on the efficacy of radiotherapy for cerebral low-grade glioma in the adult: European Organization for Research and Treatment of Cancer Study 22845 with the Medical Research Council Study BR04: An interim analysis. Intl J Rad Oncol Biol Phys 2002;52:316–24.

54. van den Bent M, Afra D, De Witte O, et al. Long-term efficacy of early versus delayed radiotherapy for low-grade astrocytoma and oligodendroglioma in adults: the EORTC 22845 randomised trial. Lancet 2005;366:985–90.
55. Papagikos MA, Shaw EG, Stieber VW. Lessons learned from randomised clinical trials in adult low-grade glioma. Lancet Oncol 2005;6:240–4.
56. Eyre HJ, Crowley JJ, Townsend JJ, et al. A randomized trial of radiotherapy versus radiotherapy plus CCNU for incompletely resected low-grade gliomas: a Southwest Oncology Group study. J Neurosurg 1993;78:909–14.
57. Shaw EG, Wang M, Coons S, et al. Final report of Radiation Therapy Oncology Group (RTOG) protocol 9802: Radiation therapy (RT) versus RT + procarbazine, CCNU, and vincristine (PCV) chemotherapy for adult low-grade glioma (LGG) (abstract). J Clin Oncol 2008;26:90s.
58. Lee Y-Y, Van Tassel P, Bruner JM, et al. Juvenile pilocytic astrocytomas: CT and MR characteristics. AJR Am J Roentgenol 1989;152:1263–70.
59. Burkhard C, Di Patre P-L, Schuler D, et al. A population-based study of the incidence and survival rates in patients with pilocytic astrocytoma. J Neurosurg 2003;98:1170–4.
60. Mamelak AN, Prados MD, Obana WG, et al. Treatment options and prognosis for multicentric juvenile pilocytic astrocytoma. J Neurosurg 1994;81:24–30.
61. Dirks PB, Jay V, Becker LE, et al. Development of anaplastic changes in low-grade astrocytomas of childhood. Neurosurgery 1994;34:68–78.
62. Brown MT, Friedman HS, Oakes J, et al. Chemotherapy for pilocytic astrocytomas. Cancer 1993;71:3165–72.
63. Kepes JJ. Pleomorphic xanthoastrocytoma: the birth of a diagnosis and a concept. Brain Pathol 1993;3:269–74.
64. Pahapill PA, Ramsay DA, Del Maestro RF. Pleomorphic xanthoastrocytoma: Case report and analysis of the literature concerning the efficacy of resection and the significance of necrosis. Neurosurgery 1996;38:822–9.
65. Giannini C, Scheithauer B, Burger P, et al. Pleomorphic xanthoastrocytoma: What do we really know about it? Cancer 1998;85:2033–45.
66. Goh S, Butler W, Thiele EA. Subependymal giant cell tumors in tuberous sclerosis complex. Neurology 2004;63:1457–61.
67. Clarke MJ, Foy AB, Wetjen N, Raffel C. Imagine characteristics and growth of subependymal giant cell astrocytomas. Neurosurg Focus 2006;20:E5.
68. Nagib MG, Haines SJ, Erickson DL, et al. Tuberous sclerosis: a review for the neurosurgeon. Neurosurgery 1984;14:93–8.
69. Sharma M, Ralte A, Arora R, et al. Subependymal giant cell astrocytoma: a clinicopathological study of 23 cases with special emphasis on proliferative markers and expression of p53 and retinoblastoma gene proteins. Pathology 2004;36:139–44.
70. Louis DN, Ohgaki H, Weistler OD, Cavenee WK. WHO Classification of Tumours of the Central Nervous System. Lyon: IARC Press; 2007.
71. Lellouch-Tubiana A, Boddaert N, Bourgeois M, et al. Angiocentric neuroepithelial tumor (ANET): a new epilepsy-related clinicopatological entity with distinctive MRI. Brain Pathol 2005;15.
72. Wang M, Tihan T, Rojiani AM, et al. Monomorphous angiocentric glioma: a distinctive epileptogenic neoplasm with features of infiltrating astrocytoma and ependymoma. J Neuropathol Exp Neurol 2005;64.
73. Tihan T, Fisher PG, Kepner JL, et al. Pediatric astrocytomas with monomorphous pilomyxoid features and a less favorable outcome. J Neuropathol Exp Neurol 1999;58:1061–8.
74. Komotar RJ, Mocco J, Carson BS, et al. Pilomyxoid astrocytoma: a review. MedGenMed 2004;6:42.
75. Fernandez C, Figarella-Branger D, Girard N, et al. Clinico-pathological features of pilomyxoid astrocytoma of the optic pathway. Neurosurgery 2003;53:544–53.
76. Chikai K, Ohnishi A, Kato T, et al. Clinico-pathological features of pilomyxoid astrocytoma of the optic pathway. Acta Neuropathol 2004;108:109–14.
77. Rodriguez FJ, Perry A, Gutmann DH, et al. Gliomas in neurofibromatosis type 1: A clinicopathologic study of 100 patients. J Neuropathol Exp Neurol 2008;67:240–9.
78. Gutmann DH, Rasmussen SA, Wolkenstein P, et al. Gliomas presenting after age 10 in individuals with neurofibromatosis type 1 (NF1). Neurology 2002;59:759–61.
79. Listernick R, Ferner RE, Liu GT, Gutmann DH. Optic pathway gliomas in neurofibromatosis-1: Controversies and recommendations. Ann Neurol 2007;61:189–98.

7 Oligodendrogliomas

JEREMY H. REES

Introduction

Oligodendrogliomas (OD) and oligoastrocytomas (OA), otherwise known as mixed gliomas, and their anaplastic variants are less common than astrocytomas (discussed in the previous chapter) but show distinctive clinical behaviour, molecular genetics and heightened responses to chemotherapy when compared with astrocytic tumors. For these reasons, there has been a considerable reawakening of interest in OD/OA over the last decade, justifying the inclusion of a separate chapter in order to specifically discuss these issues.

Because OD/OA have a variable clinical phenotype, with some growing extremely slowly and others (the anaplastic variants) behaving more aggressively, many of the clinical controversies surrounding the management of OD/OA are similar to those of astrocytomas: i.e., surveillance vs. resection, early treatment vs. delayed, and extent of tumor resection and how it correlates with prognosis. In order to avoid repetition, this chapter will focus on issues specifically relevant to OD/OA.

Frequency and Incidence

Oligodendrogliomas account for 2% to 5% of primary brain tumors and 4% to 15% of all gliomas. They occur more frequently in males and in young adults between the ages of 30 to 40 years. These tumors are increasing in incidence, partly due to improved histological diagnosis and partly because of earlier imaging diagnosis, to the point that they are nearly as frequent as their astrocytic counterparts. In our practice, we have seen 21 oligodendrogliomas and 6 oligoastrocytomas in the last year, compared with only 16 astrocytomas. These compare with 4 anaplastic oligodendrogliomas, 4 anaplastic oligoastrocytomas, and 11 anaplastic astrocytomas in the same time period.

According to data collected by the Central Brain Tumor Registry of the United States (CBTRUS 2007-2008), OD, OA, and anaplastic oligodendroglioma (AO) accounted for 5.1%, 2.8%, and 2.8% respectively of neuroepithelial tumors and 2.0%, 1.0%, and 1.1% of all primary brain tumors. Therefore low-grade oligodendroglial tumors are three times more frequent than anaplastic tumors, and in total represent 4.1% of tumors compared with 8.5% for astrocytomas.[1] Assuming a population of just over 58 million people in the United Kingdom and an incidence rate of between 15/100,000[2] and 21/100,000[3] for all primary brain tumors, there are approximately 428 new cases of OD/OA/AO per year.

Histology

The realization that oligodendrogliomas are more chemosensitive than astrocytomas has increased the enthusiasm amongst neuropathologists to search hard for evidence of oligodendroglial differentiation in biopsy and resection specimens.[4] This in turn has ignited considerable debate about the minimum criteria for OD/OA.

Oligodendrogliomas can present at any age and in any location in the brain, although they frequently occur in cortical locations in the frontotemporal lobes as partially calcified mass lesions. Macroscopically, they may be distinguished by the presence of a mucoid matrix that is softer than the firmer surrounding brain. They often infiltrate grey matter and change the appearance of the cerebral cortex. The most characteristic microscopic feature of OD are the sheets of uniformly rounded cells and perinuclear halos, giving the so-called fried egg appearance, due to a technical artifact whereby the cytoplasm swells up in paraffin sections after a delay in fixation (Figure 7-1). This is not always present, however, particularly if the tumor specimen is frozen prior to being embedded in paraffin, nor is this appearance pathognomic for OD, as it also occurs in ependymomas and central neurocytomas. The key pathological feature that distinguishes OD from astrocytomas is the fact that cell density and nuclear size and shape are much more uniform. Astrocytomas typically display considerable nuclear pleomorphism and, in particular, angulated nuclei with spindle-shaped cells. Another classic feature is the presence of a rich, thin-walled capillary network arranged in a way that resembles chicken wire. Other frequent features include calcification, either within the tumor or within the surrounding brain, and cortical invasion with perineuronal or perivascular cells, known as satellitosis.

The differential diagnosis of an oligodendroglioma includes dysembryoplastic neuroepithelial tumor (DNET), clear cell ependymoma, central neurocytoma, pilocytic astrocytoma, and reactive gliosis.

Grade II oligodendrogliomas have a low mitotic index (less than 5%), although there may be well-circumscribed foci of higher cellularity, an occasional mitosis, and cellular atypia.[5] By definition, OD cannot have "significant mitotic activity," but this is a vague term and the exact number of mitoses has not been defined,

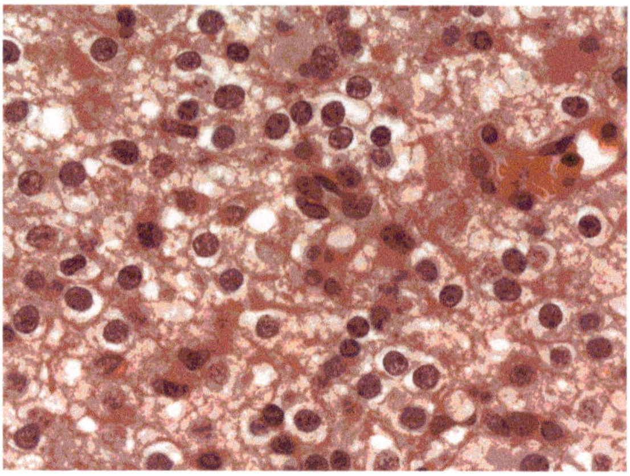

Figure 7-1 Oligodendroglioma showing characteristic rounded cell nuclei with perinuclear haloes—giving rise to the so-called fried egg appearance. Note also the network of delicate capillaries. (Courtesy Dr. Thomas Jacques, Division of Neuropathology.)

although in a recent large series, a cutoff value of 6 to 10 mitoses per high power field correlated with reduced survival.[6]

Tumors with a mixture of astrocytic and oligodendroglial components are called oligoastrocytomas (OA) or mixed gliomas, which, by definition, show divergent forms of glial differentiation. The two cell types may occur as regionally distinct and cytologically distinct populations of cells within the same tumor (Figure 7-2) or, more rarely, as intermixed populations containing cells with both astrocytic and oligodendroglial phenotypes. Many oligodendrogliomas contain GFAP-positive cells (i.e., cells of astrocytic lineage) and so the demonstration of astrocyte-like cells in an OD should not be regarded as necessarily diagnostic of an oligoastrocytoma, unless the proportion of the minority cell type exceeds some arbitrary figure ranging from 20% to 60%. Particular care should be taken when interpreting frozen specimens, as the process of freezing can change cells with an oligodendroglial morphology to cells with a more astrocytoma-like pattern with dark irregular nuclei. These tumors are regarded as morphologically ambiguous tumors and further characterization can only be carried out using molecular genetics. The variable criteria for the diagnosis of an OA has been succinctly reviewed by Burger.[7]

The grade III anaplastic OD (AO) still retains the characteristic nuclear uniformity of OD but is more cellular, and shows more nuclear atypia, frequent mitotic

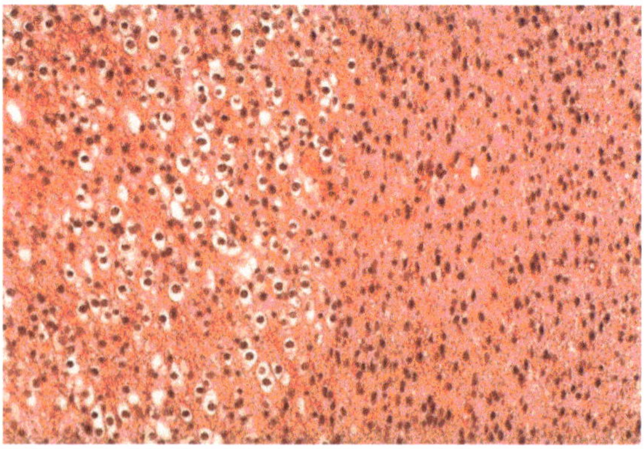

Figure 7-2 Oligoastrocytoma showing two distinct regional variations in cellular morphology, with oligodendroglial cells on the left and astrocytic cells on the right.

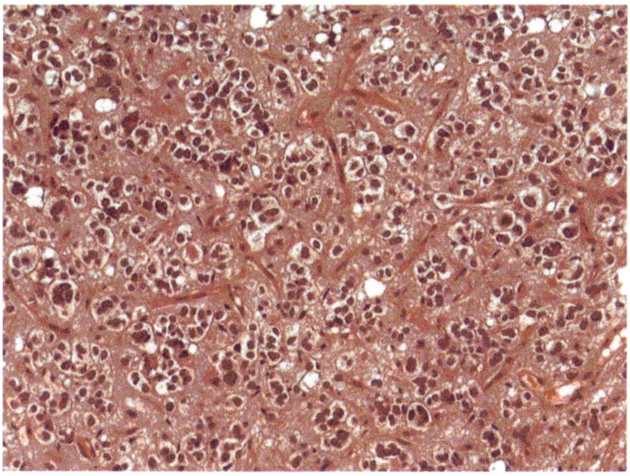

Figure 7-3 Anaplastic oligodendroglioma: lobules of oligodendroglial cells with marked cellular pleomorphism and extensive branching vasculature due to microvascular proliferation. (Courtesy Dr. Thomas Jacques.)

activity, and noticeable microvascular proliferation or hypertrophy (Figure 7-3). AO may present de novo or evolve from malignant transformation of a pure OD. Necrosis may be present and does not in itself indicate a grade IV glioma.[8] The vessels are frequently thickened and hypertrophied but do not form the glomerular tufts seen in glioblastoma multiforme (GBM). Most AOs do not evolve into GBMs; however, there are occasional cases and, in these, it is not really possible to distinguish between a "highly malignant" AO and a GBM with some oligodendroglial features. In the most recent WHO classification (2007), anaplastic oligoastrocytoma (AOA) with necrosis was reclassified as GBM-O. Recent data from a large trial of AOs and AOAs suggest that these tumors have similar survival curves to that of GBM and confirm this reclassification. Whether this tumor is a separate clinicopathological and molecular genetic entity remains to be proven.

Oligodendrogliomas have a greater propensity for leptomeningeal spread than astrocytic tumors. This occurs in about 1% to 2% of cases, with systemic metastases also being occasionally reported. This may be a consequence of the longer survival of patients as compared to other glioma subtypes and of heterozygous deletions of CDKN2A/p 16 genes.[9]

Molecular genetics

Oligodendrogliomas are associated with specific genetic abnormalities, namely loss of the short arm of chromosome 1 (1p) and the long arm of chromosome 19 (19q). This was first demonstrated 10 years ago in a genomic wide analysis,[10] and subsequently linked in retrospective studies to a durable response to a combination of procarbazine, CCNU, and Vincristine (PCV) as well as longer survival.[11,12] In contrast, response rates for patients with isolated 1p loss or no loss was less than 25%, although the presence of 1p loss may also identify other treatment-sensitive malignant gliomas, including rare GBMs (see Table 7-1).[13] The chromosomal locations involved in the favourable therapeutic response have been further narrowed down to lesions at 1p36 and 19q13.3.[14] Of the two markers, 1p has the greater specificity since 19q losses have also been reported in high-grade astrocytomas and OA.[15]

TABLE 7-1 1p and 19q Losses versus Glioma Subtypes and Primary/Recurrent Status Adapted from Smith et al. 2000[13]

Status	No. of patients	1p loss (%)	19q loss (%)	1p/19q loss (%)
Primary				
OD	36	42	58	39
OA	19	21	53	21
A	79	18	27	8
Recurrent				
OD	16	63	75	56
OA	12	42	42	33
A	18	17	39	6
Primary & Recurrent				
OD	52	48	63	44
OA	31	29	48	26
A	79	18	27	8

OD = oligodendroglioma
OA = oligoastrocytoma
A = astrocytoma

The frequency of these losses varies between different grades of glioma and different histological subtypes (see Figure 7-1). As can be seen, the 1p/19q loss is not specific to OD as it also occurs in OA and a minority of astrocytomas; however, it appears to be a statistically significant predictor of prolonged survival in patients with pure OD, irrespective of tumor grade, but not in patients with OA or astrocytomas.[16] The presence of a typical perinuclear halo in more than 50% of tumor cells and a "chicken wire" vascular pattern is seen in more than 90% of tumors showing LOH on 1p or 19q.[17]

More recently, mutations of two enzymes involved in the Krebs cycle, isocitrate dehydrogenase (IDH) 1 and 2, have been described in 84% of OD, 94% of AO, and 100% of OA and AOA, making this an even more common molecular signature than 1p19q.[18] These mutations are rarely seen in primary GBM.

Clinical Features and Natural History

Most ODs are slow-growing tumors; they usually present in adults between the ages of 30 and 50 with partial or generalized seizures. The incidence of seizures is lower in AO than in OD/OA.[19] Occasionally, they occur in older patients. In these cases, they more commonly present with symptoms of an expanding, infiltrating mass lesion (raised intracranial pressure with or without focal neurological deficits).[20] They are more likely to present as an intracerebral hemorrhage than other low-grade gliomas, probably because of their thin-walled capillary network.

ODs and other low-grade gliomas account for up to 15% of patients with medically intractable seizures.[21] Seizure control may vary and, particularly in tumors occurring in the motor strip, be resistant to anticonvulsant polypharmacy.[22] In this situation, patients may be considered for "epilepsy surgery" on symptomatic grounds rather than on pure oncological grounds. The relationship between the molecular genetics and their mode of presentation is not clear, but the clinical phenotype is presumably related in some way to the speed of growth and the duration of time that the tumor has been present in the brain. This is supported by the observation that there is an inverse relationship between tumor grade and frequency of seizures—as a general rule, the more benign the tumor, the more likely it is to be associated with intractable epilepsy.

The natural history of these tumors is variable; some grow very slowly over many years and remain essentially unchanged, while others may progress rapidly and cause significant neurological deficit (aggressive OD). On the basis of personal experience, there seem to be a group of patients with very slow-growing ODs who have a long history of epilepsy (one to two decades) and a second group who have a much shorter history of tumor growth before malignant transformation occurs. This difference in clinical behavior highlights the need for a tailor-made approach to each individual patient.

The prognosis of OD is significantly better than for astrocytomas, with a median survival of 10 years or more. As with astrocytomas, there is a wide range of survival times, presumably due to underlying genetic factors. Like other low-grade tumors, favourable prognostic factors for OD include age less than 40 years, presentation with seizures, normal neurological examination and, in some reports, extent of resection.[23,24] In a retrospective review of 106 patients with OD (n=77) and OA (n=29) from the Memorial Sloan Kettering Cancer Center in New York, the overall median time to progression was 5.0 years (0.5 –14.2) and the overall survival, 16.7 years.[25] Neither of these two markers of outcome were significantly affected by treatment.

Imaging

Oligodendrogliomas and oligoastrocytomas are space-occupying lesions that have a predilection for frontal lobes and often infiltrate up to the cortical surface. There are no specific features that distinguish OD/OA from astrocytomas, although the presence of calcification on CT scans and, specifically, a gyriform pattern (due to calcification along the cortical ribbon) is highly suggestive. MR spectroscopy may, in time, be able to distinguish OD/OA from astrocytomas; a study of 15 patients with OD and AO showed that the level of glutamine plus glutamate was significantly higher than in low-grade astrocytomas.[26] Similarly, a study of diffusion-weighted imaging (DWI) showed that ODs had significantly lower group apparent diffusion coefficient (ADC) values than astrocytomas (A) and that up to 83% of the subjects could be correctly classified into the OD and A groups by reference to an ADC histogram.[27]

These tumors can be diffusely infiltrating (Figure 7-4) or well-demarcated (Figure 7-5), and appear on MR imaging as high-signal on T2W, PD, and FLAIR sequences and as intermediate-signal or low-signal on T1W sequences. Of these, FLAIR offers superior delineation of the tumor margins and is also better at showing different tumor components, at defining the borders of a postoperative cavity, and at demonstrating local spread to white matter tracts.[28]

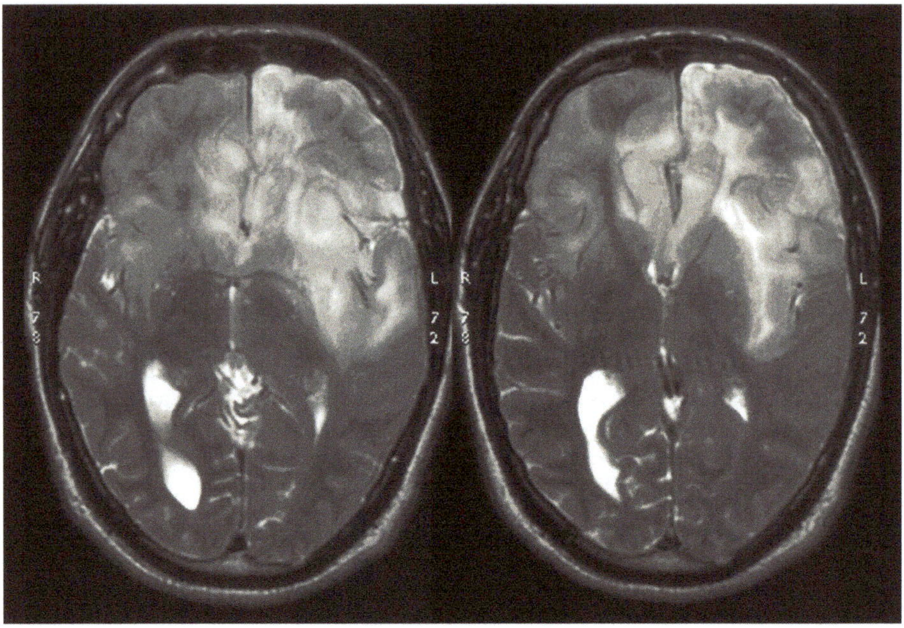

Figure 7-4 Axial T2W MRI scan showing diffuse bifrontal oligodendroglioma in a man presenting with focal motor seizures and cognitive decline.

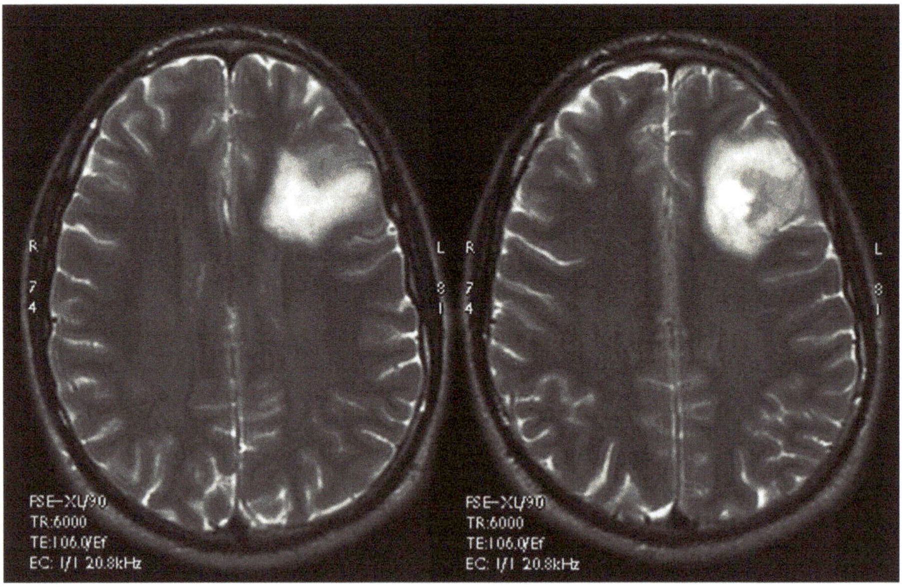

Figure 7-5 Axial T2W image of a well-demarcated left frontal oligodendroglioma in a man presenting with frontal adversive seizures.

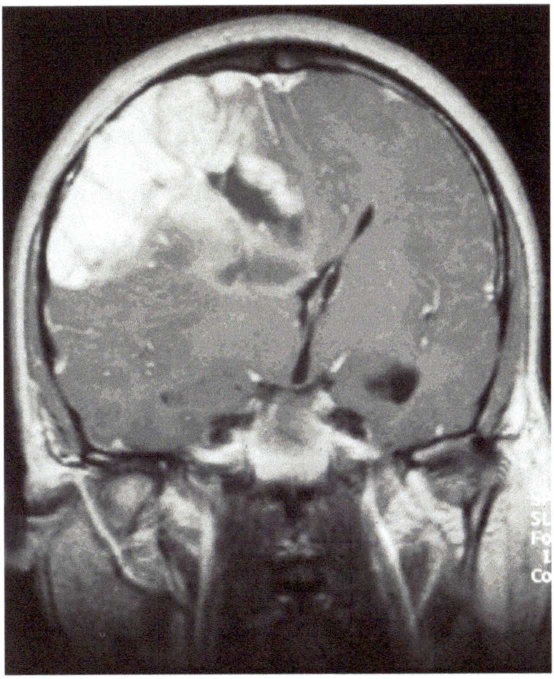

Figure 7-6 Coronal gadolinium-enhanced MRI scan in a man presenting with frontal seizures and headache. Resection revealed an anaplastic oligodendroglioma.

The presence of contrast enhancement in a glioma is often regarded as a sign of malignancy (Figure 7-6) and, in the case of OD, reduces the median survival from 11 years in nonenhancing tumors to 3 years in enhancing ones. For this reason, Daumas-Duport has suggested a grading classification for OD that includes the presence of contrast enhancement as a variable and which was found to be highly predictive of survival.[29] Contrast enhancement reflects breakdown of the blood-brain barrier and correlates with angiogenesis. In a study examining the prognostic significance of both tumor enhancement and angiogenesis in OD, 10-year survival was 83% in patients with nonenhancing tumors, compared to only 14% in enhancing tumors; 79% of the tumors showing contrast enhancement had a high tumor angiogenesis index indicating a close relationship between contrast enhancement and endothelial surface area.[30] Furthermore, a significant proportion of low-grade gliomas, and in particular OD, may display high relative cerebral blood volume (rCBV) foci on perfusion imaging not reflective of high-grade histopathology.[31]

Functional imaging, particularly using FDG-PET, has been adopted in some centers for the management of OD, in particular for determining the degree of malignancy and guiding the surgeon to the most malignant area, as well as for discrimination of recurrent tumor from radiation necrosis.[32] However, whether it provides additional information over and above that of conventional MRI sequences is debatable.

The results of imaging are vital to determining the subsequent management of a patient with a radiologically suspected low-grade glioma. However, MRI scans may be falsely reassuring. Several studies have demonstrated that contrast enhancement in gliomas is only weakly predictive of tumor grade; in a study of

314 unselected patients with both malignant and low-grade gliomas, 58 lacked contrast enhancement and, of these, approximately one third were malignant, particularly in older patients.[33] For this reason, biopsy is recommended for older patients presenting with seizures and a nonenhancing lesion, as they are more likely to be harbouring a high-grade glioma. For younger patients without neurological deficit whose tumor has not changed on a second scan 3 months after the first study, it is reasonable to adopt a watch and wait policy, although the precise scanning interval will vary according to local resources.

Imaging is therefore vital for monitoring the natural history of low-grade gliomas, particularly as these tumors are often not treated until there is clinical or radiological evidence of progression.[34] Although it is well recognized that low-grade gliomas eventually undergo malignant transformation, very little is known about their radiological history and growth rates during their "stable" phase. In a study of 27 patients with untreated OD and OA, analysis of mean tumor diameters over time showed that these tumors were continuously growing with an average slope of 4.1 mm/year.[35] We have extended this study to all types of grade II gliomas and have shown that even in nontransformers, an average growth rate of 13% per annum was observed, compared to a growth rate of transformers up until the penultimate scan (i.e., before transformation took place) of 26% per annum. This growth rate increased to 56% per annum in the final 6-month time period that included transformation, implying that low-grade gliomas that grow more rapidly in their "stable" phase are more likely to undergo malignant transformation.[36]

Management

DECISION TO TREAT

There is considerable controversy about the most appropriate first line treatment for patients with low-grade gliomas, and this has led to marked variations in practice. The therapeutic options have not changed much over the last three decades. Maximal resective surgery is advocated by some, while observation alone until progression is the choice of others and until there are randomized controlled trials (which will be almost impossible to set up), this dilemma will plague clinicians and patients alike. The therapeutic options for patients with OD/AO are further increased by the efficacy of chemotherapy in a high percentage of tumors.

As a general rule, adult patients over the age of 50 years presenting with seizures and a scan suggestive of a supratentorial low-grade glioma should undergo at least a stereotactic biopsy to confirm the diagnosis and to rule out a higher-grade tumor or a nonneoplastic lesion. As mentioned earlier, this may be deferred in a younger patient, particularly if the tumor is in an eloquent area, seizures are well-controlled, and serial imaging shows no tumor growth. Treatment of the tumor at an early stage in its natural history should be given to patients with large tumors causing symptoms of raised intracranial pressure or neurological deficits other than seizures. In patients who are otherwise well, even if the tumor is growing slightly on serial MRI studies, it is reasonable to wait until clinical deterioration or the appearance of new and substantial non-vessel gadolinium enhancement before embarking on potentially toxic and rarely curative therapies.

The decision to treat is therefore very much a matter of individual experience and will be affected by radiological interpretation and thresholds of defining "clinical deterioration" as well as by patient wishes.

SURGERY

Although surgery offers the possibility of cure in selected patients with low-grade gliomas (e.g., pilocytic astrocytomas), it is almost impossible to resect a diffusely infiltrating grade II tumor in its entirety without unacceptable neurological deficit. Although there are a large number of case series reporting retrospectively that patients with radical resections of low-grade gliomas live longer than those with partial resections or biopsies, any survival advantage may be due to patient selection and underlying tumor biology rather than the nature of the surgical procedure. More favourable results from surgery may be due to selection of young patients with good performance status who have small tumors in noneloquent regions. Even in these patients, however, recurrences at the resection margin occur some years after surgery despite an apparent gross total resection. Other arguments advanced for choosing resection over biopsy include reducing the radiotherapy treatment volume and improving the accuracy of histological diagnosis. However, whether these have any clear benefits overall is unknown.[37]

Advances in neurosurgery, including preoperative fMRI localisation of speech and motor areas, the ability to fuse this information with image-guidance data, and perioperative cortical localization using the technique of awake craniotomy, all serve to maximize the possibility of a safe resection by avoiding critical cortical structures. However, even in the most experienced hands, postoperative FLAIR imaging usually shows a small rim of residual tissue that was not seen by the surgeon, simply because tumor-infiltrated brain looks identical to normal brain. The prognostic importance of this high signal rim is not entirely clear. A recent surgical study retrospectively evaluated the survival of 170 patients with low-grade gliomas (WHO grade II astrocytomas, oligodendrogliomas, and oligoastrocytomas) and showed that gross total resection, defined as complete resection of the preoperative FLAIR signal abnormality, was associated with longer time to progression and malignant transformation than near total resections (less than 3mm signal rim around resection cavity) and subtotal resections (residual nodular FLAIR abnormality). Overall survival at 5 and 10 years was improved independently of other prognostic factors in the GTR group over the NTR/STR groups, suggesting a survival advantage from resecting all visible tumor tissue.[38] The advent of interventional MRI which permits the surgeon to assess the extent of resection perioperatively using on-table MR imaging in real time may improve the chances of a macroscopically complete resection but still will not address the problem of satellite tumor cells in radiologically normal-appearing peritumoral tissue. Furthermore, staying within the radiological margins of the tumor does not guarantee the absence of a postoperative deficit.

In contrast, CT-guided or MRI-guided stereotactic biopsy carries a very low risk of serious morbidity and mortality (1% to 2%), with a 93% chance of obtaining a definite histological diagnosis.[39]

The relationship between extent of resection (EOR) and survival is conflicting and seems to favor patients with oligodendrogliomas more than patients with astrocytomas.[40] Unfortunately, there is little data that specifically analyzes the relationship between EOR and stratifies outcome for other end points such as time to progression and malignant transformation. Furthermore, assessment of EOR in retrospective series varies from the perioperative surgical estimate to calculation of volumes from early postoperative scans. In view of these considerations, aggressive surgical resection for patients with OD should not be undertaken by neurosurgeons without careful consideration of the long natural history and heightened chemosensitivity of these tumors and the role of other therapeutic modalities. The question of resective surgery in recurrent disease is even more controversial and should be limited to situations where there is a reasonable potential for improving the function and quality of life of the patient.

RADIOTHERAPY

The use of radiotherapy as adjuvant treatment following surgery is well-established for patients with AO. In contrast, the role of radiotherapy in the treatment of patients with low-grade OD is more controversial, particularly as there are concerns over long-term radiotherapy-induced toxicity, including dementia and radiation vasculopathy. It has been suggested that patients with OD who present with intracranial hypertension and/or progressive neurological deficit benefit more from radiotherapy than those who have tumors causing seizures without neurological deficit.[41]

The radiation dose for low-grade glioma is usually 4500 to 5000 cGy, preferably with three-dimensional conformal ports.[42] The incidence of neurotoxicity may have been overestimated, as the older literature studied patients who had been given whole brain RT rather than focal RT, which is regarded as best practice nowadays. Cognitive deficits in patients with low-grade gliomas (LGG) may occur as a result of the tumor itself or as a result of the underlying seizure disorder and anticonvulsant medication, as well as the delayed effects of RT. There have been conflicting reports of late neurocognitive sequelae following RT. A recent neuropsychological cross-sectional study comparing 104 patients with LGGs who had had radiotherapy anywhere from 1 year to 22 years previously with 91 patients who had not received radiotherapy, 100 low-grade hematologic patients, and 195 healthy controls showed that overall the glioma patients had significantly lower scores on objective tests and much lower self-reported cognitive functioning than patients in both control groups. Furthermore, 34% of patients in the glioma group had moderate to severe cognitive disability compared with 22% of the hematologic controls. However, there were only slight differences in cognitive functioning between irradiated and nonirradiated glioma patients and, although a greater percentage of irradiated patients had cognitive deficits (39% vs. 29%), this difference was not statistically significant.[43] This suggests that the underlying tumor, epilepsy, and antiepileptic drugs are more important factors in causing cognitive decline than the radiotherapy itself.

Most studies addressing the efficacy of RT in OD have been retrospective and, as with low-grade astrocytomas, have reached conflicting conclusions.[44–47] It has now been established that the dose of radiotherapy used for LGGs does not influence survival. In 1985, the EORTC Radiotherapy Cooperative Group launched a randomized phase III study (EORTC 22844) comparing high-dose (59.4 Gy in 6.5 weeks) with low-dose (45 Gy in 5 weeks) radiotherapy in patients with histologically verified LGGs and found no difference in survival between the two doses.[48]

This finding has been confirmed in a more recent American study comparing survival and toxicity in patients treated with low-dose (50.4 Gy/28 fractions) and high-dose (64.8 Gy/36 fractions) radiotherapy.[49] Both 2-year and 5-year survival were better in the low-dose group, albeit not significantly, while radiation necrosis, although rare, occurred in both groups, with one fatality in each arm. The actuarial incidence at 2 years was slightly higher (5% vs. 2.5%) in the high-dose arm. A quality-of-life questionnaire revealed lower levels of functioning and higher symptom burden in patients given higher doses of RT. These group differences were statistically significant for fatigue/malaise and insomnia immediately after radiotherapy and in leisure time and emotional functioning at 7 to 15 months after randomization. These findings suggest that for conventional radiotherapy for low-grade cerebral glioma, a schedule of 45 Gy in 5 weeks not only saves valuable resources, but also spares patients a prolonged treatment at no loss of clinical efficacy.[50]

The timing of radiotherapy as either primary or adjuvant treatment (i.e., given after surgery) has now been addressed in a recently published large European study, EORTC 22845.[51] Over 300 patients with pathologically diagnosed grade II gliomas were randomized to either radiotherapy at a dose of 54 Gy in 6 weeks immediately after surgery or no treatment until tumor progression. Progression-free survival was 5.3 years in the early irradiated group compared to 3.4 years in the control group ($p<0.0001$) but there was no difference in overall survival (7.4 years vs. 7.2 years). Therefore, on present evidence adjuvant radiotherapy following incomplete tumor excision is not routinely recommended in patients without evidence of progressive disease. The doses and techniques usually employed are the same as for astrocytomas.

In the same way as with chemotherapy, loss of chromosome 1 p may also predict response to radiotherapy. Patients with 1 p LOH had significantly longer median progression-free survival after RT compared with those whose tumors had intact 1 p (55 vs. 6 months, $p<0.01$) implying a common mechanism of sensitivity to ionizing radiation and alkylating chemotherapy.[52]

CHEMOTHERAPY

Chemotherapy has traditionally been used as adjuvant treatment for high-grade gliomas, although the data in low-grade gliomas is sparse. A small study carried out in the 1980s by the Southwest Oncology Group was prematurely closed because of slow accrual after recruiting only 60 patients.[53] Patients were randomized to receive radiotherapy only following an incomplete resection or radiotherapy plus lomustine (CCNU). There was a nonsignificant trend to improved median survival in the chemotherapy arm (7.4 years vs. 4.5 years) hinting at a possible benefit, but no further prospective studies have been done in this group of patients.

CHEMOTHERAPY FOR ANAPLASTIC OLIGODENDROGLIOMA

Interest in chemotherapy as an option for treating LGGs remained low until 1994 when a National Cancer Institute of Canada study reported a 75% response rate in patients with AO treated with the familiar and previously relatively unsuccessful PCV regimen (procarbazine, lomustine (CCNU), and vincristine) (Figure 7-7).[5] Subsequently, temozolomide (TMZ) has also been found to have activity, with

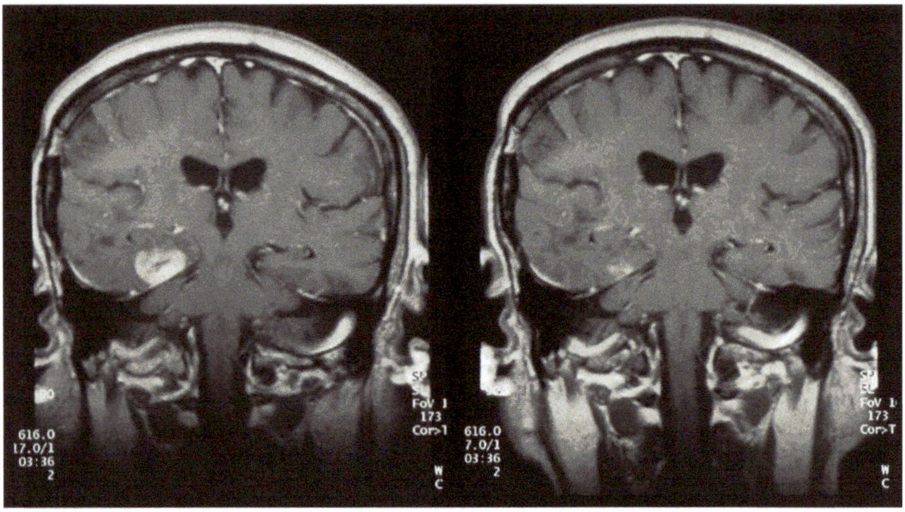

Figure 7-7 Coronal gadolinium-enhanced MRI scan showing response of right medial temporal anaplastic oligodendroglioma to two cycles of PCV.

high response rates and durable responses.[54,55] These responses correlate with loss of 1p and 19q LOH, and the presence of this unique genetic signature correlates with increased survival. The combination of 1p and 19q LOH is associated with a 100% response rate to PCV with median progression-free survival rates in excess of 31 months, and overall survival in excess of 123 months. The presence of 1p loss only without 19q conferred a high level of chemosensitivity but shorter progression-free survival and overall survival, whereas patients with an intact 1p had lower responses and shorter survival times.[56] AO may have other genetic abnormalities such as p53 or PTEN mutations, 10q LOH, or amplification of the EGFR gene,[57] but none of these appear to confer the same degree of responsiveness as 1p and 19q LOH. The relationship between 1p loss and chemosensitivity has also been shown to occur in OA, albeit to a lesser extent.[58,59]

Because of the increasing interest in chemotherapy for AO, two large prospective trials investigating the role of PCV (procarbazine, CCNU, vincristine) chemotherapy were carried out comparing neoadjuvant and adjuvant chemotherapy against radiotherapy alone. Despite the different timing of chemotherapy with regard to radiotherapy, the results were broadly similar and somewhat surprising. In the neoadjuvant study of 289 patients with pure and mixed AO, there was no benefit in terms of overall survival between the two groups (median survival 4.9 years after PCV+RT vs. 4.7 years after RT alone). There was a slight prolongation of progression-free survival in the combined treatment group (2.6 years for PCV+RT vs. 1.7 years for RT alone), but this was at the expense of considerable acute toxicity in the PCV group (65% patients had Grade 3 or 4 toxicity and one patient died). Irrespective of treatment, patients with 1p and 19q loss lived longer than other patients (greater than 7 years vs. 2.8 years).[60] Similarly, in the adjuvant study of 368 patients followed up for a median of 5 years, median survival was 40.3 months in the RT/PCV group vs. 30.6 months in the RT group alone, which was not significant. As in the neoadjuvant study, progression-free survival was longer in the RT/PCV group than the RT group (23 months vs. 13 months; $p=0.018$).[61]

Both studies identified a significant survival advantage for patients whose tumors had combined 1p/19q deletions, irrespective of treatment received. In fact, combined loss of 1p/19q is now regarded as the most important prognostic factor for anaplastic oligodendroglial tumors, with median survivals of 6 to 7 years in the presence of 1p/19q loss compared with 2 to 3 years in the absence of these codeletions. Similarly, in WHO grade II OD and OA, median survival was 10 to 15 years for 1p/19q codeleted tumors, compared to 5 to 8 years for patients without the deletion.[62]

CHEMOTHERAPY FOR LOW-GRADE OD/OA

Following some small observational studies that suggested that chemotherapy using a combination of PCV was beneficial in ordinary low-grade oligodendrogliomas[63,64] three phase II studies of TMZ have recently been published.

The first study treated 46 patients with "progressive low-grade glioma" and reported an objective response rate of 61% (complete response [CR] 24% and partial response [PR] 37%), with an additional 35% having stable disease (SD).[65] For the 20 patients with oligodendrogliomas, the response rate was 60% (CR 25%, PR 35%). Serious toxicity occurred in six patients. This study included heavily pretreated patients: 52% of the patients had had either subtotal or gross total resections, 15% had had prior radiotherapy, and 22% prior chemotherapy. Furthermore, 70% of patients had enhancing lesions on MRI scanning, suggesting a higher grade tumor.

In contrast, a single center study that only recruited untreated patients with histologically verified grade II gliomas (17 astrocytomas, 11 oligodendrogliomas and 2 mixed gliomas) showed much less impressive results. Of 29 evaluable patients, 10% had a partial response, 48% a minimal response (MR), 38% stable disease, and 4% progressive disease. The figures for the patients with OD were PR 20%, MR 30%, SD 50%, and PD 0%. The hematological toxicity was 3.5%.[66] A third study treated 60 patients with both OD and OA and reported clinical improvement in 51% of patients, particularly those with intractable seizures, and "objective radiological response" in 31% of patients (17% PR and 14% MR).[67] Interestingly the mean time to maximum tumor response was 12 months (range 5 to 20 months) and, as expected, tumor response correlated with loss of chromosome 1p.

The chemosensitivity of OD extends to gliomatosis cerebri, where there is diffuse infiltration of the brain by glioma cells, rendering surgery inappropriate and increasing the potential toxicity of large-field RT. In a recent retrospective study of 63 consecutive patients with gliomatosis cerebri (GC), oligodendroglial GC had a better prognosis in terms of progression-free and overall survival compared to astrocytic and oligoastrocytic GC, regardless of the chemotherapy regimen used.[68]

Chemotherapy is, therefore, becoming increasingly accepted as an alternative treatment for patients with OD, although the dramatic response rates seen in patients with anaplastic tumors have not yet been replicated in patients with low-grade OD. In addition, there are no studies comparing the efficacy and toxicity of chemotherapy against radiotherapy; a trial comparing these two treatment modalities is currently recruiting throughout Europe. In a recent informal survey of 30 oncologists in the United Kingdom, 50% used radiotherapy as the primary treatment modality for patients with progressive OD/OA, 10% used chemotherapy, and 40% would use either depending on the individual tumor, reflecting the considerable uncertainty about the best way of treating these tumors.

MANAGEMENT OF RECURRENT DISEASE

As indicated above, the response rates of patients with AO to PCV chemotherapy vary from 60% to 70%[69,70] to 30% to 40%[71] in patients with recurrent disease. In an EORTC phase II study of TMZ in 38 patients with recurrent OD and OA, the response rate was 53% and the median time to progression for responding patients 13.2 months.[72] This is significantly better for other recurrent high-grade gliomas and implies that about 50% of tumors remain chemosensitive even at recurrence. In exceptional circumstances, tumors may be re-irradiated; response is best seen in patients with OD who have a good performance status.[73]

BIOLOGICAL AGENTS

Targeted biological therapy is designed to modulate a specific signaling event that is thought to have a critical role in the survival, proliferation, or invasion of gliomas. There has been increasing interest in the use of targeted biological agents for the management of malignant gliomas, and results of a number of Phase I and Phase II studies using EGFR antagonists (ZD1839-gefitinib [Iressa®] and OSI774-erlotinib [Tarceva®], PDGFR inhibitors (ST1571–imatinib mesylate [Glivec®], VEGFR inhibitors (PTK787/ZK222584), and monoclonal antibodies against VEGF (bevacizumab, Avastin®) have now been carried out on patients with relapsed malignant gliomas. The data to date suggest these agents may be active in stabilizing disease progression, but partial responses are rare; it seems likely that these molecules will be used in combination with more traditional cytotoxic agents rather than in isolation. No studies of these agents have been carried out in low-grade gliomas.

Prognosis

There are a large number of prognostic factors for patients with oligodendroglial tumors, the most important of which are age, performance status, histological grade, and 1p/19q status. The effect of age is the most striking, with patients less than 40 years consistently experiencing a longer survival; in one study, patients younger than 20 years at presentation had a median survival of 17.5 years compared to 13 months in patients over 60.[74] Other clinical variables include frontal location, absence of neurological deficit at diagnosis, and presentation with seizures. Molecular prognostic factors, excluding 1p/19q status, include lower proliferative activity, loss of 10q, and EGFR amplification.

The survival times from recently published series are significantly longer than from reports from over a decade ago. The 5-year and 10-year survival figures for OD are 73% and 49%, respectively, and for AO, 63% and 33%, respectively.[75] Other studies have confirmed these figures.

Conclusions

Diffuse WHO grade II gliomas have traditionally been grouped together, but the realization that there are clinically relevant differences in chromosomal makeup and biological behavior suggests that these tumors warrant separation into distinct entities. Chemosensitivity in patients with OD, combined with the difficulties in histological diagnosis due to tumor heterogeneity emphasize the need for better molecular markers to facilitate separation of OD/OA from other types of glioma. Radiation therapy, long regarded as the standard adjuvant treatment for incompletely resected OD, is now being delayed until progression without any adverse impact on survival.

Even with aggressive multimodality treatments and the recent optimistic reports of chemosensitivity and occasionally prolonged survival in these tumors, oligodendroglioma ultimately recurs and, by and large, remains a fatal disease, as malignant transformation at the time of recurrence is the rule. What is needed now is more precise definition of the molecular pathology in order to develop better targeted therapies.

REFERENCES

1. Central Brain Tumor Registry of the United States. Primary brain tumors in the United States 1995–1999. URL: http://www.cbtrus.org/2007-2008/tables/report/2007.
2. Counsell CE, Collie DA, Grant R. Incidence of intracranial tumours in the Lothian region of Scotland 1989–90. J Neurol Neurosurg Psychiatry 1996;61:143–50.
3. Pobereskin LH, Chadduck JB. Incidence of brain tumours in two English counties: a population based study. J Neurol Neurosurg Psychiatry 2000;69:464–71.
4. Burger PC. What is an oligodendroglioma? Brain Pathol 2002;12:257–9.
5. MacDonald DR. Low-grade gliomas, mixed gliomas and oligodendrogliomas. Semin Oncol 1994;21:236–48.
6. Giannini C, Scheithauer BW, Weaver AL, et al. Oligodendrogliomas: reproducibility and prognostic value of histologic diagnosis and grading. J Neuropathol Exp Neurol 2001;60:248–62.
7. Burger OC. What is an oligodendroglioma? Brain Pathol 2002;12:257–9.
8. Burger PC, Rawlings CE, Cox EB, et al. Clinicopathologic correlations in the oligodendroglioma. Cancer 1986;59:1345–52.
9. Giordana MT, Ghimenti C, Leonardo E, et al. Molecular genetic study of a metastatic oligodendroglioma. J Neurooncol 2004;66:265–71.
10. Reifenberger J, Reifenberger G, Liu L, et al. Molecular genetic analysis of oligodendroglial tumors show preferential allelic deletions on 19 q and 1 p. Am J Pathol 1994;145:1175–90.
11. Cairncross G, Macdonald D, Ludwin S, et al. Chemotherapy for anaplastic oligodendroglioma: National Cancer Institute of Canada Clinical Trials Group. J Clin Oncol 1994;12:2013–21.
12. van den Bent MJ, Looijenga LHJ, Langenberg K, et al. Chromosomal anomalies in oligodendroglial tumours are correlated with clinical features. Cancer 2003;97:1276–84.
13. Ino Y, Zlatescu MC, Sakai H, et al. Long patient survival and therapeutic responses in histologically disparate high grade gliomas with chromosome 1 p loss. J Neurosurg 2000;92:983–90.
14. van den Bent MJ. New perspectives for the diagnosis and treatment of oligodendroglioma. Expert Rev Anticancer Ther 2001;1:348–56.
15. Smith JS, Alderete B, Minn y, et al. Localisation of common deletion regions on 1 p and 19 q in human gliomas and their association with histological subtype. Oncogene 1999;18:4144–52.
16. Smith JS, Perry A, Borell TJ, et al. Alterations of chromosome arms 1 p and 19 q as predictors of survival in oligodendrogliomas, astrocytomas and mixed oligoastrocytomas. J Clin Oncol 2000;18:636–45.
17. Watanabe T, Nakamura M, Kros JM, et al. Phenotype versus genotype correlation in oligodendrogliomas and low-grade diffuse astrocytomas. Acta Neuropathol 2002;103:267–75.
18. Yan H, Parsons W, Jin G, et al. *IDH1* and *IDH2* mutations in gliomas. N Engl J Med 2009;360:765–73.
19. Whittle IR, Beaumont A. Seizures in patients with supratentorial oligodendroglial tumours. Clinicopathological features and management considerations. Acta Neurochir (Wien) 1995;135:19–24.
20. Tucha O, Smely C, Preier M, et al. Cognitive deficits before treatment among patients with brain tumors. Neurosurgery 47:324–33.
21. Spencer DD, Spencer SS, Mattson RH, Williamson PD. Intracerebral masses in patients with intractable partial epilepsy. Neurology 1984;34:432–6.
22. Pace A, Bove L, Innocenti P, et al. Epilepsy and gliomas: incidence and treatment in 119 patients. J Exp Clin Cancer Res 1998;17:479–82.

23. Shaw EG, Scheithauer BW, O'Fallon JR, et al. Oligodendrogliomas: the Mayo clinic experience. J Neurosurg 1992;76:428–34.
24. Celli P, Nofrone I, Palma L, et al. Cerebral oligodendroglioma: prognostic factors and life history. Neurosurgery 1994;35:1018–34.
25. Olson JD, Riedel E, DeAngelis LM. Long-term outcome of low-grade oligodendroglioma and mixed glioma. Neurology 2000;54:1442–8.
26. Rijpkema M, Schuuring J, van der Meulen Y, et al. Characterization of oligodendrogliomas using short echo time 1 H MR spectroscopic imaging. NMR Biomed 2003;16:12–8.
27. Tozer DJ, Jäger HR, Danchaivijitr N, et al. Apparent diffusion coefficient histograms may predict low-grade glioma subtype. NMR Biomed 2007;20:49–57.
28. Bynevelt M, Britton J, Seymour H, et al. FLAIR imaging in the follow-up of low-grade gliomas: time to dispense with the dual echo? Neuroradiology 2001;43:129–33.
29. Daumas-Duport C, Tucker ML, Kolles H, et al. Oligodendrogliomas. Part II: A new grading system based on morphological and imaging criteria. J Neurooncol 1997;34:61–78.
30. Vaquero J, Zurita M, Morales C, et al. Prognostic significance of tumor-enhancement and angiogenesis in oligodendroglioma. Acta Neurol Scand 2002;106:19–23.
31. Lev MH, Ozsunar Y, Henson JW, et al. Glial tumor grading and outcome prediction using dynamic spin-echo MR susceptibility mapping compared with conventional contrast-enhanced MR: confounding effect of elevated rcbv of oligodendrogliomas. AJNR Am J Neuroradiol 2004;25:214–21.
32. Engelhard HH, Stelea A, Mundt A. Oligodendroglioma and anaplastic oligodendroglioma: clinical features, treatment and prognosis. Surg Nurol 2003;60:443–56.
33. Scott JN, Brasher PMA, Sevick RJ, et al. How often are nonenhancing supratentorial gliomas malignant? A population study. Neurology 2002;59:947–9.
34. Recht LD, Lew R, Smith TW. Suspected low-grade glioma: is deferring treatment safe? Ann Neurol 1992;31:431–6.
35. Mandonnet E, Delattre J-Y, Tanguy M-L, et al. Continuous growth of mean tumor diameter in a subset of grade II gliomas. Ann Neurol 2003;53:524–8.
36. Rees JH, Watt H, Jäger HR, et al. Volumes and growth rates of untreated adult low-grade gliomas indicate risk of malignant transformation. Eur J Radiol 2008; Jul 14 Epub.
37. Whittle IR. The dilemma of low-grade glioma. J Neurol Neurosurg Psychiatry 2004;75(Suppl. 2):ii31–6.
38. McGirt MJ, Chaichana KL, Attenello FJ, et al. Extent of surgical resection is independently associated with survival in patients with hemispheric infiltrating low-grade gliomas. Neurosurgery 2008;63:700–7.
39. Kondziolka D, Lunsford LD. The role of stereotactic biopsy in the management of gliomas. J Neuro-oncol 1999;42:205–13.
40. Berger MS, Rostomily RC. Low-grade gliomas: functional mapping resection strategies, extent of resection and outcome. J Neuro-oncol 1997;34:85–101.
41. Celli P, Nafrone I, Lucio Palma BS, et al. Cerebral oligodendroglioma: prognostic factors and life history. Neurosurg 1994;35:1018–35.
42. Dropcho EJ. Low-grade gliomas in adults. Curr Treat Options Neurol 2004;6:265–71.
43. Klein M, Heimans JJ, Aaronson NK, et al. Effect of radiotherapy and other treatment-related factors on mid-term to long-term cognitive sequelae in low-grade glioms. A comparative study. Lancet 2002;360:1361–8.
44. Nijjar TS, Simpson WJ, Gadalla T, et al. Oligodendroglioma. The Princess Margaret Hospital experience (1958–84). Cancer 1993;71:4002–6.
45. Wallner KE, Gonzales M, Sheline GE. Treatment of oligodendrogliomas with or without postoperative irradiation. J Neurosurg 1988;68:684–8.
46. Bullard DE, Rawlings CE, Phillips B, et al. Oligodendroglioma. An analysis of the value of radiation therapy. Cancer 1987;60:2179–88.
47. Gannett DE, Wisbeck WM, Silbergeld DL, Berger MS. The role of postoperative irradiation in the treatment of oligodendroglioma. Int J Radiat Oncol Biol Phys 1994;30:567–73.
48. Karim ABMF, Maat B, Hatlevoll R, et al. A randomized trial on dose-response in radiation therapy of low-grade cerebral glioma: European Organization for Research and Treatment of Cancer (EORTC) study 22844. Int J Radiat Oncol Biol Phys 1996;36:549–56.
49. Shaw E, Arusell R, Scheithauer B, et al. Prospective randomized trial of low- versus high-dose radiation therapy in adults with supratentorial low-grade glioma: initial report of a North Central Cancer Treatment Group/Radiation Therapy Oncology Group/Eastern Cooperative Oncology Group study. J Clin Oncol 2002;20:2223–4.
50. Curran D, Kiebert GM, Aaronson F, et al. Quality of life after radiation therapy of cerebral low-grade gliomas of the adult: results of a randomized phase III trial on dose response. Eur J Cancer 1998;34:1902–9.

51. van den Bent MJ, Afra D, de Witte O, et al. Long-term efficacy of early versus delayed radiotherapy for low-grade astrocytoma and oligodendroglioma in adults: the EORTC 22845 randomised trial. Lancet 2005;366:985–90.
52. Bauman GS, Ino Y, Ueki K, et al. Allelic loss of chromosome 1 p and radiotherapy plus chemotherapy in patients with oligodendrogliomas. Int J Radiat Oncol Biol Phys 2000;48:825–30.
53. Eyre HJ, Eltringham JR, Crowley J, et al. A randomised trial of radiotherapy versus radiotherapy plus CCNU for incompletely resected low-grade gliomas: Southwest Oncology Group study. J Neurosurg 1993;78:909–14.
54. Chinot OL, Honore S, Dufour H, et al. Safety and efficacy of temozolomide in patients with recurrent anaplastic oligodendroglioma after standard radiotherapy and chemotherapy. J Clin Oncol 2001;19:2449–55.
55. van den Bent MJ, Taphoorn MJB, Brandes AA, et al. Phase II study of first-line chemotherapy with temozolomide in recurrent oligodendroglial tumours. The European Organisation for Research and Treatment of Cancer Brain Tumour Group Study 26971. J Clin Oncol 2003;21:2525–8.
56. Cairncross JG, Ueki K, Zlatescu MC, et al. Specific genetic predictors of chemotherapeutic response and survival in patients with anaplastic oligodendrogliomas. J Natl Cancer Inst 1998;90:1473–9.
57. Ino Y, Betensky RA, Zlatescu MC, et al. Molecular subtypes of anaplastic oligodendroglioma: implications for patient management at diagnosis. Clin Cancer Research 2001;7:839–45.
58. Bissola L, Eoli M, Pollo B, et al. Association of chromosome 1 losses and negative response in oligoastrocytomas. Ann Neurol 2002;52:842–5.
59. Smith JS, Perry A, Borell TJ, et al. Alterations of chromosome arms 1 p and 19 q as predictors of survival in oligodendrogliomas, astrocytomas and mixed oligoastrocytomas. J Clin Oncol 2000;18:636–45.
60. Intergroup Radiation Therapy Oncology Group Trial 9402, Cairncross G, Berkey B, Shaw E, et al. Phase III trial of chemotherapy plus radiotherapy compared with radiotherapy alone for pure and mixed anaplastic oligodendroglioma: Intergroup Radiation Therapy Oncology Group Trial 9402. J Clin Oncol 2006;24:2707–14.
61. van den Bent MJ, Carpentier AF, Brandes AA, et al. Adjuvant procarbazine, lomustine, and vincristine improves progression-free survival but not overall survival in newly diagnosed anaplastic oligodendrogliomas and oligoastrocytomas: a randomized European Organisation for Research and Treatment of Cancer phase III trial. J Clin Oncol 2006;24:2715–22.
62. Fallon KB, Palmer CA, Roth KA, et al. Prognostic value of 1 p, 19 q, 9 p, 10 q and EGFR-FISH analyses in recurrent oligodendrogliomas. J Neuropathol Exp Neurol 2004;63:314–22.
63. Mason WP, Krol GS, DeAngelis LM. Low-grade oligodendroglioma responds to chemotherapy. Neurology 1996;46:203–7.
64. Streffer J, Schabet M, Bamberg M, et al. A role for preirradiation PCV chemotherapy for oligodendroglial brain tumors. J Neurol 2000;247:297–302.
65. Quinn JA, Reardon DA, Friedman AH, et al. Phase II trial of temozolomide in patients with progressive low-grade glioma. J Clin Oncol 2003;21:646–51.
66. Brada M, Viviers L, Abson C, et al. Phase II study of primary temozolomide chemotherapy in patients with WHO II gliomas. Annals of Oncology 2003;14:1715–21.
67. Hoang-Xuan K, Capelle L, Kujas M, et al. Temozolomide as initial treatment for adults with low-grade oligodendrogliomas or oligoastrocytomas and correlation with chromosome 1 p deletions. J Clin Oncol 2004;22:3133–8.
68. Sanson M, Cartaleat-Carel S, Taillibert, et al. Initial chemotherapy in gliomatosis cerebri. Neurology 2004;63:270–5.
69. Paleologos NA, Macdonald DR, Vick NA, Cairncross JG. Neoadjuvant procarbazine, CCNU and vincristine for anaplastic and aggressive oligodendroglioma. Neurology 1999;53:1141–3.
70. van den Bent M, Kros J, Heimans J, et al. Response rate and prognostic factors of recurrent oligodendroglioma treated with procarbazine, CCNU and vincristine chemotherapy. Neurology 1998;51:1140–5.
71. Sofietti R, Ruda R, Bradac G, Schiffer D. PCV chemotherapy for recurrent oligodendrogliomas and oligoastrocytomas. Neurosurgery 1998;43:1066–73.
72. van den Bent MJ, Taphoorn MJB, Brandes AA, et al. Phase II study of first-line chemo with temozolomide in recurrent oligodendroglial tumors: the European Organization for Research and Treatment of Cancer Brain Tumor Group Study 26971. J Clin Oncol 2003;21:2525–8.
73. Veninga T, Langendijk HA, Slotman BJ, et al. Reirradiation of primary brain tumours: survival, clinical response and prognostic factors. Radiother Oncol 2001;59:127–37.
74. Westergaard L, Gjerris F, Klinken L. Prognostic factors in oligodendrogliomas. Acta Neurochir (Wien) 1997;139:600–5.
75. Henderson KH, Shaw EG. Randomized trials of radiation therapy in adult low-grade gliomas. Semin Oncol 2001;11:145–51.

8 Pediatric Neuro-Oncology

MARK T. JENNINGS

Introduction

The predominant neoplastic diseases of the central nervous system (CNS) that arise during childhood are categorized as "low-grade" astrocytomas (AST), malignant gliomas (MG), and the "embryonal" or primitive neuroectodermal tumors (PNET), such as medulloblastoma (MBL). In addition, there are ependymomas (EPD) and oligodendrogliomas (OLG), as well as the rare primary germ cell tumors (GCT) which arise around the 3rd ventricle. The pathogenesis of each of these diseases appears complex, and is not as yet fully understood.

EPIDEMIOLOGY

The incidence of brain tumors among children (ages 0 to 14 years) is highest in the Scandinavian countries (31.4 per 10^6 per annum) followed by Western Europe, the United States of America, and New Zealand (24 to 27 per 10^6). The age-specific incidence for brain tumors is highest among children less than 5 years of age

(36 per 10^6 per annum), then declines among those 5 to 9 years (31.9 per 10^6) and 10 to 14 years (24.6 per 10^6) to the 15-19 age group (20.2 per 10^6 annually).[1–4]

Age correlates with the relative site of origin among cancers of the brain, in a pattern that is quite different than that observed among adults. Brainstem gliomas (BSG) are more common in children between 5 and 9 years of age (5.9 per 10^6 per annum) than among preschoolers (4.7 per 10^6), adolescents of 10 to 14 years (2.8 per 10^6), or older teenagers (1.7 per 10^6 per annum). Cerebellar neoplasms are similarly distributed, occurring most frequently between 5 and 9 years of age (9.7 per 10^6). By comparison, the relative distribution of tumors arising in the cerebrum gradually increases following the first 5 years of life (5.8 per 10^6 per annum) through adolescence (15 to 19 years of age) (7 per 10^6).[4] In contrast, during adulthood, the vast majority of primary CNS neoplasms are supratentorial in origin.

Reliable epidemiologic data confirm an increase in the incidence of children with gliomas between 1973 and 1992. This increase has been restricted to the AST (World Health Organization Grades I and II), with an average yearly rise of 3%. The trend has been more notable among females, in whom there has been an average annual increase of 3.9%. During this period, there was no change in the relative incidence of the other "classic" childhood CNS tumors, such as MBL and EPD.[5]

Among children and adolescents, tumors of astrocytic lineage constitute about 52% of reported cases. Other types of gliomas, such as gangliogliomas or mixed AST-OLG, contribute an additional 15.5%.[4] There are two clearly defined peaks in relative incidence, observed at five years (20.7 per 10^6 per annum) and thirteen (19.7 per 10^6) years of age.[3] After puberty, the incidence of AST and malignant astrocytomas (MA) falls to 12.3 per 10^6 annually.[1]

The PNETs comprise neoplasms considered "embryonal" in their pathogenetic derivation, and include the MBL, medulloepithelioma, pineoblastoma and the "cerebral neuroblastoma." Overall, this family of cancers comprises only 3.6% of all brain tumors.[6] As a group, the PNET constitute about 22% of primary CNS neoplasms occurring during childhood and adolescence.[4] Their relative incidence declines throughout childhood, from the peak seen among children less than 5 years of age (9.6 per 10^6 per annum), through those of 5 to 9 years of age (7.4 per 10^6), 10 to 14 years (4 per 10^6), and older adolescents (2.5 per 10^6 annually).[4] According to the National Cancer Institute's SEER data, the incidence of MBL-PNET rose 23% between 1973-1976 and 1993-1998, that is from 4 to 4.9 per 10^6 person-years (PY).[10]

Ependymomas constitute about 9% of tumors arising within the CNS during childhood and adolescence, but represent only 3% of brain tumors overall.[4,9] The relative incidence varies among age cohorts, being highest among infants, toddlers, and preschoolers (5.6 per 10^6 per annum), then falling to 1.1-1.6 per 10^6 annually among children older than 5 years of age.[1] The peak age at diagnosis is during the second year of life (8.6 per 10^6).[4]

Germ cell tumors present in three principal age periods. Congenital GCTs are typically benign teratomas, and during infancy (1 month to 3 years), endodermal sinus tumors and/or malignant teratomas predominate. Adolescence and young adulthood are usually associated with endodermal sinus tumors and embryonal carcinomas, often with teratomatous elements. In contrast to the prevalence of these nongerminomatous GCTs (NG-GCT) among the young, the majority of adult GCTs are pure germinomas.[8] In Japan, Taiwan, and South Korea, GCTs comprise 2.1% to 9.4% of primary intracranial neoplasms.[9] This is consistently higher than the 0.4% to 3.4% reported in western series.[10] In North America, origin within the brain accounts for 14% of all GCTs occurring among persons less than 20 years of age. Their relative incidence has steadily risen from 0.5 per 10^6 per annum in the 1970s to 1.5 per 10^6 in the late 1990s, which, within the industrialized countries, has suggested an environmental influence for their pathogenesis.

The observed survival rates for malignant CNS tumors diagnosed between 1973 and 1999 were grim: 50.0% at 1 year, 35.0% at 2 years, 25.6% at 5 years, and only 19.5% at 10 years from diagnosis. This translates to a mortality rate of 5.3/100,000 PY for males and 3.6/100,000 PY among females.[2]

PROPOSED ETIOLOGIC FACTORS

There is an approximately three- to nine-fold increased risk of developing a brain tumor should a family member be so affected; however, the nature of this association is not understood.[11] Allegations have been raised regarding electromagnetic waves, nitrosourea derivatives in processed meats, pesticides, and unique occupational hazards. However, no chemical agent not already known to be carcinogenic for other human tissues has been found to be uniquely associated with cancer of the brain. Neuroectodermal tissue is vulnerable to the carcinogenic effects of external-beam radiation therapy (EBRT). A strong dose-response relationship exists, as exposures higher than 2.5 Gray (Gy) are associated with a 20-fold increased carcinogenic potential.[12] The latency period for postradiation neuro-oncogenesis stretches from 12 years to 15 years (range 4 to 30 years).[13]

CLINICAL PRESENTATION

Low-Grade and Malignant Glioma

The child afflicted with a cerebral neoplasm complains of symptoms referable to its location. Cognitive impairment (15% to 20%) and seizures, either at presentation (about one third) or during the course of the illness (50% to 70%), are common problems that bring the patient to medical attention.[14] Superficial cerebral tumors may produce partial, complex partial, or secondarily generalized seizures. Symptoms of dysphasia, mental confusion, or motor deficit are predictive of significantly impaired physical, cognitive, emotional, and social function.[15] Motor or sensory compromise will reflect proximity to eloquent cortex. Deeply seated neoplasms, or those situated so as to obstruct the drainage of cerebrospinal fluid (CSF), produce headache, altered mental status, and, possibly, visual obscuration with or without localizing corticospinal tract findings. The pattern of headache, such as those which awaken the patient from sleep (10% to 32%), early morning occurrence followed by vomiting, as well as the influence of position, posture, or exercise (20% to 32%), contribute to the recognition of increased intracranial pressure. Recent onset, evolution of the headache's intensity, papilledema and/or focal deficits on exam also expedite a diagnostic investigation.[16] Brainstem gliomas are recognized by the combination of multiple cranioneuropathies, corticospinal tract findings, ataxia, and/or obstructive hydrocephalus.

Medulloblastoma

Park et al.[17] reviewed 144 patients treated at a major Canadian referral center between 1950 through 1980. The prediagnosis symptomatic interval was less than 6 weeks in 51%, and less than 12 weeks in 76%. The age at the time of diagnosis ranged from 7 weeks to 15 years. Eighty-one percent of patients were between 1 and 10 years of age. The clinical presentation was that of a posterior fossa mass, i.e., intracranial hypertension from hydrocephalus (Figure 8-1). Seventy-six percent had papilledema and 65% complained of headache. Recurrent vomiting occurred in 47%. Axial ataxia (62%), nystagmus (44%), and appendicular dysmetria (35%) were common neurologic signs. Hemorrhage into the primary tumor occurred in four, who presented with abrupt neurological deterioration.[17]

Staging evaluation is an important aspect in establishing the clinical diagnosis. Harisiadis and Chang[18] stratified patients based on tumor size ("T") and extent of metastatic spread ("M"). Spinal subarachnoid dissemination has been identified in 36% to 43% of prospectively studied patients.[19] Dissemination to the bone

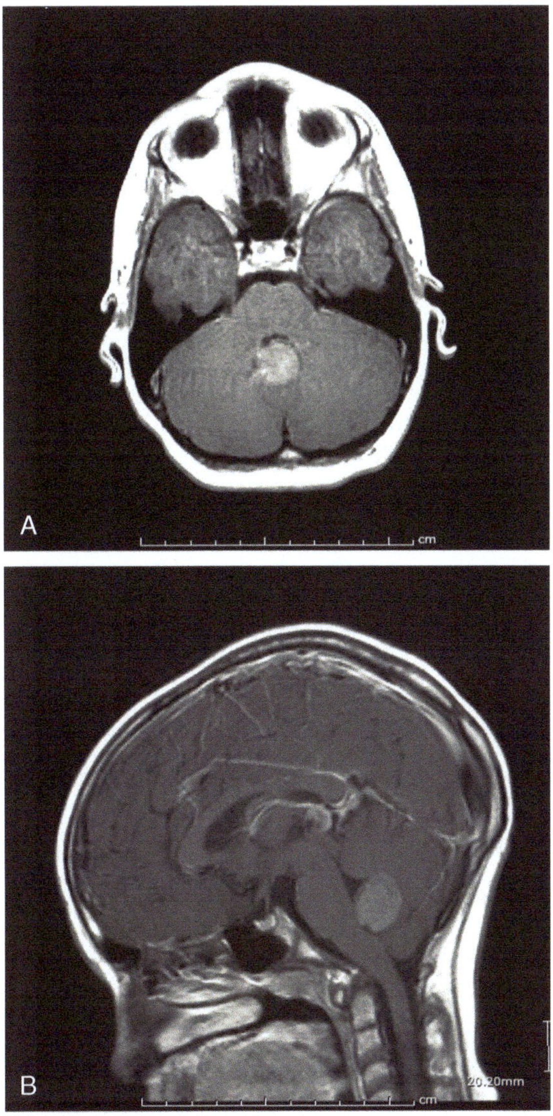

Figure 8-1 Axial **(A)** and sagittal **(B)** T1 contrast-enhanced MRI showing medulloblastoma in the posterior wall of the 4th ventricle.

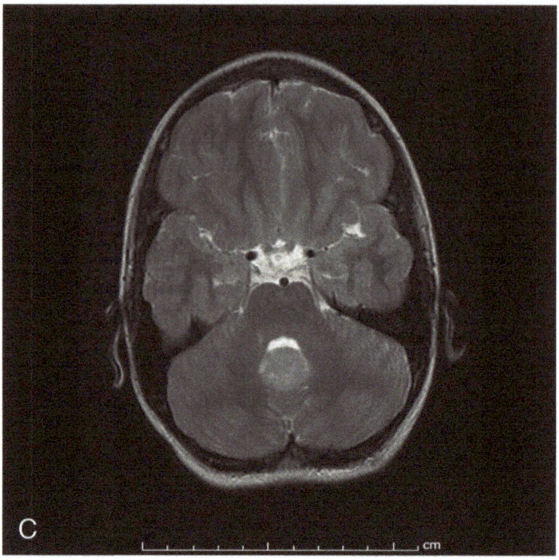

Figure 8-1—cont'd **C,** Axial T2 MRI. (Slides courtesy Susan Chi, M.D., Dana-Farber Cancer Institute and Boston Children's Hospital.)

marrow has been reported to be as high as 18% at the time of diagnosis.[19] The frequency of this complication at recurrence rises to approximately 35%.[20]

The "atypical teratoid/rhabdoid tumor" has previously been confused with the MBL. This early childhood neoplasm of the CNS arises either supra- or infratentorially and is composed of rhabdoid cells and undifferentiated small cells, with epithelial, mesenchymal, and neural elements. Overall survival (OS) periods of only 11 to 13 months have been reported following surgery and EBRT.[21,22]

Ependymoma

Supratentorial origin is more likely to be associated with corticospinal tract deficits and increased intracranial pressure at the time of presentation. Intratentorial location is frequently identified because of cranioneuropathies, ataxia, hydrocephalus, and a briefer prodrome because of the higher grade of malignancy encountered (Figure 8-2). Spinal EPDs present with back and/or radicular pain as well as lower motor neuron signs. The overall incidence of subarachnoid dissemination with intracranial EPD is reported to be approximately 10% to 22%, but this is influenced by site of origin and tumor grade. Anaplastic infratentorial tumors have a rate approaching 30%, while the incidence of spinal dissemination among the supratentorial EPD is negligible.[23]

Oligodendroglioma

A series of 37 patients demonstrated that the common presenting symptoms were seizures (43%), headache (38%), motor deficits (38%), and to a lesser degree, behavioral changes (16%). The most common site of origin was the frontal lobe (43%). Low grade histopathology (WHO grades I and II) was documented in 60%, with the remainder being grade III or IV disease.[24]

Germ Cell Tumor

Ninety-five percent of primary intracranial GCTs arise along an axis from the suprasellar cistern (37%) to the pineal gland (48%) (Figure 8-3). In one study, germinomas were found to preferentially involve the suprasellar region (57%), while 68% of NG-GCT's originated in the pineal recess ($P < .0001$). Germ-cell tumors were found in the suprasellar region in 75% of female patients; pineal involvement was more frequent (67%) among males ($P = .0001$). The age distribution peaked during early puberty. Nongerminomatous GCTs (24%) were more frequently diagnosed between birth and 9 years than were germinomas (11%)

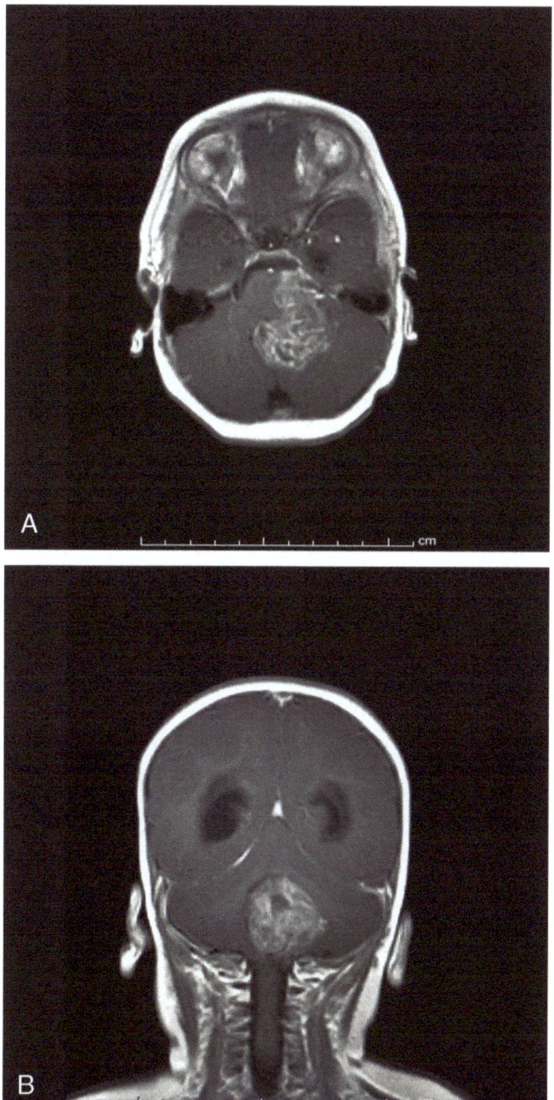

Figure 8-2 Axial **(A)** coronal **(B)** and sagittal **(C)** T1 contrast-enhanced MRI showing large ependymoma, effacing the 4th ventricle and invading into the brain stem There is associated hydrocephalus. (Slides courtesy Susan Chi, M.D., Dana-Farber Cancer Institute and Boston Children's Hospital.)

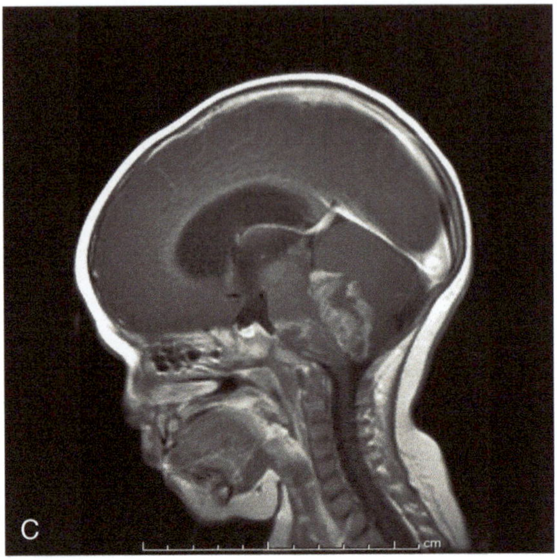

Figure 8-2—cont'd

(P < .0001). Among patients with germinomas, 35% were reported to be symptomatic for 6 months or longer, with half of these in excess of 24 months. The prodrome was much shorter among patients with NG-GCT (P = .0007).[8]

Patients with germinomas, which were commonly suprasellar, presented with chiasmal visual field defects (33%), diabetes insipidus (41%), and hypothalamic-pituitary dysfunction (33%). These neuroendocrine deficits included delay or regression of sexual development (16%), hypopituitarism (16%), and growth failure (9%). Presenting symptoms and signs among the NG-GCTs, which usually localized the lesion to the pineal recess, included hydrocephalus (47%),

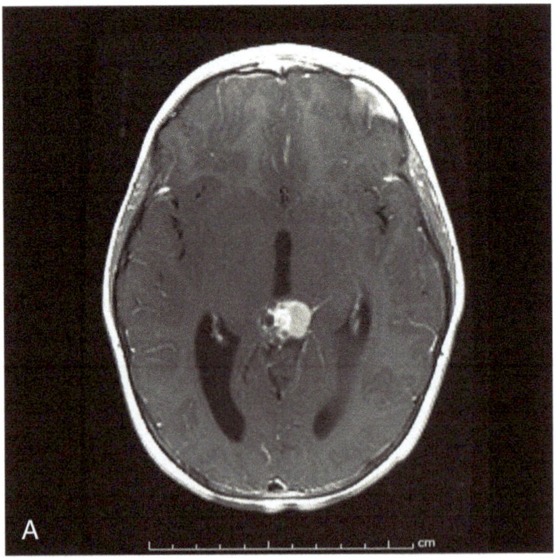

Figure 8-3 Axial **(A)** and sagittal **(B)** T1 contrast-enhanced MRI showing enhancing, partially cystic, mixed germ cell tumor. (Slides courtesy Susan Chi, M.D., Dana-Farber Cancer Institute and Boston Children's Hospital.)

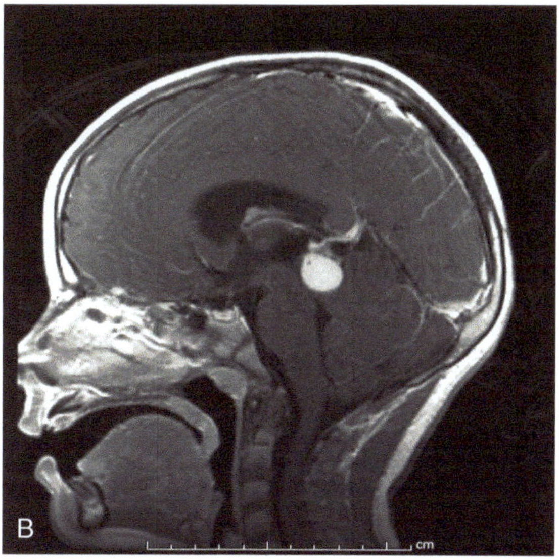

Figure 8-3—cont'd

Parinaud's sign (34%), obtundation (26%), pyramidal tract findings (21%), and ataxia (19%). Spinal cord metastases were more prevalent among patients with germinomas (11%) and endodermal sinus tumor (23%). Abdominal and pelvic metastases developed in approximately 10% of the 106 patients who were known to have received ventriculoperitoneal shunting.[8]

Choriocarcinomas were often (55%) associated with sexual precocity and increased human chorionic gonadotropin (HCG) and/or luteinizing hormone in the serum and/or CSF. Considerable effort has been made to use serological "biomarkers" such as HCG and alpha-fetoprotein (α-FP) for diagnostic, monitoring, and prognostic purposes. Among primary intracranial GCT, elevated levels of HCG have been reported among patients with choriocarcinomas, germinomas with syncytiotrophoblastic elements, embryonal carcinomas, teratomas, and endodermal sinus tumors. Alpha-fetoprotein levels are known to be raised among children with intracranial germinoma, teratoma, embryonal carcinoma, endodermal sinus tumor, and choriocarcinoma.

Brain Tumors Arising During Infancy

Primary CNS neoplasms during the first 2 years of life are considered quite uncommon in individual practice. However, they actually constitute 13% of all childhood brain tumors. The ratio between malignant (47%) and low-grade tumors is nearly equal in this age-group. Symptoms and signs are related to the site of origin, which is infratentorial in most (40% to 57%).[25] The most common symptom has been vomiting (43%), with early morning occurrence in only a third of infants. Headache may be suspected in 33% because of head banging and irritability. Gait ataxia (38%) and macrocephaly (19%) were other findings. The nonspecific nature of these symptoms contributes to the frequent delay in diagnosis. Tonsillar herniation has been documented in 43% at the time of diagnosis, presenting with head tilt (one third) or opisthotonic arching (one third), the latter has been misinterpreted as tonic seizure activity. As many as 10% of these children have presented as failure to thrive secondary to hypothalamic involvement, termed "the diencephalic syndrome."[25]

PROGNOSTIC VARIABLES

Malignant Glioma

It has proven difficult to identify biologic determinants of survival that can be conveniently assayed in a timely manner at the time of diagnosis in order to better guide the intensity of therapy. However, some attempts have been encouraging. For example, identification of the labeling index has shown an encouraging prognostic correlation with the histopathologic grade of MG, which in the future may allow stratification of pediatric subjects in clinical trials by relative risk.[26] The literature also suggests that expression of the multiple drug resistance (PgP/MDR) proteins and intratumoral hypoxia may also influence outcome.

Histopathologic Grade and Age among Malignant Astrocytomas

The Children's Cancer Group (CCG) #943 study showed the median survival among children with anaplastic astrocytomas (AAST) was greater than 6 years; among GBM patients, overall survival averaged less than 15 months (P = .012).[27] Age and histopathologic grade jointly influenced outcome. The CCG #921 study found that among children less than 24 months old, the 3-year progression-free survival (3Y-PFS) was 36%. The 3Y-PFS for patients with AAST was 44%, which was dramatically better than that for GBM (0%) (Table 8-1).[28]

Multidrug Resistance Phenotype

The PgP and MRP proteins are thought to function as ATP-dependent transmembrane transporters, which nonspecifically remove large molecular weight solutes from the brain and/or prevent hematogenously borne chemicals from entering the CNS.[29] PgP/MDR-1-associated resistance is hypothesized to function at the interface between the blood-brain and blood-tumor barriers as well as within the neoplastic cells themselves. Despite their association with progressive anaplasia and an adverse prognosis, there is actually little evidence that the PgP/MDR1 is a major mechanism of acquired resistance among MG.[29–31] Resistance to therapy appears to be a more complex phenomenon which disrupts the mechanisms of repair of genotoxic injury and/or induction of apoptosis.

The O^6-methylguanine-DNA methyltransferase (*MGMT*) enzyme's function is to counteract the cytotoxic effects of alkylating agents; its expression correlates inversely with survival among adult MG patients. Archival histopathologic specimens from 109 patients treated on the CCG Study #945 were analyzed, and 11% had overexpression of *MGMT*. The 5Y-PFS was 8.3% among these patients, in contrast to those whose tumors did not show overexpression of *MGMT* (5Y-PFS of 42%, P = .017). This adverse correlation was independent of age, histopathologic grade, tumor location, or extent of residual disease.[32]

Hypoxia and the Abrogation of Apoptosis

Intratumoral hypoxia is known to be the most significant predictor of radiotherapeutic resistance.[33] Radiation therapy has only one third the effectiveness against

TABLE 8-1 Prognostic Risk Factors Derived from Pediatric Phase III Studies of Malignant Gliomas

Study	**Factor**	**Significance**			**Reference**
CCG #943	Site of origin (deep vs. superficial)	P < .001			27
	Extent of resection	P < .001			
	Histopathologic grade (AAST vs. GBM)	P = .019			
Diagnosis	**Age**	**5Y-PFS in Relation to Extent of Resection**			**Reference**
		< 10%	*> 10%*		
CCG #945 study (131 pediatric pts)					106
MG		35%	17%	P = .006	
AAST		44%	22%	P = .055	
GBM		26%	4%	P = .046	
Diagnosis	**Age**	**1Y-PFS**	**2Y-PFS**		**Reference**
		<1.5 cm^2	*>1.5 cm^2*		
"Baby POG" (198 pediatric pts)					107
MG	Infants <24 mo	74%	65%	P < .001	
	24–36 mo	91%			

Abbreviations: 1-, 2-, and 5-year progression-free survival (5Y-PFS), Brain Tumor Cooperative Group (BTCG), Children's Cancer Group (CCG), Pediatric Oncology Group (POG), malignant glioma (MG), anaplastic astrocytoma (AAST), glioblastoma multiforme (GBM), patients (pts), months (mo).

hypoxic tumor cells that it does against well-oxygenated cells. It was previously thought that radiation-induced DNA damage required the presence of oxygen radicals. Instead, normal cells, when deprived of oxygen, will arrest in late G_1 and early S phase, in concert with hypophosphorylation of the retinoblastoma gene protein, pRB, and die through induction of apoptosis.[33] Arrest of the DNA-damaged cell at the G_1/S interface is associated with stabilization of intact wild-type *TP53* (*TP53wt*) expression, inhibition of replicative DNA synthesis, and possibly the initiation of repair. *TP53wt* appears to achieve G_1/S arrest through transcriptional regulation of at least one critical downstream target, the Cdk inhibitor $p21^{WAF1/CIP1}$. This protein inactivates cyclin D/Cdk4, D/Cdk6, and E/Cdk2 complex activity and directly inhibits PCNA, a regulatory subunit of DNA polymerase (the principal replicative DNA polymerase).[34]

Ionizing radiation also produces G_1 arrest in cells with *TP53wt* and increases *TP53* protein expression.[35] In contrast, the hypoxic regions within the tumor actually create a reservoir for malignantly transformed cells, which do not arrest at the G_1/S interface, are more likely to have mutations in the *TP53* gene (*TP53m*), and become resistant to *TP53*-induced apoptosis (Graeber et al., 1996).[36]

Stable cytoplasmic *TP53wt* expression has been shown to a favorable predictor for survival among AAST patients (P = .015). By comparison, such expression was not found among the GBM (P = .8), which by definition contain areas of necrosis.[37] Intratumoral hypoxia thus constitutes a key mechanism of clonal selection.

Furthermore, hypoxia has also been correlated with insensitivity to carmustine (BCNU) and cisplatin, independently of the putative drug resistance genes *MDR1*, *MRP*, *O^6MGMT*, or *ERCC*.[38] Here too, the acquisition of resistance appears be mediated through *TP53m*. For example, 86% of *TP53wt* positive MG cell lines have been shown to be responsive to currently available chemotherapy drugs. In contrast, there were no effective cytotoxic agents against 75% of the glioma cultures expressing *TP53m* (P = .0006). Supporting this specificity, the resistance conferred by *TP53m* is restricted to alkylators and platinators, which damage DNA, rather than against the microtubular toxins.[39]

The Molecular Basis for Multiple Models of Glioma Progression: The Tumor Suppressor Genes

There is a large literature on the nonrandom cytogenetic aberrations observed among MGs, which include gains or losses of chromosomes, as well as rearrangements. Some of these changes, such as 10q, 9p, 11p15.5-pter and 19q may be found only among AASTs and/or GBMs.[40,41] Loss of heterozygosity (LOH) analysis has correlated 17p deletions with allelic loss of the tumor suppressor gene (TSG), *TP53*.[42] Hence, it has been hypothesized that such nonrandom patterns of genetic loss can be exploited to predict the location of other as yet unknown TSGs. This in turn has generated the concept of modeling mechanisms for tumor progression.

TP53

One pathway in the evolution of the MG involves *TP53m*, which occurs in 14% to 46% of adult patients and is preferentially associated with development of the glioma (often an AAST) between 18 and 45 years of age.[42,43] Clonal expansion of *TP53m* cells have been observed from a small subpopulation within a primary AST to become the dominant cell type within a recurrent, or "secondary" MG.[44]

Alternate means of *TP53wt* inactivation exist as *TP53wt* may be complexed by the *MDM2* oncogene product. In 8% to 10% of GBM, the *MDM2* gene is amplified and overexpressed, supporting the importance of *TP53wt* in glial cell cycle dysregulation. A more recent study has identified that about 35% of gliomas demonstrate either *TP53m* or methylation of *p14(ARF)*, suggesting that *TP53wt* is controlled by down-regulation of *p14(ARF)*.[45] Inactivation of the astrocyte's apoptotic response may therefore be effected either by deletion of 17p, mutation of *TP53*, *MDM2* overpression, or hypermethylation of *p14(ARF)*, thus unmasking multiple points of vulnerability along a common pathway that permit further progression towards the endpoint of malignant transformation.[45]

PTEN

Another fraction of about 30% (23% to 62%) of adult GBM patients has been characterized by the association of LOH of chromosome 10 with epidermal growth factor receptor (EGFR) amplification. In contrast to the previous group, these patients (typically older individuals) appear to present de novo with a "primary" GBM. The LOH at 10q23 has been demonstrated in approximately 70% of GBMs, and therefore predicted to be the site of another glial TSG.[42,43] The "Mutated in

Multiple Advanced Cancers" and "Phosphatase and Tensin" gene (*MMAC/PTEN*) has been localized to chromosome 10q25 and shown to function as a phosphatidylinositol 3,4,5-triphosphate phosphatase, which modulates cell growth as well as apoptosis.[46,47]

Patients with GBM have demonstrated a significantly higher incidence of LOH at the *MMAC/PTEN* locus (72%) than did patients with AAST (29%)($P < .0001$). The clinical relevance is that patients with LOH at the *MMAC/PTEN* locus have a more adverse prognosis ($P < .0001$), even when controlled for age at surgery and histologic grade.[48] Conversely, Kaplan-Meier analysis has demonstrated significantly better survival for patients whose MG exhibited high *MMAC/PTEN* expression.[49] These results have been interpreted to implicate alteration or loss of the *MMAC/PTEN* locus as a late marker of disease progression with ominous significance.

RB

About 15% to 44% of MG patients are reported to have loss of chromosome 13 as well as LOH or partial deletions of the 13q14 allele, which suggests the possibility that the *RB* gene is also a glioma TSG. Loss of heterozygosity at the *RB* 1.20 region has not been detected among low-grade gliomas, but occurred in 20% of AAST and 32% of GBM. The presence of LOH at the *RB* 1.20 region has also been associated with an adverse prognosis, implying that loss/inactivation of pRB contributes to disease progression.[50]

Investigation suggests that aberrant function of cyclin D, Cdk4, $p16^{INK4A/MTS1}$, and/or pRB is critical for both the process of transformation and that of progression towards increasing anaplasia among glial neoplasms. Cyclin D1 was originally cloned from a human GBM cDNA library, where its transcript and 34 kD product were in abundant expression. Deletion of $p16^{INK4A/MTS1}$ and/or amplification of its target Cdk4 occur in 50% of AAST and 85% of GBM.[51,52] The coordinate deletion of both $p15^{INK4B/MTS2}$ and $p16^{INK4A/MTS1}$ among GBMs suggests that selection favors homozygous deletions of chromosome 9p21 as more efficient for the simultaneous inactivation of both Cdk inhibitors than independent intragenic mutations would be.[51] This remarkable specificity suggests that knocking out $p16^{INK4A/MTS1}$'s inhibition of cyclin D1/Cdk4-induced hyperphosphorylation of pRB marks a critical event in the progression to the most advanced grade of glioma, the GBM.[52]

Evidence is accumulating that cyclin D1 overexpression, absence of pRB expression, failure of pRB dephosphorylation, and/or pRB cleavage may also contribute to chemotherapeutic drug resistance as well, although the mechanism or mechanisms are not understood. Altered *CDKN2/p16* function has been correlated with increased sensitivity to antimetabolite agents as opposed to the alkylators, topoisomerase inhibitors, and microtubular toxins.[53]

To conclude, the genetic mechanism of glial transformation in children is not understood. In one series of 20 pediatric GBMs, 25% were associated with *TP53*m, the majority of which presented with a brief prodromal period and were considered "primary." Loss of $p16^{CDKN2/INK4A/MTS1}$ was detected in 61% of these GBMs. Overexpression of EGFR was infrequent (11%) and was coincidental with *TP53 m* in one case. Of the four GBMs, which progressed from lower-grade tumors, only one contained *TP53 m*.[54] In another series of 29 childhood MGs, 95% of cases were found to harbor an alteration in at least one member of the *TP53/MDM2/p14ARF* tumor suppressor pathway. Overexpression of *MDM2*, which downregulates *TP53* transcriptional activity, was present in 65%, and loss of *p14AFT*, which inactivates the pathway through *MDM2*, was found in 10%.[55]

Among pediatric MGs, the presence of *MMAC/PTEN* mutations has also been confirmed as a marker of an adverse outcome that is independent of patient age or histopathologic grade (III vs. IV).[56] In tumor specimens of 62 evaluable patients treated on the Children's Cancer Group (CCG) #945 protocol for children with MG (*vide infra*), alteration of *PTEN* sequence was detected in just one, in conjunction with loss of chromosome 10. Deletions of *PTEN* without mutations were found in seven additional specimens. The *PTEN* alterations were more common among GBM than other histopathologic grades (P = .0056). Although 37% (14/38) of evaluable tumors had increased EGFR expression, only one exhibited amplification of the EGFR gene. This may be interpreted to indicate that pediatric MGs differ in the mechanisms of tumorigenesis from those of adulthood.[57]

Brainstem Glioma

Favorable prognostic features include (a) protracted symptoms, (b) origin within the optic tectum, the mesencephalon, or at the cervicomedullary junction, (c) lesions which are cystic, focal, and/or dorsally exophytic, (d) onset in adulthood, and (e) neurofibromatosis type I (NF1). By comparison, the adverse markers for disease progression are diffuse pontine infiltration, a high mitotic index, a brief symptomatic prodrome, and multiple cranioneuropathies at presentation.[58]

Low-Grade Astrocytoma

Low-grade glial neoplasms (LGGN), which include AST, mixed astrocytoma-oligodendroglioma (AST-OLG), and pure OLG, constitute a heterogenous group of tumors without a predictable natural history. The 5Y-OS and 10Y-OS rates for LGGN following resection and EBRT are reported to range between 40% to 70% and 11% to 50%, respectively.[59] In a review of 461 AST patients, the 5Y-OS rate was 36%; that is a third of the predicted actuarial survival for a comparable population of unaffected individuals.[59] Only 16% of LGGN patients of any age were alive at 15 years following diagnosis.[60] Otherwise stated, the long-term survival rate among patients with LGGN is less than that of their peers suffering from acute lymphocytic leukemia.

The literature suggests that age at presentation, seizures as the sole presenting symptom, site of origin, favorable Karnofsky status, absence of contrast enhancement on imaging, histopathologic grade (i.e., pilocytic vs. diffuse) (Figure 8-4), initial tumor dimensions, extent of resection (i.e., unresectable tumor), presence of hydrocephalus, or coexistence of NF1 are the important variables that influence quality of life as well as survival.[61] The prognostic value of the labeling index has been previously reviewed.[26]

Site of Origin

It is accepted that the biology of LGGN arising within the hypothalamus, optic tectum, and cervico-medullary junction clearly differs from those arising within the pons and cerebrum. Consensus exists that gross total resection of an AST or mixed LGGN *during childhood* is adequate therapy and does not require immediate postoperative irradiation (Nishio et al., 1989).[62] Univariate analysis has

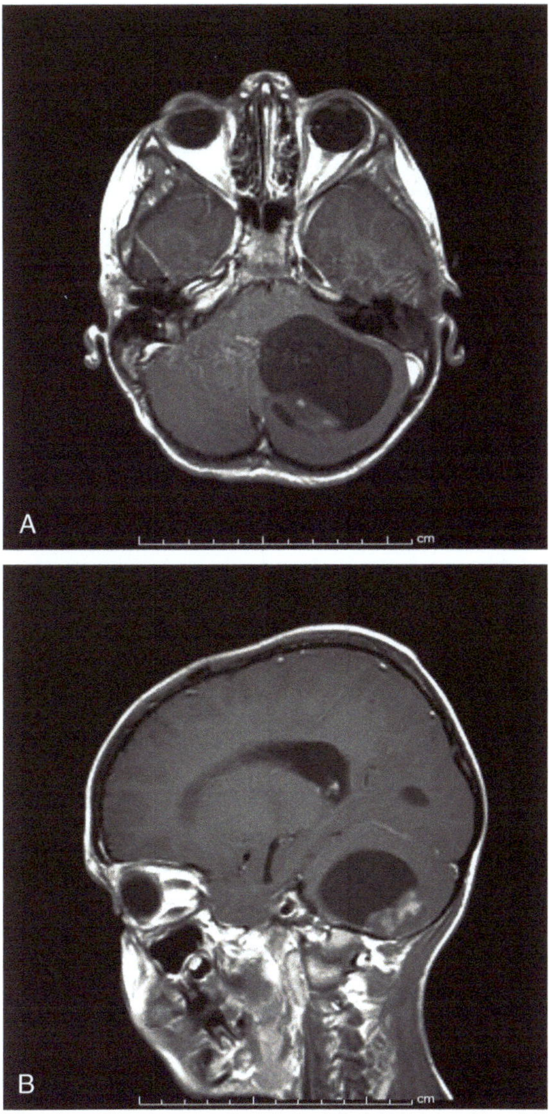

Figure 8-4 Axial **(A)** and sagittal **(B)** T1 contrast-enhanced MRI showing typical cystic left cerebellar pilocytic astrocytoma with a posterior mural nodule.

demonstrated that optic chiasmal origin and only partial resection are associated with a worsened prognosis.[63] This has influenced the controversy regarding EBRT (*vide infra*).

Neurofibromatosis

The 5Y-OS and 10Y-OS for patients with optic nerve gliomas and NF1 has been reported to be 93% and 81%, respectively. This compares favorably to survival rates of 83% and 76% at 5 and 10 years, respectively, for those children without evidence of NF1. The mean time to disease progression (TDP) was significantly

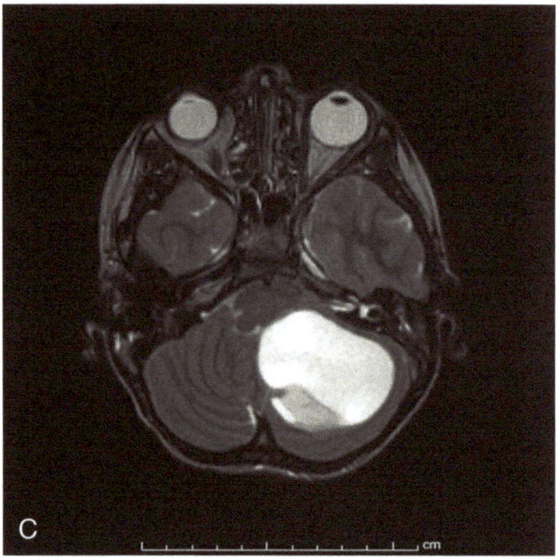

Figure 8-4—cont'd **C,** Axial T2 MRI. (Slides courtesy Susan Chi, M.D., Dana-Farber Cancer Institute and Boston Children's Hospital.)

different between the two groups (P < .01) in favor of those with NF1, although this did not impact OS.[64] However, this relative advantage does not appear to apply to patients with von Recklinghausen disease who suffer from gliomas of the cerebrum.[65]

Histopathologic Grade and Malignant Progression among Low-Grade Astrocytomas

The process of malignant transformation was studied among 11 of 65 children with LGGN. The median latency was 5.1 years, and the 15-year cumulative incidence estimate was 6.7 %. Overexpression of *TP53* was more common after progression to higher histopathologic grade. Deletions of *RB1* and/or *CDKN2A* were observed in 71% of the LGGN and 90% of their malignant successors. There were *PTEN* pathway abnormalities found in 76% of patients.[66]

Medulloblastoma and Primitive Neuroectodermal Tumor

Staging evaluation stratifies patients by tumor size ("T") and extent of metastatic spread ("M").[18] Table 8-2 summarizes its prognostic significance as derived from the European Societie Internationale Oncologie Pediatrie (SIOP) and the North American CCG study #942.[67,68] Stepwise analysis of survival among randomized patients demonstrated earlier age of onset to be the dominant adverse variable (P = .034). There were significant interactions between treatment and M stage, which support postoperative irradiation and chemotherapy among patients with advanced disease, i.e., high T and M stages (P = .004) (Table 8-2).[68]

The subsequent CCG #921 study of children with MBL (203 patients) demonstrated the significance of residual disease prior to EBRT, whether determined by extent of surgical resection (P = .023) or by evidence of metastatic tumor (M_{1-3}) (P < .003) (Table 8-2).[69,70]

TABLE 8-2 Prognostic Risk Factors Derived from Phase III Studies of Medulloblastoma

Factor	5Y-PFS	Significance	References
SIOP-I (285 pts)			67
Partial resection/biopsy		P = .01	
$T_{1,2}$ vs. $T_{3,4}$		P < .001	
CCG #942 (233 pts)			68
M-stage: M_0 vs. M_{1-3}	59% vs. 36%	P < .003	
Age: < 4 vs. ≥ 4 yrs		P = .003	
Gross total vs. partial resection		P = .07	
$T_{1,2}$ vs., $T_{3,4}$	61% vs. 52%	NS	
CCG #921 (203 pts)			69,70
Residual disease < 1.5 cm^2	78% vs. 54%	P = .023	
M_0 vs. M_{1-3}	67% vs. 43%	P < .003	
Age: < 3 yrs vs. > 3 yrs		P = .0014	
M_{1-3} + Age > 3 yrs		P = .0006	
Sick Children's Hospital of Toronto			139
Gross total vs. partial resection	93% vs. 45%	P = .0003	
Postoperative meningitis (+ vs. –)	42% vs. 69%	P = .02	
$M_{0,1}$ vs. $M_{3,4}$		P = .07	
Postoperative residual disease (+ vs. –)	42% vs. 82%	P = .02	
Postradiotherapy residual disease (+ vs. –)	44% vs. 79%	P = .04	
Supratentorial Primitive Neuroectodermal Tumors			
	3Y-PFS		
CCG #921			140,141
Pineal vs. elsewhere	61% vs. 45%	P < .03	
$M_{0,1}$ vs. $M_{3,4}$	50% vs. 0%	P < .03	
Age: < 2y vs. > 3 yrs	25% vs. 53%	P < .02	
Ependymomas			
	5Y-PFS		
Gross total vs. other resection	68% vs. 9%	P = .0001	23
Age: < 3 yrs vs. > 3 yrs	12% vs. 60%	P = .01	
Symptomatic < 1 mo vs. >1 mo	33% vs. 53%	P = .02	

Pathologic Studies

A series of 330 cases studied by the Pediatric Oncology Group (POG) found significant anaplasia among 24%, which was strongly associated with an unfortunate outcome. Diffuse or extensive anaplasia was worse than focal involvement. In contrast, extensive nodularity conferred a more favorable course.[71] Reevaluation of 347 MBL biopsies treated under the SIOP II trial confirmed that severe anaplasia conferred an adverse prognostic effect on 5-year progression-free survival (49.5%) relative to mild-moderate change (65.4%) (P = .001). This effect was magnified when the presence or absence of extensive apoptosis (P = .00216) was factored in.[72]

Drug Resistance Genes

There is evidence that the expression of the *MDR1, MRP1, LRP* and *BCRP* genes does not correlate with overall outcome among patients with MBL/PNET.[73]

Biologic Determinants of Survival

Established chromosome abnormalities include amplication of isochromosome 17q, novel amplicons, and losses as well as gains of chromosomes; these are known to occur in greater than 20% of MBL. Copy number abnormalities have been identified in specific regions of chromosomes 1, 8p, 10q, 11p, and 16q, which occur frequently among MBLs and may identify distinct subsets.[74] Furthermore, differences in DNA copy number at chromosome regions 1p12-22.1, 9p21, 19p, and chromosome 17 have been used to segregate between MBL and supratentorial PNET. The 9p21 deletions correlated with loss of CDKN2A protein expression more frequently among the PNET (P < .001). Gains of 19p were also more evident among the PNET (P = .02), whereas gains of 17q were more common among the MBL (P = .02).[75]

(i) Tumor suppressor genes. Haploinsufficiency of the 17p13.3 region is the most commonly found disrupted genetic site (35-50%) among MBLs, which may indicate the site of yet another TSG(s). This chromosomal site contains the "Hypermethylated in Cancer" gene *(HIC1)*, a transcriptional repressor, which is a frequent target of epigenetic gene silencing in MBL. *HIC1* is a direct transcriptional repressor of "Atonal Homolog 1" gene *(ATOH1)*, a proneural transcription factor essential for cerebellar development. *ATOH1* is a putative target of "(Sonic) Hedgehog" *(HH)* signaling and its expression has been shown to be required for human MBL cell growth in vitro. The *PTCH* gene, an inhibitor of *SHH* signaling, is among the characterized TSG in MBL; however, fewer than 20% of MBLs have mutations in this gene. Recent work suggests that the *HIC1* and *PTCH1* TSG cooperate to silence *ATOH1* expression during a critical phase of granule cell precursor differentiation in the cerebellum to contribute to the malignant progression to MBL.[76]

Specimens of MBL collected from 65 children treated in the SIOP/United Kingdom Children's Cancer Group *PNET3* trial were segregated into the histopathologic groups such as the large cell/anaplastic phenotype and nodular/desmoplastic variant, among others. Loss of 17p13.3 was found among 38% of samples of all variants, whereas *MYCC/MYCN* amplification (6%/8% respectively of MBLs) was significantly associated with the large cell/anaplastic phenotype. Loss of 9q22 coincided with the nodular/desmoplastic type. Together with metastatic disease at diagnosis, the large cell/anaplastic phenotype, 17p13.3 loss, or high frequency *MYC* amplification defined a high-risk group of children whose outcome was significantly worse than those without such tumor characteristics (P = .0002).[77] However, the relationships between chromosome 17 lesions with anaplastic/large cell MBL and the abnormalities in the *Sonic Hedgehog/PATCH (SHH/PTCH)* pathway with the desmoplastic variant remain controversial.[78]

The *SHH* antagonist, cyclopamine, blocked expression of the *SHH* pathway targets *PTCH1* and *GLI1*, lowered *Bcl2* levels, and increased apoptosis in MBL cells in vitro. Blockade of the *SHH* pathway sensitized MBL cells to lovastatin, a proapoptotic agent used for lowering cholesterol levels. The combination of cyclopamine and lovastatin target pathways appear crucial for MBL cell survival.[79] Agents targeting the *SHH* pathway are in clinical trials for the therapy of medulloblastomas.

Activation of the canonical WNT/Wingless *(WNT/WG)* signaling pathway occurs in up to 25% of cases of primary MBL and is associated with a favorable prognosis. Activation of *WNT/WG* was determined by evidence of *CTNNB1* mutations and/or beta-catenin nuclear stabilization. Loss of chromosome 6 has been correlated with *WNT/WG* active tumors ($P < .001$), but few other cytogenetic aberrations including chromosome 17. In contrast, *WNT/WG*-negative MBLs were found to have losses of chromosomes 17p, 8, 10, and 16, with gains of chromosomes 7 and 17q. This supports the hypothesis of independent pathways of tumorigenesis among MBL, which are of potential clinical relevance.[80]

TP73 is a member of the *TP53* TSG family that is overexpressed in a variety of tumors and mediates apoptotic responses to genotoxic stress. Biopsy samples of MBL and MBL cell lines have been reported to contain elevated levels of *TP73* RNA and increased expression of the TAp73 and DeltaNp73 protein products. Overexpression of these induced apoptosis among cultured MBL cells in vitro and sensitized them, resulting in cell death upon exposure to chemotherapeutic agents. *TAp73* RNA overexpression within biopsy samples was determined to correlate with a favorable PFS by Kaplan-Meier analysis.[81]

The 10q23.3 chromosomal region is subject to frequent allelic losses in MBL, which is the locus of the *PTEN* gene. Activation of the phosphoinosityl 3-kinase/AKT *(P13k/AKT)* signaling pathway appears to be associated with alterations of the *PTEN* gene. Proliferation of MBL cell lines has been shown to be dependent upon *P13k/AKT* signaling and inhibited by a P13K antagonist as well as by *AKT* overexpression. Reduction of *PTEN* mRNA and protein expression has been found to be correlated with *PTEN* promoter hypermethylation in 50% of 22 MBL tissue samples. This suggests that *PTEN* loss or dysregulation by the *P13k/AKT* signaling pathway may be an important mechanism of tumorigenesis for a subset of MBL.[82] In contrast, *PTEN* deletion has not been found among supratentorial PNET biopsies or cell lines.[83]

(ii) The Putative Oncogenes. The Duke group studied 31 MBL specimens for *MYCC, MYCN* and *TRKC* expression and correlated this with clinical outcome and histopathologic grading. The presence of *MYCC* mRNA was associated with shorter survival ($P = .04$) as well as with anaplasia. Regulation of *MYCC* is influenced by *WNT* signaling and *MXI1* mutations. Nuclear translocation of beta-catenin, a marker of *WNT* pathway activation, was more common among the MBLs with high *MYCC*. No *MXI1* mutations were detected in the 22 cases examined.[84]

Archival formalin-fixed, paraffin-embedded MBL samples from 78 patients treated on the prospective European multicenter HIT'91 protocol were studied for DNA amplification of *C-MYC* and *N-MYC* and mRNA expression of *C-MYC* and *TRKC*. *TRKC* and *C-MYC* mRNA expression were identified as independent prognostic factors on multivariate analysis. A favorable-risk group (eight patients), with a 7Y-PFS of 100%, possessed elevated *TRKC* and reduced *C-MYC* expression. The poor-risk group (15 patients) had metastatic disease, with high *C-MYC* and low *TRKC* mRNA expression. Their 7Y-PFS was only 33%. An intermediate-risk group of the remaining subjects showed a 7Y-PFS of 65%.[85] Not all investigators have made similar correlations.[86]

Ependymoma

Pathologic Grading

The prognostic utility of pathologic grading of ependymomas has engendered a long-standing controversy, as there has been no clear distinction in 5Y-OS rates between "benign" and "malignant" EPD. However, one recent blinded review demonstrated that the PFS at 2 years following postoperative irradiation was 84% for differentiated EPD, and 32% for specimens considered anaplastic.[87]

Site of Origin

There is a correlation between site of origin and histopathologic grade of malignancy. Approximately two thirds of supratentorial EPDs are high-grade at diagnosis, whereas those arising in the IVth ventricle tend to have a better prognosis.[88] A series of 49 patients found that 78% originated infratentorially and exhibited low grade histology.[89] Those arising in the spine and cauda equina are usually low-grade and/or myopapillary.

Extent of Surgical Resection

The CCG #921 study accessioned 20 EPD and 12 anaplastic EPD patients, of whom only three had metastatic disease at diagnosis. The prognostic variables of significance included the extent of resection (gross total vs. other, $P = .0001$) and postoperative residual disease of $< 1.5\,cm^2$ ($P < .0001$), in contrast to age, staging, or treatment, emphasizing the importance of local disease control.[90]

The French Society of Pediatric Oncology has studied the efficacy of postoperative chemotherapy, with the intent of avoiding EBRT, among 73 children less than 5 years of age with intracranial EPD. The favorable prognostic variables included supratentorial origin ($P = .0004$) and complete resection ($P = .0009$). Patients with gross total resection demonstrated a 4Y-OS of 74% in contrast to those with residual disease (35%).[91]

Univariate and Multivariate Analysis

Three prognostic factors have been identified to have a significant correlation with the 5Y-PFS. These included the extent of surgical resection ($P < .0001$), age at diagnosis ($P = .003$), and the prediagnosis symptomatic interval ($P = .02$).[23] Another multicenter retrospective study of 83 children with EPD confirmed that age of less than 3 years, identifiable postoperative residual disease, and Grade III histology were significant adverse factors for PFS in both univariate and multivariate analysis.[92]

Biologic Determinants of Survival

Overexpression of specific genes (*YAP* and *LOC374491*) and downregulation of others such as *SULT4A1*, *NF-[kappa]B2*, and *PLEK* have been implicated in determining the age of onset, relapse potential, and tumor location of pediatric EPD.[93,94] The catalytic subunit of telomerase, the human telomere reverse transcriptase (*hTERT*), which aids in uncontrolled cell proliferation, has been shown to correlate with prognosis among 65 children with EPD. Study of 87 tumors from these patients found the presence of *hTERT* to be adversely correlated with 5Y-OS (41% vs. 84% in its absence).[95]

Oligodendroglioma

The accepted favorable prognostic variables for OLG include youth (less than 21 years), low histopathologic grade, and extent of resection.[96] Multivariate analysis in a series of 51 patients aged 5 to 75 years found younger age and presentation with seizures alone to be statistically significant for a favorable outcome. Approximately one third of patients of all ages appear to be cured by aggressive treatment including surgical resection, EBRT, and chemotherapy.[96]

Biologic Determinants of Survival

In several studies of LGGN, the classic histology of the OLG has been strongly associated with 1p deletion ($P = .002$), loss of 19q ($P < .0001$), or loss of both ($P < .0001$).[97] Deletion of 9p was found in 36% (8/22), always in association with tumor necrosis and/or microvascular proliferation. In addition, epigenetic alterations of *CDKN2A* were observed in 71% of these 1p/19q/9p deleted OLG, suggesting that it may have a role in microvascular proliferation.[98] A collaborative study of 162 diffuse gliomas (52 OLG, 79 AST, and 31 AST-OLG) has demonstrated that the combined loss of 1p/19q is a statistically significant predictor ($P < .0001$) of prolonged survival among patients with pure OLG, even after adjusting for patient age and tumor grade ($P < .01$).[97]

Allelic deletions on the short arm of chromosome 1 have been correlated with chemosensitivity and a better prognosis for patients with high-grade OLG. The $p18^{INK4C}$ gene is considered to be a good candidate for the putative TSG located at the chromosome 1p32 locus. The incidence of LOH at 1p is 50% among primary OLG; mutations in the gene have been found among recurrent tumors, implicating it as a possible progression factor as well.[99] The 1p loss has been shown to be inversely related to deletions of the *CDKN2A* gene on 9p, which encodes a key cell cycle regulatory molecule $p16^{INK41}$.[100] The 19q13.3 locus is deleted in 50% to 80% of OLG. This region codes for the *p190RhoGAP* gene, which appears to suppress gliomagenesis by inducing a differentiated glial phenotype.[101]

Germ Cell Tumors

Histopathologic diagnosis

Matsutani et al.[102] performed a clinical analysis of 153 cases treated between 1963 and 1994 at the University of Tokyo Hospital, which revealed pathologic diagnosis to be the dominant prognostic determinant. The 10-year overall survival rate (10Y-OS) for germinomas was 93%. The 10Y-OS rates for mature and "malignant" teratoma were 93% and 71%, respectively. The diagnoses of embryonal carcinoma, endodermal sinus tumor, and choriocarcinoma had a 3Y-OS of 27%.[102]

Biomarker Expression

The First International Germ Cell Tumor Study observed, in a series of 71 patients, that elevated β-HCG was associated with increased risk of disease progression ($P = .06$), but did not affect OS.[103] In a Japanese study, 33 GCTs (16 germinomas, 11 β-HCG positive germinomas, 3 mixed teratoma-germinoma and 3 NG-GCT) were treated with preradiation chemotherapy. Patients with "pure germinomas" had a 86% 5Y-PFS, while germinoma patients with measurable β-HCG expression exhibited only a 44% 5Y-PFS.[104]

THERAPEUTIC EFFECTIVENESS AND CONSEQUENT PROGNOSIS

The essential clinical problem of neuro-oncology has been succinctly stated. The patient typically presents with a tumor volume of 30 to 60 gm at the time of diagnosis. This represents 3 to 6 × 10^{10} cells within the mass, of which the neurosurgeon may be able to resect 20% to 90%. Therefore, a "best-case" postoperative scenario is a residual tumor burden of 3 to 6 × 10^9 cells. EBRT achieves an approximate two-log cell kill in the treatment of MG. Conventionally dosed chemotherapy may provide an additional one-log cytoreduction. Thus the "ideal" patient completes multimodality therapy with a repository of approximately 3 to 6 × 10^6 malignant cells, which are presumably then radio- and chemo-resistant.[105] The treatment intensity concept may help to explain the patterns of failure when the strategic plan is critiqued for the relative degree of cytoreduction achieved at each sequential stage of multimodality intervention.

Malignant Gliomas

Surgical Intervention

Among newly diagnosed pediatric MG patients, the CCG #943 study demonstrated the impact of the following factors on progression free-survival. Deeply seated diencephalic MG demonstrated a median survival being less than 10 months. Patients receiving only a biopsy experienced a median survival of less than 8 months regardless of subsequent therapy. Partial resection and gross total resection were associated with better but similar long-term outcomes (Table 8-1).[27] Among children with MG treated on the CCG phase III study #945, radical surgical resection doubled the 5Y-PFS rate (P = .006) (Table 8-1).[106] Unfortunately, it has only been possible to achieve minimal postoperative residual tumor burden for 33% (19% to 45%) of newly diagnosed pediatric MG patients treated in contemporary series.[106–109]

Radiotherapy. The conventional radiotherapeutic prescription for MG usually consists of 2 Gray (Gy) fractions per day, 5 days/week to achieve total dosages of 40 to 60 Gy. (One Gray equals 100 rad.) The initial Brain Tumor Cooperative Group (BTCG) #6901 trial proved, for the first time, that surgery and conventionally fractionated EBRT (1.8 to 2 Gy) improved the median survival among adult MG patients (Table 8-3). Unfortunately, subsequent studies concluded that irradiation was therapeutic rather than curative. Responses were not improved by altering fractionation schedules or adding the radiosensitizing agents then available.[110] These studies have not been replicated among children with MG.

Chemotherapy Trials: Phase III and Phase II, Dose Intensification of Chemotherapy with Hematopoietic Support, and Chemo-radiotherapy

The Phase III Trials. The BTCG #7201 study showed that the addition of a nitrosourea, carmustine (BCNU), further improved median survival to 51 weeks (Table 8-3). One may critique the subsequent BTCG experience (studies #7501, 7702, 8001, 8301, 8420A) to say that nitrosourea-based adjuvant chemotherapy has provided a modest improvement in survival among adult patients, which was comparable to that of other single drugs or multidrug regimes. The multiagent schedules, however, had a correspondingly higher toxicity rate.[110,111]

TABLE 8-3 Selected Phase III Trials Regarding the Role of Chemotherapy for Malignant Gliomas

Treatment Arm	MS (weeks)	Survivors at 1.5 yr (%)	Significance	Reference
BTCG #7201 (358 adult pts)				110
EBRT	36	15		
EBRT + BCNU	51	27	P = .072	
		5Y-PFS		
CCG #943 (58 pediatric pts)				27
All MG				
EBRT		18%		
EBRT-CT		46%	P = .026	
GBM				
EBRT		6%		
EBRT-CT		42%	P = .011	
	TDP (mo)	**MS (mo)**	**5Y-PFS**	
CCG #945 (172 pts)	16	26	33%	108
EBRT-CCNU-	14	25	26%	
VCR-prednisone vs. *Eight in One*				
pre-/post-EBRT	14	31	33%	P = .52

Abbreviations: Brain Tumor Cooperative Group (BTCG), Children's Cancer Group (CCG), median survival (MS), years (yrs), patients (pts), external beam radiotherapy (EBRT), carmustine (BCNU), 5-year progression-free survival (5Y-PFS), chemotherapy (CT), malignant glioma (MG), glioblastoma multiforme (GBM), time to disease progression (TDP), months (mo), 5-year event free survival (5Y-EFS), radiotherapy (EBRT), lomustine (CCNU), vincristine (VCR), "*Eight in One*" (vincristine-BCNU or CCNU–methylprednisolone–procarbazine–hydroxyurea–cisplatin-cytosine arabinoside–cyclophosphamide)

The pediatric neuro-oncologic experience with the adjuvant chemotherapy of MG is less comprehensive and methodical, although more encouraging. The CCG #943 study of newly diagnosed AAST and GBM contrasted surgery with conventional EBRT against surgery, EBRT, and lomustine (CCNU) –vincristine–prednisone. The chemotherapy arm achieved a significantly better 5Y-PFS than the EBRT-only control group ($P < .05$). The impact of chemotherapy on the treatment of GBM was proven by comparison to the irradiated arm ($P = .01$).[27] These data remain the best results yet achieved with conventional EBRT and nitrosoureas for MG patients of any age (Table 8-3).

Single Agent Phase II Studies. A variety of Phase II studies have been directed at the treatment of newly diagnosed, progressive or recurrent MGs to identify promising agents for further development.[111]

Rationale for Multiagent Adjuvant Chemotherapy Regimens. The theoretic rationale for the multidrug protocols is to combine agents with activity against tumor cells traversing different phases of the cell cycle, in order to elicit an additive or synergistic cytotoxic effect. The enthusiasm for the *Eight in One* [vincristine–BCNU or CCNU–methylprednisolone–procarbazine–hydroxyurea–cisplatin–cytosine arabinoside–cyclophosphamide] chemotherapy regimen was based upon the early response rate among those children treated, following resection and prior to EBRT.[112] The CCG #945 trial for the treatment of newly diagnosed children with MA, contrasted EBRT followed by CCNU-vincristine-prednisone against the *Eight in One* chemotherapy regimen, which was administered for two courses before EBRT and with eight subsequent courses. Comparison of this complex protocol structure with a single nitrosourea found no statistical difference in outcome between the two arms, although the *Eight in One* regimen was clearly more toxic (Table 8-3).[108,113] During this period, the *Eight in One* regimen continued to be studied among infants and younger children in order to defer EBRT. (Table 8-4 gives the response rates when used in a neoadjuvant setting.)[28,107,109,113–116]

TABLE 8-4 Neoadjuvant Results with Synergistic Drug Regimens Among Newly Diagnosed Malignant Glioma Patients

Therapy	Response Rate	TDP (mo)	1Y-PFS	2Y-PFS	3Y-PRS	Reference
Eight in One						112
(22 pts)	36%					
CCG #945 (Eight in One)						113
(79 pts)	18%					
(39 infants)	24%	8			36%	28
cDDP-VP16						114
MG (4 pts)	25%	14.8				
"Baby POG"						107
MG (18 pts)	60%		54%	54%		
BSG (14 pts)	0%			28%		
VETOPEC	0%					109
(3 infants)						
HIT'88/'89	25%		65%	42%		115
MG (22 pts)						
HIT'91	35%	19				116
(17 pts)						

Abbreviations: Time to disease progression (TDP), months (mo), 1- and 2-year event-free survival (1Y-, 2Y-EFS), patients (pts), Children's Cancer Group (CCG), Pediatric Oncology Group (POG), malignant glioma (MG), brainstem glioma (BSG), carboplatin (CBDCA), etoposide (VP16), cisplatin (cDDP), "*Eight in One*" (vincristine-BCNU or CCNU–methylprednisolone–procarbazine–hydroxyurea–cisplatin-cytosine arabinoside–cyclophosphamide), *Baby POG* (alternating cyclophosphamide-vincristine and cisplatinum–etoposide), *VETOPEC* (vincristine-etoposide-cyclophosphamide × 4, followed by sequential administration of cyclophosphamide-vincristine, cisplatin-etoposide and carboplatin-etoposide), *HIT'88/89* (ifosfamide-etoposide-methotrexate, cisplatin-cytarabine, hyperfractionated radiotherapy, lomustine-carboplatin-vincristine), *HIT'91* (ifosfamide-etoposide, then methotrexate, followed by cisplatin-cytarabine, to hyperfractionated radiotherapy, and then lomustine-carboplatin-vincristine)

Chemotherapy with Putatively Synergistic Drug Combinations. Platinators and topoisomerase inhibitors are thought to have more than an additive interaction. Clinical trials against pediatric CNS tumors with a variety of drug combinations have not confirmed this, exhibiting response rates of roughly 25% (0 to 60%) and 2Y-PFS rates of 28% to 54% (Table 8-4). Further experience with multiagent chemotherapy regimens suggested greater dose-intensification prior to proceeding to irradiation. The German HIT'88/'89 protocol sequentially combined procarbazine, followed by ifosfamide and etoposide, then methotrexate, and finally cisplatin with cytarabine administered over a 7 week period. Two complete courses were administered prior to EBRT. However, the response rate among children and young adults with MA remained 25% (3/12) with a 5Y-PFS rate of 36% (Table 8-4).[115]

Myeloablative Chemotherapy with Bone Marrow Rescue. The introduction of myeloablative chemotherapy followed by autologous bone marrow transplant (ABMT) for MA has been justified by the availability of drugs exhibiting steep dose/response curves and limited nonhematologic toxicity, as well as by the rarity of metastatic spread to the bone marrow. The most recently published series showed that no significant improvement in long-term survival could be demonstrated for adult MA patients treated with myeloablative therapy and ABMT.[117] The results among pediatric MA patients have not been significantly better, although an objective critique is complicated by the small numbers of patients, heterogeneous induction regimens (even within a small series), lack of stratification by known risk factors, and equating ABMT and peripheral blood stem cell (PBSC) harvesting techniques (Table 8-5).[118–122]

Dose-Intensive Chemotherapy with Peripheral Blood Stem Cell Rescue. Multiple investigators have demonstrated that dose-dependent cytoreduction is achievable only if the inherent dose-limiting toxicity of myelosuppression can be overcome. The relatively low mitotic index of solid tumors limits the effectiveness of phase-specific agents administered intensively over a brief exposure period. Hence the ABMT regimens, which maximize the peak dose by administering ultra-high doses over a short time, have shown little in the way of sustained efficacy among MAs. Repetitive chemotherapy protocols that emphasize the concepts of peak-dose and time-intensity, have now become feasible with the development of PBSC methodology. A dose-escalation study of the chemotherapy combination of procarbazine–CCNU–vincristine with PBSC support allowed the 1.7- to 1.8-fold intensification among patients aged 2 to 35 years (Table 8-6).[123,124]

The Milan group reported 21 children with MG who were treated with induction chemotherapy consisting of cisplatin–etoposide–cyclophosphamide–vincristine–high dose methotrexate for two courses followed by high dose thiotepa with PBSC, then by focal EBRT and maintenance with CCNU-vincristine for a total duration of one year. The median time to disease progression and 4Y-PFS are shown in Table 8-6.[125]

Phase-specific Chemotherapy Agents as Radiosensitizers—"Chemoradiotherapy." The Goldie-Goldman model predicts that concomitant administration should minimize the emergence of resistance to chemotherapy and EBRT. Sequential radiochemotherapy was administered in the HIT'91 regimen to 17 children and young adults. Induction chemotherapy consisted of two courses of ifosfamide-etoposide-methotrexate and cisplatin-cytarabine, delivered over

TABLE 8-5 Results of Myeloablative Induction Regimens Among Newly Diagnosed Pediatric Malignant Glioma Patients

Treatment	No	Response Rate	MS	Reference
CPM-TT--ABMT-HF-EBRT	9	22% CR	10 mo	118
High-dose BCNU-ABMT	13	12.5%	15.6 mo	119
BCNU-TT-VP16-ABMT followed by HF-EBRT	6 BSG		11.4 mo	120

Treatment	Response	Rate	1Y-EFS	2Y-EFS	1Y-OS	2Y-OS	Reference
cDDP-CPM-VP16-VCR	MA	11%	11%	11%	56%	22%	121
followed by CBDCA-TT-VP16-ABMT	BSG	17%	33%	17%	50%	33%	
BCNU-TT-VP16-ABMT-EBRT		27%	64%	46%	73%	46%	122

Abbreviations: Number of patients (No), 1-, 2- and 3-year event-free survival (1Y-, 2Y-, 3Y-EFS), median survival (MS), cyclophosphamide (CPM), thiotepa (TT), carmustine (BCNU), cisplatin (cDDP), etoposide (VP16), carboplatin (CBDCA), vincristine (VCR), autologous bone marrow transplant (ABMT), hyperfractionated external beam radiotherapy (EBRT), complete response (CR), malignant astrocytoma (MA), brainstem glioma (BSG), months (mo)

TABLE 8-6 Results with Dose Intensification with Peripheral Stem Cell Support Among Newly Diagnosed Pediatric Malignant Glioma Patients

Treatment	Response Rate	TDP	MS	4Y-PFS	Reference
PCV-PBSC +/–EBRT	57%	9.2 mo	17 mo		123
CBDCA-VP16-CPM-TT-PBSC or CBDCA-VP16-BCNU-TT-PBSC	17%	7.2 mo			124
cDDP-VP16-VCR-(21 pts) CPM-HD/MTX x2, then HD/TT, PBSC, then EBRT then CCNU-VCR			14 mo	46%	125

Abbreviations: Time to disease progression (TDP), median survival (MS), 4-year progression-free survival (4Y-PFS), procarbazine–CCNU-vincristine (PCV), peripheral blood stem cells (PBSC), radiotherapy (EBRT), carboplatin (CBDCA), etoposide (VP16), cyclophosphamide (CPM), thiotepa (TT), carmustine (BCNU), high dose methotrexate (HD/MTX), high dose thiotepa (HD/TT), lomustine (CCNU), months (mo)

a 4-week period. Hyperfractionated EBRT was begun on day 12 of the first course and continued into the second. Maintenance chemotherapy consisted of CCNU, carboplatin, and vincristine administered every 6 weeks for eight courses. Among 11 patients with MA, there were one complete and two partial responses; overall results were not very different from the other strategies discussed above. There was no additive, acute toxicity due to the synchronous administration of radiochemotherapy among the MA patients, who had received only involved field radiotherapy (Table 8-4).[116]

Brainstem Glioma

Surgical Intervention

A de facto consensus has emerged within the CCG and POG that a biopsy is not warranted in cases of diffuse pontine glioma (DPG) with a "classical" presentation and a diagnostic MRI appearance, as the therapeutic approach employed by current multicenter protocols has not been altered by a specific pathologic diagnosis.[126]

Radiotherapy

Historically, "standard therapy" for the DPG constituted a radiotherapeutic prescription of 45 to 55 Gy, delivered in single daily fractions of 180 to 200 cGy. Unfortunately, the median time of disease progression (TDP) was only 5 to 7 months with an expected survival of 9 to 13 months. Hyperfractionation of the radiotherapy prescription should lessen the neurotoxicity. However, these hyperfractionated radiation therapy (HFEBRT) trials have used doses of 64.8, 66, 70.2, 72, and 78 Gy without significantly altering the TDP.

Previous Combination Therapy Trials

Adjuvant chemotherapy with nitrosoureas has not improved the outcome among children with BSG receiving EBRT. However, pilot studies with neo-adjuvant multiagent chemotherapy did achieve responses in terms of tumor reduction.[126,127] The *POG-8833* study of preirradiation chemotherapy and HFEBRT for BSG treated 32 evaluable, newly diagnosed patients with four induction cycles of cisplatin and cyclophosphamide followed by HFEBRT (66 Gy). While clinical responses were reported in 65%, the 1-year PFS was 16%; the median survival of 9 months was not significantly different from the previous POG experience with HFEBRT alone.[126]

The CCG Phase II trial #9941 evaluated the efficacy and toxicity of two arms of induction chemotherapy administered prior to HFEBRT. Neither the difference in postinduction response rate nor the difference in postinduction/HFEBRT response rate was statistically significant. The PFS was 17% at one year and 6% at two years. Hyperfractionated radiotherapy was also not found to consolidate the response to induction chemotherapy among those who did achieve a partial or minor response.[128]

Low-grade Glial Neoplasms

Surgical Intervention

Operative resection is the accepted standard of care for actively symptomatic patients or those with progressive disease. Analysis of 70 children with LGGN treated in a single institution demonstrated that extent of surgical resection was the dominant predictor for PFS (P = .015) and OS (P = .013). Actuarial PFS rates were 88%, 79%, and 76% at 5, 10, and 20 years, respectively, following complete removal.[129]

About 80% of infratentorial and only 18% of supratentorial LGGN are accessible enough to allow such radical resection.[59] A retrospective review of cerebellar AST demonstrated postoperative residual disease in as many as 35%.[130] Realistically, a significant percentage of children with LGGN have postoperative residual disease and are at risk for disease progression or recurrence.

This raises the related controversy of "early vs. late" surgery. This issue has been difficult to answer in the setting of multi-institutional group trials due to the selection bias toward operating on readily accessible lesions. What data exists would suggest that patients presenting with epilepsy as their sole symptom have a favorable prognosis, which is not adversely affected by waiting until disease progression.[131]

Radiotherapy

While EBRT has been the "accepted" treatment for unresectable and/or progressive disease, a quantitative determination of its contribution to disease control remains problematic.[129,132] Postoperative irradiation for adults with incompletely resected LGGN has been associated with 5Y-OS of approximately 48% and 10Y-OS of 26%, which are twice the 26% and 12% rates, respectively, reported for patients receiving surgery alone.[133] The addition of EBRT has been found to favorably influence disease control among patients older than 35 years (P = .008). However, this association between younger age at diagnosis with a lower grade of glioma and better prognosis has long been known and compromises interpretation of this data.

Recent analysis of the literature has concluded that for gliomas of the visual pathway, local tumor control with stable or improved visual function is achieved with EBRT in approximately 90% of cases. There is a consensus to employ radiotherapy in older children with progressive disease, regardless of location or histopathologic subtype.[134] Given the absence of compelling data for the use of EBRT among children, there has been increasing interest in the application of chemotherapy for unresectable, residual, or progressive disease.

Chemotherapy

Among children, single chemotherapy agents have largely been considered ineffective. The Washington group piloted a 10-week induction regimen of carboplatinum-vincristine for children with LGGN. Patients with either SD or a cytoreductive response were additionally treated with twelve cycles of carboplatinum-vincristine. Among 37 newly diagnosed patients, the overall response rate was 62%. In a subsequent report of 70 children less than 5 years of age who were treated with this combination, 57% experienced objective responses, with a PFS rate of 85% at one year and 76% at two years.[135]

The San Francisco group has proposed the *TPCV* combination (thioguanine, procarbazine, lomustine, and vincristine) in order to defer EBRT among younger children with chiasmal and hypothalamic AST. Among 41 children with a median age of 5.2 years, the median TDP was delayed to 30 months with a 5Y-OS of 83%.[136]

Medulloblastomas and Primitive Neuroectodermal Tumors

Surgical Resection

The studies reviewed in Table 8-2 have demonstrated the advantage of aggressive surgical debulking to achieve minimal residual disease among children with MBL. Several of these reach statistical significance.[67–70,137] Jakacki et al.[138] and Albright et al.[139] investigated the results of the CCG #921 study for children with pineal (Figure 8-5) and other supratentorial PNETs. Among these other supratentorial PNETs, postoperative tumor burden of greater than 1.5 cm^2 was associated with a 4Y-OS of only 13%. This was much worse than that of children with a residual of less than 1.5 cm^2, 40% of whom were alive after 4 years.[139]

Radiotherapy

For children older than 3 to 4 years of age with minimal postoperative residual disease and no evidence of dissemination, treatment with surgical resection and conventional craniospinal EBRT (tumor dose: 54 Gy; whole brain and spinal dose 36 Gy) has achieved a 5Y-PFS rate of approximately 63% (±5) (Table 8-7).[70]

Lower Craniospinal EBRT Dosimetry for Standard-Risk Therapy

There has been increasing concern regarding the neurologic and endocrinologic toxicity of neuraxis irradiation for younger children with standard risk MBL, and attempts have been made to reduce the extratumoral dosage. The SIOP sponsored a study that compared 36 Gy vs. 24 Gy craniospinal EBRT and found the 5Y-PFS was actually better for the reduced dose arm, although some patients did receive preradiation chemotherapy (Table 8-7).[140]

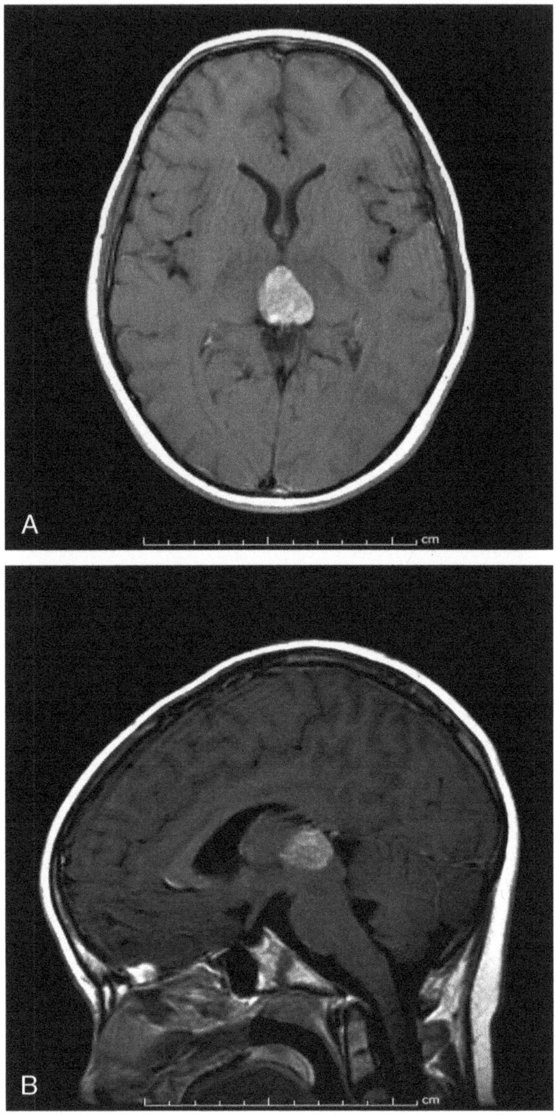

Figure 8-5 Axial **(A)** and sagittal **(B)** T1 contrast-enhanced MRI showing densely enhancing pineoblastoma. (Slides courtesy Susan Chi, M.D., Dana-Farber Cancer Institute and Boston Children's Hospital.)

A joint CCG-POG trial was performed between 1985 and 1991 to determine whether the craniospinal EBRT prescription could safely be reduced from 36 Gy to 23.4 Gy. The study was halted when preliminary information suggested that the reduced dose arm was associated with a higher early relapse and "distant failure" rate. However, subsequent follow-up studies have found that the 5Y-PFS for the standard radiation prescription arm was greater but not statistically significant when compared to the reduced dose arm (P = .08). These results remained durable at 8 years following treatment, as well.[141]

TABLE 8-7 Trials regarding the Role of Reduced Dose Craniospinal EBRT and Adjunctive Chemotherapy for Newly Diagnosed Children with Standard Risk Medulloblastoma

Reduced Dose Treatment Arm	5Y-PFS	5Y-OS	Significance	Reference
SIOP				140
36 Gy	60%			
24 Gy	69%			
CCG-POG				
36 Gy	67%		(P = .08)	141
23.4 Gy	52%			
CCG #9891				143
23.4 Gy with	78%			
CCNU-VCR-cDDP				
PCB then 35 WB				144
and 25 SP	63%	68%		
with concurrent HY				
PNET-3				145
EBRT vs.	59.8%			
CBDCA-VP16	74.2%		(P = .0366)	
alternating with CPM				
then 35 Gy				
Conformal EBRT to PF				
with 23.4 Gy	86%			146
VCR-cDDP +				
CCNU or CPM				
23.4 Gy (421 pts) then	81%	86%		147
CCNU-cDDP-VCR vs.			NS	
CPM-cDDP-VCR				
Risk Adapted EBRT (86 pts)				148
23.4 Gy with CPM and	83%			
PBSC				
Conformal EBRT to PF (86 pts)				149
with 23.4 Gy	83%			
HD CPM-cDDP-VCR				

Abbreviations: Children's Cancer Group (CCG), Pediatric Oncology Group (POG), 5-year progression-free survival (5Y-PFS), 5-year overall survival (5Y-OS), Gray (Gy), patients (pts), procarbazine (PCB), external beam radiotherapy (EBRT), whole brain (WB), spine (SP), hydroxyurea (HY), not significant (NS), peripheral blood stem cells (PBSC), lomustine (CCNU), posterior fossa (PF), high dose (HD), cisplatin (cDDP), etoposide (VP16), cyclophosphamide (CPM), vincristine (VCR), carboplatinum (CBDCA)

Encouraging results with adjuvant chemotherapy had been reported around this time by Packer et al.[142] for the treatment of "high-risk" MBL patients. The addition of eight cycles of lomustine-vincristine-cisplatinum increased the 5Y-PFS to 85%. This exceeded the survival rates being reported among "standard-risk" patients treated with EBRT alone, at the time. Therefore, the CCG initiated trial #9892 for children without significant postoperative or metastatic disease, aged 3 to 10 years, using the same adjuvant chemotherapy but with a decrease in the neuraxis radiation prescription (23.4 Gy). The 5Y-PFS of this regimen was a remarkable 78% (Table 8-7).[143]

A series of trials then examined the same reduced EBRT dosage and randomized for adjuvant chemotherapy. These results are summarized in Table 8-7, but suffice it to say that the 5Y-PFS has remained at a plateau of 80% (±6). In one study, patients with average-risk medulloblastoma were treated with 23.4 Gy of CSRT, 55.8 Gy of posterior fossa RT, plus one of two adjuvant chemotherapy regimens: lomustine (CCNU), cisplatin, and vincristine; or cyclophosphamide, cisplatin, and vincristine. Five-year event-free survival and survival was 81% ± 2.1% and 86% ± 9%, respectively. These results were comparable to those obtained with higher doses of irradiation, suggesting that reduced-dose craniospinal radiation may be feasible in children with average-risk medulloblastomas. [147]

High-Risk Medulloblastoma

This cancer would appear the prototypical target for chemotherapy, as it is characterized by a high mitotic rate, has known radiosensitivity, and has a relatively high rate of meningeal dissemination (36% to 43%) at time of diagnosis.[19]

Phase III Trials regarding the Role of Chemotherapy in Treatment of Medulloblastoma

Two parallel-designed studies conducted by the European (SIOP-1) and North American CCG (#942) have been discussed (see Prognostic Variables). The *SIOP-I* enrolled patients between 0 and 16 years during the years 1975 through 1979, and randomized between surgery and irradiation vs. surgery, EBRT, and CCNU-vincristine. Analysis at 54 months demonstrated a statistically significant advantage in outcome for the combination therapy arm (P = .005) (Table 8-8).[67]

TABLE 8-8 Phase III Trials regarding the Role of Adjunctive Chemotherapy for Newly Diagnosed Children with Medulloblastoma

Treatment Arm		5Y-PFS	Significance	Reference
SIOP-I	(285 patients)			67
All MBL	EBRT			
	EBRT-CT		P = .005	
CCG #942	(233 patients)			68
All MBL	EBRT	50%		
EBRT-CT		59%	NS	
Stage $T_{3,4}$	EBRT	0%		
	EBRT-CT	46%	P = .006	
POG	(71 patients)			150
	EBRT	57%		
	EBRT-CT	68%	P = .18	
Pts > 5 yrs	EBRT-CT		P = .05	

Abbreviations: 5-year progression-free survival (5Y-PFS), European Société Internationale d'Oncologie Pédiatrique Study I (*SIOP-I*), Children's Cancer Group (CCG), Pediatric Oncology Group (POG), external beam radiotherapy (EBRT), chemotherapy (CT), not significant (NS), patients (pts), years (yrs)

The CCG #942 accessioned patients between 2 and 16 years, during the years 1975 through 1981. Comparison was made between surgery and EBRT vs. surgery, irradiation, and adjuvant chemotherapy with CCNU-vincristine-prednisone. Among the high-risk patients, the PFS was significantly better for the EBRT-chemotherapy treated patients (P = .006) (Table 8-8).[68] The third randomized trial was a POG study comparing conventional neuraxis irradiation with/without MOPP chemotherapy (1979 to 1986), which demonstrated no advantage to adjunctive pharmacotherapy among children less than 5 years of age (Table 8-8).[150]

Multiagent Combination Chemotherapy Regimens

Preliminary studies of the *Eight in One* combination chemotherapy regimen had been encouraging in terms of response rates among MBL/PNET patients (Table 8-9). The CCG #921 protocol was designed to compare the relative efficacy of adjuvant CCNU-vincristine-prednisone for high-risk patients with this more aggressive chemotherapy

TABLE 8-9 Response and Survival Results with Neoadjuvant Chemotherapy among Infants and Children with Medulloblastoma and Primitive Neuroectodermal Tumors

Diagnosis	Age	Regimen	Response Rate	2Y-PFS	5Y-PFS	Reference
MBL (32 pts)		*Eight in One*	50%			112
CCG #921 (203 pts)		EBRT-CCNU-VCR-prednisone	63%			70
		vs.				
		Eight in One pre-/post-EBRT	45% (P = .06)			
CCG #921 (82 infants)		*Eight in One*	28%			151
MBL (8 pts)	Child	cDDP-VP16	88%			152
sPNET (3 pts)			100%			
All				76%		
MBL (6 pts)	Child	CBDCA-VP16	83%			153
MBL (4 pts)		cDDP-VP16	83%			154
PNET (2 pts)						
MBL (62 pts)	Infants	*"Baby POG"*	48%	34%		107
sPNET (36 pts)			29%	19%		
sPNET	Infants	CPM-VCR *concurrent with* CDDP-VCR	80%			155
MBL (16 pts)	Children	CBDCA-VP16	48%			156

Table continued on following page

TABLE 8-9 Response and Survival Results with Neoadjuvant Chemotherapy among Infants and Children with Medulloblastoma and Primitive Neuroectodermal Tumors—cont'd

Diagnosis	Age	Regimen	Response Rate	2Y-PFS	5Y-PFS	Reference
PNET (9 pts)						
MBL (16 pts)	Infants	*VETOPEC*	82%			109
sPNET (8 pts)			50%			
sPNET	Children	*HIT'88/'89*	57%			115,157
MBL			67%			
sPNET (50 pts)	Children	*HIT'88/'89/'91*	25%	42%		115,157,158
MBL/PNET (28 pts)		CBDCA-VP16 -HDMTX	79%			154
MBL (19 pts)			74%			
PNET (9 pts)			89%			
< 3 yrs			71%			
> 3 yrs			81%			
MBL M2–3 (68 pts)		*PNET-3*	39% CR 34% PR		35%	159

Abbreviations: 2-year progression free survival (2Y-PFS), 5-year progression free survival (5Y-PFS), patients (pts), medulloblastoma (MBL), primitive neuroectodermal tumor (PNET), Children's Cancer Group (CCG), radiotherapy (EBRT), lomustine (CCNU), vincristine (VCR), "*Eight in One*" (vincristine-BCNU or CCNU–methylprednisolone–procarbazine–hydroxyurea–cisplatin-cytosine arabinoside–cyclophosphamide), medulloblastoma (MBL), supratentorial PNET (sPNET), cisplatin (cDDP), etoposide (VP16), cyclophosphamide (CPM), vincristine (VCR), carboplatinum (CBDCA), *Baby POG* (alternating cyclophosphamide-vincristine and cisplatinum–etoposide), *VETOPEC* (vincristine-etoposide-cyclophosphamide × 4, followed by sequential administration of cyclophosphamide-vincristine, cisplatin-etoposide and carboplatin-etoposide), *HIT'88/'89'91* (ifosfamide-etoposide, then methotrexate, followed by cisplatin-cytarabine, to hyperfractionated radiotherapy, and then lomustine-carboplatin-vincristine), high-dose methotrexate (HDMTX), *PNET-3* (preradiation vincristin-etoposide-carboplatin-cyclophosphamide), metastasis stages 2-3 (M2-3), complete response (CR), partial response (PR)

regimen before and after EBRT. This study demonstrated no significant advantage for the *Eight in One* polypharmacy combination (P= .06) (Table 8-9).[70]

Synergistic Chemotherapy Studies

Platinators and topoisomerase antagonists have become increasingly popular by virtue of a putative synergistic interaction in treatment of a number of pediatric brain tumors (Table 8-9). The German *HIT'91* trial demonstrated that high dose, multiagent chemotherapy could be as effective in achieving a complete response (42-57% of patients) as irradiation (57-63%) among newly diagnosed children with MBL (Table 8-9).[157,158]

Dose Intensive Chemotherapy with Autologous Bone Marrow Transplant or Peripheral Stem Cell Rescue

Several groups have examined the feasibility, toxicity, and efficacy of dose-intensification using this approach. A collaborative study treated 53 children with newly diagnosed MBL/PNET, 19 of whom were high-risk, and 34 with average-risk disease. All patients were treated with craniospinal EBRT. Postradiotherapy chemotherapy consisted of four courses of high-dose cyclophosphamide-cisplatin-vincristine administered with PBSC or ABMT hematopoietic support. The high-risk patients additionally received topotecan in a 6-week phase II window between EBRT and this chemotherapy regimen. Early outcome analysis revealed a 2Y-PFS of 93.6% among the average-risk patients and 73.7% among high-risk subjects.[160]

The New York University Group employed five courses of cisplatin-etoposide-cyclophosphamide-methotrexate with leucovorin rescue for MBL patients with disseminated disease. Following this induction, eligible patients were treated with a single myeloablative course of chemotherapy and PBSC. The 81% complete response rate and 49% 3Y-PFS were considered encouraging enough to warrant additional trials with methotrexate.[161]

Ependymoma

Surgical Management

Historically, meaningful surgical debulking has been possible in about 42% to 62% of patients, usually those with tumors originating supratentorially or in the roof of the IVth ventricle. Not surprisingly, the 5Y-PFS rates have been poor, on the order of 23% to 45%. In recent studies, aggressive surgical resection has improved the 5Y-PFS estimates to 51% to 75%.[23,89,90,92]

Radiotherapy

There has been no study to establish the optimal dose or appropriate treatment volume for EBRT among pediatric or adult patients with EPD. Comparison between patients treated with surgery versus surgery plus EBRT has shown long-term survival rates of 17% and 40%, respectively.[162] A dose-response relationship was documented.

The requirement for craniospinal EBRT among children with anaplastic EPD has been controversial. Goldwein et al.[163] have shown that the 2Y-OS for children receiving neuroaxis irradiation was 52%, while focal irradiation was resulted in a 40% survival rate over the same period. From the perspective of long-term survival, five out of 11 children treated with craniospinal EBRT were alive at 6 years, compared to none of those treated with local EBRT.[163] Paulino et al.[89] cited the 10Y-OS rates to be 64% for patients receiving craniospinal EBRT, 60% for whole brain irradiation, and 65% for local field radiotherapy (P = 0.88).

Chemotherapy

In retrospective analysis of 83 children with EPD, adjuvant chemotherapy did not significantly alter the PFS among patients older than 3 years of age, nor did craniospinal EBRT improve the PFS for M_0 patients.[92] Duffner et al.[107] demonstrated responses and durable survival with two cycles of cyclophosphamide-vincristine among 25 infants less than 3 years of age. The *VETOPEC* regimen achieved an impressive initial response rate (Table 8-10).[109] The French Society of Pediatric Oncology has studied the efficacy of postoperative chemotherapy, in hopes of avoiding EBRT among 73 children less than 5 years of age with intracranial EPD. The regimen consisted of seven cycles of three courses,

TABLE 8-10 Neoadjuvant Results with Synergistic Drug Regimens Among Newly-Diagnosed Ependymoma Patients

Regimen	Response Rate	TDP	2Y-EFS	4Y-EFS	Reference
"Baby POG" (48 pts)	48%		42%		107
VETOPEC (14 pts)	86%				109
PCZ-CBDCA, (73 pts) cDDP-VP16, CPM-VCR				22%	91

Abbreviations: Time to disease progression (TDP), 2- and 4-year event-free survival (2Y-, 4Y-EFS), *Baby POG* (alternating cyclophosphamide - vincristine and cisplatinum – etoposide), *VETOPEC* (vincristine-etoposide-cyclophosphamide x 4, followed by sequential administration of cyclophosphamide-vincristine, cisplatin-etoposide and carboplatin-etoposide), procarbazine (PCZ), carboplatinum (CBDCA), cisplatinum (cDDP), etoposide (VP16), cyclophosphamide (CPM), vincristine (VCR)

alternating two drugs at each course (procarbazine–carboplatin, etoposide–cisplatin, cyclophosphamide–vincristine) over 1½ years. Unfortunately, there were no complete or partial responses observed. While the 4Y-OS was 59%, only 23% of those surviving evaded irradiation (Table 8-10).[91] Disappointingly, dose intensification using PBSC with cyclophosphamide–etoposide–vincristine, with or without cisplatinum, has achieved response rates of only 16% among children with EPD less than 6 years of age.[121]

Oligodendroglioma

General principles regarding the management of LGGN apply to low-grade OLG as well. Radical or gross total resection, when feasible, improves long-term survival. There continue to be controversies over the timing of surgical intervention, especially among epilepsy patients who are being successfully managed medically, as well as over the role of EBRT.

The combination of procarbazine-CCNU-vincristine (PCV) is regarded as the "gold standard" for chemotherapy due to the remarkable responses seen among anaplastic, progressive, and recurrent OLG. Neoadjuvant administration of PCV for anaplastic OLG has achieved meaningful cytoreduction for 52% to 70%; the remaining patients proceeded to EBRT because of chemoresistance or toxicity.[164,165] Phase II examination of temozolamide has also resulted in impressive response rates (53%, with greater than 50% cytoreduction) among chemotherapy-naïve OLG patients at recurrence. The median time to further progression was 10.4 months for all patients, but 13.2 months for those responding to drug treatment.[166]

Germ Cell Tumors

Surgical Intervention

In Japan, it has been the practice to first irradiate a pineal tumor thought to be a germinoma with 20 Gy ("the radiation test"), and then, if the tumor regressed, to continue radiotherapy. If there was no reduction in tumor size, only then was surgical excision to be considered.[167] Over time, aggressive surgical resection has proven itself to be an important determinant of survival, as evidenced in the largest single series of patients (number 153) reported by the University of Tokyo.[102]

The pendulum has swung back again, because of the increasing effectiveness of nonsurgical therapies. If the appropriate neuroradiographic findings and biomarker serologic studies are present, the Japanese and Korean Societies for Pediatric Neurosurgery advocate a minimally invasive surgical procedure, such as neuroendoscopic or stereotactic biopsy, to be followed by platinum-based chemotherapy and/or targeted EBRT.[167] It is only among cases demonstrating a poor response to "trial therapy" that surgical intervention is then reconsidered to debulk the tumor and clarify the pathologic diagnosis.[168]

External Beam Radiotherapy

Among patients with known germinomas, combined surgical resection and radiotherapeutic intervention improved 10Y-OS rates from 69% to 93%.[102] The typical radiotherapy prescription today consists of a primary tumor dose of 50 to 55 Gy, with 36 Gy to the neuraxis. Subsequent controversy regarding the treatment of germinomas has centered on the issues of dosimetry and the indication for craniospinal radiotherapy. As germinomas of the CNS proved to be as radiosensitive as those of the testis, it was shown that those without evident CSF dissemination could be controlled with involved field radiotherapy alone.[102,169,170] In contrast, there is no debate regarding the necessity of treating NG-GCT with a full radiotherapy prescription to the tumor (50 to 55 Gy) and craniospinal axis (36 to 40 Gy) due to their significantly higher rate of metastasis and recurrence.[8,168,169] Unfortunately, the NG-GCTs remain refractory to radiation prescriptions even greater than 50 Gy.

Chemotherapy

A number of reports investigating the role of chemotherapy in the management of GCT have been encouraging (Table 8-11).[103,171–174]

The practice of the University of Tokyo has been to rank GCT patients by relative risk: (*i*) mixed germinoma and teratoma, (*ii*) mixed GCT with predominance of germinoma or teratoma with some *"pure malignant tumor"* (embryonal carcinomas, endodermal sinus tumors, and choriocarcinomas), and (*iii*) mixed tumors with predominance of *"pure malignant tumor."* Surgery and radiotherapy produce a 10Y-OS rate of 91.7% among germinoma patients. In the intermediate prognostic group, combination chemotherapy (cisplatin-vinblastine-bleomycin, cisplatin-etoposide, or carboplatin-etoposide) and EBRT has been shown to significantly reduce the risk of disease recurrence when compared to irradiation alone ($P = .049$). The high-risk patients did relatively better with chemotherapy than with only EBRT, although the difference was not statistically significant.[102]

The First International Germ Cell Tumor Study proposed a chemotherapy-only regimen of carboplatin, etoposide, and bleomycin. This study accessioned 45 patients with germinoma and 26 with NG-GCT, of whom 68 were considered evaluable. The protocol for germinoma patients, who achieved a complete response after four induction courses, prescribed two additional cycles. Those subjects with a lesser response were treated with a chemotherapy regimen fortified by cyclophosphamide then followed by EBRT. A complete response was achieved in 57% of patients after four induction courses of chemotherapy, and an

TABLE 8-11 Complete Response Rates to Induction Chemotherapy among Newly Diagnosed Germinomas and Non-Germinomatous Germ Cell Tumor Patients

Study/Agents	Course 2 4 6	EBRT	2Y-OS	4Y-PFS 5Y-PFS	Reference
Germinomas					
CBCDA (11 pts)	45%	63%	yes	25 mo	171
1st IGCTS CBCDA-VP16-BLM (45 pts)		84%	no	84%	103
NG-GCT					
1st IGCTS CBCDA-VP16-BLM (26 pts)		78%	no	62%	103
cDDP-VP16 (18 pts)	42%	94%	67%		174
2nd IGCTS cDDP-VP16-CPM-BLM (20 pts)	94%	92%		36%	173
All GCT					
1st IGCTS CBCDA-VP16-BLM (68 pts)	57%	81%	no		103
CG/IS cDDP-VP16-IFOS (19 pts)	16%	42%			172

Abbreviations: external beam radiotherapy (EBRT), 2-year overall survival (2Y-OS), 4- and 5- year progression-free survival (4Y-, 5Y-PFS), germ cell tumors (GCT), nongerminatous germ cell tumors (NG-GCT), International Germ Cell Tumor Study (IGCTS), Cooperative German/Italian Study (CG/IS), carboplatin (CBDCA), cisplatin (cDDP), etoposide (VP16), bleomycin (BLM), cyclophosphamide (CPM), ifosfamide (IFOS), patients (pts), months (mo)

additional 24% were left with no evident disease after intensified chemotherapy or "second-look surgery." Thus, a significant majority were rendered disease-free without irradiation (Table 8-11). Thirty-nine percent of patients remained in complete remission over a median follow-up of 31 months.[103]

The Cooperative German/Italian Study accepted the classic neuroradiographic appearance with elevated biomarkers (β-HCG and/or α-FP) as diagnostic entry criteria. Nineteen patients (16 males) were placed into the study. The therapeutic design consisted of two induction courses of PEI (cisplatinum–etoposide-ifosfamide); patients responding to chemotherapy were to receive an additional two courses. Nonresponders and those with progressive disease were to be advanced to surgical resection, if feasible, prior to craniospinal EBRT (30 Gy with a tumor boost of 24 Gy). Thirteen of 16 with elevated α-FP and/or β-HCG had normalization of biomarker levels following the second course of PEI induction chemotherapy, which paralleled objective neuroradiographic evidence of a cytoreductive effect in ten. Increasing response rates were seen with further chemotherapy (Table 8-11). Seventeen of the patients survived, of whom 81% remain in remission over a median follow-up interval of 11 months (range 7 to 39 months).[172]

The Second International CNS Germ Cell Study Group employed two courses of cisplatin–etoposide–cyclophosphamide–bleomycin to assess chemosensitivity in a group of 20 patients with NG-GCT. The study design planned that participants achieving a complete response would receive two additional courses of carboplatin–etoposide–bleomycin and another cycle of the original treatment regimen. Those not reaching or sustaining this underwent "second-look surgery" and/or EBRT. A greater than 50% tumor cytoreduction was achieved in a remarkable majority of patients (Table 8-11). The median PFS for subjects with a complete response was 62 months compared with patients with lesser responses, who demonstrated a mean PFS of 23 months. Regrettably, 69% of evaluable patients suffered from progressive disease during or following chemotherapy.[173]

Infant Brain Tumors

Long-term survival among infants with malignant tumors has been approximately 24%, in comparison those with "benign" tumors fare better (73%).[175] While effective at disease control, the neurotoxicity of irradiation is unacceptable. In one study of 78 infants, 80% of those treated with surgery and chemotherapy had a satisfactory functional outcome in contrast to those who required irradiation prior to 24 months of age (42%). Only 21 of 39 survivors had little or no neurologic/cognitive deficit.[175] An early study among babies with MG, supratentorial PNET, and anaplastic EPD showed an encouraging response rate to cisplatinum-etoposide with a median survival of 34 months (Table 8-12).[176]

Studies of infants with Malignant Astrocytomas

The *"Baby POG"* protocol design consisted of alternating cycles of cyclophosphamide-vincristine and cisplatinum-etoposide.[107] This combination yielded "very encouraging" results among infants with MA and DPG, which exceeded the responses seen at the time among older children treated with postoperative EBRT alone (PFS 20%), irradiation with CCNU–vincristine–prednisone, or the *Eight in One* regimen before and after EBRT (Table 8-4).[27,107] Experience with *Eight in One* combination, the *VETOPEC* regimen (vincristine-etoposide-cyclophosphamide for four courses, followed by sequential administration of cyclophosphamide-vincristine, cisplatin-etoposide, and carboplatin-etoposide), and the more recently reported *BBSFOP* Protocol (seven cycles of three drug pairs: carboplatin-procarbazine, cisplatin-etoposide, cyclophosphamide-vincristine) is shown in Table 8-12.[28,109,177] None of these has emerged as clearly superior.

Infants with Standard and High-Risk Medulloblastoma, Primitive Neuroectodermal Tumor and Ependymoma

The "Baby POG" study of alternating cyclophosphamide-vincristine and cisplatinum-etoposide yielded both responses and durable remissions for young children with MBL (Table 8-12).[107] The CCG study #921 administered the *Eight in One* regimen; many of the infants, with different tumor types, were able to avoid irradiation (Table 8-12).[151] The concurrently-administered combination of cisplatin-cyclophosphamide-etoposide-vincristine has been considered very active in infants with newly diagnosed CNS tumors, particularly supratentorial PNETs, with a response rate of approximately 80% in this high risk subgroup (Table 8-12).[155] More recent studies have acknowledged 3Y-PFS rates of less than

TABLE 8-12 Results with Neoadjuvant, Synergistic Chemotherapy Agents among Infants with Malignant Brain Tumors

Diagnosis	Agents	Response Rate	TDP	2Y-PFS	3Y-PFS	5Y-PFS	Reference
All (8 pts)	cDDP-VP16	50%	17.5 mo				176
All	*"Baby POG"*	39%		37%			107
MG (18 pts)		60%		54%			
BSG (14 pts)		0%		28%			
MBL (62 pts)		48%		34%			
sPNET (36 pts)		29%		19%			
EPD (48 pts)		48%		42%			
sPNET	CPM-VCR concurrent with CDDP-VCR	80%					155
MBL	*Eight in One*			22%			151
MBL, M0				29%			
MBL, M1-3				11%			
sPNET				55%			
EPD				26%			
MG (39 pts)	*Eight in One* after two courses	24%	8 mo	36%			28
Overall	*VETOPEC*	64%			11%		109
MG (3 pts)		0%					
MBL (16 pts)		82%					
sPNET (8 pts)		50%					

TABLE 8-12 Results with Neoadjuvant, Synergistic Chemotherapy Agents among Infants with Malignant Brain Tumors—cont'd

Diagnosis	Agents	Response Rate	TDP	2Y-PFS	3Y-PFS	5Y-PFS	Reference
EPD (14 pts)		86%					
Overall (43 pts) CPM-VCR-	CPM-VCR-						178
GTR	CBDCA-VP16					82%	
PTR	IV & IT MTX					50%	
M2-3						33%	
Overall (15 pts) *HDC-PBSC*			52%				180
MG (21 pts < 5 yrs)	*BBSFOP*					35%	177
MBL (21 pts < 3 yrs)	*Head Start I/II* followed by PBSC						181
All						52%	
GTR						64%	
PTR						29%	
Desmoplastic						67%	
Classical MBL						42%	

Abbreviations: time to disease progression (TDP), 2- and 3-year progression-free survival (2Y-, 3Y-PFS), cisplatinum (cDDP), etoposide (VP16), months (mo), cyclophosphamide (CPM), vincristine (VCR), carboplatinum (CBDCA), *Baby POG* (alternating cyclophosphamide-vincristine and cisplatinum–etoposide), *Eight in One* (vincristine-BCNU or CCNU–methylprednisolone–procarbazine–hydroxyurea–cisplatin-cytosine arabinoside–cyclophosphamide), *VETOPEC* (vincristine-etoposide-cyclophosphamide × 4, followed by sequential administration of cyclophosphamide-vincristine, cisplatin-etoposide and carboplatin-etoposide), intravenous and intrathecal methotrexate (IV& IT MTX), gross total resection (GTR), partial tumor resection (PTR), metastasis stage 2-3 (M2-3), *HDC* (cisplatin-cyclophosphamide-etoposide-vincristine × 3, then carboplatin-thiotepa × 3 followed by peripheral blood stem cells) (PBSC), *BBSFOP* (7 cycles of three drug pairs: carboplatin/procarbazine, cisplatin/etoposide, cyclophosphamide/vincristine), *Head Start* (vincristine-cisplatin-cyclophosphamide-etoposide × 5, myeloablation with carboplatin-thiothepa-etoposide), malignant glioma (MG), brainstem glioma (BSG), medulloblastoma (MBL), supratentorial PNET (sPNET), ependymoma (EPD), patients (pts), years (yrs)

50% with the *Eight in One* regimen and the VETOPEC regimen among babies with MBL and PNET.[109,159] The addition of intrathecal and intravenous methotrexate to the platinator-cyclophosphamide-etoposide-vincristine structure appeared to make a difference among the younger infants with identifiable postoperative disease, however (Table 8-12).[178]

The POG study #9233 was the first to compare conventionally dosed versus dose-intensive induction chemotherapy among infants with newly diagnosed MBL (101 patients) and EPD (84 eligible patients). Induction consisted of cyclophosphamide-vincristine and cisplatin-etoposide, with the investigational arm receiving a relative dose intensification of 1.8. The MBL patients showed no difference in PFS (P = .67) between the two arms. The subjects with EPD found that dose intensification was advantageous in terms of PFS (P = .003).[179]

Dose-Intensive Chemotherapy with Autologous Stem Cell Rescue

A series of 15 children less than 38 months of age with newly diagnosed malignant CNS tumors was reported using high-dose chemotherapy with PBSC followed by selective EBRT. Three courses of cisplatin-cyclophosphamide-etoposide-vincristine were succeeded by three cycles of carboplatin-thiotepa with reinfusion of PBSC. Ten patients are disease-free at a median of 18 months; five received EBRT (Table 8-12). There were no toxicity-related deaths.[180]

The "*Head Start*" *I* and *II* protocols administered postoperative induction chemotherapy with vincristine-cisplatin-cyclophosphamide-etoposide for five cycles. Myeloablative chemotherapy with carboplatin-thiotepa-etoposide was supported with PBSC. Irradiation was used only at relapse. A series of 21 children with nonmetastatic MBL were studied. The 5Y-PFS rates are shown in Table 8-12; gross total resection and desmoplastic morphology were associated with especially favorable results. Most survivors (71%) and 52% of the whole cohort avoided EBRT. Mean intellectual function among these patients remained within the average range for the majority tested.[181]

LONG-TERM COMPLICATIONS OF DISEASE AND THERAPY

Cognitive, Behavioral, and Functional Sequelae

Hirsch et al.[182] noted that only 12% of MBL survivors retained IQs above 90; in addition, 93% displayed behavioral disorders. Especially severe deficits appear to be associated with earlier age at irradiation and adjuvant chemotherapy.[183] The frequency and causation of intellectual deficits of such magnitude consequent to therapeutic irradiation have been disputed.[184] Comparable deficits are not seen among children with posterior fossa AST, for whom surgical resection constituted adequate therapy.[185]

Prospective evaluation of PNET/MBL patients who received whole brain EBRT has demonstrated progressive decrease of 14 points in full-scale intelligence quotient (FSIQ) during the two years after treatment (P = .001). Children less than 7 years at time of diagnosis have declined to a median FSIQ of 82 (range 50-98), compared to 103 (range 92-133) for the older children. Children less than 5 years of age suffered a mean reduction of 25 points in FSIQ (P < .02).[183]

One series of 34 children with MBL (30) and EPD (4) treated with EBRT examined the long-term cognitive effects of therapy. Twelve children received reduced-dose and 21 patients conventionally dosed cranial irradiation; all received an additional boost to the posterior fossa. Standardized neuropsychological testing revealed a 2-4 point annual decline in intelligence scores. Intellectual function declined more rapidly during the first few years after therapy and more gradually thereafter. Significant deterioration in visual-motor integration, visual memory, verbal fluency, and executive functioning were the dominant findings.[186] Another investigation examined the late effects of reduced dose neuraxis EBRT (23.4 Gy craniospinal with 32.4 Gy boost to the posterior fossa) with adjuvant chemotherapy among 43 children with standard risk MBL. The rate of decline in FSIQ was –4.3 points per year, –4.2 points for verbal and –4.0 for nonverbal function annually ($P < .001$ for all three). Patients less than seven years of age ($P = .016$), females ($P = .008$), and children with higher baseline scores were more adversely affected.[187]

Retrospective investigation of 1,607 patients who survived a brain tumor during childhood demonstrated that 17% had a neurosensory impairment. Relative to their siblings, there was a significant increased risk for hearing impairment ($P < .0001$), legal blindness in one or both eyes ($P < .0001$), cataracts ($P < .0001$), and diplopia ($P < .0001$). Incoordination (49%), motor control difficulties (26%), and seizure disorders (25%) were other common neurologic problems. Irradiation of the frontal lobe to 50 or more Gy increased the risk for motor deficits ($P < .05$). Cerebral irradiation to more than 30 Gy doubled the risk of a subsequent seizure disorder.[188]

Radiation Toxicity and Necrosis

Of the long-term effects, radionecrosis is progressive, irreversible, dose-dependent, and potentially fatal. It occurs in about 3% to 14% of EBRT-treated patients; the incidence is increasing as duration of survival and imaging techniques improve. The latency interval is between 6 and 36 months in 78% of cases (range: 2 months to 19 years). Clinical features include focal seizures, encephalopathy, dementia, signs of increased intracranial pressure, and new focal neurologic deficits.[189] Positron emission tomography is the best noninvasive test currently available for distinguishing radionecrosis from recurrent neoplasm.[190]

Cerebrovascular Disease

Another late sequela of EBRT that is recognized among children is the occurrence of cerebrovascular accidents. The latency for ischemic complications may vary between 2 and 24 years. Radiation-induced thrombosis of the carotid and intracranial arteries may present as transient ischemic attacks as well as acute infarction.[189,191] Long-term survivors of pediatric brain tumors are forty times more likely to experience a stroke than siblings.[192]

Neuroendocrine Sequelae

Children treated with craniospinal EBRT are at risk for growth failure secondary to growth hormone deficiency, as well as primary, secondary, and/or tertiary hypothyroidism.[193] Growth hormone deficiency is the most common form of pituitary insufficiency to follow irradiation.[194] Chemical evidence of hypothyroidism occurs in 25% to 50% of patients following EBRT to the head and neck, although not all will be symptomatic. Primary hypothyroidism was found in 24% (71% of which had received craniospinal treatment), compensated hypothyroidism in 73%, and central hypothyroidism in 6%. Chemotherapy was not found to affect thyroid function.[195] This may be a progressive process which requires replacement years following EBRT.

Conclusions

Irradiation and chemotherapy are now the "standard of care" for "high-risk" pediatric brain tumor patients with an appropriate functional status. The early excitement (and hubris) of Phase III trials has faded, with more interest being subsequently paid to combination and neoadjuvant chemotherapy. The concept of dose-intensive escalation with alkylators and epiphyllotoxins for disease control continues to hold theoretic promise but must be regarded as unproven, given the paucity of trials utilizing protracted treatment schedules with PBSC support. Short-term myeloablative chemotherapy with ABMT rescue appears to have little or nothing to offer in the treatment of neoplastic diseases with a relatively low mitotic index. Sequential and/or alternating "chemoradiotherapy" appears attractive as a means of locoregional control but there has been relatively little experience with this approach. However, there are a number of effective chemotherapeutic agents, which may also be valid radiosensitizers in the appropriate setting. Antagonizing angiogenesis seems intuitively appealing; however, intratumoral hypoxia constitutes a very important mechanism for promoting resistance to treatment against both chemotherapy and EBRT. The intrinsic and selected-for mechanisms of therapeutic resistance are poorly understood and appear intimately related to the pathogenetic events of malignant transformation itself. These are obvious fields for investigation in order to develop a future generation of genetically based therapies.[196]

REFERENCES

1. Smith MA, Gurney JG, Gloeckler, et al. Cancer among adolescents 15–19 years old. In: Reis LAG, Smith MA, Berney JG, et al. editors. Cancer Incidence and Survival Among Children and Adolescents: United States SEER Program 1975–1995. Bethesda MD: National Cancer Institute SEER Program; NIH Pub. No. 99–4649, 1999. p. 157–64.
2. CBTRUS. Statistical Report: Primary Brain Tumors in the United States, 1995–1999. Published by the Central Brain Tumor Registry of the United States; 2002.
3. Ries LAG, Bercy CL, Bunin GR. In: Reis LAG, Smith MA, Berney JG, et al. editors. Cancer Incidence and Survival Among Children and Adolescents: United States SEER Program 1975–1995. Bethesda MD: National Cancer Institute SEER Program; 1999. p. 1–15. NIH Pub. No. 99–4649.
4. Gurney JC, Smith MA, Bunin GR. CNS and miscellaneous intracranial and intraspinal neoplasms. In: Reis LAG, Smith MA, Berney JG, et al. editors. Cancer Incidence and Survival Among Children and Adolescents: United States SEER Program 1975–1995. Bethesda MD: National Cancer Institute SEER Program; 1999. p. 51–63. NIH Pub. No. 99–4649.
5. Hjalmars U, Kulldorff M, Wahlqvist Y, et al. Increased incidence rates but no space-time clustering of childhood astrocytoma in Sweden, 1973–1992: a population-based study of pediatric brain tumors. Cancer 1999;85:2077–90.
6. Polednak AP, Flannery JT. Brain, other central nervous system, and eye cancer. Cancer 1995;75:330–7.

7. McNeil DE, Cote TR, Clegg L, et al. Incidence and trends in pediatric malignancies medulloblastoma/primitive neuroectodermal tumor: a SEER update. Med Pediatr Oncol 2002;39:190–4.
8. Jennings MT, Gelman R, Hochberg F. Intracranial germ cell tumors: natural history and pathogenesis. J Neurosurg 1985;63:155–67.
9. Araki C, Matsumoto S. Statistical reevalution of pinealoma and related tumors in Japan. J Neurosurg 1969;30:146–9.
10. Jellinger K. Primary intracranial germ cell tumours. Acta Neuropathol 1973;25:291–306.
11. Grossman SA, Osman M, Hruban R, et al. Central nervous system cancers in first-degree relatives and spouses. Cancer Investig 1999;17:299–308.
12. Ron E, Modan B, Boice JD, et al. Tumors of the brain and nervous system after radiotherapy in childhood. N Engl J Med 1988;319:1033–9.
13. Shapiro S, Mealy Jr J, Sartorius C. Radiation-induced intracranial malignant gliomas. J Neurosurg 1989;71:77–82.
14. McKeran RO, Thomas DGT. The clinical study of gliomas. In: Thomas DGT, Graham DL, editors. Brain Tumors: Scientific Basis, Clinical Investigation and Current Therapy. Baltimore; 1980. p. 194–230.
15. Osoba D, Aaronson NK, Muller M, et al. Effect of neurological dysfunction on health-related quality of life in patients with high-grade glioma. J Neuro-Oncol 1997;34:263–78.
16. Forsythe P, Posner JB. Headaches in patients with brain tumors: a study of 111 patients. Ann Neurol 1992;32:289 (Abstr.).
17. Park TS, Hoffman HJ, Hendrick EB, et al. Medulloblastoma: clinical presentation and management. J Neurosurg 1983;58:543–52.
18. Harisiadis L, Chang CH. Medulloblastoma in children: a correlation between staging and results of treatment. Int J Radiat Oncol Biol Phys 1997;2:833–41.
19. Allen JC, Epstein F. Medulloblastoma and other primary malignant neuroectodermal tumors of the CNS. The effect of patients' age and extent of disease on prognosis. J Neurosurg 1982;57:446–51.
20. Chatty EM, Earle KM. Medulloblastoma. A report of 201 cases with emphasis on the relationship of histologic variants to survival. Cancer 1971;28:977–83.
21. Burger PC, Yu I-T, Tihan T, et al. Atypical teratoid/rhabdoid tumor of the central nervous system: a highly malignant tumor of infancy and childhood frequently mistaken for medulloblastoma: a Pediatric Oncology Group study. Amer J Surg Pathol 1998;22:1083–92.
22. Packer RJ, Biegel JA, Blaney S, et al. Atypical teratoid/rhabdoid tumor of the central nervous system: report on workshop. J Ped Hematol/Oncol 2002;24:337–42.
23. Pollack IF, Gerszten PC, Martinez AJ, et al. Intracranial ependymomas of childhood: long-term outcome and prognostic factors. Neurosurgery 1995;37:655–66.
24. Allam A, Radwi A, El Weshi A, et al. Oligodendroglioma: an analysis of prognostic factors and treatment results. Amer J Clin Oncol 2000;23:170–5.
25. Gordon GS, Wallace SJ, Neal JW. Intracranial tumours during the first two years of life: presenting features. Arch Dis Child 1995;73:345–7.
26. Pollack IF, Hamilton RL, Burnham J, et al. Impact of proliferation index on outcome in childhood malignant gliomas: results in a multiinstitutional cohort. Neurosurgery 2002;50:1238–44.
27. Sposto R, Ertel IJ, Jenkin RDT, et al. The effectiveness of chemotherapy for treatment of high grade astrocytoma in children: results of a randomized trial. J Neuro-Oncol 1989;7:165–77.
28. Geyer JR, Finlay JL, Boyett JM, et al. Survival in infants with malignant astrocytomas. A report of the Children's Cancer Group. Cancer 1995;75:1045–50.
29. Ashmore SM, Thomas DGT, Darling JL. Does p-glycoprotein play a role in clinical resistance of malignant astrocytoma?. Anticancer Drugs 1999;10:861–72.
30. Goldstein LJ. Clinical reversal of drug resistance. Curr Probl Cancer 1995;19:65–124.
31. Valera ET, Lucio-Eterovic AK, Neder L, et al. Quantitative PCR analysis of the expression profile of genes related to multiple drug resistance in tumors of the central nervous system. J Neuro-Oncol 2007;85:1–10.
32. Pollack IF, Hamilton RL, Sobol RW, et al. O6-methylguanine-DNA methyltransferase expression strongly correlates with outcome in childhood malignant gliomas: results from the CCG-945 cohort. J Clin Oncol 2006;24:3431–7.
33. Green SL, Giaccia AJ. Tumor hypoxia and the cell cycle: implications for malignant progression and response to therapy. The Cancer Journal 1998;4:214–23.
34. Hainaut P. The tumor suppressor protein p53: a receptor to genotoxic stress that controls cell growth and survival. Curr Opin Oncol 1995;7:76–82.

35. Kastan MB, Onyekwere N, Sidransky D, et al. Participation of p53 protein in cellular response to DNA damage. Cancer Res 1991;51:6304–11.
36. Graeber TC, Osmanian C, Jacks T, et al. Hypoxia-mediated selection of cells with diminished apoptotic potential in solid tumors. Nature 1996;379:88–91.
37. Kyritsis AP, Bondy ML, Hess KR, et al. Prognostic significance of p53 immunoreactivity in patients with glioma. Clin Cancer Res 1995;1:1617–22.
38. Liang BC. Effects of hypoxia on drug resistance phenotype and genotype in human glioma cell lines. J Neuro-Oncol 1996;29:149–55.
39. Iwadate Y, Tagawa M, Fujimoto S, et al. Mutation of the p53 gene in human astrocytic tumours correlates with increased resistance to DNA-damaging agents but not to antimicrotubule anti-cancer agents. Brit J Cancer 1998;77:547–51.
40. Bigner SH, Mark J, Bullard DE, et al. Chromosomal evolution in malignant human gliomas starts with specific and usually numerical deviations. Cancer Genet Cytogenet 1986;22:121–35.
41. Ransom DT, Ritland SR, Moertel CA, et al. Correlation of cytogenetic analysis and loss of heterozygosity studies in human diffuse astrocytomas and mixed oligo-astrocytomas. Genes Chromosomes Cancer 1992;5:357–74.
42. Lang FF, Miller DC, Koslow M, et al. Pathways leading to glioblastoma multiforme: a molecular analysis of genetic alterations in 65 astrocytic tumors. J Neurosurg 1994;81:427–36.
43. von Deimling A, Louis DN, von Ammon K, et al. Molecular genetic evidence for two distinct subsets of glioblastoma multiforme. Clin Neuropathol 1992;11:265–6.
44. Sidransky D, Mikkelsen T, Schwechheimer D, et al. Clonal expansion of p53 mutant cells is associated with brain tumour progression. Nature 1992;355:846–7.
45. Yin D, Xie D, Hofmann WK, et al. Methylation, expression, and mutation analysis of the cell cycle control genes in human brain tumors. Oncogene 2002;21:8372–8.
46. Li J, Yen C, Liaw D, et al. PTEN, a putative protein tyrosine phosphate gene mutated in human brain, breast and prostate cancer. Science 1997;275:1943–7.
47. Steck PA, Pershouse MA, Jasser SA, et al. Identification of a candidate tumour suppressor gene, MMAC1, at chromosome 10q23.3 thi is mutated in multiple advanced cancers. Nature Genet 1997;15:356–62.
48. Lin H, Bondy ML, Langford LA, et al. Allelic deletion analyses of MMAC/PTEN and DMBT1 loci in gliomas: relationship to prognostic significance. Clin Cancer Res 1998;4:2447–57.
49. Sano T, Lin H, Chen X, et al. Differential expression of MMAC/PTEN in glioblastoma multiforme: relationship to localization and prognosis. Cancer Res 1999;59:1820–4.
50. Henson JW, Schnitker BL, Correa KM, et al. The retinoblastoma gene is involved in malignant progression of astrocytomas. Ann Neurol 1994;36:714–21.
51. Kamb A, Gruis NA, Weaver-Feldhaus J, et al. A cell cycle regulator potentially involved in the genesis of many tumor types. Science 1994;264:436–40.
52. Schmidt EE, Ichimura K, Reifenberger G, et al. CDKN2 (p16/MTS1) gene deletion or CDK4 amplification occurs in the majority of glioblastomas. Cancer Res 1994;54:6321–4.
53. Iwadate Y, Mochizuki S, Fujimoto S, et al. Alteration of CDKN2/p16 in human astrocytic tumors is related with increased susceptibility to antimetabolite anticancer agents. Int J Oncol 2000;17:501–5.
54. Sure U, Ruedi D, Tachibana O, et al. Determination of p53 mutations, EGFR overexpression, and loss of p16 expression in pediatric glioblastomas. J Neuropathol & Exper Neurol 1997;56:782–9.
55. Sung T, Miller DC, Hayes RL, et al. Preferential inactivation of the p53 tumor suppressor pathway and lack of EGFR amplication distinquish de novo high grade pediatric astrocytomas from de novo adult astrocytomas. Brain Pathol 2000;10:249–59.
56. Raffel C, Frederick L, O'Fallor JR, et al. Analysis of oncogene and tumor suppressor gene alterations in pediatric malignant astroytomas reveals reduced survival for patients with PTEN mutations. Clin Cancer Res 1999;5:4085–90.
57. Pollack IF, Hamilton RL, James CD, et al. Rarity of PTEN deletions and EGFR amplification in malignant gliomas of childhood: results from the Children's Cancer Group 945 cohort. J Neurosurg 2006;105(Suppl. 5):418–24.
58. Albright AL, Guthkelch AN, Packer RJ, et al. Prognostic factors in pediatric brainstem gliomas. J Neurosurg 1986;65:751–775.
59. Laws ER, Taylor WR, Bergstralh EJ, et al. The neurosurgical management of low-grade astrocytoma. Clin Neurosurg 1985;33:575.
60. Sheline GE. The role of radiation therapy in the treatment of low-grade gliomas. Clin Neurosurg 1986;33:563.

61. Janny P, Cure H, Mohr M, et al. Low grade supratentorial astrocytomas: management and prognostic factors. Cancer 1994;73:1937–45.
62. Nishio S, Takeshia I, Fujii K, et al. Supratentorial astrocytic tumours of childhood: a clinicopathologic study of 41 cases. Acta Neurochir (Wien) 1989;101:3–8.
63. Fernandez C, Figarella-Branger D, Girard N, et al. Pilocytic astrocytomas in children: prognostic factors – a retrospective study of 80 cases. Neurosurgery 2003;53:544–55.
64. Deliganis AV, Geyer JR, Berger MS. Prognostic significance of type 1 neurofibromatosis (von Recklinghausen disease) in childhood optic glioma. Neurosurgery 1996;38:1114–8.
65. Micheli R, Giordano L, Balestrini MR. Cerebral tumors in children with neurofibromatosis type 1. Minerva Pediatr 1996;48:89–97.
66. Broniscer A, Baker SJ, West AN, et al. Clinical and molecular characteristic of malignant transformation of low-grade glioma in children. J Clin Oncol 2007;25:682–9.
67. Tait DM, Thorton-Jones H, Bloom HJG, et al. Adjuvant chemotherapy for medulloblastoma: the first multi-centre control trial of the International Society of Paediatric Oncology (SIOP). Eur J Cancer 1990;26:464–9.
68. Evans AE, Jenkin RDT, Sposto R, et al. The treatment of medulloblastoma: results of a prospective randomized trial of radiation therapy with and without CCNU, vincristine and prednisone. J Neurosurg 1990;72:572–82.
69. Albright AL, Wisoff JH, Zeltzer PM, et al. Effects of medulloblastoma resections on outcome in children: a report from the Children's Cancer Group. Neurosurgery 1996;38:265–71.
70. Zeltzer PM, Boyett JM, Finlay JL, et al. Metastasis stage, adjuvant treatment, and residual tumor are prognostic factors for medulloblastoma in children: conclusions from the Children's Cancer Group 921 randomized phase III study. J Clin Oncol 1999;17:832–45.
71. Eberhart CG, Kepner JL, Goldthwaite PT, et al. Histologic grading of medulloblastomas. A Pediatric Oncology Group study. Cancer 1992;94:552–60.
72. Giangaspero F, Wellek S, Masuoka J, et al. Stratification of medulloblastoma on the basis of histopathological grading. Acta Neuropath 2006;112:5–12.
73. Valera ET, Lucio-Eterovic AK, Neder L, et al. Quantitative PCR analysis of the expression profile of genes related to multiple drug resistance in tumors of the central nervous system. J Neuro-Oncol 2007;85:1–10.
74. Lo KC, Rossi MR, Eberhart CG, et al. Genome wide copy number abnormalities in pediatric medulloblastoma as assessed by array comparative genome hybridization. Brain Pathol 2007;17:282–96.
75. Pfister S, Remke M, Toedt G, et al. Supratentorial primitive neuroectodermal tumors of the central nervous system frequently harbor deletions of the CDKN2A locus and other genomic aberrations distinct from medulloblastomas. Genes Chromosome Cancer 2007;46:839–51.
76. Briggs KJ, Corcoran-Schwartz IM, Zhang W, et al. Cooperation between the Hic1 and Ptch1 tumor suppressors in medulloblastoma. Genes Dev 2008;22:770–85.
77. Lamont JM, McManamy CS, Pearson AD, et al. Combined histopathological and molecular cytogenetic stratification of medulloblastoma patients. Clin Cancer Res 2004;10:5482–93.
78. Ellison E. Classifying the medulloblastoma: insights from morphology and molecular genetics. Neuropathol Appl Neurobiol 2002;278:257–82.
79. Bar EE, Stearns D. New developments in medulloblastoma treatment: the potential of a cycopamine-lovastatin combination. Expert Opinion Investig Drugs 2008;17:185–95.
80. Clifford SC, Lusher ME, Lindsey JC, et al. Wnt/Wingless pathway activation and chromosome 6 loss characterize a distinct molecular subgroup of medulloblastomas associated with a favorable prognosis. Cell Cycle 2006;5:2666–70.
81. Castellino RC, De Bortoli M, Lin LL, et al. Overexpressed TP73 induces apoptosis in medulloblastoma. BMC Cancer 2007;7:127.
82. Hartmann W, Digon-Sontgerath B, Koch A, et al. Phosphatidyl 3'±-kinase/AKT signaling is activated in medulloblastoma proliferation and associated with reduced expression of PTEN. Clinical Cancer Res 2006;12:3019–27.
83. Inda MM, Mercapide J, Munoz J, et al. PTEN and DMBT1 homozygous deletion and expression in medulloblastoma and primitive neuroectodermal tumors. Oncol Reports 2004;12:1341–7.
84. Eberhart CG, Kratz J, Wang Y, et al. Histopathological and molecular prognostic markers in medulloblastoma: c-myc, N-myc, trkc, and anaplasia. J Neuropath Exp Neurol 2004;63:441–9.
85. Grotzer MA, von Hoff K, von Buieren AO, et al. Which clinical and biological tumor markers proved predictive in the prospective multicenter trial HIT'91 – implications for investigating childhood medulloblastoma. Klin Padiatr 2007;219:312–7.

86. Gajjar A, Hernan R, Kocak M, et al. Clinical, histopathologic, and molecular markers of prognosis: toward a new disease risk stratification system for medulloblastoma. J Clin Oncol 2004;22:984–93.
87. Merchant TE, Jenkins JJ, Burger PC, et al. The influence of histology on the time to progression after irradiation for localized ependymoma in children. Int J Radiat Oncol Biol Phys 1999;45:235 (Abstr. 169).
88. Nazar GB, Hoffman HJ, Becker LE, et al. Infratentorial ependymomas in childhood: prognostic factors and treatment. J Neurosurg 1990;72:408–17.
89. Paulino AC, Wen B-C, Buatti JM, et al. Intracranial ependymomas: an analysis of prognostic factors and patterns of failure. Amer J Clin Oncol 2002;25:117–22.
90. Robertson PL, Zeltzer PM, Boyett JM, et al. Survival and prognostic factors following radiation therapy and chemotherapy for ependymomas in children: a report of the Children's Cancer Group. J Neurosurg 1998;88:695–703.
91. Grill J, Le Deley M-C, Gambarelli D, et al. Postoperative chemotherapy without irradiation for ependymoma in children under 5 years of age: a multicenter trial of the French Society of Pediatric Oncology. J Clin Oncol 2001;19:1288–96.
92. Horn B, Heideman R, Geyer R, et al. A multi-institutional retrospective study of intracranial ependymoma in children: identification of risk factors. J Pediatr Hemat Oncol 1999;21:203–11.
93. Sowar K, Straessle J, Donson AM, et al. Predicting which children are at risk for ependymoma relapse. J Neurooncol 2006;78:41–6.
94. Modena P, Lualdi E, Facchinetti F. Identification of tumor-specific molecular signatures in intracranial ependymoma and association with clinical characteristics. J Clin Oncol 2006;24:5223–33.
95. Tabori U, Ma J, Carter M, et al. Human telomere reverse transcriptase expression predicts progression and survival in pediatric intracranial ependymoma. J Clin Oncol 2006;24:1522–8.
96. Feigenberg SJ, Amdur RJ, Morris C, et al. Oligodendroglioma: does deferring treatment compromise outcome? Amer J Clin Oncol 2003;26:e60–6.
97. Smith JS, Perry A, Borell TJ, et al. Alterations of chromosome arms 1p and 19q as predictors of survival in oligodendrogliomas, astrocytomas and mixed oligoastrocytomas. J Clin Oncol 2000;18:636–45.
98. Godfraind C, Rousseau E, Ruchoux M-M, et al. Tumour necrosis and microvascular proliferation are associated with 9p deletion and CDKNA2 alterations in 1p/19q-delected oligodendrogliomas. Neuropathol Appl Neurobiol 2003;29:462–71.
99. He J, Hoang-Xuan K, Marie Y, et al. P18 tumor suppressor gene and progression of oligodendrogliomas to anaplasia. Neurology 2000;55:867–9.
100. Pohl U, Cairncross JG, Louis DN. Homozygous deletions of the CDKN2C/pinh4c gene on the short arm of chromosome 1 in anaplastic oligodendrogliomas. Brain Pathology 1999;9:639–43.
101. Wolf RM, Draghi N, Liang X, et al. P190rhogap can act to inhibit PDGF-induced gliomas in mice: a putative tumor suppressor encoded on human chromosome 19q13.3. Genes Dev 2003;17:476–87.
102. Matsutani M, Sano K, Takakura K, et al. Primary intracranial germ cell tumors: a clinical analysis of 153 histologically verified cases. J Neurosurg 1997;86:446–55.
103. Balmaceda C, Heller G, Rosenblum M, et al. Chemotherapy without irradiation – a novel approach for newly diagnosed CNS germ cell tumors: results of an international cooperative trial. J Clin Oncol 1996;14:2908–15.
104. Aoyama H, Shirato H, Ikeda J, et al. Induction chemotherapy followed by low-dose involved field radiotherapy for intracranial germ cell tumors. J Clin Oncol 2002;20:857–65.
105. Shapiro WR. Treatment of neuroectodermal brain tumors. Ann Neurol 1982;12:231–7.
106. Wisoff JH, Boyett JM, Berger MS, et al. Current neurosurgical management and the impact of the extent of resection in the treatment of malignant gliomas of childhood: a report of the Children's Cancer Group trial No. CCG-945. J Neurosurg 1998;90:1147–8.
107. Duffner PK, Horowitz ME, Krischer JP, et al. Postoperative chemotherapy and delayed radiotherapy in children less than three years of age with malignant brain tumors. N Engl J Med 1993;328:1725–31.
108. Finlay JL, Boyett JM, Yates AJ, et al. Randomized phase III trial in childhood highgrade astrocytoma comparing vincristine, lomustine, and prednisone with the eight drugs in 1 day regimen. J Clin Oncol 1995;13:112–23.
109. White L, Kellie S, Gray E, et al. Postoperative chemotherapy in children less than 4 years of age with malignant brain tumors: promising initial response to a VETOPEC-based regimen. J Ped Hem Onc 1998;20:125–30.

110. Shapiro WR. Therapy of adult malignant brain tumors: what have the clinical trials taught us?. Seminars Oncol 1986;13:38–45.
111. Jennings MT, Iyengar S. Pharmacotherapy of malignant astrocytomas of children and adults. CNS Drugs 2001;15:719–43.
112. Pendergrass TW, Milstein JM, Geyer JR, et al. Eight drugs in one day chemotherapy for brain tumors: experience with 107 children and rationale for preradiation chemotherapy. J Clin Oncol 1987;5:1221–31.
113. Finlay JL, Geyer JR, Turski PA, et al. Pre-irradiation chemotherapy in children with high-grade astrocytoma: tumor response to two cycles of the "8-drugs-in-1-day" regimen. A Children's Cancer Group study, CCG-945. J Neuro-Oncol 1994;21:255–65.
114. Kellie SJ, Kovnar EH, Kun LE, et al. Neuraxis dissemination in pediatric brain tumors: response to preirradiation chemotherapy. Cancer 1992;69:1061–6.
115. Kühl J, Müller HL, Berthold F, et al. Preradiation chemotherapy with children and young adults with malignant brain tumors: results of the German pilot trial HIT'88/'89. Klin Paediatr 1998;210:227–33.
116. Urban C, Benesch M, Pakisch B, et al. Synchronous radiochemotherapy in unfavorable brain tumors of children and young adults. J Neuro-Oncol 1998;39:71–80.
117. Abrey LE, Rosenblum MK, Papadopoulos E, et al. High dose chemotherapy with autologous stem cell rescue in adults with malignant primary brain tumors. J Neuro-Oncol 1999;44:147–53.
118. Kedar A, Maria BL, Graham-Pole J, et al. High-dose chemotherapy with marrow reinfusion and hyperfractionated irradiation for children with high-risk brain tumors. Med Pediatr Oncol 1994;23:428–36.
119. Bouffet E, Khelfaoui F, Philip I, et al. High-dose carmustine for high-grade gliomas in childhood. Cancer Chemother Pharmacol 1997;39:376–9.
120. Dunkel IJ, Garvin Jr JH, Goldman S, et al. High dose chemotherapy with autologous bone marrow rescue for children with diffuse pontine gliomas. J Neuro-Oncol 1998;37:67–73.
121. Mason WP, Grovas A, Halpern S, et al. Intensive chemotherapy and bone marrow rescue for young children with newly diagnosed malignant brain tumors. J Clin Oncol 1998;16:210–21.
122. Grovas AC, Boyett JM, Lindsley K, et al. Regimen-related toxicity of myeloablative chemotherapy with BCNU, thiotepa and etoposide followed by autologous stem cell rescue for children with newly diagnosed glioblastoma multiforme: report from the Childrens Cancer Group. Med Pediatr Oncol 1999;33:83–7.
123. Jakacki RI, Jamison C, Mathews VP, et al. Dose-intensification of procarbazine, CCNU (lomustine), vincristine (PCV) with peripheral blood stem cell support in young patients with gliomas. Med Pediatr Oncol 1998;31:483–90.
124. Jakacki RI, Jamison C, Heifetz SA, et al. Feasibility of sequential high-dose chemotherapy and peripheral blood stem cell support for pediatric central nervous system malignancies. Med Pediatr Oncol 1997;29:553–9.
125. Massimino M, Gandola L, Luksch R, et al. Sequential chemotherapy, high dose thiotepa, circulating progenitor cell rescue and radiotherapy for childhood high grade glioma. Neuro-Oncol 2005;7:41–8.
126. Kretschmar CS, Tarbell NJ, Barnes PD, et al. Pre-irradiation chemotherapy and hyperfractionated radiation therapy 66 Gy for children with brain stem tumors. Cancer 1993;72:1404–13.
127. Pakisch B, Urban C, Slavc I, et al. Hyperfractionated radiotherapy and polychemotherapy in brain stem tumors in children. Child's Nerv Syst 1992;8:215–8.
128. Jennings MT, Sposto R, Vezina LG, et al. Preradiation Chemotherapy in Primary High Risk Brain Stem Tumors: CCG-9941, a Phase II Study of the Children's Cancer Group. J Clin Oncol 2002;20:3431–7.
129. Pollack IF, Claassen D, al-Shboul Q, et al. Low-grade gliomas of the cerebral hemispheres in children: an analysis of 71 cases. J Neurosurg 1995;82:536–47.
130. Smoots DW, Geyer JR, Lieberman DM, et al. Predicting disease progression in childhood cerebellar astrocytoma. Childs Nerv Syst 1998;14:636–48.
131. Rudoler S, Corn BW, Werner-Wasik M, et al. Patterns of tumor progression after radiotherapy for low-grade gliomas: analysis from the computed tomography/magnetic resonance imaging era. Amer J Clin Oncol 1998;21:23–7.
132. West CGH, Gattamaneni R, Blair V. Radiotherapy in the treatment of low-grade astrocytomas. I. A survival analysis. Child's Nerv Syst 1995;11:438–42.
133. Berger MS, Leibel SA, Bruner JM, et al. Primary central nervous system tumors of the supratentorial compartment. In: Levin VA, editor. Cancer in the Nervous System. New York: Churchill Livingstone; 1996.

134. Kortmann RD, Timmermann B, Taylor RE, et al. Current and future strategies in radiotherapy of childhood low-grade glioma of the brain. Part I: Treatment modalities of radiation therapy. Strahlentherapie und Onkologie 2003;179:509–20.
135. Packer RJ, Allen JC, Phillips PC, et al. Efficacy of chemotherapy for children with newly diagnosed progressive low-grade gliomas. San Francisco: Child Neurology Society Meeting; 1994 (Abstr. 435).
136. Prados M, Levin V, Edwards MSB, et al. Combination chemotherapy as primary therapy for pediatric low grade gliomas. BTRC Protocol 8422, Sixth Internatl Symposium on Pediatric Neuro-Oncology, Houston; 1994. (Abstr.)
137. Jenkin RDT, Goddard K, Armstrong D, et al. Posterior fossa medulloblastoma in childhood: treatment results and a proposal for a new staging system. Int J Radiat Oncol Biol Phys 1990;19:165–274.
138. Jakacki RI, Zeltzer PM, Boyett JM, et al. Survival and prognostic factors following radiation and/or chemotherapy for primitive neuroectodermal tumors of the pineal region in infants and children: a report of the Children's Cancer Group. J Clin Oncol 1995;13:1377–83.
139. Albright AL, Wisoff JH, Zeltzer P, et al. Prognostic factors in children with supratentorial (nonpineal) primitive neuroectodermal tumors: a neurosurgical perspective from the Children's Cancer Group. Pediatr Neurosurg 1995;22:1–7.
140. Bailey CC, Gnekow A, Wellek S, et al. Prospective randomized trial of chemotherapy given before radiotherapy in childhood medulloblastoma. International Society of Paediatric Oncology (SIOP) and the (German) Society of Paediatric Oncology (GPO): SIOP I. Med Pediatr Oncol 1995;25:166–78.
141. Thomas PRM, Deutsch M, Kepner JL, et al. Low stage medulloblastoma: final analysis of trial comparing standard-dose with reduced-dose neuraxis irradiation. J Clin Oncol 2000;18:3004–11.
142. Packer RJ, Sutton LN, Elterman R, et al. Outcome for children with medulloblastoma treated with radiation and cisplatin, CCNU and vincristine chemotherapy. J Neurosurg 1994;81:690–8.
143. Packer RJ, Goldwein J, Nicholson HS, et al. Treatment of children with medulloblastoma with reduced dose craniospinal radiation therapy and adjuvant chemotherapy. A Childrens Cancer Group study. J Clin Oncol 1999;17:2127–36.
144. Levin VA, Rodriguez LA, Edwards MS, et al. Treatment of medulloblastoma with procarbazine, hydroxyurea, and reduced radiation doses to whole brain and spine. J Neurosurg 1988;68:383–7.
145. Taylor RE, Bailey CC, Robinson K, et al. Results of a randomized study of preradiation chemotherapy versus radiotherapy alone for non-metastatic medulloblastoma: the International Society of Paediatric Oncology/United Kingdom Children's Cancer Study Group PNET-3 study. J Clin Oncol 2003;21:1581–91.
146. Douglas JG, Barker JL, Ellenbogen RG, et al. Concurrent chemotherapy and reduced-dose cranial spinal irradiation followed by conformal posterior fossa tumor bed boost for average-risk medulloblastoma: efficacy and patterns of failure. Int J Radiat Oncol Biol Phys 2004;58:1161–4.
147. Packer RJ, Gajjar A, Vezina G, et al. Phase III study of craniospinal radiation therapy followed by adjuvant chemotherapy for newly diagnosed average risk medulloblastoma. J Clin Oncol 2006;24:4202–8.
148. Gajjar A, Chintagumpala M, Ashley D, et al. Risk-adapted craniospinal radiotherapy followed by high-dose chemotherapy and stem-cell rescue in children with newly diagnosed medulloblastoma. Lancet Oncol 2006;7:813–20.
149. Merchant TE, Kun LE, Krasin MJ, et al. Multi-institution prospective trial of reduced dose craniospinal irradiation (23.4 Gy) followed by conformal posterior fossa (36 Gy) and primary site irradiation (55.8 Gy) and dose-intensive chemotherapy for average-risk medulloblastoma. Int J Radiat Oncol Biol Phys 2008;70:782–7.
150. Krischer JP, Ragab A, Kun L, et al. Nitrogen mustard, vincristine, procarbazine, and prednisone as adjuvant chemotherapy in the treatment of medulloblastoma. J Neurosurg 1991;74:905–9.
151. Geyer JR, Zeltzer PM, Boyett JM, et al. Survival of infants with primitive neuroectodermal tumors or malignant ependymomas of the CNS treated with eight drugs in one day: A report of the Children's Cancer Group. J Clin Oncol 1994;12:1607–15.
152. Kovnar E, Kellie S, Horowitz M, et al. Preirradiation cisplatin and etoposide in the treatment of high-risk medulloblastoma and other malignant embryonal tumors of the central nervous system: a phase II study. J Clin Oncol 1990;8:330–6.
153. Castello MA, Clerico A, Deb G, et al. High-dose carboplatinum in combination with etoposide (JET regimen) for childhood brain tumors. Am J Ped Hem-Onc 1991;12:297–300.

154. Kellie SJ, Wong CK, Pozza LD, et al. Activity of postoperative carboplatin, etoposide, and high-dose methotrexate in pediatric CNS embryonal tumors: results of a phase II study in newly diagnosed children. Med Pediatr Oncol 2002;39:168–74.
155. Geyer R. Intensive chemotherapy pilot for infants with malignant brain tumors. Proc Amer Soc Clin Oncol 1993;12:417.
156. Heideman RL, Kovnar EH, Kellie SJ, et al. Preirradiation chemotherapy with carboplatin and etoposide in newly diagnosed embryonal pediatric CNS tumors. J Clin Oncol 1995;13:2247–54.
157. Timmermann B, Kortmann R-D, Kühl J, et al. Role of radiotherapy in the treatment of supratentorial primitive neuroectodermal tumors in childhood: results of the prospective German Brain Tumor trials HIT 88/89 and 91. J Clin Oncol 2002;20:842–9.
158. Kortmann R-D, Kühl J, Timmerman B, et al. Postoperative neoadjuvant chemotherapy before radiotherapy as compared to immediate radiotherapy followed by maintenance chemotherapy in the treatment of medulloblastoma in childhood: results of the German prospective randomized trial HIT '91. Int J Radiat Oncol Biol Phys 2000;46:269–79.
159. Taylor RE, Bailey CC, Robinson KJ, et al. Outcome for patients with metastatic (M2-3) medulloblastome treated with SIOP/KUCCSF PNET-3 chemotherapy. Europ J Cancer 2005;41:727–34.
160. Strother D, Ashley D, Kellie SJ, et al. Feasibility of four consecutive high-dose chemotherapy cycles with stem cell rescue for patients with newly diagnosed medulloblastoma or supratentorial primitive neuroectodermal tumor: results of a collaborative study. J Clin Oncol 2001;19:2696–704.
161. Chi SN, Gardner SL, Levy AS, et al. Feasibility and response to induction chemotherapy intensified with high dose methotrexate for young children with newly diagnosed disseminated medulloblastoma. J Clin Oncol 2005;22:4881–7.
162. Mork SJ, Loken AC. Ependymoma – a follow up study of 101 cases. Cancer 1977;40:907–15.
163. Goldwein JW, Corn BW, Finlay JL, et al. Is craniospinal irradiation required to cure children with malignant (anaplastic) intracranial ependymoma? Cancer 1991;67:2766–71.
164. Paleologos NA, Macdonald DR, Vick NA, et al. Neoadjuvant procarbazine, CCNU and vincristine for anaplastic and aggressive oligodendroglioma. Neurology 1999;53:1141–3.
165. Buckner JC, Gesme Jr D, O'Fallon JR, et al. Phase II trial of procarbazine, lomustine and vincristine as initial therapy for patients with low grade oligodendroglioma or oligoastrocytoma: efficacy and associations with chromosomal abnormalities. J Clin Oncol 2003;21:251–5.
166. van den Bent MJ, Taphoorn MJB, Brandes AA, et al. Phase II study of first-line chemotherapy with temozolamide in recurrent oligodendroglial tumors: the European Organization for Research and Treatment of Cancer Brain Tumor Group Study 26971. J Clin Oncol 2003;21:2525–8.
167. Oi S, Matsuzawa K, Choi J-U, et al. Identical characteristics of the patient populations with pineal region tumors in Japan and in Korea and therapeutic modalities. Child's Nerv Syst 1998;14:36–40.
168. Choi J-U, Kim D-S, Chung S-S, et al. Treatment of germ cell tumors in the pineal region. Child's Nerv Syst 1998;14:41–8.
169. Shibamoto Y, Abe M, Yamashita J, et al. Treatment results of intracranial germinoma as a function of the irradiated volume. Int J Radiat Oncol Biol Phys 1988;15:285–90.
170. Wolden SL, Wara WM, Larson DA, et al. Radiation therapy for primary intracranial germ cell tumors. Int J Radiat Oncol Biol Phys 1995;32:943–9.
171. Allen JC, DaRosso RC, Donahue B, et al. A phase II trial of preirradiation carboplatin in newly diagnosed germinoma of the central nervous system. Cancer 1994;74:940–4.
172. Calaminus G, Andreussi L, Garrè M-L, et al. Secreting germ cell tumors of the central nervous system (CNS). First results of the cooperative German/Italian pilot study (CNS sGCT). Klin Pädiatr 1997;209:222–7.
173. Kellie SJ, Boyce H, Dunkel IJ, et al. Primary chemotherapy for intracranial nongerminomatous germ cell tumors: results of the Second International CNS Germ Cell Study Group protocol. J Clin Oncol 2004;22:846–53.
174. Robertson PL, DaRosso RC, Allen JC. Improved prognosis of malignant intracranial non-germinoma germ cell tumors with multimodality therapy. J Neuro-Oncol 1997;32:71–80.
175. Cohen BH, Packer RJ, Siegel KR, et al. Brain tumors in children under 2 years: treatment, survival and long-term prognosis. Pediatr Neurosurg 1993;19:171–9.
176. Strauss LC, Killmond TM, Carson BS, et al. Efficacy of postoperative chemotherapy using cisplatin plus etoposide in young children with brain tumors. Med Ped Oncol 1991;19:16–21.
177. Dufour C, Grill J, Lellouch-Tubiana A, et al. High-grade glioma in children under 5 years of age: a chemotherapy only approach with the BBSFOP protocol. Europ J Cancer 2006;42:2939–45.
178. Rutkowski S, Bode U, Deinlein F, et al. Treatment of early childhood medulloblastoma by postoperative chemotherapy alone. New Engl J Medicine 2005;352:978–86.

179. Strother D, Kepner J, Aronin P, et al. Dose-intensive (DI) chemotherapy (CT) prolongs event-free survival (EFS) for very young children with ependymoma (EP). Results of Pediatric Oncology Group (POG) study 9233. Proc Am Soc Clin Oncol 2000;19:585a (Abstr 2302).
180. Thorarinsdotter HK, Rood B, Kamani N, et al. Outcome in children < 4 years of age with malignant central nervous systems tumors treated with high dose chemotherapy and autologous stem cell rescue. Pediatr Blood Cancer 2007;48:278–84.
181. Dhall G, Grodman H, Ji L, et al. Outcome of children less than three years old at diagnosis with non-metastatic medulloblastoma treated with chemotherapy on the "Head Start" I and II protocols. Pediatr Blood Cancer 2008;50:1169–75.
182. Hirsch JF, Reiner D, Czernichew R, et al. Medulloblastoma in childhood: survival and functional results. Acta Neurochir 1979;48:1–15.
183. Packer RJ, Sutton LN, Atkins TE, et al. A prospective study of cognitive function in children receiving whole brain radiotherapy and chemotherapy: 2-year results. J Neurosurg 1989;70:707–13.
184. Mulhern RK, Kun LE. Neuropsychologic function in children with brain tumors. III: interval changes in the six months following treatment. Med Ped Oncol 1985;13:318–24.
185. Riva D, Pantaleoni C, Milani N, et al. Impairment of neuropsychological functions in children with medulloblastomas and astrocytomas in the posterior fossa. Child's Nerv Syst 1989;5:107–10.
186. Spiegler BJ, Bouffet E, Greenberg ML, et al. Change in neurocognitive functioning after treatment with cranial radiation in childhood. J Clin Oncol 2004;22:706–13.
187. Ris DM, Packer R, Godlwein J, et al. Intellectual outcome after reduced-dose radiation therapy plus adjuvant chemotherapy for medulloblastoma: a Children's Cancer Group study. J Clin Oncol 2001;19:3470–6.
188. Packer RJ, Gurney JG, Punyko JA, et al. Long-term neurologic and neurosensory sequelae in adult survivors of a childhood brain tumor: childhood cancer survivor study. J Clin Oncol 2003;21:3255–61.
189. Rottenberg DA, Chernik NL, Deck MDF, et al. Cerebral necrosis following radiotherapy of extracranial neoplasms. Ann Neurol 1977;1:339–57.
190. Di Chiro G, Oldfield E, Wright DC, et al. Cerebral necrosis after radiotherapy and/or intrarterial chemotherapy for brain tumors: PET and neuropathologic studies. Amer J Radiol 1988;50:189–97.
191. Mitchell WG, Fishman LS, Miller JH, et al. Stroke as a late sequela of cranial irradiation for childhood brain tumors. J Child Neurol 1991;6:128–33.
192. Anderson NE. Late complications of childhood central nervous system tumour survivors. Current Opinion Neurol 2003;16:677–83.
193. Samaan NA, Bakdash MM, Caderao JB, et al. Hypopituitarism after external irradiation: evidence for both hypothalamic and pituitary origin. Ann Int Med 1975;83:771–7.
194. Dickenson WP, Berry DH, Dickenson L, et al. Differential effects of cranial radiation on growth hormone response to arginine and insulin infusion. J Pediatr 1978;92:754–7.
195. Schmeigelow M, Feldt-Rasmussen U, Rasmussen AK, et al. A population-based study of thyroid function after radiotherapy and chemotherapy for childhood brain tumor. J Clin Endocr & Metabol 2003;88:136–40.
196. Jennings MT, Iyengar S. Pharmacotherapy of malignant astrocytomas of children and adults: current strategies and future trends. CNS Drugs 2001;15:719–43.

9 Primary CNS Lymphoma

M. SIERRA DEL RIO • A. ROUSSEAU •
CAROLE SOUSSAIN • HOANG-XUAN KHE

Introduction

Primary CNS lymphomas (PCNSL) are extranodal malignant lymphomas arising within the brain, eyes, leptomeninges, or spinal cord in the absence of systemic lymphoma at the time of diagnosis. The incidence of PCNSL in western countries is 5 per 1 million person-years. Currently PCNSL are estimated to account for up to 1% of non-Hodgkin lymphomas (NHL) and 3% to 5% of all primary brain tumors. After a continual increase over the past two decades,[1] epidemiologic data suggest a recent decrease in the incidence of PCNSL, particularly among young patients suffering from acquired immunodeficiency syndrome, and probably associated with the development of new active antiviral drugs. In contrast, the incidence remains high among older patients (over 60 years), most of whom are immunocompetent.[2] The reason for the rising incidence of PCNSL among the immunocompetent population is obscure. PCNSL is also of interest because it is one of the only primary malignant brain tumors whose prognosis has improved considerably over the past two decades due to advances in treatment strategy. Although the prognosis remains poor for the majority of the patients, a substantial minority, representing approximately 20% to 30% of cases, can hope to be cured. Because long-term survivors are at increased risk of developing severe delayed cognitive dysfunction, future treatment should be aimed at improving the efficacy of treatment while limiting the risk of neurotoxicity. This review focuses on PCNSL in the immunocompetent population.

Pathology and Pathogenesis

In immunocompetent patients, all but 5% of PCNSLs are diffuse large B-cell lymphomas (DLBCL).[3] Since they are morphologically indistinguishable from systemic DLBCL, the WHO classification of tumors of hematopoietic and lymphoid tissues does not recognize PCNSL as a separate entity.[4] The remaining cases of PCNSL are T-cell lymphomas (2% to 5%)[5] or, in rare instances, low-grade B-cell lymphomas of the lymphoplasmocytic (Waldenström macroglobulinemia), follicular, or mucosa-associated lymphoid tissue (MALT) type.[6] Little is known about the tumorigenesis of PCNSL. In contrast to immunocompromised patients, the Epstein-Barr virus (EBV) does not appear to be involved in the pathogenesis of PCNSL in immunocompetent patients. The site of origin of lymphoma cells, the biological mechanisms involved in the neoplastic transformation of the lymphoid cells, and their intriguing confinement within the CNS during the course of the disease have yet to be elucidated. Indeed, the CNS does not contain resident lymphocytes under normal circumstances and lacks lymphatic vessels. However, recent evidence suggests that T and B cells enter the CNS under physiological conditions, and it has been hypothesized that PCNSL may originate from B cells derived from systemic lymphoid tissues and normally trafficking in and out of the CNS.[7] PCNSL could derive from a benign CNS inflammatory process through a monoclonal proliferation of B cells. Another hypothesis is that PCNSL might represent the metastasis of an occult systemic lymphoma, eradicated by an intact immune system but escaping within the immune-privileged CNS. Analysis of clonally rearranged immunoglobulin heavy chain (IgH) genes revealed identical dominant PCR products in bone marrow aspirates, blood samples and tumor specimens from some PCNSL patients, suggesting that subclinical systemic disease can be detected at initial diagnosis, which supports a systemic origin of the tumor in these cases.[8] In addition, B cell tropism for CNS might be acquired (before or after the oncogenic events) through specific interactions between selective homing receptors and their ligands expressed on CNS endothelial cells, as suggested by the distinctive angiotropism of CNS lymphoma cells.[9,10]

It also remains unclear whether the dismal outcome of PCNSL compared to systemic DLBCL is attributable to the immune-privileged cerebral location or reflects a specific aggressive intrinsic biologic behavior. Recently, expression profiling and genomic screening have provided new insights into understanding the poor prognosis of PCNSL. Based on lymphochip cDNA microarrays, two distinct gene expression profiles have been identified among systemic DLBCLs, indicative of different stages of B-cell differentiation. One subgroup expressed genes characteristic of germinal center B cells (GCB subgroup) whereas the other expressed genes normally induced during in vitro activation of peripheral blood B cells (ABC subgroup). Interestingly, patients with the GCB signature had a significantly better outcome than those with the ABC profile.[11] PCNSLs have been shown to frequently expresses BCL6[12] and to carry an extremely high load of somatic mutations of immunoglobulin genes and in several oncogenes demonstrating aberrant ongoing hypermutation.[13–15] Since such an ongoing hypermutation and BCL6 expression are considered as germinal center markers, it has been postulated that the cell of origin of PCNSL passed through the GC microenvironment and that these neoplasms correspond to the GCB subgroup as defined for

DLBCL. However, recent immunoprofiling[16] and gene expression studies using cDNA microarrays[17,18] demonstrated that PCNSL may exhibit characteristics associated with both ABC and GCB subtypes. Thus, PCNSL may correspond to an overlapping B-cell differentiation time slot, i.e., late GC/early post-GC stage.

Pangenomic analyses of chromosomal imbalances by comparative genomic hybridization (CGH) have shown frequent chromosome 6q loss (60% to 75%) in PCNSL.[19–21] Nakamura et al.[22] refined the candidate region suspected to contain a lymphoma-related tumor suppressor gene in the 6q22–23 locus by a fine LOH deletion mapping of 6q in PCNSL. The *PTPRK* gene seems a relevant candidate gene, since it is involved in the regulation of cell contact and adhesion, and a loss of protein expression was observed in most (76%) of the PCNSLs tested. It belongs to the protein tyrosine phosphatase superfamily of enzymes. Further studies to identify gene mutations and/or rearrangements are needed to ascertain the involvement of PTPRK in PCNSL tumorigenesis. Interestingly, the authors showed that chromosome 6q loss was found at a significantly higher rate in PCNSL than in systemic DLBCL and was correlated with shorter survival.[22] An independent study of 75 newly diagnosed HIV-negative PCNSLs investigated by interphase FISH analysis has confirmed the frequent 6q22 chromosome deletion, with a prevalence of 45%, and its negative impact on overall survival.[23] Chromosome 6q loss would therefore represent a prognostic marker in PCNSL. Otherwise, the BCL6 gene has been found mutated and its chromosomal locus (3q27) recurrently involved by translocations (20%), suggesting that BCL6 activation through genomic rearrangements may play a role in PCNSL pathogenesis.[23–25] BCL6 is frequently expressed in PCNSL, but there are conflicting data on its prognostic value as an immunohistochemical marker.[16,26–29] These results provide evidence for an alternative pathogenesis in PCNSL compared to DLBCL explaining, in part, differences in clinical behavior and prognosis.

Diagnosis and Workup

The clinical presentation of PCNSL includes focal symptoms and raised intracranial pressure. Changes in behavior and personality as well as confusion frequently occur in the elderly. The deep location of PCNSL explains why seizures are less frequent than in other brain tumors.[30,31] CT scans and MRI typically show solitary (two thirds of cases) or multiple (one third of cases) periventricular, homogeneously-enhancing lesions (Figures 9-1 and 9-2).[32–34] PCNSL is potentially associated with a large spectrum of radiological presentations and can simulate inflammatory (sarcoidosis, multiple sclerosis) or postinfectious diseases (ADEM) or other brain tumors (meningiomas, malignant gliomas, gliomatosis cerebri, brain metastases).[35–37] The diagnosis may be difficult to establish, especially with the presence of nonenhancing infiltrating lesions (occurring in about 10% of cases) (Figure 9-3),[38,39] or dural-based masses (Figure 9-4)[40,41]; perfusion MRI shows a much lower relative cerebral blood volume than that seen in malignant gliomas, and distinct signal-time intensity curves reflecting rapid leakage of contrast medium into the interstitial space.[42] Similarly magnetic resonance spectroscopy at short echo times show massive elevations of lipid resonances in PCNSL, not usually seen in high-grade gliomas.[43,44] Steroid-induced response, observed in approximately 40% of cases, is classic but not the rule and should not be used

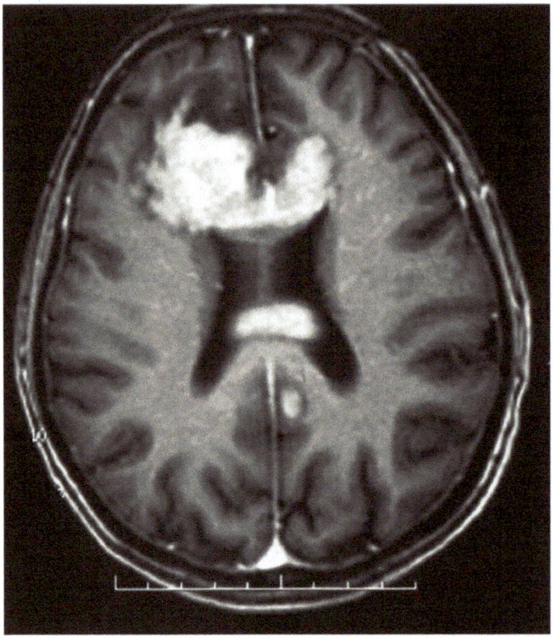

Figure 9-1 MRI T1-weighted sequence with gadolinium: Typical aspect of PCNSL presenting as a homogeneously enhancing space-occupying lesion located in the corpus callosum.

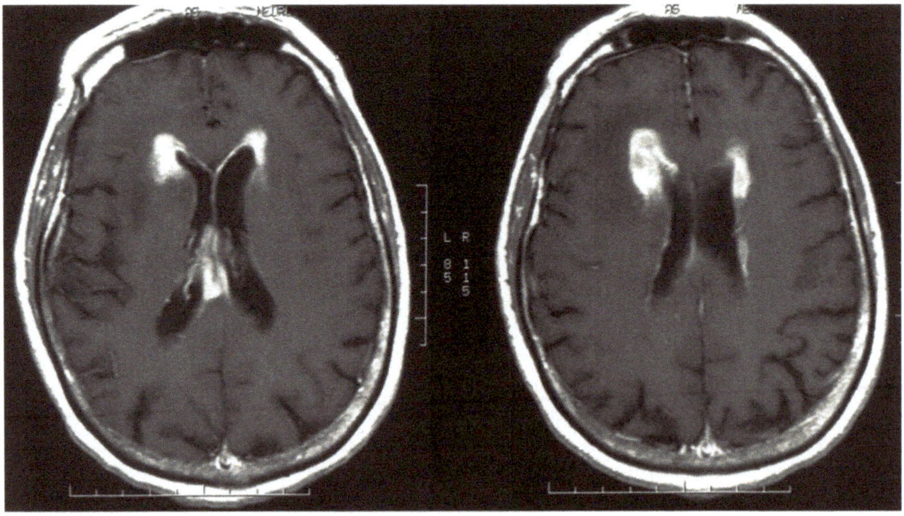

Figure 9-2 MRI T1-weighted sequence with gadolinium: PCNSL presenting as periventricular and subependymal tumoral infiltration.

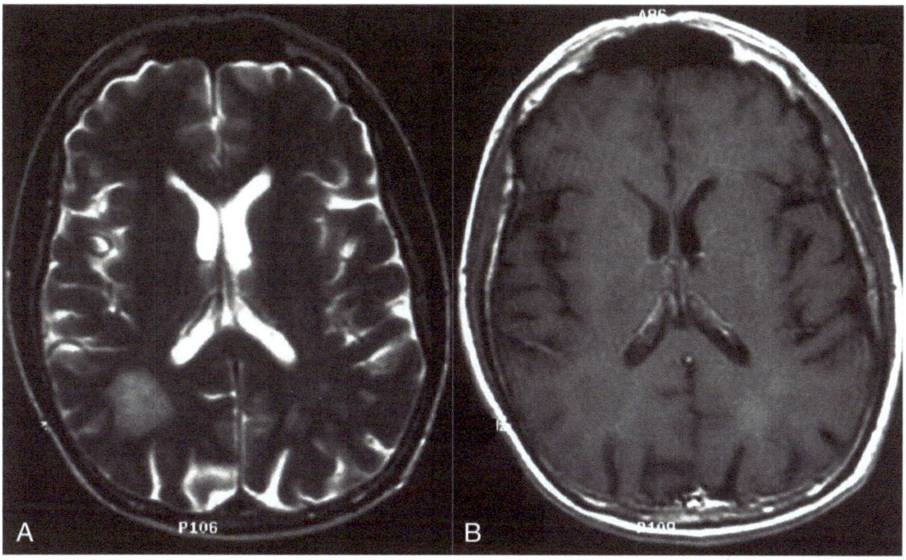

Figure 9-3 **A,** MRI T2-weighted sequence. **B,** T1-weighted sequence with gadolinium: Non enhancing PCNSL.

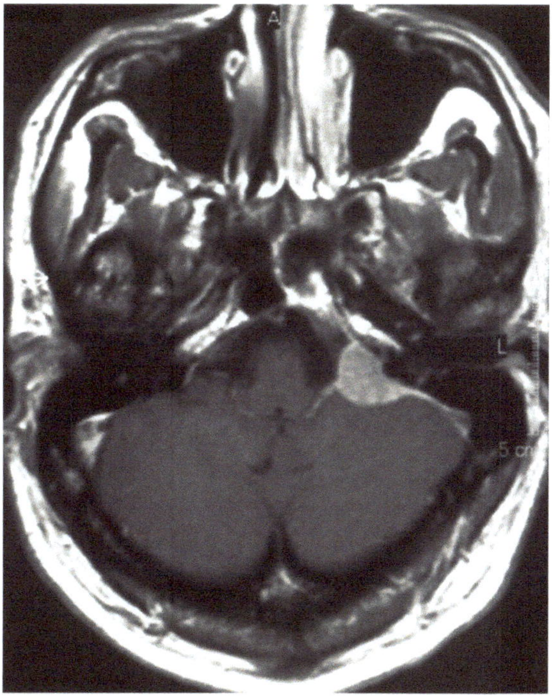

Figure 9-4 MRI T1-weighted sequence with gadolinium: PCNSL of the posterior fossa mimicking a meningioma.

as a diagnostic test since it may prevent a pathological confirmation of the diagnosis. Rarely, spontaneous disappearance of lesions has been reported, hence the term "ghost tumors."[45,46] Ring enhancement, frequently seen in immunodeficient patients, is a pattern rarely seen in immunocompetent patients. However, none of these signs are specific, and diagnosis relies on the pathological study of a tumor sample. Cerebral biopsy can be avoided when lymphomatous cells are discovered in the cerebrospinal fluid (10% to 30% of patients) or in a vitreous-body biopsy (uveitis, sometimes asymptomatic, is present in 10% to 20% of cases at diagnosis). The current recommended staging evaluation for PCNSL includes body CT scans and bone marrow biopsy.[47] In fact, systemic involvement is so rare at onset that extensive staging is not recommended by some authors, the only required examinations being HIV testing, chest radiography, analysis of cerebrospinal fluid, ocular slit-lamp examination, and a careful clinical assessment. However, in a recent retrospective study, 7% of patients were found to have systemic NHL by staging FDG body PET when body CT scans and bone marrow biopsies were negative.[48] This higher incidence of systemic lymphoma than reported in prior series suggests that occult lymphoma may be more common than recognized previously. These findings warrant prospective validation, since the identification of a systemic site of the lymphoma has important implications in the management of PCNSL.

Treatment Options

TREATMENT OF NEWLY DIAGNOSED PCNSL

Age and performance status are the main independent prognostic factors consistently identified in a large number of studies.[49–51] As PCNSL is a highly radiosensitive and chemosensitive infiltrative tumor, surgery is therefore restricted to diagnostic biopsy. Although the tumor appears on MRI as a unique contrast-enhancing lesion in the majority of the immunocompetent patients, whole-brain radiotherapy (WBRT) is recommended based on the microscopically diffuse nature of PCNSL. Despite a high rate of response, RT alone has shown a limited survival benefit in PCNSL with a median overall survival (OS) duration of 10 to 18 months and a 5-year survival rate of less than 5%.[52] The only phase II trial of radiotherapy (conducted by the RTOG) delivered a total dose of 40 Gy with an additional 20-Gy boost to contrast-enhancing lesions and reported an overall survival of 11.6 months.[53] Interestingly, most of the relapses occurred in sites that had received the maximum RT dose. These disappointing results have led to the use of chemotherapy in combination with WBRT. Since the 1990s, numerous convergent phase II studies have shown that the addition of high-dose methotrexate (MTX)-based chemotherapy to RT substantially improves survival compared with RT alone (median survival: 2 to 4 years; 5-year survival rate: 20% to 40%).[54–69] In contrast, adding the CHOP regimen (standard chemotherapy for systemic lymphoma) to RT did not appear to improve survival compared with RT alone. This may reflect the poor central nervous system penetration of the chemotherapy agents included in these regimens. The optimal dose of irradiation postchemotherapy has never been prospectively investigated. Doses between 20 and 50 Gy to the whole brain (WB) with or without a tumor bed boost are currently used, with most of the protocols using a total dose of 40-45 Gys without a boost. For patients who achieve a complete response after high-dose MTX-based chemotherapy, it still remains unclear whether consolidation with WBRT improves disease control or survival. A subset analysis from a phase II trial that included 25 patients aged less than 60 years who achieved CR after initial chemotherapy and received either 45 Gy or 30.6 Gy as consolidation treatment showed a significantly higher recurrence and lower overall survival rate in the reduced dose RT group.[61] Other studies did not share this observation. In two multicenter retrospective analyses, no differences were noted regarding disease-free or overall survival between patients in CR receiving WBRT as consolidation treatment or at the time of relapse.[70,71] In the Memorial Sloan Kettering Cancer Center (MSKCC) experience, consolidation treatment with WBRT improved failure-free survival but not overall survival in complete-responding patients after MTX-based therapy, but increased the rates of neurotoxicity.[72]

In order to reduce neurotoxicity, several groups have explored the efficacy of various high-dose MTX-based chemotherapy regimens as initial treatment for newly diagnosed PCNSL. These studies converge to suggest that chemotherapy alone and deferred radiotherapy strategy allows comparable results in terms of survival to those reported for combined chemoradiotherapy, with better neurocognitive and quality of life outcomes.[73–79] This supports the comparison of these approaches in a prospective randomized trial. While high-dose MTX is undoubtedly a key drug for PCNSL chemotherapy, interest in adding other agents to MTX exists in the scientific community. Two prospective phase II trials have investigated the efficacy of high-dose MTX (8 g/m^2) as a single drug therapy,[77,78] and similarly demonstrated a clearly shorter PFS (13 months) than that achieved with a polychemotherapy regimen. This suggests that other cytotoxic agents should be used with high-dose MTX in a chemotherapy-alone approach. However the optimal combination remains to be established. Alkylating agents able to effectively penetrate the CNS would be preferred. Concerning the optimal "high dose" of MTX to deliver, although there is no clear evidence of a dose response, a dose of greater than 3 g/m^2 in a rapid infusion is recommended.[80] In addition, this dose generally yields cytotoxic levels in the cerebral spinal fluid, thus theoretically avoiding the need to administer intrathecal chemotherapy for leptomeningeal coverage. In practice, when intravenous high dose MTX (>3 g/m^2) is used, several authors recommend adding intrathecal CT only in cases of positive CSF cytology and withholding it in the absence of detectable subarachnoid disease.[81]

DELAYED NEUROTOXICITY

WBRT, high-dose MTX chemotherapy, and the combination of both treatments expose the patients to delayed neurotoxicity. This complication can occur as early as 3 months after the treatment and is characterized by attention deficit, memory impairment, ataxia, and urinary incontinence, potentially ultimately leading to dementia. Imaging shows confluent diffuse white matter changes and later cortical-subcortical atrophy. The physiopathology of this complication remains poorly understood; loss of oligodendrocyte progenitors and oxidative stress have been suggested as potential mechanisms. Lai et al.[82] reported a well-documented series of five autopsied cases who died of treatment-related leukoencephalopathy. All had combined treatment and were in tumor remission. In addition to white matter rarefaction and spongiosis, fibrotic thickening of small vessels in the deep white matter and atherosclerosis of intracranial large vessels were systematically found, suggesting that a vascular process may be also an important component of this white matter injury. The risk of neurotoxicity increases sharply with patient age. In the elderly population (patients over age 60), virtually all long-term survivors will develop delayed neurotoxicity with its devastating consequences on quality of life and mortality.[83] In the younger population (patients under age 60), the exact incidence of this complication is more difficult to determine. Cognitive dysfunctions are usually less severe and occur later than in the elderly population, although they may interfere with quality of life.[64] An update of the MSKCC experience providing long-term data (median follow-up of 115 months) reported a 26% rate of neurotoxicity in surviving patients younger than 60 years (versus 75% in the elderly).[68] However, this should be regarded as a minimum estimate in the absence of a psychometric evaluation. A series of 19 consecutive young patients (median age: 44 years) treated in a European clinical trial and in complete remission for a mean time of 24 months after combined therapy were investigated by an extensive neuropsychological evaluation.[84] Cognitive impairments were found in 63% of patients (including 21% with severe cognitive deficits); only 42% of the patients had resumed work, and 67% had white matter abnormalities and cortical atrophy detectable by MRI. Although this study suffers from the absence of available baseline data at the completion of the treatment to assess the potential contribution of the tumor to cognitive dysfunction, it suggests that the incidence of delayed neurotoxicity after combined therapy is largely underestimated in young patients, albeit less severe than in the elderly. These results contrast sharply with a prospective neuropsychological study performed by Fliessbach et al.[84] in a series of 23 patients successfully treated with a high-dose MTX-based chemotherapy without radiotherapy. Comparison between baseline evaluation at completion of the treatment and at the last follow-up (median: 44 months) showed a good preservation of cognitive functions, although one third of the patients demonstrated some degree of white matter changes at the MRI. This latter point confirmed some previously published reports showing that MTX-related leukoencephalopathy is a frequent but not necessarily universal accompaniment to deterioration of cognitive performance.[86] The significantly better preservation of neurocognitive functions and quality of life observed in patients treated with chemotherapy alone as compared with those who received combined treatment was also supported by Correa et al.[87] in a retrospective comparative neuropsychometric analysis of 28 patients from a single institution. The incorporation of systematic psychometric and quality of life evaluations with an appropriate standardized test battery is recommended for all future prospective trials.[88] Interestingly, some functional polymorphisms interfering with the methionine metabolism might influence MTX neurotoxicity.[89,90]

TREATMENT IN THE ELDERLY

Elderly patients (i.e., ≥ 60 years of age), who experience a very poor prognosis and a high vulnerability to the delayed neurotoxicity, represent an important subgroup, accounting for approximately half of all cases of PCNSL. However, prospective trials specifically devoted to older patients are scarce. Most of the available data come from retrospective studies. In the elderly, PCNSLs exhibit a low radiosensitivity;

the RTOG Phase II trial reported a short median survival of 7.6 months with RT alone.[53] The high risk of neurotoxicity observed with the combined chemoradiotherapy approach (see above) prompted several authors to defer radiotherapy in this population. The only multicenter phase II focusing on patients older than 60 and evaluating chemotherapy alone as initial treatment was conducted by the EORTC. The regimen consisted of high-dose MTX (1 g/m^2) plus lomustine (CCNU), procarbazine, and intrathecal chemotherapy (MTX, cytarabine). The intent-to-treat response rate and median survival were 48% and 14.3 months respectively.[98] Although this study showed less favorable results than those reported by other published studies (MS ranging from 18 to 34 months),[68,74,75,95–100] it led, nevertheless, to the same conclusions and confirmed that chemotherapy alone is a valuable approach for treating elderly patients with PCNSL. Since median PFS was similar to the other studies, the lower OS may be explained by the salvage therapy. Hence, in the EORTC trial, only a small minority of patients were treated by WBRT at relapse. Altogether, chemotherapy alone appears to be more effective than RT alone and considerably reduces the risk of neurotoxicity (up to 8% of cases) as compared with that expected with combined treatment, allowing a substantial proportion of patients to reach prolonged remission without the need for consolidation radiotherapy and preserving their quality of life. Future protocols for the elderly should focus on defining the optimal chemotherapy regimen.

INTENSIVE CHEMOTHERAPY (ICT) WITH AUTOLOGOUS STEM-CELL TRANSPLANTATION (ASCT)

Intensive chemotherapy (ICT) with autologous stem-cell transplantation (ASCT) is the standard treatment for chemosensitive relapsing systemic NHL. Because ICT is expected to improve the BBB crossing, allowing cytotoxic agents to reach the brain at higher doses, this strategy has been evaluated for PCNSL. This procedure was first evaluated in refractory and recurrent cerebral and intraocular lymphoma with promising results in a single institutional pilot study.[101] The protocol consisted of an induction cytarabine-etoposide combination (CYVE regimen) followed by high-dose chemotherapy with thiotepa, busulfan, and cyclophosphamide (TBC regimen). These results have been recently confirmed in a multicenter phase II trial using the same regimen including 43 patients.[102] Twenty-seven patients (62% by intention-to-treat analysis) completed the full ICT-ASCT procedure, including 15 patients responsive and 12 nonresponsive to CYVE-induction salvage chemotherapy. Twenty-six of 27 patients achieved a complete response with prolonged remission; the median PFS and overall survival were 41 and 58 months respectively. Interestingly, all but one patient (in whom the disease was refractory to the salvage chemotherapy) achieved a complete response after ICT-ASCT (Figure 9-2). The intent-to-treat median PFS and overall survival of the whole population of this trial were 11 and 18 months. Altogether, these results compare favorably with those yet reported by other salvage treatments, including second line conventional chemotherapy regimens[103,104] and radiotherapy alone.[105,106] The favorable impact of ICT-ASCT on survival, regardless of the chemosensitivity status before IC, contrasts with the situation in relapsing systemic NH lymphomas, suggesting that ICT-ASCT might overcome resistance mediated by the BBB.

Several studies have evaluated ICT-ASCT as first-line treatment in newly-diagnosed PCNSL. BEAM protocol (BCNU, etoposide, cytarabine, and melphalan) or thiotepa-based chemotherapy were used as conditioning regimens, and increased the rate of complete remission after high-dose MTX-based induction chemotherapy. However, three of these trials included whole brain radiotherapy at the end of the procedure, making the analysis of the specific contribution of IC-ASCT to the encouraging survival results questionable. Subsequently, in order to minimize the risk of neurotoxicity, Illerhaus et al.[112] modified their initial protocol by increasing the number of chemotherapy cycles and augmenting the thiotepa dose within the conditioning regimen while restricting WBRT only to patients not in complete response after finishing chemotherapy. In addition, they delivered ICT-ASCT to all of their patients, irrespective of their response to high-dose MTX. The preliminary results of this pilot study support the hypothesis that WBRT may not be necessary to cure many patients in CR after ICT-ASCT. The only trial that did not combine radiotherapy with ICT-ASCT used an induction high-dose MTX-cytarabine chemotherapy followed by an intensive BEAM regimen.[107] The results were disappointing, with a short median event-free survival (9.3 months). This suggests that the drugs were used at suboptimal doses and that more aggressive regimens, including agents such as thiotepa and busulfan that penetrate the CNS, rather than standard lymphoma regimens may be warranted. This may be illustrated by encouraging results reported by Cheng et al.[108] using the TBC pretransplant conditioning regimen without WBRT in a small series of 7 patients, with a median event-free survival that had not been reached at 24 months.

The evaluation of the neurocognitive tolerance of this approach is an important issue. Soussain et al.[101,102] observed a 10% to 30% rate of neurotoxicity in relapsing patients treated by ICT-ASCT as salvage therapy, especially in the older and preirradiated patients. In the studies using a combined approach, i.e., ICT-ASCT followed by WBRT, for newly diagnosed PCNSL, the reported rates of severe neurotoxicity range from 0 to 20%.[110–112] In contrast, this was not reported in the two studies using ICT-ASCT without WBRT as primary treatment.[107,108] Further prolonged neurocognitive followup with psychometric evaluation is clearly needed. Neurotoxicity seems influenced by age of the patient, prior treatment (especially radiotherapy), and the CNS safety profile of the drug used. It remains to be determined whether ICT-ASCT can represent an interesting alternative option to radiotherapy as consolidation treatment.

SALVAGE TREATMENT

Although combined treatment has considerably improved the prognosis of PCNSL, one should not forget that about one third of the patients are refractory to initial treatment and that the majority of the patients who have achieved a complete remission will subsequently relapse. As discussed above, the most promising results have been reported with ICT-ASCT. Conventional second-line chemotherapy, such as temozolomide (TMZ),[104] topotecan,[113] intraarterial carboplatin,[114] and high dose cytarabine combined with etoposide and ifosfamide[103] have been also shown to be potentially active in relapsed PCNSL. These latter treatments achieved objective response rates (26% to 37%), 1-year PFS (13% to 22%) and 1-year overall survival (25% to 41%). Although the activity of TMZ and topotecan as single agents is modest in relapsed tumors, their role as part of a first-line MTX-based combination merits further investigation,[99] particularly because of their relatively good safety profile. MTX reinduction may also yield to new remission in some patients who have previously achieved a prolonged remission with high-dose MTX-based chemotherapy.[115] Two studies recently evaluated the activity and tolerance of WBRT delivered in relapsing PCNSL previously treated with high dose MTX-based CT alone as initial treatment.[105,106] Interestingly, the response rate was high (70%) and the median survival from relapse ranged from 11 to 16 months, quite similar to what we would expect with WBRT as initial treatment.[53] This suggests a preservation of radiation sensitivity at recurrence after high-dose MTX. Delayed neurotoxicity occurred in 15% to 22%, raising the possibility that when RT is deferred after high-dose MTX, the risk of neurotoxicity compared to immediate postchemotherapy irradiation is significantly lower.

IMMUNOTHERAPY BY ANTI-CD20 ANTIBODIES

Because most of PCNSLs are neoplastic B cells expressing the CD20 surface antigen, the chimeric monoclonal antibody rituximab is a potentially active treatment for this disease. It has been successfully used in systemic diffuse large B-cell lymphomas, in association with the CHOP regimen. However, the potential efficacy of rituximab in CNS tumors when delivered intravenously is limited by its high molecular weight, which prevents its penetration into the CNS through an intact blood-brain barrier. Pharmacokinetic studies have estimated that the CSF levels of rituximab are approximately 0.1% of matched serum levels after intravenous administration.[116] Schulz et al.[117] reported their experience using direct intraventricular/intrathecal administration of rituximab (10 to 40 mg), allowing them to reach a higher continuous concentration in the CSF, in a series of six patients. The only relevant toxicity was an acute reversible paraparesis associated with back pain related to a rapid tumor cell lysis in the CSF. An objective response was observed in all four patients with leptomeningeal disease, while no response was obtained in the two patients suffering from parenchymal tumor mass. Rubenstein et al.[118] conducted a phase I study in recurrent CNS lymphoma and found that intraventricular rituximab monotherapy (10 to 25 mg) was feasible and effective. They reported a cytologic response in six of nine patients with lymphomatous meningitis. Interestingly, two out of three patients with concurrent intraocular lymphoma and one out of five with brain parenchymal lymphoma exhibited an objective response. These preliminary results suggest that intraventricular/intrathecal rituximab can be safely delivered and may have a role in the management of leptomeningeal and ocular disease, rather than in parenchymal tumors of PCNSL.

Intravenous rituximab has been used in combination with a high-dose MTX-based chemotherapy regimen (MPVA) as initial treatment before WBRT for newly diagnosed PCNSL,[69] and with temozolomide as salvage treatment for recurrent parenchymal CNS lymphomas.[119,120] Both combinations were well-tolerated except for a higher rate of neutropenia seen when rituximab was added to MPVA, and were associated with improved survival. However, the specific contribution of intravenous rituximab on these results remains speculative.

Conclusions

The prognosis of PCNSL has considerably improved over the past two decades. Currently, appropriate treatment of PCNSL can lead to prolonged remission, frequently with remarkable patient recovery compatible with an active life.

A minority of patients can even hope to be cured. Long-term survivors are at increased risk of developing severe delayed cognitive dysfunction that may seriously compromise their quality of life. Future treatment should therefore improve the efficacy while minimizing the risk of neurotoxicity. In the elderly (over 60 years of age), there is growing evidence for proposing a chemotherapy-alone approach with less toxic regimens, and to defer or avoid radiotherapy. In the younger patients, the main questions addressed to clinical trials should focus on defining the optimal chemotherapy regimen, the role of radiotherapy as consolidation treatment in complete responders to chemotherapy, and the place of intensive chemotherapy with ASCT as part of the primary treatment. Prospective standardized neuropsychological testing is warranted in all clinical trials. New strategies will benefit not only from advances in the management of NHL outside the CNS, but also from the better understanding of the specific PCNSL tumorigenesis.

REFERENCES

1. Olson JE, Janney CA, Rao RD, et al. The continuing increase in the incidence of primary central nervous system non-Hodgkin lymphoma: a surveillance, epidemiology, and end results analysis. Cancer 2002;95:1504–10.
2. Kadan-Lottick NS, Skluzacek MC, Gurney JG. Decreasing incidence rates of primary central nervous system lymphoma. Cancer 2002;95:193–202.
3. Camilleri-Broët S, Martin A, Moreau A, et al. Primary central nervous system lymphomas in 72 immunocompetent patients: pathologic findings and clinical correlations. Groupe Ouest Est d'étude des Leucémies et Autres Maladies du sang (GOELAMS). Am J Clin Pathol 1998;110:607–12.
4. Swerdlow SH, Campo E, Harris NL, et al. World Health Organization Classification of Tumours. Pathology and genetics of tumours of haematopoietic and lymphoid tissues. In: WHO press, editors. WHO classification of tumours of Haematopoietic and Lymphoid Tissues. 4th ed Lyon: IARC; 2008.
5. Shenkier TN. Unusual variants of primary central nervous system lymphoma. Hematol Oncol Clin North Am 2005;19:651–64 vi.
6. Tu PH, Giannini C, Judkins AR, et al. Clinicopathologic and genetic profile of intracranial marginal zone lymphoma: a primary low-grade CNS lymphoma that mimics meningioma. J Clin Oncol 2005;23:5718–27.
7. Uccelli A, Aloisi F, Pistoia V. Unveiling the enigma of the CNS as a B-cell fostering environment. Trends Immunol 2005;26:254–9.
8. Jahnke K, Hummel M, Korfel A, et al. Detection of subclinical systemic disease in primary CNS lymphoma by polymerase chain reaction of the rearranged immunoglobulin heavy-chain genes. J Clin Oncol 2006;24:4754–7.
9. Alter A, Duddy M, Hebert S, et al. Determinants of human B cell migration across brain endothelial cells. J Immunol 2003;170:4497–505.
10. Smith JR, Braziel RM, Paoletti S, et al. Expression of B-cell-attracting chemokine 1 (CXCL13) by malignant lymphocytes and vascular endothelium in primary central nervous system lymphoma. Blood 2003;101:815–21.
11. Alizadeh AA, Elsen MB, Davis RE, et al. Distinct types of diffuse large B cell lymphoma identified by gene expression profiling. Nature 2000;403:503–11.
12. Larocca LM, Capello D, Rinelli A, et al. The molecular and phenotypic profile of primary central nervous system lymphoma identifies distinct categories of the disease and is consistent with histogenetic derivation from germinal center-related B cells. Blood 1998;1011–9.
13. Thompsett AR, Ellison DW, Stevenson FK, et al. V_H gene sequences from primary central nervous system lymphomas indicate derivation from highly mutated germinal center B cells with ongoing mutational activity. Blood 1999;5:1738–46.
14. Montesinos-Rongen M, Küppers R, Schlüler D, et al. Primary central nervous system lymphomas are derived from germinal-center B cells and show a preferential usage of the *V4–34* gene segment. Am J Pathol 1999;155:2077–86.

15. Montesinos-Rongen M, Van Roost D, Schaller C, et al. Primary diffuse large B-cell lymphomas of the central nervous system are targeted by aberrant somatic hypermutation. Blood 2004;103:1869–75.
16. Camilleri-Broët S, Crinière E, Broët P, et al. A uniform activated B-cell-like immunophenotype might explain the poor prognosis of primary central nervous system lymhpomas: analysis of 83 cases. Blood 2006;107:190–6.
17. Rubinstein JL, Fridlyand J, Shen A, et al. Gene expression and angiotropism in primary CNS lymphoma. Blood 2006;107:3716–23.
18. Montesinos-Rongen M, Brunn A, Bentink S, et al. Gene expression profiling suggests primary central nervous system lymphomas to be derived from a late germinal center B cell. Leukemia 2008;22:400–5.
19. Weber T, Weber RG, Kaulich K, et al. Characteristic chromosomal imbalances in primary central nervous system lymphomas of the diffuse large B-cell type. Brain Pathol 2000;10:73–84.
20. Harada K, Nishizaki T, Kubota H, et al. Distinct primary central nervous system lymphoma defined by comparative genomic hybridization and laser scanning cytometry. Cancer Genet Cytogenet 2001;125:147–50.
21. Boonstra R, Koning A, Mastik M, et al. Analysis of chromosomal copy number changes and oncoprotein expression in primary central nervous system lymphomas: frequent loss of chromosome arm 6q. Virchows Arch 2003;443:164–9.
22. Nakamura M, Kishi M, Sakaki T, et al. Novel tumor suppressor loci on 6q22–23 in primary central nervous system lymphomas. Cancer Res 2003;63:737–41.
23. Cady FM, O'Neill BP, Law ME, et al. Del(6)(q22) and BCL6 rearrangements in primary CNS lymphoma are indicators of an aggressive clinical course. J Clin Oncol 2008;26:4814–9.
24. Montesinos-Rongen M, Zühlke-Jenisch R, Gesk S, et al. Interphase cytogenetic analysis of lymphoma-associated chromosomal breakpoints in primary diffuse large B-cell lymphomas of the central nervous system. J Neuropathol Exp Neurol 2002;61:926–33.
25. Schwindt H, Akasaka T, Zühlke-Jenisch R, et al. Chromosomal translocations fusing the BCL6 gene to different partner loci are recurrent in primary central nervous lymphoma and may be associated with aberrant somatic hypermutation or defective class switch recombination. J Neuropathol Exp Neurol 2006;65:776–82.
26. Chang CC, Kampalath B, Schultz C, et al. Expression of p53, c-Myc, or Bcl-6 suggests a poor prognosis in primary central nervous system diffuse large B-cell lymphoma among immunocompetent individuals. Arch Pathol Lab Med 2003;127:208–12.
27. Braaten KM, Betensky RA, de Leval L, et al. BCL-6 expression predicts improved survival in patients with primary central nervous system lymphoma. Clin Cancer Res 2003;9:1063–9.
28. Lin CH, Kuo KT, Chuang SS, et al. Comparison of the expression and prognostic significance of differentiation markers between diffuse large B-cell lymphoma of central nervous system origin and peripheral nodal origin. Clin Cancer Res 2006;12:1152–6.
29. Levy O, Deangelis LM, Filippa DA, et al. Bcl-6 predicts improved prognosis in primary central nervous system lymphoma. Cancer 2008;112:151–6.
30. Bataille B, Delwail V, Menet E, et al. Primary intracerebral malignant lymphoma: report of 248 cases. J Neurosurg 2000;92:261–6.
31. Ferreri AJM, Reni M. Primary central nervous system lymphoma. Crit Rev Oncol Hematol 2007;63:257–68.
32. Clifford RJ, Reese DF, Scheithauer BW. Radiographic findings in 32 cases of primary CNS lymphoma. AJNR 1986;146:271–6.
33. Koeller KK, Smirniotopoulos JG, Jones RV. Primary central nervous system lymphoma: radiologic-pathologic correlation. Radiographics 1997;17:1497–526.
34. Bühring U, Herrlinger U, Krings T, et al. MRI features of primary central nervous system lymphomas at presentation. Neurology 2001;57:393–6.
35. DeAngelis LM. Primary central nervous system lymphoma imitates multiple sclerosis. J Neurooncol 1990;9:177–81.
36. Herrlinger U, Schabet M, Bitzer M, et al. Primary central nervous system lymphoma: from clinical presentation to diagnosis. J Neurooncol 1999;43:219–26.
37. Ayuso-Peralta L, Ortí-Pareja M, Zurdo-Hernández M, et al. Cerebral lymphoma presenting as a leukoencephalopathy. J Neurol Neurosurg Psychiatry 2001;71:243–6.
38. De Angelis LM. Cerebral Lymphoma Presenting as a Nonenhancing Lesion on Computed Tomographic/Magnetic Resonance Scan. Ann Neurol 1993;33:308–11.

39. Kanai R, Shibuya M, Hata T, et al. A case of 'lymphomatosis cerebri' diagnosed in an early phase and treated by whole brain radiation: case report and literature review. J Neurooncol 2008;86:83–8.
40. Benouaich A, Delord JP, Danjou M, et al. Primary dural lymphoma: a report of two cases with review of the literature. Rev Neurol 2003;159:652–8.
41. Bódi I, Hussain A, Gullan RW, et al. January 2003: 56-year-old female with right frontal tumor of the dura. Brain Pathol 2003;13:417–8.
42. Hartmann M, Heiland S, Harting I, et al. Distinguishing of primary cerebral lymphoma from high-grade glioma with perfusion-weighted magnetic resonance imaging. Neuroscience Lett 2003;338:119–22.
43. Harting I, Hartmann M, Jost G, et al. Differentiating primary central nervous system lymphoma from glioma in humans using localised proton magnetic resonance spectroscopy. Neurosci Lett 2003;342:163–6.
44. Taillibert S, Guillevin R, Menuel C, et al. Brain lymphoma: usefulness of the magnetic resonance spectroscopy. Neuro Oncol 2008;86:225–9.
45. Weller M. Glucocorticoid treatment of primary CNS lymphoma. J Neurooncol 1999;43:237–9.
46. Mathew BS, Carson KA, Grossman SA. Initial response to glucocorticoids. A potentially important prognosis factor in patients with Primary CNS lymphoma. Cancer 2006;106:383–7.
47. Abrey LE, Batchelor T, Ferreri AJM, et al. Report of an International Workshop to Standardize baseline Evaluation and Response Criteria for Primary CNS Lymphoma. J Clin Oncol 2005;23:5034–43.
48. Mohile NA, DeAngelis LS, Abrey LE. The utility of body FDG PET in staging primary central nervous system lymphoma. Neuro Oncol 2008;10:223–8.
49. Ferreri AJ, Blay JY, Reni M, et al. Prognostic scoring system for primary CNS lymphomas: the International Extranodal Lymphoma Study Group experience. J Clin Oncol 2003;21:266–72.
50. Bessell EM, Graus F, Lopez-Guillermo A, et al. Primary non-Hodgkin's lymphoma of the CNS treated with CHOD/BVAM or BVAM chemotherapy before radiotherapy: long-term survival and prognostic factors. Int J Radiat Oncol Biol Phys 2004;59:501–8.
51. Abrey LE, Ben-Porat L, Panageas KS, et al. Primary central nervous system lymphoma: the Memorial Sloan-Kettering Cancer Center prognostic model. J Clin Oncol 2006;24:5711–5.
52. Bessell EM, Hoang-Xuan K, Ferreri AJ, et al. Primary central nervous system lymphoma: biological aspects and controversies in management. Eur J Cancer 2007;43:1141–52.
53. Nelson DF, Martz KL, Bonner H, et al. Non-Hodgkin's lymphoma of the brain: can high dose, large volumen radiation therapy improve survival? Report on a prospective trial by the Radiation Therapy Oncology Group (RTOG) 1992. Int J Radiat Oncol Biol Phys 1992;23:9–17.
54. Gabbai AA, Hochberg FH, Linggood RM, et al. High-dose methotrexate for non-AIDS primary central nervous system lymphoma. Report of 13 cases. J Neurosurg 1989;70:190–4.
55. De Angelis LM, Yahalom J, Thaler HT, et al. Combined modality therapy for primary CNS lymphoma. J Clin Oncol 1992;10:635–43.
56. Glass J, Gruber ML, Cher L, et al. Preirradiation methotrexate chemotherapy of primary central nervous system lymphoma: long-term outcome. J Neurosurg 1994;81:188–95.
57. Blay JY, Bouhour D, Carrie C, et al. The C5R protocol: a regimen of high-dose chemotherapy and radiotherapy in primary cerebral non-Hodgkin's lymphoma of patients with no known cause of immunosuppression. Blood 1995;15(86):2922–9.
58. Glass J, Shustik C, Hochberg FH, et al. Therapy of primary central nervous system lymphoma with preirradiation methotrexate, cyclophosphamide, doxorubicin, vincristine, and dexamethasone (MCHOD). J Neurooncol 1996;30:257–65.
59. Brada M, Hjiyiannakis D, Hines F, et al. Short intensive primary chemotherapy and radiotherapy in sporadic primary CNS lymphoma (PCL). Int J Radiat Oncol Biol Phys 1998;40:1157–62.
60. O'Brien P, Roos D, Pratt G, et al. Phase II multicenter study of brief single-agent methotrexate followed by irradiation in primary CNS lymphoma. J Clin Oncol 2000;18:519–26.
61. Bessell EM, López-Guillermo A, Villá S, et al. Importance of radiotherapy in the outcome of patients with primary CNS lymphoma: an analysis of the CHOD/BVAM regimen followed by two different radiotherapy treatments. J Clin Oncol 2002;20:231–6.
62. DeAngelis LM, Seiferheld W, Schold SC, et al. Combination chemotherapy and radiotherapy for primary central nervous system lymphoma: Radiation Therapy Oncology Group Study 93–10. J Clin Oncol 2002;20:4643–8.
63. Poortmans PM, Kluin-Nelemans HC, Haaxma-Reiche H, et al. High-dose methotrexate-based chemotherapy followed by consolidating radiotherapy in non-AIDS-related primary central

nervous system lymphoma: European Organization for Research and Treatment of Cancer Lymphoma Group Phase II Trial 20962. J Clin Oncol 2003;21:4483–8.
64. Omuro AM, DeAngelis LM, Yahalom J, et al. Chemoradiotherapy for primary CNS lymphoma: an intent-to-treat analysis with complete follow-up. Neurology 2005;64:69–74.
65. Korfel A, Martus P, Nowrousian MR, et al. Response to chemotherapy and treating institution predict survival in primary central nervous system lymphoma. Br J Haematol 2005;128:177–83.
66. Ferreri AJ, Dell'Oro S, Foppoli M, et al. MATILDE regimen followed by radiotherapy is an active strategy against primary CNS lymphomas. Neurology 2006;66:1435–8.
67. Abrey LE, Yahalom J, De Angelis L. Treatment of primary CNS lymphoma: the next step. J Clin Oncol 2000;18:3144–50.
68. Gavrilovic IT, Hormigo A, Yahalom J, et al. Long-term follow-up of high-dose methotrexate-based therapy with and without whole brain irradiation for newly diagnosed primary CNS lymphoma. J Clin Oncol 2006;24:4570–4.
69. Shah GD, Yahalom J, Correa DD, et al. Combined immunochemotherapy with reduced whole-brain radiotherapy for newly diagnosed primary CNS lymphoma. J Clin Oncol 2007;25(30):4730–5.
70. Reni M, Ferreri AJ. Therapeutic management of refractory or relapsed primary central nervous system lymphomas. Ann Hematol 2001;80(Suppl. 3):B113–7.
71. Ferreri AJ, Reni M, Pasini F, et al. Multicenter study of treatment of primary CNS lymphoma. Neurology 2002;58:1513–20.
72. Ekenel M, Iwamoto FM, Ben-Porat LS, et al. Primary central nervous system lymphoma: the role of consolidation treatment after a complete response to high-dose methotrexate-based chemotherapy. Cancer 2008;113:1025–31.
73. Neuwelt EA, Goldman DL, Dahlborg SA, et al. Primary CNS lymphoma treated with osmotic blood-brain barrier disruption: prolonged survival and preservation of cognitive function. J Clin Oncol 1991;9:1580–90.
74. McAllister LD, Doolittle ND, Guastadisegni PE, et al. Cognitive outcomes and long-term follow-up results after enhanced chemotherapy delivery for primary central nervous system lymphoma. Neurosurgery 2000;46:51–60.
75. Pels H, Schmidt-Wolf IG, Glasmacher A, et al. Primary central nervous system lymphoma: results of a pilot and phase II study of systemic and intraventricular chemotherapy with deferred radiotherapy. J Clin Oncol 2003;21:4489–95.
76. Sandor V, Stark-Vancs V, Pearson D, et al. Phase II trial of chemotherapy alone for primary CNS and intraocular lymphoma. J Clin Oncol 1998;16:3000–6.
77. Batchelor T, Carson K, O'Neill A, et al. Treatment of primary CNS lymphoma with methotrexate and deferred radiotherapy: a report of NABTT 96–07. J Clin Oncol 2003;21:1044–9.
78. Herrlinger U, Küker W, Uhl M, et al. NOA-03 trial of high-dose methotrexate in primary central nervous system lymphoma: final report. Ann Neurol 2005;57:843–7.
79. Omuro AM, Taillandier L, Chinot O, et al. Methotrexate (MTX), procarbazine and CCNU for primary central nervous system lymphoma (PCNSL) in patients younger than 60: Can radiotherapy (RT) be deferred? J Clin Oncol 2006;24: abstract 1551.
80. Hiraga S, Arita N, Ohnishi T, et al. Rapid infusion of high-dose methotrexate resulting in enhanced penetration into cerebrospinal fluid and intensified tumor response in primary central nervous system lymphomas. Neurosurgery 1999;91:221–30.
81. Khan RB, Shi W, Thaler HT. Is intrathecal methotrexate necessary in the treatment of primary CNS lymphoma? J Neurooncol 2002;58:175–8.
82. Lai R, Abrey LE, Rosenblum MK, et al. Treatment-induced leukoencephalopathy in primary CNS lymphoma: a clinical and autopsy study. Neurology 2004;62:451–6.
83. Abrey LE, DeAngelis LM, Yahalom J. Long term survival in primary CNS lymphoma. J Clin Oncol 1998;16:859–63.
84. Harder H, Holtel H, Bromberg JE, et al. Cognitive status and quality of life after treatment for primary CNS lymphoma. Neurology 2004;62:544–7.
85. Fliessbach K, Helmstaedter C, Urbach H, et al. Neuropsychological outcome after chemotherapy for primary CNS lymphoma: a prospective study. Neurology 2005;64:1184–8.
86. Fliessbach K, Urbach H, Helmstaedter C, et al. Cognitive performance and magnetic resonance imaging findings after high-dose systemic and intraventricular chemotherapy for primary central nervous system lymphoma. Arch Neurol 2003;60:563–8.
87. Correa DD, DeAngelis LM, Shi W, et al. Cognitive functions in survivors of primary central nervous system lymphoma. Neurology 2004;62:548–55.

88. Correa DD, Maron L, Harder H, et al. Cognitive functions in primary central nervous system lymphoma: literature review and assessment guidelines. Ann Oncol 2007;18:1145–51.
89. Linnebank M, Pels H, Kleczar N, et al. MTX-induced white matter changes are associated with polymorphisms of methionine metabolism. Neurology 2005;64:912–3.
90. Linnebank M, Moskau S, Jurgens A, et al. Association of genetic variants of methionine metabolism with MTX-induced CNS white matter changes in patients with primary central nervous system lymphoma. Neuro Oncol 2008 Sep 22.
91. Schultz C, Scott C, Sherman W, et al. Preirradiation chemotherapy with Cyclophosphamide, doxorubicin, vincristine, and Dexamethasone (CHOD) for PCNSL: Initial report of Radiation Therapy Oncology Group (RTOG) protocol 88–06. J Clin Oncol 1996;14:556–64.
92. O'Neill BP, O'Fallon JR, Earle JD, et al. Primary central nervous system non-Hodgkin's lymphoma: survival advantages with combined initial therapy ?. Int J Radiat Oncol Biol Phys 1995;33: 663–73.
93. Desablens B, Gardembas M, Haie-Meder C, Primary CNS lymphoma. Long-term results of the GOELAMS LCP88 trial with focus on neurological complications among 152 patients. Ann Oncol 1999;10(Suppl. 3):14.
94. Bessell EM, Graus F, Lopez-Guillermo A, et al. CHOD/BVAM regimen plus radiotherapy in patients with primary CNS non-Hodgkin's lymphoma. Int J Radiat Oncol Biol Phys 2001;50: 457–64.
95. Freilich RJ, Delattre JY, Monjour A, et al. Chemotherapy without radiation therapy as initial treatment for primary CNS lymphoma in older patients. Neurology 1996;46:435–9.
96. Ng S, Rosenthal MA, Ashley D, et al. High-dose methotrexate for primary CNS lymphoma in the elderly. Neuro Oncol 2000;2:40–4.
97. Juergens A, Pels H, Schlegel U, et al. A Primary central nervous system lymphoma: results of a pilot and phase II study of systemic and intraventricular chemotherapy with deferred radiotherapy – Final report. J Neurol 2006;253(II/23–II24) abstract O95.
98. Hoang-Xuan K, Taillandier L, Chinot O, et al. Chemotherapy alone as initial treatment for primary CNS lymphoma in patients older than 60 years: a multicenter phase II study (26952) of the European Organization for Research and Treatment of Cancer Brain Tumor Group. J Clin Oncol 2003;21:2726–31.
99. Omuro AM, Taillandier L, Chinot O, et al. Temozolomide and methotrexate for primary central nervous system lymphoma in the elderly. J Neurooncol 2007;85:207–11.
100. Gerstner ER, Zhu JJ, Engler DA, et al. High dose methotrexate for elderly patients with primary central nervous system lymphoma. Neuro Oncol 2008; Aug 29.
101. Soussain C, Suzan F, Hoang-Xuan K, et al. Results of intensive chemotherapy followed by hematopoietic stem-cell rescue in 22 patients with refractory or recurrent primary CNS lymphoma or intraocular lymphoma. J Clin Oncol 2001;19:742–9.
102. Soussain C, Hoang-Xuan K, Taillandier L, et al. Intensive chemotherapy followed by hematopoietic stem-cell rescue for refractory and recurrent primary CNS and intraocular lymphoma: Société Française de Greffe de Moëlle Osseuse-Thérapie Cellulaire. J Clin Oncol 2008;26:2512–8.
103. Arellano-Rodrigo E, López-Guillermo A, Bessell EM, et al. Salvage treatment with etoposide (VP-16), ifosfamide and cytarabine (Ara-C) for patients with recurrent primary central nervous system lymphoma. Eur J Haematol 2003;70:219–24.
104. Reni M, Mason W, Zaja F, et al. Salvage chemotherapy with temozolomide in primary CNS lymphomas: preliminary results of a phase II trial. Eur J Cancer 2004;40:1682–8.
105. Nguyen PL, Chakravarti A, Finkelstein DM, et al. Results of whole-brain radiation as salvage of methotrexate failure for immunocompetent patients with primary CNS lymphoma. J Clin Oncol 2005;23:1507–13.
106. Hottinger AF, DeAngelis LM, Yahalom J, et al. Salvage whole brain radiotherapy for recurrent or refractory primary CNS lymphoma. Neurology 2007;69:1178–82.
107. Abrey LE, Moskowitz CH, Mason WP, et al. Intensive methotrexate and cytarabine followed by high-dose chemotherapy with autologous stem-cell rescue in patients with newly diagnosed primary CNS lymphoma: an intent-to-treat analysis. J Clin Oncol 2003;21:4151–6.
108. Cheng T, Forsyth P, Chaudhry A, et al. High-dose thiotepa, busulfan, cyclophosphamide and ASCT without whole-brain radiotherapy for poor prognosis primary CNS lymphoma. Bone Marrow Transplant 2003;31:679–85.
109. Colombat P, Lemevel A, Bertrand P, et al. High-dose chemotherapy with autologous stem cell transplantation as first-line therapy for primary CNS lymphoma in patients younger than 60 years: a multicenter phase II study of the GOELAMS group. Bone Marrow Transplant 2006;38:417–20.

110. Montemurro M, Kiefer T, Schüler F, et al. Primary central nervous system lymphoma treated with high-dose methotrexate, high-dose busulfan/thiotepa, autologous stem-cell transplantation and response-adapted whole-brain radiotherapy: results of the multicenter Ostdeutsche Studiengruppe Hamato-Onkologie OSHO-53 phase II study. Ann Oncol 2007;18:665–71.
111. Illerhaus G, Marks R, Ihorst G, et al. High-dose chemotherapy with autologous stem-cell transplantation and hyperfractionated radiotherapy as first-line treatment of primary CNS lymphoma. J Clin Oncol 2006;24:3865–70.
112. Illerhaus G, Müller F, Feuerhake F, et al. High-dose chemotherapy and autologous stem-cell transplantation without consolidating radiotherapy as first-line treatment for primary lymphoma of the central nervous system. Haematologica 2008;93:147–8.
113. Fischer L, Thiel E, Klasen HA, et al. Response of relapsed or refractory primary central nervous system lymphoma (PCNSL) to topotecan. Neurology 2004;62:1885–7.
114. Tyson RM, Siegal T, Doolittle ND, et al. Current status and future of relapsed primary central nervous system lymphoma (PCNSL). Leuk Lymphoma 2003;44:627–33.
115. Plotkin SR, Betensky RA, Hochberg FH, et al. Treatment of relapsed central nervous system lymphoma with high-dose methotrexate. Clin Cancer Res 2004;10:5643–6.
116. Rubenstein JL, Combs D, Rosenberg J, et al. Rituximab therapy for CNS lymphomas: targeting the leptomeningeal compartment. Blood 2003;101:466–8.
117. Schulz H, Pels H, Schmidt-Wolf I, et al. Intraventricular treatment of relapsed central nervous system lymphoma with the anti-CD20 antibody rituximab. Haematologica 2004;89:753–4.
118. Rubenstein JL, Fridlyand J, Abrey L, et al. Phase I study of intraventricular administration of rituximab in patients with recurrent CNS and intraocular lymphoma. J Clin Oncol 2007;25: 1350–6.
119. Wong ET, Tishler R, Barron L, et al. Immunochemotherapy with rituximab and temozolomide for central nervous system lymphomas. Cancer 2004;101:139–45.
120. Enting RH, Demopoulos A, DeAngelis LM, et al. Salvage therapy for primary CNS lymphoma with a combination of rituximab and temozolomide. Neurology 2004;63:901–3.

10 Management of Intramedullary Spinal Cord Tumors

NICHOLAS H. POST • PAUL R. COOPER

Intramedullary spinal cord tumors (IMSCTs) are rare, a fact that is reflected by the paucity of large case series in the literature. Published accounts on the management of IMSCTs consist primarily of case reports and a handful of small case series. Current management strategies, therefore, are largely founded upon past experience, and expert opinion.[1] The earliest expert opinion on the treatment of IMSCTs dates back to 1911 with a serendipitous observation in the operating room by Elsberg, who unintentionally made a myelotomy in the posterior spinal cord while opening the dura, resulting in the extrusion of tumor tissue. Realizing his error, he closed the wound without an attempt at tumor resection. One week later, the incision was reopened and a well-defined tissue plane was noted, which permitted total tumor resection. **The patient, severely quadraparetic prior to surgery, was able to ambulate without assistance and use a typewriter eight months following the procedure.**[2] Based upon his experience, Elsberg advocated the following two stage method for resection of IMSCTs:

"If, then, after laminectomy and incision of the dura the surgeon finds that he has to deal with an intramedullary growth, he should make a short incision about 1 cm in length in the posterior median column. . . . The incision, made in the manner we have already described, should be deep enough to divide the pia and the substance of the column down to the tumor. The tumor will then begin to bulge through the incision. No matter how markedly the tumor protrudes, the surgeon must not attempt to remove the growth for fear of grave injury to the cord. The operation must be concluded for the time being, the dura left wide open, and the muscles, fascia and skin carefully closed, as if the operation was definitely ended. The actual removal of the tumor is left for a second operation.

"After about a week the wound is reopened, and the tumor, which will in all probability be found outside the cord, can be removed by dividing the few adhesions which remain. When the tumor has been removed and all bleeding controlled, the dura, muscles, fascia, and skin are closed in the usual manner."[3]

During the first half of the twentieth century, other surgeons did not share Elsberg's early success. In 1969 Schneider asserted that when an intramedullary tumor is encountered that is not obviously cystic in a patient with little or no neurological deficit, "the dura is left open with no attempt made to perform a myelotomy or procure a biopsy."[4] Until recently IMSCTs were treated with biopsy or subtotal removal followed by irradiation—a therapy that is usually associated with early tumor recurrence and progressive neurological impairment.[5] The evolution of diagnostic and surgical technologies now permits a more aggressive surgical role in the management of IMSCTs.

With MRI, IMSCTs are diagnosed more frequently, and in earlier stages of their disease progression.[1] It has been shown that preoperative neurological function is the most important predictor of patient outcome following surgery for an IMSCT,[6,7] and in this respect early detection with MRI is extremely helpful. Improved operative technologies such as neurophysiologic monitoring, the ultrasonic aspirator, and carbon dioxide laser have also facilitated the resection of IMSCTs.[8] These recent surgical advances, in light of poor results in tumors treated solely with radiation and chemotherapy, have led many to advocate complete surgical resection, whenever possible, as the standard of care.[1,5,8–10]

Epidemiology and Presentation of Specific Intramedullary Spinal Cord Tumors

EPENDYMOMAS

Spinal ependymomas arise from the ependymal rests in the vestigial central canal, and, as a result, are centrally located within the spinal cord.[11] Ependymomas are the most common IMSCT in adults, comprising 40% of a large series compiled by Fischer and Brotchi.[12] In children, they are the second most common primary IMSCT (28%), second only to astrocytomas.[13] However, there were no ependymomas in a series of IMSCTs in children under 3 years of age.[14] There is an equal distribution among males and females. They occur throughout the spinal cord, but are most common in the cervical region.[12,15] Myxopapillary ependymomas are a distinct subtype occurring in the conus medullaris and cauda equina, and have a slight male predominance.[16] Genetic studies have suggested a possible link between neurofibromatosis type 2 and the development of spinal ependymomas.[17,18] Families predisposed to the development of ependymal tumors have been shown to have a loss of heterozygosity on chromosome 22.[19]

These tumors are slow growing, with an average interval of 16 months between the onset of symptoms and diagnosis.[15] Sixty-five percent of patients present with complaints of radiculopathy or regional neck pain accompanied by minimal motor or sensory deficit. Because these slowly growing tumors compress rather than invade adjacent neural tissue, they can take up a considerable volume within the spinal cord without causing significant motor deficit. Parasthesias and other sensory phenomena result from compression of the crossing spinothalamic fibers. Within the corticospinal tract, hand fibers are located medially and leg fibers are located laterally. A centrally located cervical IMSCT or associated cyst, therefore, may produce weakness and atrophy of the small hand muscles from anterior horn cell compression before lower extremity dysfunction becomes apparent. Cervical lesions rarely present with bowel or bladder dysfunction.[15] Myxopapillary tumors arising from the conus, however, can compress sacral anterior horn cells and adjacent nerve roots in the cauda equina, resulting in bowel or bladder dysfunction in 20 to 25% of cases.[16]

ASTROCYTOMAS

Astrocytomas are a heterogeneous group of infiltrating tumors, resembling astrocytes, that occur in both the brain and spinal cord. They are categorized in an ascending grading scale based upon histopathological evidence of anaplasia. Characteristics of higher-grade lesions include vascular hyperplasia, mitotic figures, cellularity, and presence of giant cells. Necrosis is indicative of glioblastoma multiforme, the most extreme category of malignancy.

Juvenile pilocytic astrocytomas (JPA) are a unique subclass of astrocytomas. Generally speaking, low-grade astrocytomas fall into two categories: World Health Organization (WHO) grades I and II. Pilocytic astrocytomas are WHO grade I tumors, while protoplasmic, gemistiocytic, fibrillary, and mixed astrocytomas are classified as WHO grade II. Separation of pilocytic astrocytomas into their own grade reflects the fact that they have a different prognosis and clinical course. The 10-year survival rate in patients with a pilocytic spinal cord astrocytoma is 81%, while the 10-year survival rate drops to 15% in patients with diffuse fibrillary astrocytomas.[20]

Astrocytomas are the most common pediatric IMSCT, representing 59% of the tumors in a compilation of 13 pediatric series.[13] In adults, they are second to ependymomas in frequency, accounting for about 20% of tumors.[12,21] Unlike intracranial astrocytomas, spinal cord astrocytomas are usually low-grade lesions in both children and adults. High-grade lesions (WHO grades III and IV) comprise only 10% to 15% of pediatric tumors and a modestly higher proportion in adults.[22,23] There is a slight male predominance,[12,20] and the cervical area is most frequently affected, followed closely by the thoracic region. These lesions span an average of six spinal levels, but total spinal cord involvement has been described.[24] Genetic studies have shown a potential association between neurofibromatosis type I and the development of spinal astrocytomas.[17,18,25]

In contrast to ependymomas, astrocytomas are often infiltrative lesions that occupy an eccentric location within the spinal cord. Presenting symptoms typically consist of regional back or neck pain and sensory disturbances including dysesthesias and loss of sensation, unilateral or bilateral in nature, as well as motor deficit. In the pediatric population, pain remains the most common symptom, but gait deterioration, motor regression, torticollis, and kyphoscoliosis are common presenting findings.[26] Symptoms resulting from low-grade lesions usually evolve over months to years.[27,28] High-grade astrocytomas, however, present with a more rapid decline in motor function with progression to significant disability in only 3 to 5 months.[22,28]

GANGLIOGLIOMAS

Gangliogliomas are neoplasms containing both neoplastic neuronal and glial cells. They account for approximately 1.1% of all spinal neoplasms. Ten percent of intracranial gangliogliomas undergo malignant degeneration. Such malignant change is believed to be due to the glial component of the tumor. How this data regarding intracranial gangliogliomas translates to spinal cord gangliogliomas is unclear. They mainly occur in children and young adults, with both sexes affected in equal proportion.[29–31] Symptoms include pain and weakness of the extremities, while examination findings may include myelopathy and kyphoscoliosis. Symptoms and imaging characteristics fail to distinguish these from other glial tumors.[29–31]

HEMANGIOBLASTOMAS

Hemangioblastomas consist of thin-walled blood vessels interspersed with large, pale stromal cells. They represent 3% to 11% of IMSCTs, with a slight male predominance.[32] Up to one third of cases occur in association with von Hippel-Lindau (VHL) disease. VHL disease occurs in both an autosomal dominant and a sporadically inherited fashion. The autosomal dominant form results from a mutation of a tumor suppressor gene on chromosome 3p.[33]

Hemangioblastomas involving the spinal cord are occasional manifestations of VHL disease,[34] and multiple lesions may be present, particularly in the posterior fossa. Symptom onset is typically in the fourth decade of life and the mean age at surgery is 40 years; childhood presentation is rare.[35] The most frequent locations are thoracic (55%) and cervical (40%). Cyst formation occurs in 87% of cases.[35]

Hemangioblastomas differ from ependymomas and astrocytomas in that they generally are found on the dorsal or dorsolateral surface of the spinal cord. As a result, they often present with complaints of proprioceptive loss in addition to pain and sensory deficits.[35]

LYMPHOMAS

Intramedullary spinal cord lymphoma is an unusual entity. It is most commonly seen as part of a multifocal central nervous system lymphoma, or in patients immunosuppressed from AIDS or other causes.[36] Pathologic studies have demonstrated that the vast majority of primary spinal cord lymphomas are of the non-Hodgkin B-cell variety.[37,38] Reports of T-cell lymphomas involving the spinal cord are rare.[39] Presentation can range from myelopathy to paresis,[40,41] and can progress rapidly over a period of days to weeks.

LIPOMAS

Intramedullary spinal lipomas, excluding those associated with dysraphism, comprise just 1% of all IMSCT. These tumors consist of ordinary adipose tissue, and are believed to arise from rests of ectopic tissue.[42] Lipomas are often densely adherent to surrounding neural tissue, precluding complete resection.[43]

Most patients present in the second to fourth decade in life and there is no gender predilection.[44] Clinical presentation is that of a slowly progressive myelopathy (58%), a syringomyelic syndrome (9.5%), or a Brown-Séquard syndrome (6.5%), with the remaining 26% having atypical features.[42] Lipomas tend to have long indolent courses, followed by a rapid decline in neurological function.[43,44] In females, neurological deterioration may follow pregnancy and delivery.[45]

CAVERNOUS ANGIOMAS

Cavernous angiomas, while not true neoplasms, can form mass lesions in the spinal cord parenchyma, and should be considered in the differential diagnosis of intramedullary spinal mass lesions. Commonly known as cavernomas, they represent 1% to 3% of IMSCTs. Cavernomas are angiographically occult vascular malformations consisting of a collection of enlarged vascular spaces surrounded by a rim of gliosis, without intervening neural tissue.[46] Both sporadic and familial forms are recognized. The familial form is inherited in an autosomal dominant fashion and is associated with multiple angiomas.[47,48] Molecular analysis has shown that a gene mutation in CCM1, encoding the KRIT1 protein, is largely responsible for the hereditary form of cavernous angiomas.[49,50]

Cavernomas can cause progressive myelopathy due to repeated hemorrhage, resulting in reactive gliosis.[51,52] A large sudden hemorrhage, albeit uncommon, can lead to catastrophic neurological deterioration, and surgery is the only effective treatment.[46] Asymptomatic patients do not benefit from surgical intervention. Once a patient becomes symptomatic, however, progressive neurological deterioration from repetitive hemorrhage is the rule and surgical intervention is advisable in most cases.[52]

METASTASES

In a large postmortem study, intramedullary spinal cord metastases were found in only 2% of 627 patients with systemic cancer.[53] Other accounts estimate that metastases comprise 2% to 8% of all IMSCTs.[54,55] The incidence of intracerebral metastases in cancer patients, in contrast, has been estimated at 25% to 35%.[56] Because of the comparatively small volume of the spinal cord relative to the brain, metastases to the spinal cord are much less common.[57] The most common sources of intramedullary spinal cord metastases are the lung and breast. The mechanism of metastatic spread to the spinal cord is thought to be hematogenous rather than direct invasion, since metastases to the spinal cord are not always associated with disease in the adjacent tissues.[53,58,59] The diagnosis of spinal cord metastasis carries a grave prognosis, and 80% of patients die within three months. The presenting symptoms consist of pain and weakness. Rapid neurological deterioration is observed in almost half of all patients, progressing to cord hemisection or transection syndromes over days to weeks.[59]

Diagnostic Imaging

PLAIN X-RAYS

Plain x-rays have little place in the modern diagnosis of IMSCTs and are unremarkable in the majority of cases. However, an enlarged spinal canal with scalloping of the vertebral bodies, medial pedicle erosion, and thinning of the laminae may be seen.[60] These findings are consistent with any long-standing intradural tumor that thins and remodels the surrounding bone and are not specific for IMSCTs.

Scoliosis is frequently seen in children with IMSCTs, often with the apex of the curvature to the left rather than the right. Dextroscoliosis, where the apex of the curvature is to the right, is more common in patients with idiopathic scoliosis. Although scoliosis is unusual in older adults, it may be the presenting symptom in young adults with asymptomatic onset of tumor growth during childhood. Plain x-rays are also valuable in assessing alignment as the presence of preoperative kyphosis or scoliosis may necessitate early fusion to prevent progressive deformity.[61]

COMPUTED TOMOGRAPHY AND CT MYELOGRAPHY

Prior to the advent of MRI, CT myelography was the primary imaging modality for the diagnosis of suspected spinal cord tumors. It can demonstrate spinal cord widening but cannot be used to confidently determine its cause. Although neoplastic lesions will enhance after the intravenous administration of iodinated contrast, plain contrast CT will not identify the type of intramedullary spinal cord tumor or distinguish between tumor-associated cysts and syringomyelia. In the past, delayed CT scanning was sometimes used to demonstrate uptake of water-soluble contrast within the center of the spinal cord, which is typical of tumor-associated cysts and syringomyelia.

SPINAL ANGIOGRAPHY

Spinal angiography may be considered when MRI suggests a hemangioblastoma (Figure 10-1). Although angiography will delineate the location of the vessels that supply and drain the hemangioblastoma, the vascular supply is generally evident at surgery and we have not found angiography to be important in the planning or execution of surgery. Cavernous angiomas are angiographically occult vascular lesions and, when suspected, angiography is not indicated.

MAGNETIC RESONANCE IMAGING (MRI)

MRI performed before and after gadolinium administration has become the imaging modality of choice in the diagnosis of IMSCT. Images are first obtained in the sagittal plane, followed by axial scans at the levels of the suspected abnormality. T2-weighted sequences define cystic structures and areas of edema in the spinal cord as regions of hyperintensity. Furthermore, cysts and regions of edema in the cord that do not contain tumor will not enhance after the administration of gadolinium, whereas most glial neoplasms and hemangioblastomas will enhance. The intravenous administration of gadolinium-DTPA with T1 and T2 imaging sequences, therefore, can help distinguish tumor from cyst or edema.

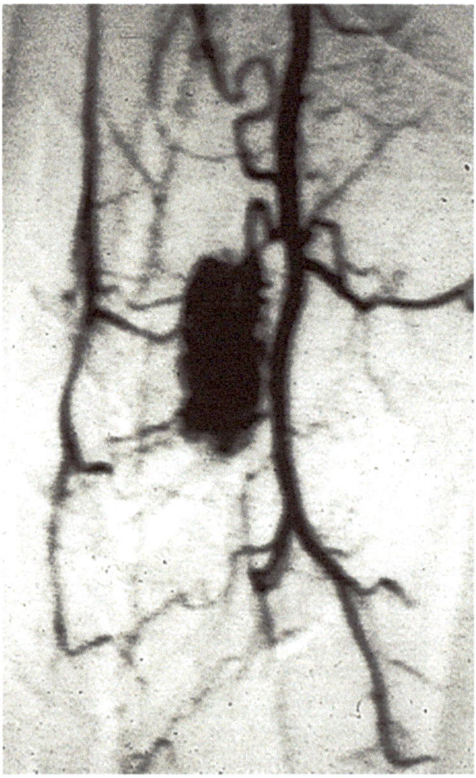

Figure 10-1 Hemangioblastoma appearance on spinal angiography. Note the impressive tumor blush of this extremely vascular tumor.

MR spectroscopy may allow for more definitive diagnosis in the future, although there are significant susceptibility artifacts because of the close proximity of tissues with different magnetic susceptibilities, such as spinal cord, CSF, bone, and muscle. Currently, this precludes evaluation by MR spectroscopy because magnetic field homogeneity is necessary for this technique.[55]

Ependymomas

Ependymomas typically occupy the central regions of the spinal cord. They are characteristically isointense on T1-weighted images, hyperintense on T2-weighted images, and administration of gadolinium yields a strongly enhancing mass that is well defined from adjacent spinal cord. Cystic areas and regions of prior hemorrhage produce mixed signal intensity. Tumor-associated cysts are commonly seen at the rostral and caudal extremes of the tumor (Figure 10-2). Prior hemorrhage can produce a hypointense cap of hemosiderin on T2-weighted images, which is pathognomonic of ependymoma.[62,63] The propensity of ependymomas to hemorrhage is attributed to their vascular connective tissue stroma.[63]

Astrocytomas

Astrocytomas may occupy the central regions of the spinal cord, or they may have an eccentric location. They are iso- to slightly hypointense on T1-weighted images, and hyperintense on T2-weighted images. Astrocytomas enhance to variable degrees after administration of gadolinium, typically to a lesser degree than ependymomas, and they are not as well defined from surrounding normal cord (Figure 10-3). Tumor-associated cysts are common, as is the case with ependymomas.

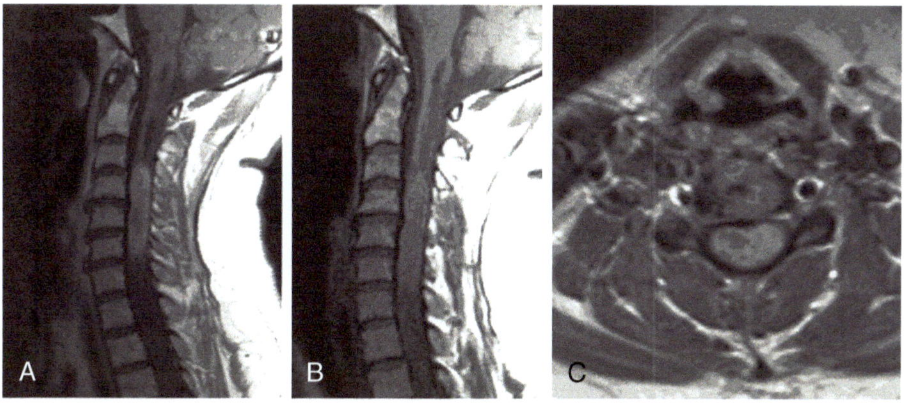

Figure 10-2 MRI appearance of an ependymoma. A, Sagittal T1-weighted imaging without gadolinium. **B,** Sagittal T1-weighted imaging with gadolinium. **C,** Axial T1-weighted imaging with gadolinium. Administration of gadolinium reveals a well-circumscribed strongly enhancing mass that is centrally located in the cord parenchyma on axial imaging. Note the cystic areas above and below the enhancing tumor.

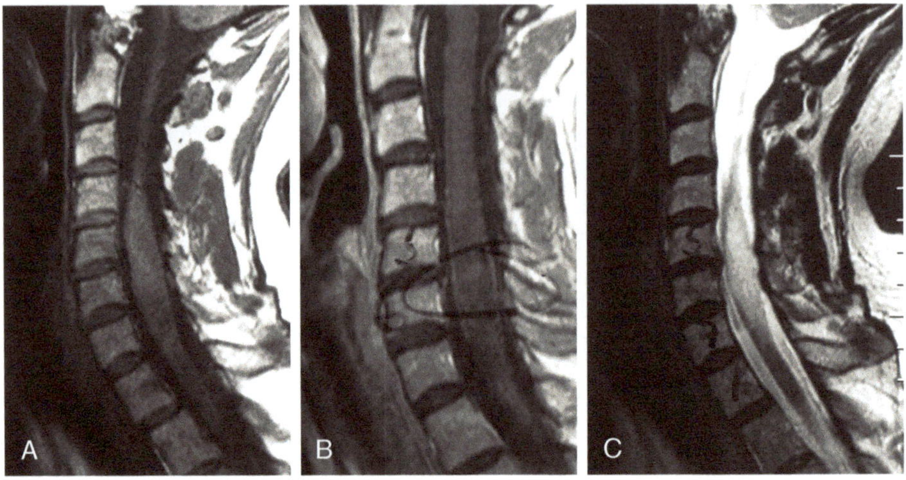

Figure 10-3 **MRI appearance of a low-grade astrocytoma. A,** Sagittal T1-weighted image. **B,** Sagittal T1-weighted image after gadolinium administration. **C,** Sagittal T2-weighted image. Note the thickened cord with a small degree of enhancement upon administration with gadolinium. T2-weighted imaging demonstrates mild edema within the cord.

Hemangioblastoma

This appears as an intensely enhancing tumor nodule following the administration of gadolinium. Tumor-associated cysts are frequently larger than the tumor and do not enhance. These cysts may extend for multiple spinal levels, and contain protein-rich fluid, which is hyperintense on T2-weighted images. The lesions are usually located on the posterior or posterolateral surface of the spinal cord (Figure 10-4). Because patients with von Hippel-Lindau syndrome commonly

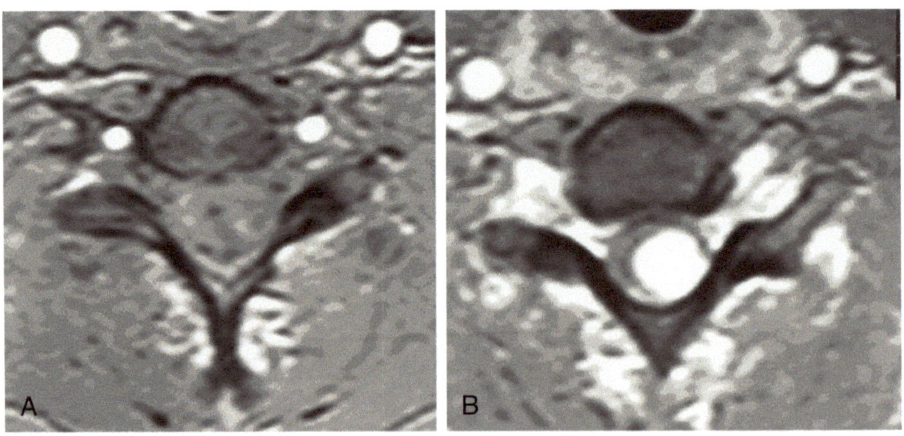

Figure 10-4 **MRI appearance of a hemangioblastoma. A,** Axial T1-weighted image without gadolinium. **B,** Axial T1-weighted image with gadolinium. Note the location on the posterolateral surface of the cord as well as the intense enhancement with gadolinium administration. **C,** Sagittal T1 with contrast demonstrating the large enhancing nodule on the dorsal aspect of the cord with a small cystic structure beneath.

have multiple lesions, the entire neuraxis should be imaged in the search for additional tumors.

Lipomas

Lipomas are hyperintense on T1-weighted images, hypointense on T2-weighted images, and do not enhance with the administration of gadolinium.

Cavernous Angiomas

Cavernous angiomas contain hemorrhagic regions of differing ages. CT scan can also demonstrate calcific areas in the lesion. MRI reveals a T2 rim of low intensity surrounding a region of variegated T2 signal intensity (Figure 10-5). Multiple lesions may be present, particularly in familial cases.

Multiple Sclerosis

MS plaques are found in the white matter, are iso- to hypointense on T1-weighted images, and are hyperintense on T2-weighted images (Figure 10-6). During active demyelination, MS plaques may enhance upon administration of gadolinium. In cases of acute MS, a follow-up MRI in 4 to 6 weeks will show lessening mass effect, diminution of enhancement, and a decreased hyperintensity on T2-weighted images.

Several key features help differentiate MS from IMSCTs on MRI. First, MS plaques usually span one to two spinal levels, whereas IMSCTs span multiple levels. Second, MS plaques are wedge-shaped and peripherally located in the

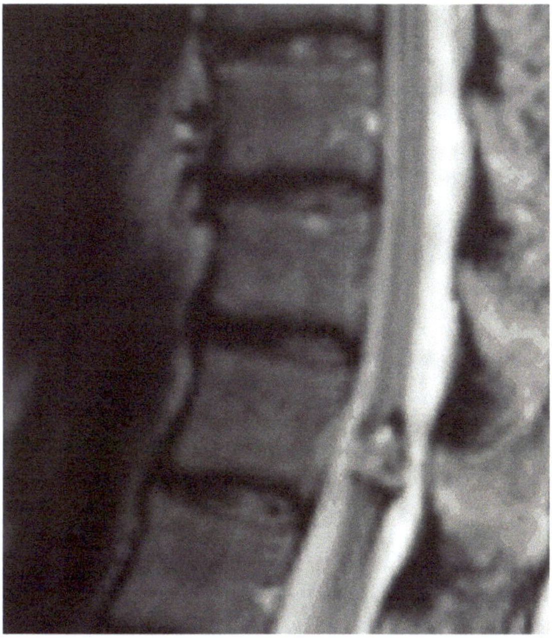

Figure 10-5 MRI appearance of a cavernous angioma. This T2-weighted sagittal image demonstrates a rim of hypointensity (known as a hemosiderin ring) surrounding a mass with an irregular border and heterogeneous T2 signal characteristics.

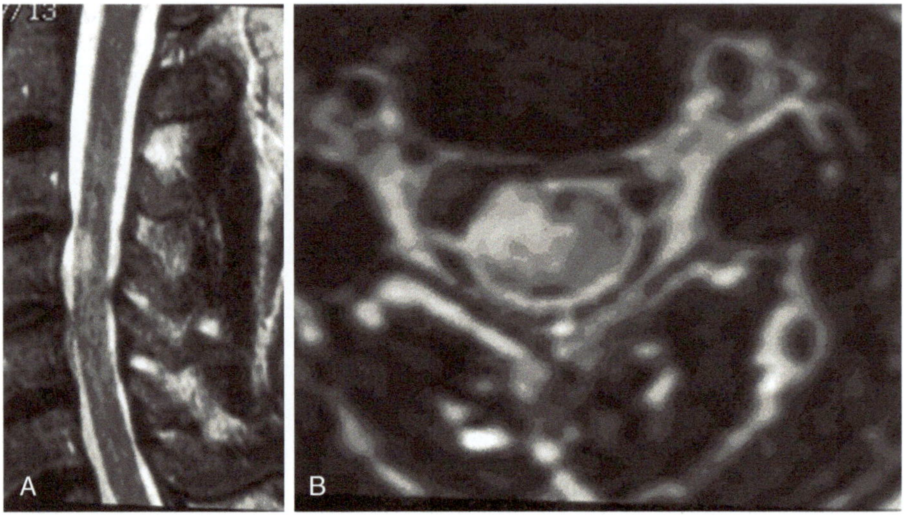

Figure 10-6 MRI appearance of multiple sclerosis. A, T2-weighted sagittal image. **B,** T2-weighted axial image. Note that the signal abnormality is restricted to a single level, as well as the absence of spinal cord enlargement. Also characteristic is the quadrantic involvement of the spinal cord on axial imaging.

white matter tracts, while IMSCTs tend to have a central location, displacing or invading surrounding white matter. Third, MS does not widen the spinal cord like IMSTs. Lastly, IMSCTs frequently have tumor-associated cysts, whereas cysts never accompany an MS plaque.

Differential Diagnosis

MULTIPLE SCLEROSIS

Multiple sclerosis (MS) affecting the spinal cord results in the following clinical findings: Lhermitte sign, limb weakness (usually asymmetric spastic paraparasis), and sensory dysfunction.[64] The presence of oligoclonal bands in the CSF will help confirm the diagnosis of MS.[65] Important clues differentiating MS from IMSCT can be obtained in a detailed history. IMSCTs often result in a gradual, steady deterioration in neurological function. MS, with the exception of the primary progressive variety (PPMS), typically follows a relapsing and remitting course.[64] IMSCTs are usually accompanied by pain, whereas MS myelitis is usually painless.

SARCOIDOSIS

Sarcoidosis is a multisystemic granulomatous disease that affects the spinal cord in only 0.43% of patients.[66] Spinal sarcoidosis can present with progressive myelopathy and sphincter dysfunction if the conus is involved.[67–69] On MRI, spinal sarcoid often demonstrates regional enlargement of the spinal cord along with patchy, multifocal enhancing nodules in the spinal parenchyma.[67,70] Most patients with sarcoid affecting the central nervous system have systemic disease, with the lungs and thoracic lymph nodes almost always affected. Bronchial biopsy or bronchialveolar lavage is useful to establish the diagnosis.[70–72] Elevated angiotensin-converting enzyme levels in both the serum and the CSF can be helpful in confirming the diagnosis.[70,73] Definitive diagnosis, however, is made only with a spinal cord biopsy. The mainstay of treatment is a prolonged course of corticosteroids, but other immunosuppressants such as cyclosporine and methotrexate are useful adjuncts in refractory cases.[72,74,75]

SYRINGOMYELIA

Syringomyelia, a cystic cavitation within the spinal cord that occurs following trauma or in association with Chiari malformations, may be confused with the cystic component of some intramedullary spinal cord tumors. A syrinx widens the spinal cord and clinically presents with slowly progressive deficits, classically affecting spinothalamic sensory modalities before dorsal columns. It can be difficult to distinguish from a slow growing IMSCT by history and neurological examination. After the administration of gadolinium, tumor tissue adjacent to the cyst will enhance whereas there will be no enhancement in syringomyelia. Tonsillar or brainstem herniation is seen with a cervical syrinx associated with a Chiari malformation but does not occur with IMSCTs.[76]

INFECTION

A variety of infectious agents can mimic intramedullary spinal cord tumors. Parasitic infections such as *Angiostrongylus catonensis* and *Schistosoma haematobium* can mimic spinal cord tumors both in clinical presentation and MRI imaging.[77–79] Toxoplasmosis and tuberculosis of the spinal cord resembling an IMSCT, likewise, have been described.[77,80]

Surgical Management

GOALS

The objectives of surgical intervention are to achieve total tumor removal while preserving or improving neurological function, and to obtain a tissue diagnosis. The infiltrating nature of some lesions, however, may make total removal impossible without an unacceptable loss of neurological function. In such instances, subtotal resection may still be a worthwhile goal to obtain a definitive diagnosis and to reduce tumor mass in preparation for adjunctive therapy. In children, radical resection is preferable and radiation treatment, with its deleterious effects upon the developing nervous system, is deferred.

SELECTION OF OPERATIVE CANDIDATES

The natural history of IMSCTs is that of progressive neurological deficit and early operative intervention is desirable, as postoperative functional outcome is closely correlated with the severity of the patient's preoperative deficit.[14,81]

Ideal surgical candidates are ambulatory patients with minimal neurological deficit. Even patients with significant deficit may still derive benefits from surgery with preservation of sphincter function or retention of the ability to position in bed. Patients with complete loss of neurological function are not appropriate surgical candidates.

Although early surgical intervention is recommended, surgical candidates must maintain realistic expectations of surgical outcomes. Published postoperative results suggest that 10% to 40% of patients remain stable, 40% to 80% improve, and 10% to 20% worsen neurologically.[82,83] It is reasonable, therefore, to defer surgery in a patient with very mild symptoms. Should serial examinations (approximately every 3 to 6 months) demonstrate decline in neurological function, both patient and physician might become more accepting of the surgical risks.

Tumor histology, as suggested on MRI, must also be considered when counseling a patient. Ependymomas are often well defined from surrounding neural elements, and their resection is less likely to be associated with permanent worsening of neurological function. Astrocytomas, on the other hand, infiltrate surrounding neural structures and their removal poses greater risk.

PERIOPERATIVE MANAGEMENT

Imaging studies are analyzed to precisely delineate the tumor's solid and cystic components and to distinguish these from spinal cord edema. The levels and extent of the anticipated laminectomy are noted. We place patients on high-dose corticosteroids every 6 hours for 24 hours prior to surgery. Corticosteroid administration is continued in the postoperative period at the same dose for 48 hours, and gradually tapered over the next 5 days. This patient population is at increased risk for deep venous thrombosis and pulmonary embolism due to lack of mobility. If lower extremity motor deficits exist, Doppler studies of the deep lower extremity venous system are performed and a removable vena caval filter is placed in all patients with deep venous thrombosis. If the deep venous system is normal, anti-embolism compression stockings are placed immediately prior to operation and continued in the postoperative period until the patient is ambulatory.

EVOKED POTENTIAL MONITORING

Most surgeons employ evoked potential monitoring in the hope that intraoperative data will guide the extent of the surgical resection and predict postoperative deficits. Somatosensory evoked potentials (SSEPs) are used to monitor the integrity of the dorsal columns and spinothalamic tracts. Significant intraoperative changes in SSEPs are demonstrated to be predictive of postoperative neurological deficits.[84] Their usefulness in improving outcome, however, may be limited.[85] Furthermore, preoperative neurological deficit may result in failure to obtain baseline readings. Variability in user skill and equipment error can be other causes for unsatisfactory physiologic data. Most important, however, neurological damage can result in the brief, 10 to 60 second delay between the time of spinal cord injury and evoked potential changes generated from computer averaging techniques. Such neurological injury may be irreversible, in contrast to evoked potential changes seen in the course of scoliosis surgery, which are usually reversible by repositioning of the instrumentation.

Motor evoked potentials (MEPs) are a newer technique used to assess the integrity of the corticospinal tracts during IMSCT surgery and provide "real time" intraoperative data. Utilizing scalp electrodes in combination with epidural electrodes, the presence of MEPs is believed to correlate better with surgical outcome than the preoperative neurological exam.[86] One surgical group reports the use of a 50% decline in the amplitude of MEPs as a mark at which to interrupt dissection.[87] The benefit of this technique was limited, however, by the fact that MEPs could not be measured in a large proportion of patients, many of whom had baseline neurological compromise and stood to benefit most from such monitoring.[88] Kothbauer et al. believe that evoked potential monitoring is an essential adjunct to surgery.[87] The use of evoked potential monitoring allows prediction of outcome after surgery.[86] However, controlled case studies supporting the efficacy of evoked potential monitoring in preventing neurological deterioration and improving the outcome from surgery are lacking. In short, there is little downside to the use of evoked potentials and we routinely employ both MEP and SSEP monitoring, but we are not convinced by our own experience or data from the literature that monitoring results in improved outcome.

OPERATIVE TECHNIQUE

The patient is placed prone, and a laminectomy is performed at the level of the tumor. Ultrasound is utilized to visualize the extent of the tumor, to confirm the adequacy of the laminectomy, and to identify any tumor-associated cysts. The dura is then opened, starting above the most superior portion of the tumor and proceeding to the inferior extent of the tumor. The opening of the dura is important and CSF pressure dynamics must be taken into account. CSF pressure above the tumor is greater than below the tumor, and release of CSF from the subarachnoid space distal to the inferior margin of the tumor could exacerbate this pressure differential, potentially leading to downward herniation of the spinal cord with devastating neurological consequences.

After the dura is opened, the midline of the cord is identified and a myelotomy is made between the dorsal columns. The myelotomy is extended to the superior and inferior poles of the tumor and the pial surfaces of the dorsal columns are then gently retracted with fine sutures, exposing the posterior extent of the tumor. At this time a biopsy is obtained, and the periphery of the tumor is examined for a cleavage plane between tumor and cord. If a cleavage plane is found, as may be the case with juvenile pilocytic astrocytomas, complete resection should be attempted. If no cleavage plane exists, the tumor is likely infiltrating, and complete resection is likely to be associated with exacerbation of neurological deficit.

When a tumor is found that is well defined from normal spinal cord, complete resection is attempted. The central region of the tumor is removed with an ultrasonic aspirator and the cleavage plane is developed around the periphery. In this fashion the tumor is folded in upon itself with minimal retraction on the surrounding normal cord. The dissection along the anterior aspect of the tumor must be done with great care, as the tumor often lies in close proximity to the anterior spinal artery from which it receives its blood supply. When the anterior surface of the tumor is dissected from its anterior vascular attachments, hemostasis is obtained and the wound is closed in layers. Often the dura is closed using a fascial graft to allow for any postoperative swelling of the spinal cord. This is particularly important in patients with an infiltrating tumor, when resection has been limited.

Since the laminectomies employed in the treatment of IMSCTs rarely compromise the architecture of the facet joints, development of deformity is uncommon and instrumentation is not routinely placed at the time of initial IMSCT resection. Even when a laminectomy must span many vertebral levels, postoperative spinal stability is rarely a concern. Furthermore, instrumentation can lead to artifact on the MRI that degrades the quality of postoperative imaging, making it difficult to assess both extent of resection and tumor recurrence. Nonetheless, a small subset of patients will develop kyphotic deformity requiring instrumentation; the management of these patients is discussed in the section on postoperative complications.

Postoperative Complications

INCREASED NEUROLOGICAL DEFICIT

Deterioration of motor function in the immediate postoperative period is reported in most series. These deficits generally are followed by recovery over a period of days to months. However, approximately 20% of patients experience a permanent increase in their deficits.[6,15,28,82,87,89] Progressive deterioration in the postoperative period suggests spinal cord compression by hematoma or spinal cord swelling and compression by the dura in a patient with significant amounts of residual tumor who did not undergo duraplasty.

Patients with more severe motor deficits preoperatively are less likely to sustain recovery and are more likely to experience further deterioration than those with lesser degrees of impairment. Because most astrocytomas infiltrate neural tissue, resection of astrocytomas (with the exception of juvenile pilocytic astrocytomas) inevitably results in injury to functional neural tissue. For this reason, increased permanent postoperative deficit is more common with astrocytomas than with ependymomas. Innocenzi reports that at discharge from the hospital, the proportion of children with neurological deterioration from their preoperative status was greater in those with astrocytomas than those with ependymomas.[90]

Loss of proprioception can occur as a result of injury to the dorsal columns from the myelotomy, and is more likely with larger tumors and longer myelotomies.[21] The spinothalamic tracts also may be injured during dissection at the lateral margins of a centrally placed tumor. Intraoperative somatosensory evoked potentials can provide an early warning of disturbance to either the dorsal columns or the spinothalamic tracts. Dysesthesia, hyperesthesias, and anesthesia are feared complications of surgery. Their presence may render a functional extremity useless and prevent a patient with minimal or no motor deficit from returning to a former occupation or resuming a normal social life. In general, sensory deficits resolve within 3 months after surgery, after which point any residual deficit is usually fixed. Motor deficits, however, are not fixed and can continue to gradually improve beyond the 3-month postoperative window.[91]

SPINAL DEFORMITY

In children, deformities of the thoracic and lumbar spine may represent the initial manifestation of an IMSCT months or years before the appearance of neurological signs and symptoms.[92] It is unclear whether the exacerbation of these deformities following operation results from the effects of the tumor or of laminectomy. Whether present preoperatively or not, progressive postoperative kyphoscoliosis of the thoracic spine and swan-neck deformity of the cervical spine are seen with great frequency in children, but are rare in adults if not present preoperatively.[13,93] The incidence varies with the spinal level involved; the cervical area is affected more frequently than the thoracic area and lumbar deformity is exceptional.[94]

Deformity may occur as a consequence of laminectomy and loss of the support of the posterior elements, from radiation, or from tumor-induced paraspinal muscle weakness. In the cervical spine, flexion deformity is the usual pattern and may progress to result in spinal cord compression and neurological deficit. Kyphoscoliosis of the thoracic spine does not typically produce neurological deficit but, if untreated, may eventually result in respiratory compromise.

Osteoplastic laminotomy is favored in children to retard or prevent the development of kyphoscoliosis.[95] In the cervical spine, early fusion at the first sign of flexion deformity is indicated. Progression of kyphoscoliosis may be a sign of tumor recurrence, and this is not prevented by laminoplasty.[26] Thus, appropriate follow-up to identify early development of spinal deformities is an essential part of the postoperative management. In the thoracic and lumbar spine, instrumentation and fusion are indicated when progressive deformity is recognized and the presence of recurrent tumor is ruled out.

CEREBROSPINAL FLUID FISTULA

Leakage of CSF from the wound can complicate any surgery in which the dura is violated. Wounds, in previously unoperated patients, have an excellent vascular supply and well-defined tissue planes that promote rapid wound healing, and CSF leakage is uncommon. The postoperative course in patients who have had multiple surgeries, who have received radiation, or who are malnourished is more often complicated by CSF leakage. In all patients who have had prior operation and radiation, plastic surgical assistance in wound closure is essential. Often, rotational flaps of tissue from regions not previously irradiated are required. Insertion of a lumbar drain postoperatively provides an alternative route for the egress of CSF, minimizing the chances of CSF fistulas.

MORTALITY

Mortality was once significant for IMSCT surgery. Large series in the past 15 years, however, report minimal or no operative mortality.[15,21,96]

Radiation Therapy

Radiation is reserved for cases of subtotal removal, recurrence, and otherwise inoperable infiltrating tumors. It is inappropriate for use in ependymomas which are almost always totally resectable. Radiation results in arachnoiditis as well as gliosis and fibrosis within the neoplasm, obscuring the cleavage plane between tumor and cord. Furthermore, the microvasculature of the spinal cord is obliterated by radiation, further increasing its sensitivity to surgical manipulation.[83] Numerous surgeons have noted an association between poor postoperative outcome and preoperative radiation therapy.[82,83] Radiation therefore increases the difficulty and risk of surgery substantially, and is reserved for use when surgery is not felt to be beneficial. The use of postoperative radiation therapy has not been validated in a prospective, controlled study, but many reports describe its beneficial effects upon recurrence and survival.[20,97] There is disagreement regarding its utility in instances where gross total resection is accomplished.

Recently, a new technique for delivering radiation has been developed, called the Cyberknife. The Cyberknife is a machine that administers image-guided frameless stereotactic robotic radiosurgery. A linear accelerator is mounted on a robotic arm, and internal anatomic markers act as fiducials that are registered to the radiotherapy plan at the time of treatment. This machine is able to treat irregular volumes with multiple overlapping radiation beams. The theoretical advantage of stereotactic radiosurgery is that it permits a very high dose of radiation to be administered to the tumor, while minimizing exposure of surrounding tissues. Unfortunately the spinal cord's small volume and extreme sensitivity to radiation negate these potential benefits of the Cyberknife.

The use of the Cyberknife to treat IMSCTs is experimental, and only two cases are reported in the literature. Ryu et al. describe the treatment of a hemangioblastoma and a cavernous angioma with total radiation doses approaching 25 Gy.[98] Both of these intramedullary lesions, however, are extremely amenable to surgical resection, and we question the use of radiation in their treatment. Recent reports have only demonstrated that the Cyberknife is a feasible and safe treatment modality.[98,99] Further study is needed to compare the efficacy of Cyberknife to other existing treatments. The Cyberknife will still result in radiation changes to the spinal cord, making surgery difficult.

LOW-GRADE ASTROCYTOMA

There is considerable controversy regarding the use of radiation therapy in cases of low-grade astrocytomas. Kopelson recommended radiation for all low-grade astrocytomas without regard to the extent of resection.[100] Epstein et al., however, concluded that radiation should be reserved for cases where subtotal resection is performed,[28] and in a subsequent study by this group, they concluded that less than 80% resection was associated with a significantly worse prognosis.[28,101] While Guidetti et al. did not find any consistent benefit from radiation therapy, others contend that postoperative radiation therapy will reduce the relapse rate after partial resection of low-grade gliomas.[102–105] Given the changes in the architecture of the spinal cord following radiation therapy, however, it should be reserved for instances when surgery is no longer a treatment option.

For astrocytomas in adults, total resection is usually difficult, because astrocytomas are infiltrative and poorly defined from the normal spinal cord. For low-grade astrocytomas we prefer to follow patients with MRI and consider radiation when imaging shows tumor growth. However, others have reported that subtotal removal followed by 45 Gy given in a local field will result in satisfactory motor function and survival in low-grade astrocytomas in adults.[103]

MALIGNANT ASTROCYTOMAS

The outcome of patients with high-grade intramedullary gliomas remains dismal in spite of the progress in neurosurgical and radiotherapy techniques, and it is not clear that radiation therapy beneficially affects survival or retards the onset of neurological impairment. Aggressive radiotherapy in doses that cause "radiation cordotomy" has been reported by Cohen et al. to result in an occasional survival at 4 years after the initial surgery.[27,103,106] Radiation cordotomy may be one option for patients with high-grade astrocytomas who have already poor motor function at the level of the thoracic or conus medullaris, providing that the malignant nature of the tumor is histologically confirmed.

EPENDYMOMAS

Gross total resection is the most efficacious treatment in the management of ependymomas, and radiation therapy is unnecessary if complete removal has been accomplished. Patients who have had incomplete removal should be followed closely with frequent MRI and treated with reoperation rather than radiation for recurrence. In one large series, radiotherapy had no effect on disease progression or recurrence when patients with and without radiotherapy were compared.[107] Although Isaacson et al. recommended up to a total dose of 50.40 Gy in 1.80 Gy fractions for residual benign ependymomas using local fields,[108] we disagree with the use of radiation therapy for this benign, potentially curable tumor.

SIDE EFFECTS OF RADIATION

Radiation to IMSCTs is a potential hazard to the spinal cord, bone growth, fertility, and the gastrointestinal tract. The spinal cord has a tolerance dose reported as 45 to 50 Gy in conventional fractionation, considerably lower than the brain. Doses of more than 50 Gy have been proposed,[106] but such treatment is not recommended because of the risk of radiation myelopathy. The tolerance of the spinal cord in children may be lower than in adults. Isaacson et al. recommended reducing radiation dose in children by 10%.[22] Because of the harmful effect of radiation therapy on development in children, most authorities do not irradiate pediatric patients who are believed to have had a gross total resection of their tumors.

Chemotherapy

Chemotherapy has become a subject of interest in the pediatric population, since children are more sensitive than adults to the deleterious effects of radiation. Treatment protocols for intramedullary gliomas are based upon regimens currently used for intracranial neoplasms.[109–111] Two small case series have demonstrated some promise. Lowis et al. report their experience in two pediatric patients with WHO grade II and III astrocytomas using carboplatin and vincristine. Both patients improved neurologically, and the disappearance of contrast-enhancing tumor was noted on follow-up MRI.[112] Doireau et al. reported progression-free intervals ranging from 16 to 59 months in five of eight children with predominantly low-grade glial tumors treated using a six drug chemotherapy regimen including carboplatin, procarbazine, vincristine, cyclophosphamide, etoposide, and cisplatin.[113] While chemotherapy has shown some promise, the reported numbers of patients treated are small, and there is lack of comparison with other treatment groups. A multicenter study will be necessary to define efficacy and the ideal chemotherapy drug regimen.

Outcome

Long-term postoperative neurological outcome correlates most closely with the preoperative functional status. Significant neurological improvement rarely occurs in the face of long-standing deficit, and even if there is some improvement in patients who are severely impaired, change in the clinical functional grade is exceptional.[21]

EPENDYMOMAS

The outcome for ependymomas is generally good. There is a clear relationship between the extent of resection and the rate of recurrence and survival.[15,96] Gross total resection is attainable, and, when achieved, recurrence is rare. Hoshimaru reports that in 36 patients with spinal cord ependymomas at a mean postoperative follow-up of 56 months, 39% were neurologically improved, 47% were stable, and only 14% worse, using McCormick's functional status scale.[15,114]

The histological grade of ependymomas does not appear to affect outcome.[115] In cases of gross total removal, radiation therapy is withheld, as surgery for recurrence is feasible and less difficult to accomplish in a nonradiated field. If postoperative imaging reveals significant residual tumor that is resectable, reoperation should be undertaken. Tumors that have been subtotally resected are followed with serial MRI scans and treated with reoperation when there is evidence of tumor growth.

ASTROCYTOMAS, GRADE I AND II

Although low-grade astrocytomas are categorized as "benign," recurrences occur and neurological outcomes are generally far less satisfactory than is the case with ependymomas. Tumor recurrence is associated with progressive neurological deficit, and eventual paraplegia or quadriplegia. Patients with tumor recurrence can encounter numerous health problems that affect the life expectancy of debilitated and immobile individuals such as septicemia, pulmonary emboli, and pneumonia.[116] Five-year survival was 57% in a series of 21 patients, 18 of whom had a pathological grade of I or II.[117] In another series, 4 of 11 patients with grade I or II astrocytomas died within the follow-up period and only four of these were not worse in functional grade as compared with their preoperative status.[96]

A correlation between extent of resection and tumor recurrence is controversial and poorly demonstrated in the literature.[6,20,117,118] The infiltrating nature of these tumors complicates the assessment of extent of resection, subjecting the surgeon's estimates to inaccuracy. Even when a surgeon believes that a gross total resection was accomplished and MRI fails to demonstrate residual tumor, tumor fragments most likely remain.[119] Cristante notes that 16 of 22 low-grade astrocytomas radically or "quasiradically" resected were tumors that had a discrete tumoral plane, and most had a fibrillary histology with adjacent cystic areas.[21]

Histological subtype is also reported to have prognostic value, as those with pilocytic features enjoy better outcomes than those with the diffuse fibrillary subtype.[20] This probably accounts, at least in part, for the more favorable prognosis for the pediatric age group seen by Sandler, as the pilocytic tumors represent a larger proportion of their tumors.[117]

ASTROCYTOMAS, GRADE III AND IV

The prognosis for high-grade astrocytomas (WHO grades III and IV), like their intracranial counterparts, is extremely poor, and all patients will eventually die as a consequence of progressive disease. Like patients with malignant intracranial astrocytomas, widespread leptomeningeal metastases and hydrocephalus are common, occurring in 58% of patients.[27] The terminal event in many malignant astrocytomas is tumor growth to the cervicomedullary area with respiratory paralysis. Pulmonary embolus and pneumonia may prove fatal to patients bedridden by progressive disease.

Surgical intervention usually results in worsened or, at best, the same level of neurological function. Median survival after surgery for a grade IV tumor is 6 months, and length of survival does not correlate with the extent of resection.[27,28] A series of pediatric patients (median age of 11) fared slightly better, with a median survival of 13 months.[120]

GANGLIOGLIOMAS

Gangliogliomas, like ependymomas, are amenable to surgical cure. Recurrences, however, occur in 25% to 33% of cases, at which point a second resection is pursued. Histological grading has been undertaken but does not significantly correlate with outcome. Adjuvant chemotherapy or radiation is not recommended.[14,31]

LIPOMAS

Attempted total resection of lipomas will result in poor outcome, with worsening of postoperative motor function, although preoperative pain is generally relieved. Resection of the central portion of the lesion without ever visualizing adjacent neural tissue is the best strategy and will usually result in maintenance or improvement in neurological function. Adjuvant therapy is not recommended.

CAVERNOUS ANGIOMA

The results of resection of cavernous angiomas have been favorable. Although a transient increase in neurological deficit may occur in the immediate period after surgery, long-term follow-up shows that most have a modest improvement in symptomatology. Pain and paresthesias are much more likely to improve than motor deficits. Recurrence is not a concern if total resection is achieved.

Conclusions

Intramedullary spinal cord tumors represent a treatment challenge in many respects. A wide variety of pathologies can result in intramedullary spinal cord lesions, and most of these pathologies have very similar clinical presentations. The advent of MRI has played a critical role in the evaluation and management of intramedullary spinal lesions. MRI not only permits early diagnosis, but also provides insight into the pathology of the lesion via its signal and enhancement characteristics.

Radiation and chemotherapeutic treatments of IMSCTs remain controversial, leaving surgery as the mainstay of treatment. The safety of modern surgical intervention has been improved through better patient selection and intraoperative neurophysiologic monitoring, as well as surgical devices such as the microscope, ultrasonic aspirator, and carbon dioxide laser. Unfortunately, infiltrative glial tumors are not completely resectable, and surgery is of little or no benefit in individuals with high-grade astrocytomas.

REFERENCES

1. Brotchi J. Intrinsic spinal cord tumor resection. Neurosurgery 2002;50(5):1059–63.
2. Elsberg CA, BE. The operability of intramedullary tumors of the spinal cord. A report of two operations with remarks upon the extrusion of the spinal cord. Am J Med Sci 1911;142:636–47.
3. CA, E. Diagnosis and Treatment of Surgical Diseases of the Spinal Cord and Its Membranes. 1916.
4. Schneider R. Intraspinal Tumors. In: Schneider R, editor. Correlative Neurosurgery. Springfield, Ill: Charles C. Thomas; 1969. p. 444–63.
5. Cooper PR, Epstein F. Radical resection of intramedullary spinal cord tumors in adults. Recent experience in 29 patients. J Neurosurg 1985;63(4):492–9.
6. Samii M, Klekamp J. Surgical results of 100 intramedullary tumors in relation to accompanying syringomyelia. Neurosurgery 1994;35(5):865–73; discussion 873.
7. Chang UK, et al. Surgical outcome and prognostic factors of spinal intramedullary ependymomas in adults. J Neurooncol 2002;57(2):133–9.
8. Jallo GI, Freed D, Epstein F. Intramedullary spinal cord tumors in children. Childs Nerv Syst 2003;19(9):641–9.
9. Bowers DC, Weprin BE. Intramedullary Spinal Cord Tumors. Curr Treat Options Neurol 2003;5(3):207–12.
10. Chamberlain MC. Ependymomas. Curr Neurol Neurosci Rep 2003;3(3):193–9.
11. Moser FG, et al. Ependymoma of the spinal nerve root: case report. Neurosurgery 1992;31(5): 962–4; discussion 964.
12. Fischer G, BJ, Chignier A, et al. Clinical Material. In: B.J, Fischer G, editors. Intramedullary Spinal Cord Tumors. Stuttgart: Thieme; 1996. p. 10–20.
13. Reimer R, Onofrio BM. Astrocytomas of the spinal cord in children and adolescents. J Neurosurg 1985;63(5):669–75.
14. Constantini S, et al. Intramedullary spinal cord tumors in children under the age of 3 years [see comments]. J Neurosurg 1996;85(6):1036–43.
15. McCormick PC, et al. Intramedullary ependymoma of the spinal cord. J Neurosurg 1990;72(4):523–32.
16. Schweitzer JS, Batzdorf U. Ependymoma of the cauda equina region: diagnosis, treatment, and outcome in 15 patients. Neurosurgery 1992;30(2):202–7.
17. Roos KL, Muckway M. Neurofibromatosis. Dermatol Clin 1995;13(1):105–11.
18. Lee M, et al. Intramedullary spinal cord tumors in neurofibromatosis. Neurosurgery 1996; 38(1):32–7.
19. Yokota T, et al. A family with spinal anaplastic ependymoma: evidence of loss of chromosome 22q in tumor. J Hum Genet 2003;48(11):598–602.

20. Minehan KJ, et al. Spinal cord astrocytoma: pathological and treatment considerations. J Neurosurg 1995;83(4):590–5.
21. Cristante L, HH. Surgical management of intramedullary spinal cord tumors: functionaloutcome and sources of morbidity. Neurosurgery 1994;35:69–76.
22. Allen JC, et al. Treatment of high-grade spinal cord astrocytoma of childhood with "8-in- 1" chemotherapy and radiotherapy: a pilot study of CCG-945. Children's Cancer Group. J Neurosurg 1998;88(2):215–20.
23. McCormick PC, SB. Intramedullary tumors in adults. Neurosurg Clin North Am 1998; (1)687–700.
24. Epstein F, Epstein N. Surgical management of holocord intramedullary spinal cord astrocytomas in children. J Neurosurg 1981;54(6):829–32.
25. Yagi T, et al. Intramedullary spinal cord tumour associated with neurofibromatosis type 1. Acta Neurochir (Wien) 1997;139(11):1055–60.
26. Constantini S, EF. Intraspinal Tumors in infants and Children. In: YJ, editor. Neurological Surgery, vol. 4. Philadelphia: WB Saunders; 1996. p. 3123–33.
27. Cohen AR, et al. Malignant astrocytomas of the spinal cord. J Neurosurg 1989;70(1):50–4.
28. Epstein FJ, Farmer JP, Freed D. Adult intramedullary astrocytomas of the spinal cord. J Neurosurg 1992;77(3):355–9.
29. Hamburger C, Buttner A, Weis S. Ganglioglioma of the spinal cord: report of two rare cases and review of the literature. Neurosurgery 1997;41(6):1410–5; discussion 1415–6.
30. Miller DC, Lang FF, Epstein FJ. Central nervous system gangliogliomas. Part 1: Pathology. J Neurosurg 1993;79(6):859–66.
31. Lang FF, et al. Central nervous system gangliogliomas. Part 2: Clinical outcome. J Neurosurg 1993;79(6):867–73.
32. Murota T, Symon L. Surgical management of hemangioblastoma of the spinal cord: a report of 18 cases. Neurosurgery 1989;25(5):699–707; discussion 708.
33. Nelson JS. Inhereted Tumor Syndromes Involving The Nervous System. In: Nelson JS, et al., editors. Principles and Practice of Neuropathology. New York: Oxford University Press; 2003. p. 448–58.
34. Wizigmann-Voos S, Plate KH. Pathology, genetics and cell biology of hemangioblastomas. Histol Histopathol 1996;11(4):1049–61.
35. Brotchi J, FG. Treatment. In: Fischer BJ, G, editors. Intramedullary Spinal Cord Tumors. Stuttgart: Thieme; 1996. p. 60–84.
36. Landan I, Gilroy J, Wolfe DE. Syringomyelia affecting the entire spinal cord secondary to primary spinal intramedullary central nervous system lymphoma. J Neurol Neurosurg Psychiatry 1987;50(11):1533–5.
37. Hautzer NW, Aiyesimoju A, Y. Robitaille, "Primary" spinal intramedullary lymphomas: a review. Ann Neurol 1983;14(1):62–6.
38. McDonald AC, Nicoll JA, Rampling R. Intramedullary non-Hodgkin's lymphoma of the spinal cord: a case report and literature review. J Neurooncol 1995;23(3):257–63.
39. Lee DK, et al. Multifocal primary CNS T cell lymphoma of the spinal cord. Clin Neuropathol 2002;21(4):149–55.
40. Bekar A, et al. A case of primary spinal intramedullary lymphoma. Surg Neurol 2001; 55(5): 261–4.
41. Caruso PA, et al. Primary intramedullary lymphoma of the spinal cord mimicking cervical spondylotic myelopathy. AJR Am J Roentgenol 1998;171(2):526–7.
42. Mrabet A, et al. [Cervicobulbar intramedullary lipoma. Apropos of a case with review of the literature]. Neurochirurgie 1992;38(5):309–14.
43. Jarmundowicz W, Sakowski J, Wilska E. [Own experience in surgical treatment of intramedullary spinal cord lipomas]. Neurol Neurochir Pol 1998;32(4):969–78.
44. Lee M, et al. Intramedullary spinal cord lipomas. J Neurosurg 1995;82(3):394–400.
45. Fujiwara F, et al. Intradural spinal lipomas not associated with spinal dysraphism: a report of four cases. Neurosurgery 1995;37(6):1212–5.
46. Cristante L, HD. Hermann, Radical excision of intramedullary cavernous angiomas [see comments]. Neurosurgery] 1998;43(3):424–30; discussion 430–1.
47. Zabramski JM, et al. The natural history of familial cavernous malformations: results of an ongoing study. J Neurosurg 1994;80(3):422–32.
48. Rigamonti D, et al. Cerebral cavernous malformations. Incidence and familial occurrence. N Engl J Med 1988;319(6):343–7.

49. Laberge-le Couteulx S, et al. Truncating mutations in CCM1, encoding KRIT1, cause hereditary cavernous angiomas. Nat Genet 1999;23(2):189–93.
50. Sahoo T, et al. Mutations in the gene encoding KRIT1, a Krev-1/rap1a binding protein, cause cerebral cavernous malformations (CCM1). Hum Mol Genet 1999;8(12):2325–33.
51. Deutsch H, JG, Faktorovich A, Epstein F. Spinal intramedullary cavernoma: clinical presentation and surgical outcome. J Neurosurg 2000;93(Suppl. 1):65–70.
52. Zevgaridis D, MR, Hamburger C, Steiger HJ, Reulen HJ. Cavernous haemangiomas of the spinal cord. A review of 117 cases. Acta Neurochir (Wien) 1999;141:237–45.
53. Costigan DA, Winkelman MD. Intramedullary spinal cord metastasis. A clinicopathological study of 13 cases. J Neurosurg 1985;62(2):227–33.
54. Chigasaki H, PJ. A long term follow-up study of 128 cases of intramedullary spinal cord tumors. Neurol Med Chir(Tokyo) 1968;10:25–66.
55. Edelson RN, DM, Posner JB. [Intramedullary spinal cord metastasis]. Neurology 1979;22: 1222–31.
56. Kehrli P. [Epidemiology of brain metastases.] Neurochirurgie 1999;45(5):357–63.
57. McCormick PC, SB. Spinal Cord Tumors in Adults. In: Y, JR, editors. Neurological Surgery. Philadelphia: WB Saunders; 1996. p. 3102–22.
58. Jellinger K, et al. Intramedullary spinal cord metastases. J Neurol 1979;220(1):31–41.
59. Grem JL, Burgess J, Trump DL. Clinical features and natural history of intramedullary spinal cord metastasis. Cancer 1985;56(9):2305–14.
60. Thorpe JW, et al. Spinal MRI in patients with suspected multiple sclerosis and negative brain MRI. Brain 1996;119(Pt 3):709–14.
61. Malis LI. Intramedullary spinal cord tumors. Clin Neurosurg 1978;25:512–39.
62. Fischer G, BJ. Intramedullary Spinal Cord Tumors. Stuttgart: Thieme; 1996.
63. Fine MJ, et al. Spinal cord ependymomas: MR imaging features. Radiology 1995;197(3): 655–8.
64. Miller J. Multiple Sclerosis. In: Rowland L, editor. Merritt's Neurology. Philadelphia; Lippincott Williams and Wilkins; 2000.
65. Feasby TE, et al. Spinal cord swelling in multiple sclerosis. Can J Neurol Sci 1981;8(2):151–3.
66. Vighetto A, et al. Intramedullary sarcoidosis of the cervical spinal cord. J Neurol Neurosurg Psychiatry 1985;48(5):477–9.
67. Pascuzzi RM, et al. Sarcoid myelopathy. J Neuroimaging 1996;6(1):61–2.
68. Morimoto T, et al. [Spinal cord sarcoidosis without abnormal shadows on chest radiography or chest CT diagnosed by transbronchial lung biopsy]. Nihon Kokyuki Gakkai Zasshi 2001;39(11):871–6.
69. Prelog K, Blome S, Dennis C. Neurosarcoidosis of the conus medullaris and cauda equina. Australas Radiol 2003;47(3):295–7.
70. Peltier J, et al. [Sarcoidosis revealed by a spinal cord lesion]. Rev Neurol (Paris) 2004;160(4 Pt 1):452–5.
71. Pierre-Kahn V, et al. [Intramedullary spinal cord sarcoidosis. Case report and review of the literature]. Neurochirurgie 2001;47(4):439–41.
72. Vinas FC, Rengachary S. Diagnosis and management of neurosarcoidosis. J Clin Neurosci 2001;8(6):505–13.
73. Tahmoush AJ, et al. CSF-ACE activity in probable CNS neurosarcoidosis. Sarcoidosis Vasc Diffuse Lung Dis 2002;19(3):191–7.
74. Zajicek JP. Neurosarcoidosis. Curr Opin Neurol 2000;13(3):323–5.
75. Jallo GI, et al. Intraspinal sarcoidosis: diagnosis and management. Surg Neurol 1997;48(5): 514–20; discussion 521.
76. Schubeus P, et al. Spinal cord cavities: differential-diagnostic criteria in magnetic resonance imaging. Eur J Radiol 1991;12(3):219–25.
77. Cohen-Gadol AA, et al. Spinal cord biopsy: a review of 38 cases. Neurosurgery 2003;52(4): 806–15; discussion 815–6.
78. Petjom S, et al. Angiostrongylus cantonensis infection mimicking a spinal cord tumor. Ann Neurol 2002;52(1):99–101.
79. Samandouras G, King A, Kellerman AJ. Schistosoma haematobium presenting as an intrinsic conus tumour. Br J Neurosurg 2002;16(3):296–300.
80. Mehren M, et al. Toxoplasmic myelitis mimicking intramedullary spinal cord tumor. Neurology 1988;38(10):1648–50.
81. Schwartz TH, MP. Intramedullary ependymomas: clinical presenttion, surgical treatment strategies and prognosis. J Neurooncol 2000;47:211–8.

82. Brotchi J, et al. A survey of 65 tumors within the spinal cord: surgical results and the importance of preoperative magnetic resonance imaging. Neurosurgery 1991;29(5):651–6; discussion 656–7.
83. Xu QW, et al. Aggressive surgery for intramedullary tumor of cervical spinal cord. Surg Neurol 1996;46(4):322–8.
84. Kearse Jr LA, et al. Loss of somatosensory evoked potentials during intramedullary spinal cord surgery predicts postoperative neurologic deficits in motor function [corrected]. [published erratum appears in J Clin Anesth 1993 Nov-Dec;5(6):529.] J Clin Anesth 1993;5(5):392–8.
85. Adams DC, et al. Monitoring of intraoperative motor-evoked potentials under conditions of controlled neuromuscular blockade [see comments]. Anesth Analg 1993;77(5):913–8.
86. Murota T, SL. Surgical management of hemangioblastoma of the spinal cord: a report of 18 cases. Neurosurgery 1989;25:699–708.
87. Kothbauer K, Deletis V, Epstein FJ. Intraoperative spinal cord monitoring for intramedullary surgery: an essential adjunct [see comments]. Pediatr Neurosurg 1997;26(5):247–54.
88. JS. Comment. Neurosurgery 1997;41:1336.
89. Herrmann HD, Neuss M, Winkler D. Intramedullary spinal cord tumors resected with CO2 laser microsurgical technique: recent experience in fifteen patients. Neurosurgery 1988;22(3):518–22.
90. Innocenzi G, et al. Intramedullary astrocytomas and ependymomas in the pediatric age group: a retrospective study. Childs Nerv Syst 1996;12(12):776–80.
91. Fischer G, BJ. Functional Results. In: Fischer BJ, G, editors. Intramedullary Spinal Cord Tumors. Stuttgart: Thieme; 1996. p. 85–90.
92. Houten JK, Weiner HL. Pediatric intramedullary spinal cord tumors: special considerations. J Neurooncol 2000;47(3):225–30.
93. DeSousa AL, et al. Intraspinal tumors in children. A review of 81 cases. J Neurosurg 1979;51(4):437–45.
94. Yasuoka S, Peterson HA, MacCarty CS. Incidence of spinal column deformity after multilevel laminectomy in children and adults. J Neurosurg 1982;57(4):441–5.
95. Abbott R, FN, Wisoff JH, Epstein FJ. Osteoplastic laminotomy in children. Pediatr Neurosurg 1992;18:153–6.
96. Cooper PR. Outcome after operative treatment of intramedullary spinal cord tumors in adults: intermediate and long-term results in 51 patients. Neurosurgery 1989;25(6):855–9.
97. O'Sullivan C, et al. Spinal cord tumors in children: long-term results of combined surgical and radiation treatment. J Neurosurg 1994;81(4):507–12.
98. Ryu SI, et al. Image-guided hypo-fractionated stereotactic radiosurgery to spinal lesions. Neurosurgery 2001;49(4):838–46.
99. Gerszten PC, et al. CyberKnife frameless stereotactic radiosurgery for spinal lesions: clinical experience in 125 cases. Neurosurgery 2004;55(1):89–98; discussion 98–9.
100. Kopelson G, et al. Management of intramedullary spinal cord tumors. Radiology 1980;135(2):473–9.
101. Constantini S, MD, Allen JC, Rorke LB, Freed D, Epstein FJ. Radical excision of intramedullary spinal cord tumors: surgical morbidity and long-term follow-up evaluation in 164 children and young adults. J Neurosurg 2000;93:(Suppl. 2):183–93.
102. Jyothirmayi R, MJ, Nair MK, Rajan B. Conservative surgery and radiotherapy in the treatment of spinal cord astrocytoma. J Neurooncol 1997;33:205–22.
103. Shirato H, KT, Hida K, Koyanagi I, Iwasaki Y, Miyasaka K, et al. The role of radiotherapy in the management of spinal cord glioma. Int J Rad Oncol Biol Phys 1995;33:323–8.
104. Whitaker SJ, et al. Postoperative radiotherapy in the management of spinal cord ependymoma. J Neurosurg 1991;74(5):720–8.
105. Guidetti B, Mercuri S, Vagnozzi R. Long-term results of the surgical treatment of 129 intramedullary spinal gliomas. J Neurosurg 1981;54(3):323–30.
106. McLaughlin MP, BJ, Marcua RB, Maria BL, Mickle PJ, Kedar A. Outcome after radiotherapy of primary spinal cord glial tumors. Rad Oncol Invest 1998;6:276–80.
107. Sgouros S, MC, Jackowski A. Spinal ependymomas-the value of postoperative radiotherapy for residual disease contro. Br J Neurosurg 1996;10:559–66.
108. Isaacson SR. Radiation therapy and the management of intramedullary spinal cord tumors. J Neurooncol 2000;47(3):231–8.
109. Finlay JL, et al. Randomized phase III trial in childhood high-grade astrocytoma comparing vincristine, lomustine, and prednisone with the eight-drugs-in-1-day regimen. Childrens Cancer Group. J Clin Oncol 1995;13(1):112–23.

110. Balmaceda C. Chemotherapy for intramedullary spinal cord tumors. J Neurooncol 2000; 47(3):293–307.
111. Packer RJ, et al. Carboplatin and vincristine for recurrent and newly diagnosed low-grade gliomas of childhood. J Clin Oncol 1993;11(5):850–6.
112. Lowis SP, et al. Chemotherapy for spinal cord astrocytoma: can natural history be modified? Childs Nerv Syst 1998;14(7):317–21.
113. Doireau V, et al. Chemotherapy for unresectable and recurrent intramedullary glial tumours in children. Brain Tumours Subcommittee of the French Society of Paediatric Oncology (SFOP). Br J Cancer 1999;81(5):835–40.
114. Hoshimaru M, et al. Results of microsurgical treatment for intramedullary spinal cord ependymomas: analysis of 36 cases. Neurosurgery 1999;44(2):264–9.
115. Rawlings CEd, et al. Ependymomas: a clinicopathologic study. Surg Neurol 1988;29(4):271–81.
116. DeVivo MJ, et al. Cause of death for patients with spinal cord injuries. Arch Intern Med 1989;149(8):1761–6.
117. Sandler HM, et al. Spinal cord astrocytomas: results of therapy [see comments]. Neurosurgery 1992;30(4):490–3.
118. Hardison HH, et al. Outcome of children with primary intramedullary spinal cord tumors. Childs Nerv Syst 1987;3(2):89–92.
119. Epstein F. Surgical management of intramedullary spinal cord tumors: functional outcome and sources of morbidity (Comments). Neurosurgery 1994;35:69–76.
120. Merchant TE, et al. High-grade pediatric spinal cord tumors [In Process Citation]. Pediatr Neurosurg 1999;30(1):1–5.

11 Extraaxial Brain Tumors

NADER POURATIAN • ASHOK R. ASTHAGIRI • DAVID SCHIFF • JASON P. SHEEHAN

Introduction

Extraaxial brain tumors (EBTs) include an array of tumors that arise from structures and tissues directly adjacent to the brain, including the meninges, nerve sheaths, and the pituitary gland, which give rise to meningiomas, schwannomas, and pituitary adenomas, respectively. As a group, they account for over 50% of all brain tumors diagnosed in the United States and, therefore, a large proportion of brain tumors seen by neurologists and neurosurgeons.[1] In fact, meningiomas (which account for 32.1% of all brain tumors) are the most common brain tumor diagnosed in patients greater than 34 years of age and pituitary adenomas (8.4% of all brain tumors) are the most common brain tumor diagnosed in patients between 20 and 34 years of age.[1] While these tumors are usually benign, they can be associated with significant morbidity and, rarely, mortality, because of their prevalence and occasionally malignant behavior. In this chapter, we discuss the current management of extraaxial brain tumors, with particular emphasis on the three major types of EBTs, including meningiomas, schwanommas, and pituitary adenomas. General principles of diagnosis, management, and treatment can be extrapolated to other EBTs, such as craniopharygiomas and chordomas. We consider recent advances in the diagnosis and treatment of these tumors that have either impacted or may prospectively impact the management of patients.

Incidence and Epidemiology

EBTs account for three out of the four most common primary brain tumors diagnosed in the United States. According to the Central Brain Tumor Registry of the United States (CBTRUS), the incidence of EBTs is 8.3 cases per 100,000 person-years.[1] Meningiomas, with an incidence of 5.3 per 100,000 person-years, are the single most common brain tumor histology diagnosed in the United States, occurring in nearly twice as many patients as high-grade gliomas. The incidence of meningiomas is 2.2 times greater in females than males. Despite their classical presentation in middle-aged women, the incidence steadily increases with age (i.e., greatest incidence in the 85+ age group). While there is no reported racial predilection in the United States, there is an increased incidence in the Polynesian population, who more frequently have multiple and larger tumors than other populations.[2]

Nerve sheath tumors and pituitary tumors are the third and fourth most common brain tumors after meningiomas and glioblastoma (accounting for 9.0% and 8.4% of brain tumors, respectively). Although these tumors are the most common brain tumors diagnosed in patients 20 to 34 years of age, their incidence actually peaks in the 65 to 74-year-old age group. Neither tumor has different gender-specific incidence rates, but pituitary tumors are significantly more likely to be diagnosed in blacks, whereas vestibular schwannomas are significantly more likely to be identified in whites.[1]

Like gliomas, the incidence of EBTs has increased steadily over the last decade, presumably due to an increased rate of diagnosis rather than a true increase in incidence.[3] The increased availability and use of neuroimaging modalities have significantly increased the detection of incidental intracranial pathologies, including meningiomas and vestibular schwannomas.[4] The increased incidence is also partially attributed to an increased willingness of the medical community to pursue a diagnosis and treatment in older patients.[5]

Many risk factors have been suggested for EBTs. Of these, radiation exposure is the only universally accepted factor placing people at risk for meningioma induction.[6] This concept gained wide acceptance after Modan and colleagues retrospectively discovered a four-fold increase in the incidence of meningiomas among children treated with the Kienbock-Adamson protocol for tinea capitis, a low dose radiation treatment targeting the scalp.[7] Low-dose radiation-induced meningiomas are those associated with exposure to less than 10 Gy, but meningiomas have been induced by as little as 1 to 2 Gy. Higher radiation doses are associated with a decrease in latency of meningioma induction.[8]

Other risk factors for meningiomas have also been explored. One of the early postulates was that head injury caused meningiomas. Associations between head trauma (especially in young males 10 to 19 years of age) and meningiomas have been reported, with a latency of 15 to 24 years.[9,10] The evidence supporting this hypothesis is inconsistent and the seemingly conflicting data leaves no definitive proof of a causal relationship between head injury and the subsequent development of meningiomas. The female predilection of meningiomas suggests that female sex hormones may also be a risk factor for tumorigenesis. This theory was bolstered by the identification of estrogen and progesterone receptors on subsets of meningiomas. Tumors expressing progesterone receptors (PR+) behave in a more benign clinical fashion and are less likely to recur. Those expressing estrogen receptors or lacking progesterone receptors display more frequent genotypic alterations and karyotype abnormalities consistent with more aggressive meningiomas.[11] Despite these findings, the evidence that exogenous hormones affect tumor frequency is mixed. Blitshteyn and colleagues retrospectively reviewed records from 355,318 women at the Mayo Clinic between 1993 and 2003 and found that women with either current or past hormone replacement therapy (HRT) had a 2.2-fold risk of developing meningiomas.[12] A much smaller population-based case-control study failed to find such an association.[13] The fact that receptor status affects gene expression profiles, particularly of those near the *NF2* gene locus, which has been implicated in meningioma tumorigenesis, suggests that further examination into the effect of female sex hormones may be warranted.[14] Increased body mass index (BMI) has also been associated with a greater incidence of meningiomas.[15,16] The association between increased BMI and meningioma incidence may be mediated by aromatase in adipose tissue which increases circulating estrogen levels.

Recently, many studies have studied the impact of mobile phone use on tumor incidence. Hardell and colleagues performed a meta-analysis of such studies and concluded that there is a slight statistically significant increased risk for development of glioma (odds ratio [OR] = 2.0, 95% confidence interval [CI] = 1.2 to 3.4) and vestibular schwanomma (OR = 2.4, 95% CI = 1.1 to 5.3), but not meningiomas, using a greater than or equal to 10 years latency period.[17]

Presentation

Besides those tumors discovered incidentally, EBTs most often present with headache, focal neurologic deficit, or seizures (in up to 50% of patients). Tumors produce symptoms by one of four major mechanisms: (1) local pressure from tumor mass and/or edema disrupting function of adjacent normal tissue; (2) intracranial hypertension due to mass, ventricular outlet obstruction (e.g., posterior fossa meningiomas), or dural venous sinus obstruction (e.g., parasagittal meningiomas); (3) compression, infiltration, and destruction of neurons; and (4) hypersecretory syndromes, specifically in the case of functional pituitary adenomas, due to overproduction of pituitary hormones.

The precise symptomatology with which a tumor presents depends on its location and size. The most common locations of meningiomas in descending order of frequency are: convexity, parasagittal, sphenoid and middle cranial fossa, frontal base and posterior fossa, cerebellar convexity, cerebellopontine angle, intraventricular, and clivus. Schwannomas arise most commonly from the vestibular component of the vestibulocochlear nerve (>90%), sensory division of the trigeminal nerve (1% to 10%), facial nerve (1%), nerves of the jugular foramen (glossopharyngeal, vagus, and spinal accessory nerve), hypoglossal nerve, extraocular nerves, and the olfactory nerve. The various syndromes with which EBTs present are outlined in Tables 11-1 through 11-3.

Because EBTs are generally benign, slow-growing tumors, the insidious onset of symptoms related to EBTs may conceal the diagnosis for years. The patient's

TABLE 11-1 Meningioma Location and Associated Typical Clinical Presentations

Parasagittal and falcine meningiomas	*Anterior 1/3*	Headache and mental status changes
	Middle 1/3	Jacksonian seizures and progressive hemiparesis
	Posterior 1/3	Headache, visual symptoms, seizures, or mental status changes
Sphenoid wing meningiomas	*Lateral / pterional*	Similar to convexity tumors
	Middle 1/3 (alar)	Hemiparesis / dysphasia
	Medial (clinoidal)	Visual acuity/field disturbance due to optic nerve compression, proptosis, cranial nerve dysfunction (III,IV,V,VI)
Olfactory groove		Foster-Kennedy syndrome (anosmia, ipsilateral optic atrophy with contralateral papilledema), frontal lobe syndromes / mental status changes, urinary incontinence, seizure
Tuberculum sella / suprasellar		Visual acuity/field disturbance, anosmia, hydrocephalus, endocrinologic syndromes
Cavernous sinus		Cranial nerve deficits (III,IV,V,VI)
Cerebellopontine angle		Hearing loss, facial pain / numbness / weakness / spasm, headaches, cerebellar signs
Foramen magnum		Unilateral cervical pain, extremity motor and sensory loss (clockwise involvement), cold and clumsy hands with intrinsic hand atrophy
Petroclival		Hearing loss, vertigo, tinnitus, facial pain, diplopia, cranial nerve deficits (V,VI,VII,VII)

TABLE 11-2 Intracranial Schwannomas: Typical Clinical Presentation

Vestibular	Unilateral sensory hearing loss, tinnitus, disequilibrium
Trigeminal	Trigeminal nerve dysfunction (numbness, pain), headache, diplopia, hearing loss/tinnitus
Facial	Hearing loss, facial paralysis (may be acute), facial pain, hemifacial spasm, tinnitus, vertigo
Jugular foramen	Cranial nerve palsies (IX,X,XI)
Accessory nerve	Chronic neck and shoulder pain, muscle spasms
Hypoglossal	Headache, cranial nerve dysfunction (IX,X,XI), limb weakness

TABLE 11-3 Pituitary Adenomas: Typical Clinical Presentation

Nonfunctioning adenoma	Headache, bitemporal hemianopia, diplopia, dysmenorrhea, fatigue
Prolactinoma	Amenorrhea, lactation, impotence
Cushing disease	Weight gain, hypertension, diabetes mellitus, moon facies, supraclavicular fat pads, central obesity, facial plethora, abdominal striae, muscle weakness, osteoporosis
Acromegaly	Increasing hand/foot size, prominent brow/jaw, diabetes mellitus, carpal tunnel syndrome
TSH-secreting adenoma	Signs and symptoms consistent with hyperthyroidism

presenting symptoms and imaging characteristics critically impact management: both neurosurgeons and neurologists are likely to recommend surgical intervention in patients presenting with signs and symptoms attributable to mass effect or intracranial hypertension but may consider observation or other minimally invasive neurosurgical approaches for asymptomatic patients.

Diagnosis

Proper identification of tumor type and thorough imaging characterization is critical prior to rendering any treatment, especially in light of options for minimally invasive treatments, such as stereotactic radiosurgery. Even for those contemplating microsurgical excision, it is advantageous for the treating neurosurgeon to have detailed knowledge of an individual patient's unique anatomy (structural and vascular) and tumor extension.

MENINGIOMAS

The classic radiographic features of meningiomas include presence of a broad dural base, dural tails, diffuse contrast enhancement, and the presence of an arachnoid plane.[18] These criteria can help distinguish between a CP angle meningioma and a vestibular schwannoma (Figure 11-1). Using these classic criteria, MRI has a sensitivity and specificity of 98% and 97%, respectively. However, the sensitivity and positive-predictive value of conventional MRI drops significantly in high-grade (i.e., atypical and malignant) meningiomas.[19] MR spectroscopy, which displays distinct peaks for various intratumoral metabolites including choline, creatine, N-acetyl-aspartate (NAA), and lactate, can more definitively identify meningiomas by identifying an alanine peak (unique to meningiomas) and an increased glutamate/creatine ratio.[20] Moreover, atypical meningiomas (WHO grade II) are much more likely to have a lactate peak (a marker of proliferation) than WHO grade I tumors.[21]

MR venograms, which assess the patency of dural-based blood sinuses (e.g., superior sagittal sinus in parasagittal/falcine meningiomas), have also become

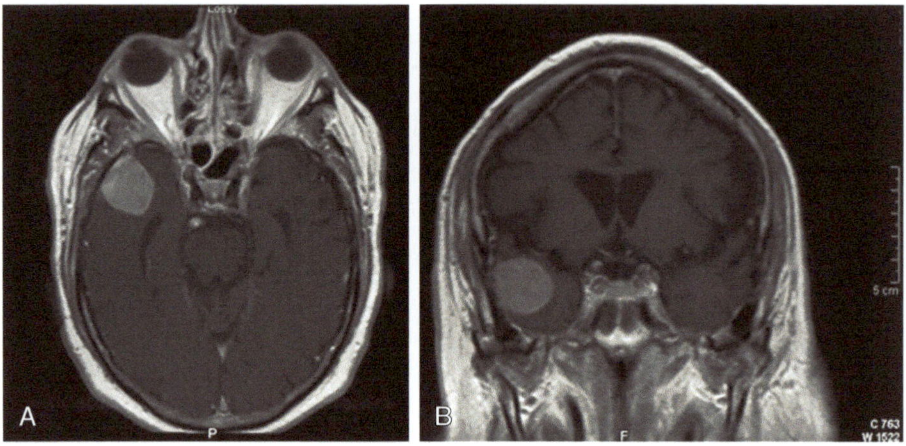

Figure 11-1 Axial **(A)** and coronal **(B)** T1-weighted postcontrast MRIs of a patient with a meningioma. This middle cranial fossa meningioma demonstrates a broad-based dural attachment.

vital for guiding timing of treatment and preoperative planning. Cerebral venous anatomy can be challenging to assess noninvasively. It is critical for the surgeon to assess anatomic variation and patency in order to know which veins must be protected during surgery. As such, cerebral angiography remains the gold standard for assessing arterial supply and venous outflow; it has the added benefit of allowing for direct preoperative tumor embolization.

SCHWANNOMAS

The imaging evaluation of schwannomas includes conventional MR sequences with contrast. Like meningiomas, schwanommas are extraaxial lesions that enhance diffusely. In contrast, schwannomas generally do not have dural tails but rather follow the course of cranial nerves along the skull base, such as into the internal auditory meatus and Meckel's cave (Figure 11-2). Besides imaging appearance, brainstem auditory evoked responses (BAERs) are a critical diagnostic test for management planning. While for large tumors with brainstem compression it is nearly impossible to preserve hearing, with smaller tumors there is a great interest to preserve functional hearing.

PITUITARY TUMORS

Pituitary tumors are the most common tumor of the sellar region, accounting for over 90% of such lesions. Unlike other EBTs, because of the hypervascularity of the pituitary gland, microadenomas (i.e., pituitary adenomas < 10mm) are often identified by their lack of contrast enhancement while the remainder of the gland enhances briskly (Figure 11-3). Still, in some cases, especially in Cushing disease, an adenoma cannot be identified on MRI despite biochemical evidence of an ACTH-secreting pituitary adenoma. Dynamic pituitary MRI, which uses multiple sequential image acquisition following gadolinium intravenous contrast,

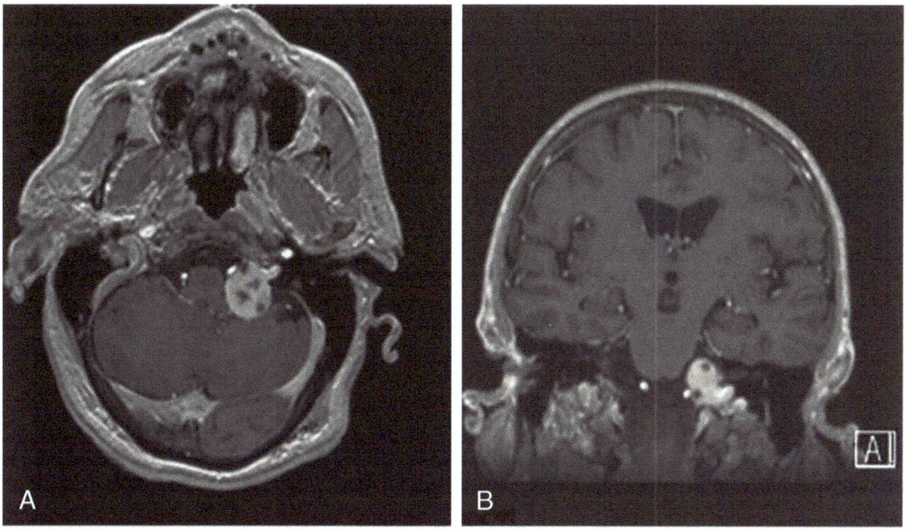

Figure 11-2 Axial **(A)** and coronal **(B)** T1-weighted postcontrast MRIs of a patient with a vestibular schwannoma. Vestibular schwannoma demonstrates typical extension into the internal audititory canal.

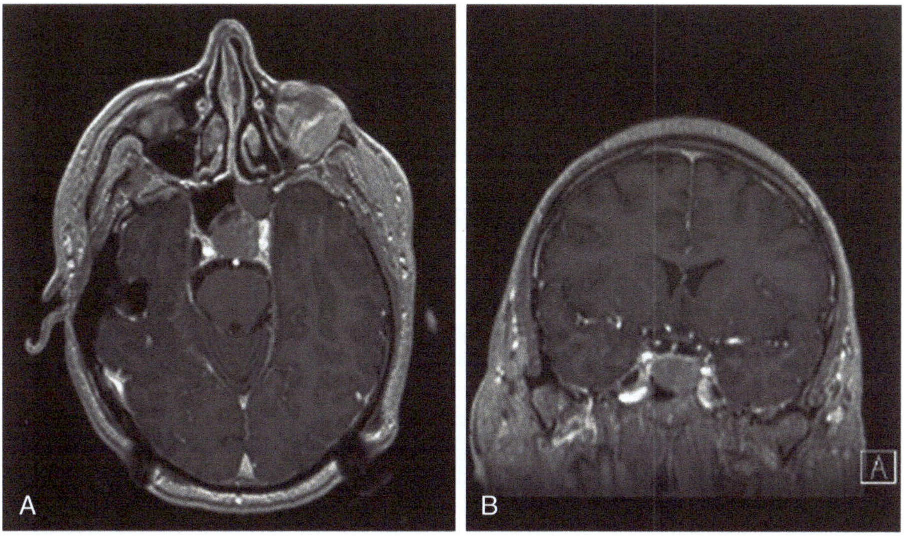

Figure 11-3 Axial **(A)** and coronal **(B)** T1-weighted postcontrast MRIs of a patient with a nonfunctioning pituitary adenoma.

significantly increases adenoma detection to nearly 100%, a rate much higher than the 50% to 60% rate reported for nondynamic MRI.[22]

In addition to imaging, all patients with sellar or suprasellar lesions need thorough biochemical evaluation of their hypothalamic-pituitary axis, which can provide insight into the nature of an otherwise seemingly nonfunctional pituitary tumor. In addition to biochemical evaluation of circulating hormone levels in the peripheral blood, inferior petrosal sinus sampling (IPSS) has become an integral part of the evaluation of patients with suspected Cushing disease. Comparing central-to-peripheral ratios of ACTH levels at baseline and in response to corticotrophin releasing hormone (CRH) (≥ 2.0 and ≥ 3.0, respectively) is very sensitive for confirming a "central" etiology for Cushing syndrome, or Cushing disease.[23]

Management

The management of EBTs may include: (1) observation, (2) open microsurgery, (3) stereotactic radiosurgery, (4) fractionated radiotherapy (XRT), or fractionated stereotactic radiotherapy (FSRT), (5) chemotherapy, or combinations thereof. Again, discussion of management is limited to the three most common EBTs: meningiomas, vestibular schwanommas, and pituitary adenomas, but general principles can be extrapolated to other EBTs.

OBSERVATION

Expectant management potentially provides patients with an overall improved quality of life (QOL) for the duration of the disease by not exposing them to the morbidity associated with other treatment paradigms.[24] The morbidity of surgery can be quite significant; in one study, among patients older than age 70 years who underwent operation for asymptomatic meningioma, the neurological morbidity rate was 23.3%.[25] Expectant management is therefore particularly pertinent to older patients with incidentally discovered and asymptomatic tumors.

The majority of incidental meningiomas show minimal growth. This is particularly true for heavily calcified meninigiomas. Thus, they may be observed without surgical intervention unless specific symptoms appear. Tumor growth is associated with patient age, with tumors in younger patients having a shorter doubling time than in older patients. While radiological features, such as calcification or T2 signal hypointensity or isointensity, may predict decreased growth potential, initial tumor size does not correlate with growth rate.[26] Despite minimal growth in most tumors, asymptomatic tumors must be followed: in one study of 40 patients with incidental meningiomas, 33% of tumors grew during a mean follow-up of 32 months, and 36% of patients had symptomatic progression.[27]

Like incidental meningiomas, there is a place for expectant management of schwannomas. Small and medium-sized vestibular schwannomas that are found incidentally (accounting for approximately 10% of all vestibular schwannomas and found in up to 0.02% of the general population) may have a more benign nature and be less likely to require intervention.[28,29] In one series, conservatively managed schwannomas either did not grow or regressed in 42% of patients and had an overall average growth rate of 0.91 mm per year.[30] Conservative management can be successful in up to 85% of patients selected for expectant management.[31] First-year growth rate is an good predictor of future growth, and therefore must be monitored, if tumors are to be managed conservatively, to determine whether intervention will be necessary.[32] The indications for intervention should be based on a combination of rapid tumor growth with the development of symptoms.[30]

In patients older than 65 years with vestibular schwannomas, these tumors may not require surgical intervention.

Incidental pituitary tumors, or pituitary "incidentalomas," can also be managed without surgical intervention. Patients with pituitary incidentalomas usually follow a benign course for at least 6 years, not requiring neurosurgical intervention as long as clinical observation is continued.[33] Generally, only those that are greater than 10 mm (macroadenomas) enlarge or cause complications and may require closer clinical observation or upfront surgery. Regardless of size, patients who are treated conservatively should undergo biochemical assessment and ophthalmological examination, since occult endocrine dysfunction or visual field defects may be present at the time a pituitary incidentaloma is detected.[33–35]

Expectant management carries other risks, including malignant degeneration, interval tumor growth making subsequent resection more difficult, and development of an irreversible neurologic deficit. Close clinical, biochemical and radiologic monitoring is necessary if expectant management is pursued.

MICROSURGICAL RESECTION

With the exception of prolactin-secreting pituitary adenomas, surgical resection is the mainstay of treatment of EBTs, because most are benign tumors for which surgical resection can be "curative," and because surgical excision secures a tissue diagnosis.

Meningiomas

The importance of complete surgical excision for meningiomas has been well documented for over 50 years. In 1957, Simpson retrospectively reviewed the postoperative course of 265 patients with meningiomas, 55 of whom experienced recurrences (21%). Patients with a gross total resection of tumor, dural attachments, and abnormal bone (grade I excision) had a recurrence rate of 9%, those with gross total excision with coagulation of dural attachments (grade II) had a recurrence rate of 19%, those with gross total excision without coagulation of dural attachments (grade III) had a recurrent rate of 29%, and those with partial resection (grade IV) had a recurrence rate of 44%.[36] These recurrence rates most likely are underestimates since this study was conducted in the pre-CT and pre-MRI era. Nonetheless, these findings highlight the fact that surgical excision is the most important factor in the prevention of recurrence. Tumors that cannot be totally excised because of their adjacency to critical structures such as cranial nerves and sinuses (e.g., medial sphenoid wing, petroclival, clinoidal, and tentorial-based tumors, and posterior parasagittal lesions, respectively) therefore are at highest risk for tumor recurrence. The highest recurrence rates are found for patients with sphenoid wing meningiomas(>20%), parasagittal meningiomas (8% to 24%), and suprasellar meningiomas (5% to 10%). In contrast, convexity meningiomas, which are relatively easily excisable, have reported recurrence-free rates at 5,10, and 15 years of 93%, 80%, and 68%, respectively.[37] Other risk factors for recurrence include histopathologic findings of increased mitosis/Ki-67 labeling index, focal necrosis, nuclear pleomorphism, prominent nucleoli, syncytial tumors, the presence of brain invasion, and loss of 1p36.1-p34.[38,39] Interestingly, "high-risk tumors" occur more frequently at the brain surface than at the cranial base, suggesting that the tendency of cranial base meningiomas to recur depends on surgical rather than biological factors.[40]

The morbidity of microsurgical excision, like extent of resection, is intimately related to tumor location. Easily accessible tumors, such as convexity, lateral and middle third sphenoid wing meningiomas, and anterior third parasagittal and falcine meningiomas, are amenable to complete resection and associated with low morbidity (10% of patients with neurologic sequelae) and mortality (0 to 3%). Neurologic sequelae associated with these resections typically manifest secondary to compromise of adjacent cerebrovascular structures, immediate postoperative edema, and epilepsy. Tumors of the skull base, tentorium, foramen magnum, and other difficult locations are associated with significantly higher morbidity and mortality due to associations with cranial nerves and proximal cerebral vessels. Permanent neurologic deficit ascribed to cranial nerve dysfunction has been reported in a wide range (18% to 86%).[41] The highest of these complication rates are typically associated with petroclival and cavernous sinus meningiomas, especially in cases where a complete resection is performed. Preoperative embolization has led to decreased morbidity in patients in whom the tumor blood supply may be difficult to access at the time of surgery.

Despite improvements in microsurgical techniques, image guidance and perioperative critical/medical care, mortality rates in large series remain at 1% to 14%.[42,43] Factors increasing mortality include poor preoperative clinical condition, compressive symptoms from tumor, older age, incomplete tumor removal, pulmonary embolism, and intracranial hemorrhage.[44]

Vestibular Schwannomas

The introduction of the operating microscope, more sensitive diagnostic imaging, and intraoperative facial and cochlear monitoring have steadily decreased the morbidity and mortality associated with resection of vestibular schwannomas. In a meta-analysis of 16 studies including 5005 patients undergoing microsurgery for sporadic unilateral vestibular schwannomas, tumor resection was complete in 96% of cases, with a mortality rate of 0.63%. The most common nonneurologic complication was cerebrospinal fluid leak, which occurred in 6.0% of patients.[45] The challenge of surgical resection lies in preserving facial nerve and auditory function. Detailed evaluation of individual large series shows preservation of facial nerve function is inversely proportional to tumor size. Indeed, when evaluating facial nerve preservation after resection of intracanalicular lesions alone, multiple studies have reported 100% postoperative grade I House-Brackmann function.[46,47] Resection of small tumors (<2.0 cm), medium sized tumors (2.0 to 3.9 cm), and large tumors (>4.0 cm) is associated with a 95%–97%, 61%–73%, and 28%–57% preservation of grade I or II House-Brackmann function, respectively.[48–50] The suboccipital and translabyrinthine approaches afford comparable and excellent results as compared to the middle fossa approach in which increased manipulation of the superiorly located facial nerve in the internal auditory canal may account for a higher risk to facial nerve function.

The importance of preserving serviceable ipsilateral hearing is also paramount. Risk to serviceable auditory function is directly related to tumor size and operative approach. Functional ipsilateral hearing is retained in 29% to 60% of cases, primarily among tumors less than 3 cm in size, with a precipitous decline in hearing preservation rates in larger tumors.[47,51,52] Resection of purely intracanalicular tumors is associated with a 57% to 82% preservation of ipsilateral serviceable auditory function.[46,47] The translabyrinthine approach, on the other hand, with its destruction of the otic capsule, is not compatible with hearing preservation but is often necessary to approach large CP angle tumors that otherwise would require excessive retraction and manipulation of the cerebellum.

Pituitary Adenomas

Surgical decompression remains the treatment of choice for nonfunctioning pituitary adenomas as well as for symptomatic craniopharyngiomas and Rathke cleft cysts. With the exception of craniopharyngiomas, the most common surgical approach to these tumors is a transsphenoidal procedure. Transsphenoidal surgery yields low morbidity and mortality rates, and leads to improvement in visual symptoms in 87% to 90% of cases.[53] The recent development of the endoscopic transsphenoidal approach to the pituitary region offers potential advantages over traditional surgical approaches because of its minimal invasiveness and panoramic visualization. The wider operating field of vision and angled views increase the likelihood of a more thorough and safer tumor removal and preservation of normal gland. Despite its advantages, the endoscopic approach does not allow for three-dimensional visualization and requires the surgeon to operate at an increased working distance. Moreover, the improved visualization requires a larger sellar opening, which makes it more difficult to repair CSF leaks when they occur. For suprasellar tumors that are difficult to resect transsphenoidally, a variety of transcranial approaches (pterional, subfrontal, anterior interhemispheric, and transcallosal) allow adequate visualization and decompression of the optic nerves and chiasm. Variations of the pterional craniotomy include resection of the orbital rim and zygoma to provide a more basal view and better access to suprasellar tumors.

Apart from prolactinomas, surgical resection remains the primary treatment for functional pituitary adenomas. Surgical excision is successful in the majority of patients, with long-term remission rates for Cushing disease ranging from 50% to 98%, for acromegaly ranging from 50% to 85%, and for TSH adenomas ranging from 80% to 91%.[54–57] Although pharmacological therapy with a dopamine agonist is the primary and most efficacious treatment for prolactinomas, 10% to 20% of patients fail medical therapy, either because they are intolerant of the drugs (e.g., nausea, headache, fatigue, orthostatic hypotension, and depression) or because their tumors are refractory to pharmacological therapy (despite increasing doses).[58,59] In these cases, transsphenoidal surgery can obtain remission in up to 91% of patients with microprolactinomas.[60]

Following surgery, new endocrine deficits have been reported in up to 40% of patients.[61] Immediate postoperative polyuria (diabetes insipidus) may occur in up to 30% of patients, but the majority of cases resolve within the first week following surgery. Delayed hyponatremia, occurring most often 7 to 10 days after surgery, is evident in 1% to 9% of patients.[62] Worsening of preoperative visual function is seen in 1% to 4% of patients. Anatomic complications include nasal septal perforations (7%) and chronic sinusitis. Postoperative cerebrospinal fluid leaks and meningitis occur in 0.5% to 3.9% of cases.[61,63] Adrenal insufficiency often follows surgery, and patients may require steroid replacement therapy for 6 to 12 months postoperatively.[61]

In 10% to 20% of pituitary adenoma patients, tumors recur within 10 years following surgical intervention.[18,64] Subtotal resection and cavernous sinus invasion are prognostic of recurrence.[18] Patients with functional adenomas need to be followed carefully for recurrence, which can occur more than 10 years after surgery. In acromegalics who have undergone transsphenoidal surgery, up to 8% of patients recur within 10 years, of whom up to 80% again achieve remission with repeat transsphenoidal surgery.[65] Recurrence rates for Cushing disease generally range between 5% and 15%, with a median time to recurrence of 33 to 59 months.[55,66,67]

RADIOSURGERY

Stereotactic radiosurgery (SRS) allows relatively safe treatment of those EBTs for which surgical resection is associated with exceedingly high rates of morbidity and mortality or in which surgical resection fails to achieve remission. SRS, which includes Gamma Knife surgery (GKS), modified linear accelerator-based technologies (LINAC), and the proton beam devices, delivers a high dose of radiation in 1 to 5 sessions to a stereotactically-defined target by converging multiple beams of ionizing radiation. By creating a steep radiation dose fall-off around the target, SRS minimizes damage to surrounding structures. Like fractionated radiotherapy, SRS takes advantage of the natural difference in susceptibility of pathological and normal tissue due to differences in mitotic activity. By delivering the radiation dose in less than or equal to 5 sessions, SRS improves the biological effectiveness of the target dose by 2.5 to 3 times that of the same dose delivered in a fractionated manner. Little is known about the pathophysiological mechanisms of SRS-mediated tumor control at the cellular level. Tumor control is mediated, at least in part, by inducing DNA damage and apoptosis in proliferating cells and altering the microvascular supply of tumors. For example, reduced blood flow has been seen over time in meningiomas after GKS.[68–70] SRS does not, however, generally cause tumor necrosis (which requires higher radiation doses than are typically used). The radiobiology of SRS is fundamentally different from that of fractionated radiation therapy, and this difference appears in part to be due to vascular changes following radiosurgery.

Meningiomas

The efficacy and relative safety of SRS have dramatically changed its indications. While it was once thought that microsurgical resection should always precede SRS, SRS is now considered a reasonable first-line treatment for surgically inaccessible lesions that possess the typical imaging characteristics of meningiomas. For example, in patients with parasagittal meningiomas less than 3 cm in maximal diameter (<15 cc), no progressive neurological sequelae, and minimal associated peritumoral edema, radiosurgery is a reasonable first choice. Patients with atypical findings on MRI or CT, however, should undergo surgery to obtain a histological diagnosis. For patients with larger lesions or those with progressive neurological symptoms, resection followed by radiosurgery can be performed. SRS can be used to treat residual tumor attached to still patent vascular or neural structures, allowing less radical microsurgical resection and a lower incidence of morbidity. For GKS, a distance of at least 5 mm between the tumor and the optic apparatus is ideal. With a thin cut stereotactic planning MRI and plugging, GKS can be used to treat lesions within 2 mm of the optic apparatus.

Most groups use a prescription dose of 15 to 20 Gy. In determining dose, one must not only consider tumor dose but also the radiation tolerance of adjacent structures, including cranial nerves and vasculature. Lower doses of 13 or 14 Gy are therefore often used for treating cavernous sinus meningiomas, due to the adjacency of critical structures such as the optic apparatus. Some argue that a lower margin dose of 12 Gy affords the same degree of tumor control with a reduced risk of complications.[71] Unacceptably high rates of failure to control tumor growth have been reported with margin doses of 10 Gy or less.[72]

Outcomes for GKS treatment of skull base meningiomas have been reported extensively. Most reports have a median follow-up of approximately 3 years and report tumor control rates between 91% and 100%, with tumor shrinkage reported in 23% to 73% of treated skull base meningiomas.[73–76] Treatment success is associated with tumor volumes less than 10.0 cc, female gender, a high conformality index, and dural tail inclusion in the treatment plan.[77] Kondziolka and colleagues additionally note that local tumor progression after radiosurgery is related to a history of prior resection and multiple meningiomas.[78]

While SRS appears to work very well for typical meningiomas, the results for atypical and malignant meningiomas are less favorable. Harris and colleagues reported 5-year progression-free survival rates of 83% and 72% for atypical and malignant meningiomas, respectively.[79] Kreil and colleagues reported less favorable results, reporting 5-year actuarial control rate of 49% in atypical meningiomas and 0% in malignant meningiomas.[80] Five-year overall survival rates vary between 59% and 76% in patients with atypical meningiomas and 0% and 59% in patients with malignant meningiomas.[79,81,82]

In addition to radiographic control, SRS can often improve cranial nerve function after treatment of skull base meningiomas. Pollock and colleagues reported that 12 out of 38 patients who presented with cranial neuropathies associated with cavernous sinus meningiomas had improvement in cranial nerve function on follow-up.[83] Roche and colleagues reported similar success in GKS-treated petroclival meningiomas: 13 out of 32 patients treated with GKS for petroclival meningiomas had clinical improvement in cranial nerve dysfunction.[75] Kreil and colleagues reported that 96% of patients with skull-based meningiomas treated with GKS had improved or stable neurological status, with improvement noted in a broad range of areas including vision and other cranial nerve functions, hemiparesis, ataxia, vertigo, seizures, and exophthalmus.[71]

Vestibular Schwannomas

Like meningiomas, SRS is used both as a first-line treatment and as a treatment of residual or progressive disease in patients with schwannomas. High rates of tumor control have been reported with a margin dose of 12 Gy, although some suggest a margin dose as low as 10 Gy may be adequate.[84] In order to obtain an adequate margin dose and a maximum dose within accepted limits (20 to 25 Gy), only tumors measuring up to 30 mm should be treated with SRS (although treatment of tumors up to 40 mm has been reported).[85] Hasegawa and colleagues have reported an 87% to 92% 10-year progression-free survival (PFS).[86] Failure of treatment usually occurred within 3 years. Tumor volume thresholds of both 8 ml and

15 ml as well as tumors not compressing the brainstem and deviating the fourth ventricle have been identified as prognostic factors for PFS.[86,87] The outcome in terms of postradiosurgical volume reduction in patients who had prior microsurgery is worse than those who were primarily treated with Gamma Knife surgery. This difference is often attributed to increased difficulty with accurate targeting in those who have undergone prior microsurgery. Patients who fail SRS for vestibular schwannomas, either due to tumor enlargement or radiation-related edema, usually require further surgical intervention, including resection or shunting.

As with microsurgery, the safety of SRS must consider hearing preservation and facial nerve palsies. When tumors are treated with a marginal dose of 13 Gy or less, the hearing preservation rate is 58% to 68%, transient facial palsy develops at a rate of 1%, and facial numbness develops at a rate of 2%.[86,87] Hearing loss usually occurs within the first 2 years of treatment, but may occur up to 8 years after treatment. The trigeminal nerve is affected in a variety of ways in 33% of patients; a mild hypesthesia is most common. The dose to the brainstem is a more informative predictor of postradiosurgical cranial neuropathy than the length of the nerve that is irradiated; prior resection increases the risk of late cranial neuropathies after radiosurgery.[84]

Pituitary Adenomas

For pituitary adenomas, radiosurgery can be administered postoperatively as adjuvant therapy to inhibit recurrent growth, or later, when clinical symptoms, laboratory results, or radiographic signs indicate recurrence. It is rarely, if ever, used as first-line treatment. It may also be utilized postoperatively to treat known residual tumor following incomplete resection. Radiosurgery is meant not only to prevent tumor growth, but also to normalize hormone overproduction in functional adenomas.

Most series define tumor control as either an unchanged or decreased volume on follow-up radiological imaging studies. A weighted average tumor control rate for all published series detailing such findings and encompassing a total of 1283 patients was 96%, with results of individual studies ranging between 83% and 100%.[88]

Endocrine outcomes after SRS for pituitary adenomas are reasonable and demonstrate a role for SRS in the management of these tumors. In the largest series of patients treated with GKS for Cushing disease (N=90), endocrine remission was achieved in 54% of patients at an average of 13 months after treatment. Recurrence occurred in 20% of patients after an average of 27 months.[89] Remission rates for acromegaly treated with SRS vary between 20% and 96% in studies with at least 10 patients with 2 years of follow-up.[88] Results for prolactinomas treated with SRS are just as variable, with remission rates varying between 0% and 84%.[88] Some of the variability in outcomes for acromegaly and prolactinomas may be attributable to the use of somatostatin analogues and dopamine agonists, respectively. Three separate reports have found a negative association between endocrine remission and the use of medical therapy at the time of SRS.[90–92] These medical therapies for secretory pituitary adenomas likely not only reduce hormone synthesis and secretion but also reduce the metabolism and cell cycling of these tumors, thereby making them less susceptible to radiation effects. Therefore, in preparation for radiosurgery, many centers now recommend a temporary cessation of antisecretory medications in the perioperative time period (starting 2 months before SRS). Stopping antisecretory medication is not without risks, possibly allowing the adenoma to enlarge and thereby increasing the risk of radiosurgery to adjacent structures (e.g., the optic apparatus), necessitating a lower prescription dose, and making effective radiosurgical treatment more difficult.

Hypopituitarism in the postradiosurgical population is multifactorial in etiology and related to radiosurgery as well as age-related changes and prior treatments (e.g., microsurgery and radiotherapy). The true rate of delayed hypopituitarism at our radiosurgical center is approximately 20% to 30%. Long-term endocrine follow-up after SRS is therefore necessary.

Complications of SRS

The overall complication rate of SRS for EBTs is low (5% to 10%), and includes cranial neuropathies (accounting for the majority of the morbidity), vascular injuries (including, for example, carotid artery stenosis), posttreatment edema, cyst formation, and induction of new tumors. The risk of mortality with SRS is essentially zero.

Cranial neuropathies, accounting for approximately 75% of the overall 8.4% rate of complications reported by Pollock and colleagues include, in order of decreasing frequency, trigeminal, abducens, optic, oculomotor, facial, and vestibulocochlear palsies.[93] Of all the cranial nerves, the optic and acoustic nerves are the most sensitive to radiation. Recommendations for upper limits of radiation to the optic apparatus range from 8 to 14.1 Gy. The cranial nerves in the cavernous sinus are relatively robust and less susceptible to adverse radiation effects. Neuropathies have not been seen with doses up to 40 Gy. Pollock and Stafford reported that 5 out of 49 patients treated with GKS for cavernous sinus meningiomas had new or worsened trigeminal dysfunction and one patient had new oculomotor palsy; it is unclear whether this is due to radiation effects or tumor progression.[83] On the other hand, 12 of 38 patients reported improvements in cranial nerve function. In our series of over 350 pituitary adenomas treated with GKS, eight cases of cranial nerve palsies have been identified.[89,92] The cavernous carotid artery is rarely injured by SRS, but many have recommended limiting the dose to the carotid artery, when possible, to <30 Gy.

Symptomatic perilesional edema after GKS occurs in 1% to 25% of patients.[71,94] In general, symptoms occur 1 to 6 months after treatment; patients complain of severe headache that can be managed with oral corticosteroids. Edema formation is far less likely in posterior fossa lesions and more likely in parasagittal or superficially-located tumors. Limiting the margin dose to 14 or 18 Gy may reduce the risk of edema.

Symptomatic cyst formation has also been reported after GKS of meningiomas in approximately 1% to 3 % of cases.[82,95] All affected patients have undergone prior surgery and some require further surgery for treatment of symptomatic cysts. Postirradiation cysts have been attributed to degenerative and secretory changes, radiation-induced ischemic necrosis, and intratumoral hemorrhage.[95]

Radiation-induced tumors are a known complication of both fractionated radiotherapy and radiosurgery, although their incidence is greater with the former. Two cases of glioblastoma multiforme have been reported after GKS for meningiomas.[96,97] Given the total number of meningiomas treated with GKS, this is an extremely rare event and should not necessarily temper the use of GKS in cases where GKS is indicated. Ironically, patients with radiation therapy-induced meningiomas have been successfully treated with radiosurgery.

RADIATION THERAPY

In addition to SRS, conventional radiation therapy is used as an adjunctive treatment for some EBTs, with excellent efficacy in many cases. XRT and FSRT are applicable in cases where tumors are too large to be treated by SRS or when adjacency of critical structures (e.g., optic nerve) precludes the use of SRS. For lesions greater than 3 cm in greatest dimension, the risks of radiation necrosis and cranial neuropathy make SRS a less viable option. Likewise, while the optic apparatus can tolerate 54 Gy of fractionated radiation, it can only withstand a single dose of up to 8 to 12 Gy. Similarly, the brainstem's fractionated radiation tolerance is far greater (60 Gy) than the single dose tolerance (about 10 to 20 Gy).

Meningiomas

Results for XRT and FSRT of meningiomas in patients who are not appropriate candidates for SRS are comparable to those reported for SRS. In one series of 317 patients with a mean tumor volume of 33.6 ml treated with FSRT (using 57.6 Gy in 1.8 Gy fractions), tumor control was achieved in 97% of patients (including patients treated for recurrent disease) with a mean follow-up of 5.7 years.[98] Earlier time to progression was associated with larger tumor volumes (>60 ml) and atypical histology. The side effect profile is similar to that reported for SRS. Grade 3 toxicity was reported in only 2.2% of patients (affecting the optic apparatus and trigeminal nerve). Other side effects may include other cranial neuropathies, brainstem injury, encephalomalacia, or radionecrosis. Nonetheless, the current rate and profile of complications represents a substantial improvement over the side effect profile reported in earlier series using less precise conventional radiation therapy.

Vestibular Schwannomas

FSRT for vestibular schwannomas has gained in popularity because it carries the advantages of both conventional radiotherapy and SRS, sparing adjacent normal tissues (brainstem, cerebellum, cranial nerves) while killing tumor cells. Five-year PFS after FSRT (usually 54 Gy in 1.8 Gy fractions) has been reported to be 93% to 98%, on par with that reported for SRS.[87,99,100] Large tumor size at the time of treatment is predictive of a need for future neurosurgical intervention.[87] After 2.5 years, 25% of patients had objective hearing loss.[99,100] Incidentally, neurofibromatosis patients are more susceptible to hearing loss after FSRT for vestibular schwannomas than patients with sporadic tumors. Facial nerve function is preserved in 91% to 97% of patients 2.5 to 3 years after FSRT.[87,99]

Pituitary Adenomas

XRT and FSRT remains an important tool in the armamentarium for treatment of sellar lesions because these tumors often abut the optic apparatus, excluding the use of SRS. Enthusiasm has waned due to a slow rate of hormone normalization and an increased incidence of complications. Like SRS, XRT is used to treat both postoperative residual disease as well as recurrent or progressive disease. Long-term tumor control rates (in a study of 411 patients) have been reported as high as 94% and 88% at 10 and 20 years, respectively, after 45 to 50 Gy in 25 to 30 fractions.[101] Recently, differences in 10-year control rates have been reported between nonfunctional and functional adenomas (98% and 73%, respectively, p=0.0083) and depending on whether the cavernous sinus is involved.[101,102] Moreover, improved survival is noted in patients treated with stereotactic RT compared to those in whom two-field or three-field techniques were used. Clinical improvement (e.g., of headache and visual disturbance) has been reported in up to 72% of patients, related to tumor shrinkage, with greatest size reduction seen after 3 years.[103]

In addition to radiographic control, one must also consider the rate of hormone normalization. In one series, hormone hypersecretion improved in 67% of patients after conventional RT (regardless of the type of functional adenoma), with growth hormone-secreting adenomas being the most responsive.[103] In Cushing disease, XRT has been reported to result in remission in up to 83% of patients. There is nonetheless a wide range of endocrine remission rates reported following XRT and FSRT for secretory adenomas. Hormone normalization, when it occurs, generally is seen later than with radiosurgery.

The most common side effect or complication of RT, as with SRS, is hypopituitarism, which occurs in approximately 22% to 50% of patients.[101,102] Other complications noted include seizures, visual loss, strokes, and induction of glioblastoma 12 years after RT.[101,102] These rates of serious complications appear higher than with SRS.

CHEMOTHERAPY

Because of the largely benign nature of EBTs, chemotherapy has never been a major treatment modality for these tumors. Nonetheless, extensive investigations have been conducted, especially with respect to meningiomas and pituitary adenomas.

Meningiomas

Hormone receptor antagonists have been explored as possible chemomodulatory agents for the treatment of meningiomas. Trials of mifepristone, a progesterone receptor antagonist, have been ineffective or only partially successful in producing tumor regression.[104,105] Likewise, blockage of estrogen receptors with tamoxifen has shown little benefit.[106] Despite these failed studies, recent confirmation that receptor status affects gene expression profiles may stimulate new interest in this avenue of chemotherapy for meningiomas.[14]

Unlike hormone receptor anatagonists, hydroxyurea remains a chemotherapeutic option for the treatment of meningiomas, especially in patients for whom other options (i.e., repeat surgery or who have already been radiated) may not exist. Hydroxyurea can arrest progression of unresectable or recurrent benign meningiomas, with 93% PFS in benign meningiomas.[107]

Investigations into the genetic and molecular underpinning of these tumors have led the way to many theoretical opportunities for chemotherapeutic intervention.

Studies of meningiomas have found a chromosomal aberration on the long arm of chromosome 22 in 50% to 72% of cases, which involved the tumor suppressor NF-2 gene loci in up to 60% of sporadic meningiomas.[108] These mutations/deletions are not consistent across all meningiomas, being identified in as few as 26% of meningiomas in one series, underscoring the notion that non-NF2 mechanisms are also important,[109,110] and making these genes less attractive targets for chemotherapy. Other targets of interest that are critical in cellular signaling in meningiomas have been identified as potential targets, including epidermal growth factors receptor (EGFR), transforming growth factor alpha (TGF-alpha), ras protein cascades, Ras-Raf-1-MEK-1-MAPK pathway, and PKC pathways.[111] Inhibitors of many of these pathways are being explored primarily in glioblastoma models as well as in meningiomas (e.g., imatinib, sunitinib). There has also been considerable interest in the role of cyclooxygenase inhibitors on meningioma proliferation, largely due to the availability of these drugs. Although there is no evidence of COX-2 amplification in meningiomas, COX-2 inhibitors have been shown to inhibit cell growth and induce apoptosis in meningiomas and have been shown to reduce mean tumor growth rate by 66% in mouse xenograft models.[112,113] Further investigation into the therapeutic benefits of COX inhibitors may be warranted.

Pituitary Adenomas

In the absence of complications necessitating immediate surgery, such as apoplexy, hydrocephalus, or a cerebrospinal fluid leak, pharmacotherapy with dopamine agonists is considered the first-line treatment approach for prolactin-secreting adenomas. Dopamine agonists (bromocriptine, cabergoline) effectively normalize prolactin levels in as many as 89% of patients.[114] These medications decrease tumor volume by at least 50% in more than two-thirds of patients within the first several months of therapy, resulting in visual field improvements in all but 10% of patients. Quinagolide and cabergoline, both selective DA receptor subtype-2–selective agonists, have also been effective in reducing prolactin secretion and tumor size in adult patients with prolactinomas, even in those with a previous poor responsive or intolerance to bromocriptine. Cabergoline, with a longer half-life and weekly dosing, is noted for its tolerability and high compliance rates. For women who wish to maintain fertility, bromocriptine and cabergoline appear safe, without a significant increase in birth defects.

Although surgery is the primary treatment for all other pituitary adenomas, recent reports highlight impressive advancements in the pharmacologic treatment of growth hormone-secreting, TSH-secreting, and ACTH-secreting adenomas. Traditionally, the two options for medical therapy of growth hormone-secreting tumors have been dopamine agonists and somatostatin analogues. Dopamine agonists provide symptomatic relief in the majority of patients but normalize IGF-1 levels in only about 20% to 40% of cases. Somatostatin analogues (octreotide, sandostatin-LAR, lanreotide, lanreotide-SR) can normalize IGF-1 levels in up to 60% of patients and have a more favorable side-effect profile compared to dopamine agonists.[115] The recently introduced GH receptor antagonist, pegvisomant, has normalized IGF-1 levels in 75% to 85% of patients with refractory disease, although reported experience with its administration for greater than 2 years remains limited.[116]

Medical therapy for Cushing disease, in those who fail surgical and/or radiation therapy, has largely focused on inhibiting peripheral steroid production with ketoconazole. Ketoconazole, an antifungal agent, normalizes urinary free cortisol in approximately 50% of patients.[117] More recently, however, the somatostatin analogue pasireotide and the dopamine agonist cabergoline (and their combination) have shown promise in the medical therapy of Cushing disease. TSH-secreting adenomas can also be responsive to dopaminergic agonists and somatostatin analogues. Cytotoxic chemotherapy has occasionally provided modest benefit in pituitary carcinoma.[118]

Conclusions

Despite their generally being benign lesions, EBTs can cause significant symptoms, morbidity, and even mortality. The management is complex and must be decided based upon the clinical and radiologic attributes of the patient. There is a place for conservative management, particularly for asymptomatic lesions that are discovered incidentally and remain static on serial imaging. Historically, symptomatic lesions required microsurgical excision. While this is still generally true, minimally invasive management strategies, such as SRS, can now be considered even without tissue diagnosis when the diagnostic evaluation is unambiguous. Radiosurgery can often relieve tumor-related symptoms (e.g., cranial neuropathies) and halt progression. Nevertheless, microsurgical excision remains a mainstay of treatment and management of all EBTs (with the exception of prolactinomas). EBTS presenting in patients symptomatic due to mass effect should generally be resected, especially in the subset of patients harboring tumors that are relatively low risk for resection, with a goal of complete resection. Fractionated radiation therapy appears to be playing less of a role with these tumors, as most patients undergo a resection, radiosurgery, or a combination of the two. Medical management also has a role, particularly in secretory pituitary adenomas. Ultimately, the long-term management of patients with EBTs will require close neurological, radiological, and biochemical surveillance.

REFERENCES

1. CBTRUS. Statistical Report: Primary Brain Tumors in the United States, 2000–2004. Published by the Central Brain Tumor Registry of the United States. 2008.
2. Olson S, Law A. Meningiomas and the Polynesian population. ANZ J Surg 2005;75:705–9.
3. Hoffman S, Propp JM, McCarthy BJ. Temporal trends in incidence of primary brain tumors in the United States, 1985–1999. Neuro Oncol 2006;8:27–37.
4. Vernooij MW, Ikram MA, Tanghe HL, Vincent AJ, Hofman A, Krestin GP, et al. Incidental findings on brain MRI in the general population. N Engl J Med 2007;357:1821–8.
5. Claus EB, Black PM. Survival rates and patterns of care for patients diagnosed with supratentorial low-grade gliomas: data from the SEER program, 1973–2001. Cancer 2006;106:1358–63.
6. Umansky F, Shoshan Y, Rosenthal G, Fraifeld S, Spektor S. Radiation-induced meningioma. Neurosurg Focus 2008;24:E7.
7. Modan B, Baidatz D, Mart H, Steinitz R, Levin SG. Radiation-induced head and neck tumours. Lancet 1974;1:277–9.
8. Mack EE, Wilson CB. Meningiomas induced by high-dose cranial irradiation. J Neurosurg 1993;79:28–31.

9. Phillips LE, Koepsell TD, van Belle G, Kukull WA, Gehrels JA, Longstreth Jr WT. History of head trauma and risk of intracranial meningioma: population-based case-control study. Neurology 2002;58:1849–52.
10. Preston-Martin S, Pogoda JM, Schlehofer B, Blettner M, Howe GR, Ryan P, et al. An international case-control study of adult glioma and meningioma: the role of head trauma. Int J Epidemiol 1998;27:579–86.
11. Pravdenkova S, Al-Mefty O, Sawyer J, Husain M. Progesterone and estrogen receptors: opposing prognostic indicators in meningiomas. J Neurosurg 2006;105:163–73.
12. Blitshteyn S, Crook JE, Jaeckle KA. Is there an association between meningioma and hormone replacement therapy? J Clin Oncol 2008;26:279–82.
13. Custer B, Longstreth Jr WT, Phillips LE, Koepsell TD, Van Belle G. Hormonal exposures and the risk of intracranial meningioma in women: a population-based case-control study. BMC Cancer 2006;6:152.
14. Claus EB, Park PJ, Carroll R, Chan J, Black PM. Specific genes expressed in association with progesterone receptors in meningioma. Cancer Res 2008;68:314–22.
15. Aghi MK, Eskandar EN, Carter BS, Curry Jr WT, Barker 2nd FG. Increased prevalence of obesity and obesity-related postoperative complications in male meningioma patients. Clin Neurosurg 2007;54:236–40.
16. Benson VS, Pirie K, Green J, Casabonne D, Beral V. Lifestyle factors and primary glioma and meningioma tumours in the Million Women Study cohort. Br J Cancer 2008;99:185–90.
17. Hardell L, Carlberg M, Soderqvist F, Hansson Mild K. Meta-analysis of long-term mobile phone use and the association with brain tumours. Int J Oncol 2008;32:1097–103.
18. Chang EF, Zada G, Kim S, Lamborn KR, Quinones-Hinojosa A, Tyrrell JB, et al. Long-term recurrence and mortality after surgery and adjuvant radiotherapy for nonfunctional pituitary adenomas. J Neurosurg 2008;108:736–45.
19. Julia-Sape M, Acosta D, Majos C, Moreno-Torres A, Wesseling P, Acebes JJ, et al. Comparison between neuroimaging classifications and histopathological diagnoses using an international multicenter brain tumor magnetic resonance imaging database. J Neurosurg 2006;105:6–14.
20. Hazany S, Hesselink JR, Healy JF, Imbesi SG. Utilization of glutamate/creatine ratios for proton spectroscopic diagnosis of meningiomas. Neuroradiology 2007;49:121–7.
21. Buhl R, Nabavi A, Wolff S, Hugo HH, Alfke K, Jansen O, et al. MR spectroscopy in patients with intracranial meningiomas. Neurol Res 2007;29:43–6.
22. Friedman TC, Zuckerbraun E, Lee ML, Kabil MS, Shahinian H. Dynamic pituitary MRI has high sensitivity and specificity for the diagnosis of mild Cushing's syndrome and should be part of the initial workup. Horm Metab Res 2007;39:451–6.
23. Oldfield EH, Doppman JL, Nieman LK, Chrousos GP, Miller DL, Katz DA, et al. Petrosal sinus sampling with and without corticotropin-releasing hormone for the differential diagnosis of Cushing's syndrome. N Engl J Med 1991;325:897–905.
24. Yano S, Hamada J, Kai Y, Todaka T, Hara T, Mizuno T, et al. Surgical indications to maintain quality of life in elderly patients with ruptured intracranial aneurysms. Neurosurgery 2003;52:1010–5; discussion 1015–1016.
25. Kuratsu J, Kochi M, Ushio Y. Incidence and clinical features of asymptomatic meningiomas. J Neurosurg 2000;92:766–70.
26. Nakamura M, Roser F, Michel J, Jacobs C, Samii M. The natural history of incidental meningiomas. Neurosurgery 2003;53:62–70 discussion; 70–61.
27. Niiro M, Yatsushiro K, Nakamura K, Kawahara Y, Kuratsu J. Natural history of elderly patients with asymptomatic meningiomas. J Neurol Neurosurg Psychiatry 2000;68:25–8.
28. Jeyakumar A, Seth R, Brickman TM, Dutcher P. The prevalence and clinical course of patients with 'incidental' acoustic neuromas. Acta Otolaryngol 2007;127:1051–7.
29. Lin D, Hegarty JL, Fischbein NJ, Jackler RK. The prevalence of "incidental" acoustic neuroma. Arch Otolaryngol Head Neck Surg 2005;131:241–4.
30. Rosenberg SI. Natural history of acoustic neuromas. Laryngoscope 2000;110:497–508.
31. Deen HG, Ebersold MJ, Harner SG, Beatty CW, Marion MS, Wharen RE, et al. Conservative management of acoustic neuroma: an outcome study. Neurosurgery 1996;39:260–4; discussion 264–266.
32. Tschudi DC, Linder TE, Fisch U. Conservative management of unilateral acoustic neuromas. Am J Otol 2000;21:722–8.
33. Donovan LE, Corenblum B. The natural history of the pituitary incidentaloma. Arch Intern Med 1995;155:181–3.

34. Feldkamp J, Santen R, Harms E, Aulich A, Modder U, Scherbaum WA. Incidentally discovered pituitary lesions: high frequency of macroadenomas and hormone-secreting adenomas—results of a prospective study. Clin Endocrinol (Oxf) 1999;51:109–13.
35. Oyama K, Sanno N, Tahara S, Teramoto A. Management of pituitary incidentalomas: according to a survey of pituitary incidentalomas in Japan. Semin Ultrasound CT MR 2005;26:47–50.
36. Simpson D. The recurrence of intracranial meningiomas after surgical treatment. J Neurol Neurosurg Psychiatry 1957;20:22–39.
37. Morimura T, Takeuchi J, Maeda Y, Tani E. Preoperative embolization of meningiomas: its efficacy and histopathological findings. Noshuyo Byori 1994;11:123–9.
38. Kim YJ, Ketter R, Henn W, Zang KD, Steudel WI, Feiden W. Histopathologic indicators of recurrence in meningiomas: correlation with clinical and genetic parameters. Virchows Arch 2006;449:529–38.
39. Boker DK, Meurer H, Gullotta F. Recurring intracranial meningiomas. Evaluation of some factors predisposing for tumor recurrence. J Neurosurg Sci 1985;29:11–7.
40. Ketter R, Rahnenfuhrer J, Henn W, Kim YJ, Feiden W, Steudel WI, et al. Correspondence of tumor localization with tumor recurrence and cytogenetic progression in meningiomas. Neurosurgery 2008;62:61–9; discussion 69–70.
41. DeMonte F, Smith HK, al-Mefty O. Outcome of aggressive removal of cavernous sinus meningiomas. J Neurosurg 1994;81:245–51.
42. Kallio M, Sankila R, Hakulinen T, Jaaskelainen J. Factors affecting operative and excess long-term mortality in 935 patients with intracranial meningioma. Neurosurgery 1992;31:2–12.
43. Pertuiset B, Farah S, Clayes L, Goutorbe J, Metzger J, Kujas M. Operability of intracranial meningiomas. Personal series of 353 cases. Acta Neurochir (Wien) 1985;76:2–11.
44. Jaaskelainen J. Seemingly complete removal of histologically benign intracranial meningioma: late recurrence rate and factors predicting recurrence in 657 patients. A multivariate analysis. Surg Neurol 1986;26:461–9.
45. Yamakami I, Uchino Y, Kobayashi E, Yamaura A. Conservative management, gamma-knife radiosurgery, and microsurgery for acoustic neurinomas: a systematic review of outcome and risk of three therapeutic options. Neurol Res 2003;25:682–90.
46. Haines SJ, Levine SC. Intracanalicular acoustic neuroma: early surgery for preservation of hearing. J Neurosurg 1993;79:515–20.
47. Samii M, Matthies C, Tatagiba M. Intracanalicular acoustic neurinomas. Neurosurgery 1991;29:189–98; discussion 198–189.
48. Ebersold MJ, Harner SG, Beatty CW, Harper Jr CM, Quast LM. Current results of the retrosigmoid approach to acoustic neurinoma. J Neurosurg 1992;76:901–9.
49. Ojemann RG. Management of acoustic neuromas (vestibular schwannomas) (honored guest presentation). Clin Neurosurg 1993;40:498–535.
50. Sekhar LN, Gormley WB, Wright DC. The best treatment for vestibular schwannoma (acoustic neuroma): microsurgery or radiosurgery? Am J Otol 1996;17:676–82; discussion 683–679.
51. Nadol Jr JB, Chiong CM, Ojemann RG, McKenna MJ, Martuza RL, Montgomery WW, et al. Preservation of hearing and facial nerve function in resection of acoustic neuroma. Laryngoscope 1992;102:1153–8.
52. Baldwin DL, King TT, Morrison AW. Hearing conservation in acoustic neuroma surgery via the posterior fossa. J Laryngol Otol 1990;104:463–7.
53. Jane Jr JA, Laws Jr ER. The surgical management of pituitary adenomas in a series of 3,093 patients. J Am Coll Surg 2001;193:651–9.
54. Losa M, Mortini P, Franzin A, Barzaghi R, Mandelli C, Giovanelli M. Surgical management of thyrotropin-secreting pituitary adenomas. Pituitary 1999;2:127–31.
55. Hammer GD, Tyrrell JB, Lamborn KR, Applebury CB, Hannegan ET, Bell S, et al. Transsphenoidal microsurgery for Cushing's disease: initial outcome and long-term results. J Clin Endocrinol Metab 2004;89:6348–57.
56. Sonino N, Zielezny M, Fava GA, Fallo F, Boscaro M. Risk factors and long-term outcome in pituitary-dependent Cushing's disease. J Clin Endocrinol Metab 1996;81:2647–52.
57. Laws ER. Surgery for acromegaly: evolution of the techniques and outcomes. Rev Endocr Metab Disord 2008;9:67–70.
58. Colao A, Vitale G, Cappabianca P, Briganti F, Ciccarelli A, De Rosa M, et al. Outcome of cabergoline treatment in men with prolactinoma: effects of a 24-month treatment on prolactin levels, tumor mass, recovery of pituitary function, and semen analysis. J Clin Endocrinol Metab 2004;89:1704–11.

59. Verhelst J, Abs R, Maiter D, van den Bruel A, Vandeweghe M, Velkeniers B, et al. Cabergoline in the treatment of hyperprolactinemia: a study in 455 patients. J Clin Endocrinol Metab 1999;84:2518–22.
60. Kreutzer J, Buslei R, Wallaschofski H, Hofmann B, Nimsky C, Fahlbusch R, et al. Operative treatment of prolactinomas: indications and results in a current consecutive series of 212 patients. Eur J Endocrinol 2008;158:11–8.
61. Ciric I, Ragin A, Baumgartner C, Pierce D. Complications of transsphenoidal surgery: results of a national survey, review of the literature, and personal experience. Neurosurgery 1997;40:225–36; discussion 236–227.
62. Kelly DF, Laws Jr ER, Fossett D. Delayed hyponatremia after transsphenoidal surgery for pituitary adenoma. Report of nine cases. J Neurosurg 1995;83:363–7.
63. Davis JR, Farrell WE, Clayton RN. Pituitary tumours. Reproduction 2001;121:363–71.
64. Laws Jr ER, Fode NC, Redmond MJ. Transsphenoidal surgery following unsuccessful prior therapy. An assessment of benefits and risks in 158 patients. J Neurosurg 1985;63:823–9.
65. Kurosaki M, Luedecke DK, Abe T. Effectiveness of secondary transnasal surgery in GH-secreting pituitary macroadenomas. Endocr J 2003;50:635–42.
66. Bochicchio D, Losa M, Buchfelder M. Factors influencing the immediate and late outcome of Cushing's disease treated by transsphenoidal surgery: a retrospective study by the European Cushing's Disease Survey Group. J Clin Endocrinol Metab 1995;80:3114–20.
67. Utz AL, Swearingen B, Biller BM. Pituitary surgery and postoperative management in Cushing's disease. Endocrinol Metab Clin North Am 2005;34:459–78, xi.
68. Marekova M, Vavrova J, Vokurkova D, Psutka J. Modulation of ionizing radiation-induced apoptosis and cell cycle arrest by all-trans retinoic acid in promyelocytic leukemia cells (HL-60). Physiol Res 2003;52:599–606.
69. Tsuzuki T, Tsunoda S, Sakaki T, Konishi N, Hiasa Y, Nakamura M, et al. Tumor cell proliferation and apoptosis associated with the Gamma Knife effect. Stereotact Funct Neurosurg 1996;66(Suppl. 1):39–48.
70. Hawighorst H, Engenhart R, Knopp MV, Brix G, Grandy M, Essig M, et al. Intracranial meningeomas: time- and dose-dependent effects of irradiation on tumor microcirculation monitored by dynamic MR imaging. Magn Reson Imaging 1997;15:423–32.
71. Kreil W, Luggin J, Fuchs I, Weigl V, Eustacchio S, Papaefthymiou G. Long term experience of gamma knife radiosurgery for benign skull base meningiomas. J Neurol Neurosurg Psychiatry 2005;76:1425–30.
72. Ganz JC, Backlund EO, Thorsen FA. The results of Gamma Knife surgery of meningiomas, related to size of tumor and dose. Stereotact Funct Neurosurg 1993;61(Suppl. 1):23–9.
73. Pendl G, Schrottner O, Eustacchio S, Feichtinger K, Ganz J. Stereotactic radiosurgery of skull base meningiomas. Minim Invasive Neurosurg 1997;40:87–90.
74. Subach BR, Lunsford LD, Kondziolka D, Maitz AH, Flickinger JC. Management of petroclival meningiomas by stereotactic radiosurgery. Neurosurgery 1998;42:437–43; discussion 443–435.
75. Roche PH, Pellet W, Fuentes S, Thomassin JM, Regis J. Gamma knife radiosurgical management of petroclival meningiomas results and indications. Acta Neurochir (Wien) 2003;145:883–8; discussion 888.
76. Liscak R, Kollova A, Vladyka V, Simonova G, Novotny Jr J. Gamma knife radiosurgery of skull base meningiomas. Acta Neurochir Suppl 2004;91:65–74.
77. DiBiase SJ, Kwok Y, Yovino S, Arena C, Naqvi S, Temple R, et al. Factors predicting local tumor control after gamma knife stereotactic radiosurgery for benign intracranial meningiomas. Int J Radiat Oncol Biol Phys 2004;60:1515–9.
78. Kondziolka D, Levy EI, Niranjan A, Flickinger JC, Lunsford LD. Long-term outcomes after meningioma radiosurgery: physician and patient perspectives. J Neurosurg 1999;91:44–50.
79. Harris AE, Lee JY, Omalu B, Flickinger JC, Kondziolka D, Lunsford LD. The effect of radiosurgery during management of aggressive meningiomas. Surg Neurol 2003;60:298–305; discussion 305.
80. Malik I, Rowe JG, Walton L, Radatz MW, Kemeny AA. The use of stereotactic radiosurgery in the management of meningiomas. Br J Neurosurg 2005;19:13–20.
81. Ojemann SG, Sneed PK, Larson DA, Gutin PH, Berger MS, Verhey L, et al. Radiosurgery for malignant meningioma: results in 22 patients. J Neurosurg 2000;93(Suppl. 3):62–7.
82. Stafford SL, Pollock BE, Foote RL, Link MJ, Gorman DA, Schomberg PJ, et al. Meningioma radiosurgery: tumor control, outcomes, and complications among 190 consecutive patients. Neurosurgery 2001;49:1029–37; discussion 1037–1028.
83. Pollock BE, Stafford SL. Results of stereotactic radiosurgery for patients with imaging defined cavernous sinus meningiomas. Int J Radiat Oncol Biol Phys 2005;62:1427–31.

84. Foote KD, Friedman WA, Buatti JM, Meeks SL, Bova FJ, Kubilis PS. Analysis of risk factors associated with radiosurgery for vestibular schwannoma. J Neurosurg 2001;95:440–9.
85. Inoue HK. Low-dose radiosurgery for large vestibular schwannomas: long-term results of functional preservation. J Neurosurg 2005;102(Suppl.):111–3.
86. Hasegawa T, Fujitani S, Katsumata S, Kida Y, Yoshimoto M, Koike J. Stereotactic radiosurgery for vestibular schwannomas: analysis of 317 patients followed more than 5 years. Neurosurgery 2005;57:257–65; discussion 257–265.
87. Chan AW, Black P, Ojemann RG, Barker 2nd FG, Kooy HM, Lopes VV, et al. Stereotactic radiotherapy for vestibular schwannomas: favorable outcome with minimal toxicity. Neurosurgery 2005;57:60–70; discussion 60–70.
88. Sheehan JP, Jagannathan J, Pouratian N, Steiner L. Stereotactic radiosurgery for pituitary adenomas: a review of the literature and our experience. Front Horm Res 2006;34:185–205.
89. Jagannathan J, Sheehan JP, Pouratian N, Laws ER, Steiner L, Vance ML. Gamma Knife surgery for Cushing's disease. J Neurosurg 2007;106:980–7.
90. Landolt AM, Haller D, Lomax N, Scheib S, Schubiger O, Siegfried J, et al. Octreotide may act as a radioprotective agent in acromegaly. J Clin Endocrinol Metab 2000;85:1287–9.
91. Landolt AM, Lomax N. Gamma knife radiosurgery for prolactinomas. J Neurosurg 2000;93(Suppl. 3):14–8.
92. Pouratian N, Sheehan J, Jagannathan J, Laws Jr ER, Steiner L, Vance ML. Gamma knife radiosurgery for medically and surgically refractory prolactinomas. Neurosurgery 2006;59:255–66; discussion 255–266.
93. Pollock BE. Stereotactic radiosurgery for intracranial meningiomas: indications and results. Neurosurg Focus 2003;14:e4.
94. Singh VP, Kansai S, Vaishya S, Julka PK, Mehta VS. Early complications following gamma knife radiosurgery for intracranial meningiomas. J Neurosurg 2000;93(Suppl. 3):57–61.
95. Shuto T, Inomori S, Fujino H, Nagano H, Hasegawa N, Kakuta Y. Cyst formation following gamma knife surgery for intracranial meningioma. J Neurosurg 2005;102(Suppl.):134–9.
96. Loeffler JS, Niemierko A, Chapman PH. Second tumors after radiosurgery: tip of the iceberg or a bump in the road? Neurosurgery 2003;52:1436–40; discussion 1440–1432.
97. Yu JS, Yong WH, Wilson D, Black KL. Glioblastoma induction after radiosurgery for meningioma. Lancet 2000;356:1576–7.
98. Milker-Zabel S, Zabel A, Schulz-Ertner D, Schlegel W, Wannenmacher M, Debus J. Fractionated stereotactic radiotherapy in patients with benign or atypical intracranial meningioma: long-term experience and prognostic factors. Int J Radiat Oncol Biol Phys 2005;61:809–16.
99. Horan G, Whitfield GA, Burton KE, Burnet NG, Jefferies SJ. Fractionated conformal radiotherapy in vestibular schwannoma: early results from a single centre. Clin Oncol (R Coll Radiol) 2007;19:517–22.
100. Fuss M, Debus J, Lohr F, Huber P, Rhein B, Engenhart-Cabillic R, et al. Conventionally fractionated stereotactic radiotherapy (FSRT) for acoustic neuromas. Int J Radiat Oncol Biol Phys 2000;48:1381–7.
101. Brada M, Rajan B, Traish D, Ashley S, Holmes-Sellors PJ, Nussey S, et al. The long-term efficacy of conservative surgery and radiotherapy in the control of pituitary adenomas. Clin Endocrinol (Oxf) 1993;38:571–8.
102. Snead FE, Amdur RJ, Morris CG, Mendenhall WM. Long-term outcomes of radiotherapy for pituitary adenomas. Int J Radiat Oncol Biol Phys 2008;71:994–8.
103. Sasaki R, Murakami M, Okamoto Y, Kono K, Yoden E, Nakajima T, et al. The efficacy of conventional radiation therapy in the management of pituitary adenoma. Int J Radiat Oncol Biol Phys 2000;47:1337–45.
104. Lamberts SW, Tanghe HL, Avezaat CJ, Braakman R, Wijngaarde R, Koper JW, et al. Mifepristone (RU 486) treatment of meningiomas. J Neurol Neurosurg Psychiatry 1992;55:486–90.
105. Grunberg SM, Weiss MH, Spitz IM, Ahmadi J, Sadun A, Russell CA, et al. Treatment of unresectable meningiomas with the antiprogesterone agent mifepristone. J Neurosurg 1991;74:861–6.
106. Goodwin JW, Crowley J, Eyre HJ, Stafford B, Jaeckle KA, Townsend JJ. A phase II evaluation of tamoxifen in unresectable or refractory meningiomas: a Southwest Oncology Group study. J Neurooncol 1993;15:75–7.
107. Hahn BM, Schrell UM, Sauer R, Fahlbusch R, Ganslandt O, Grabenbauer GG. Prolonged oral hydroxyurea and concurrent 3d-conformal radiation in patients with progressive or recurrent meningioma: results of a pilot study. J Neurooncol 2005;74:157–65.
108. Dumanski JP, Rouleau GA, Nordenskjold M, Collins VP. Molecular genetic analysis of chromosome 22 in 81 cases of meningioma. Cancer Res 1990;50:5863–7.

109. Drummond KJ, Zhu JJ, Black PM. Meningiomas: updating basic science, management, and outcome. Neurologist 2004;10:113–30.
110. Perry A, Cai DX, Scheithauer BW, Swanson PE, Lohse CM, Newsham IF, et al. Merlin, DAL-1, and progesterone receptor expression in clinicopathologic subsets of meningioma: a correlative immunohistochemical study of 175 cases. J Neuropathol Exp Neurol 2000;59:872–9.
111. Johnson MD, Sade B, Milano MT, Lee JH, Toms SA. New prospects for management and treatment of inoperable and recurrent skull base meningiomas. J Neurooncol 2008;86:109–22.
112. Ragel BT, Jensen RL, Gillespie DL, Prescott SM, Couldwell WT. Celecoxib inhibits meningioma tumor growth in a mouse xenograft model. Cancer 2007;109:588–97.
113. Ragel BT, Asher AL, Selden N, MacDonald JD. Self-assessment in neurological surgery: the SANS wired white paper. Neurosurgery 2006;59:759–65; discussion 765–756.
114. Webster J. Dopamine agonist therapy in hyperprolactinemia. J Reprod Med 1999;44:1105–10.
115. Castinetti F, Morange I, Jaquet P, Conte-Devolx B, Brue T. Ketoconazole revisited: a preoperative or postoperative treatment in Cushing's disease. Eur J Endocrinol 2008;158:91–9.
116. Alexandraki KI, Grossman AB. Pituitary-targeted medical therapy of Cushing's disease. Expert Opin Investig Drugs 2008;17:669–77.
117. Kienitz T, Quinkler M, Strasburger CJ, Ventz M. Long-term management in five cases of TSH-secreting pituitary adenomas: a single center study and review of the literature. Eur J Endocrinol 2007;157:39–46.
118. Lopes MB, Scheithauer BW, Schiff D. Pituitary carcinoma: diagnosis and treatment. Endocrine 2005;28:115–21.

12 Medical Complications in the Management of Brain Tumors

ROBIN GRANT

Introduction

Patients with brain tumors present with neurological symptoms in a variety of different ways, usually either to their primary physician or to an emergency department. This chapter will look at their symptomatic management, prophylactic perioperative care, complications indirectly related to the tumor and its effects, complications from medical treatment, and neurological and psychiatric postoperative complications. The medical complications of radiation therapy and chemotherapy or other treatments are dealt with in other chapters.

Symptomatic Management

SYMPTOMS

Headaches are present in 50% of patients at hospital presentation, although less than 10% of all patients have the "classical" headache of raised intracranial pressure.[1] Patients with headaches are more likely to have larger tumors.[2] The brain parenchyma does not contain pain fibers. Blood vessels, dura, and choroid plexus do have sensory nerve endings, and pain from stretching of these structures causes vascular or referred pain. In general, patients with supratentorial tumors have headaches referred frontally (cranial nerve V), and those with tumors involving the posterior fossa have headaches referred to the occipitocervical region (cranial nerves IX and X).

Sadly, the headaches associated with tumors have very few good discriminating features. Papilledema is found at some stage in more than 50% of patients with headache; however, less than 15% are identified as having papilledema at first presentation.[1,3] Some patients with midline shift do not have any headache.[2] The headache of tonsillar herniation is maximal in the neck and occiput and may be associated with nuchal rigidity and painful extensor spasms of the spine and limbs. These may mimic a generalized tonic seizure, but are not associated with loss of consciousness. Seizures are the first symptom of an intracerebral tumor in 21% of patients.Their frequency increases to 26.5% by hospital presentation, and approximately 50% of patients seize at some stage during the illness.[4]

By the time of hospital presentation, 81% of patients have some neurological signs on examination. The most common signs are unilateral focal motor or sensory signs involving the limbs; dysphasia; or impairment of memory and/or cognition. Neurological impairments are more common with increasing age, and older patients are more likely to have multiple and more severe impairments.[5] Some authors have identified subtle cognitive problems in as many as 91% of patients with brain tumors before surgery.[6] Anxiety is present in 17% to 30% prior to surgical operation; this may be more common in patients with right hemisphere tumors.[7–9] Clinical depression reaching the DSM-IV criteria for major depressive disorder occurs in 19% to 38% of patients with a brain tumor and has been found to be the single most important independent predictor of quality of life.[10] Depression is most common in women and those with a past or family history of psychiatric disorder.[7,11] Patients with left hemisphere tumors reported significantly more memory problems and depressive symptoms.[12] If the depression is severe, suicide is a real risk.

MANAGEMENT OF SYMPTOMS

Steroids have been shown to improve symptoms and neurological impairments and to reduce cerebral edema seen on imaging. In many patients with primary CNS lymphoma, and occasional patients with malignant glioma, the tumor can disappear on imaging. Steroids are not indicated in patients without significant symptoms or without cerebral edema seen on imaging, since the side effects of steroids are likely to outweigh any benefit.[13] Patients with focal neurological deficits, and without symptoms or signs of raised intracranial pressure, respond well to dexamethasone 4 mg/day. This dose is as effective as 8 mg/day or 16 mg/day and has fewer side effects.[14] If patients have symptomatic raised intracranial pressure or a significant shift seen on imaging studies, or in cases where herniation is suspected, an initial dose of 12 to 16 mg intravenously may be followed by 16 mg orally each day, until the tumor has been decompressed surgically or until a maximum benefit has been achieved. The dose should then be titrated downwards to the minimum effective dose. Steroids should be avoided after 6 pm because of the common side effect of insomnia. A clinical response to steroids was found in 37% of patients with a primary brain tumor at the time of diagnosis, 40% of patients with symptoms during radiotherapy, and 6% of patients after completion of radiotherapy.[13] The frequency of improvement in symptoms was similar in patients with brain metastases.

In patients with symptoms suggesting impending clinical herniation, who do not respond to steroids, fluid restriction and mannitol 0.5 to 1.0 g/kg (with the higher doses being effective up to 6 hours) to produce an osmotic diuresis and decrease the formation of CSF by removal of sodium and water from the brain will commonly be effective. This is a temporary solution which should be followed by urgent surgical tumor resection or cyst drainage.

There is an uncommon phenomenon sometimes found in patients with large mass lesions, in which paroxysmal neurological symptoms are triggered by standing. The attacks may occur despite dexamethasone therapy, but the addition of acetazolomide will often promptly stop symptoms.[15] Patients with dysphasia, dysarthria and dysphagia and dysphonia should be assessed by a speech therapist and a swallowing assessment should be performed where indicated. Patients with hemiparesis or gait problems should be assessed by a physiotherapist and given advice regarding gait, mobility, and prevention of deep vein thrombosis. Resective surgery will lead to further improvements in many patients, often after an early postoperative worsening. Postoperative neurological deterioration occurs in 30% of patients undergoing resection and 36% who were biopsied.[5] The postoperative nonneurological complication rate is highest for complete (9.7%) or partial resection (8%), and lowest for stereotactic biopsy (3.8%).

Where imaging has revealed an intracranial tumor and the patient presents with seizures, the patient should receive the advice of the neuro-oncology multidisciplinary team about seizure control and treatment of the tumor. The seizure threshold will be lowered by poor sleep, irregular diet, anxiety, noncompliance with medications, and the use of certain medications (e.g., antipsychotics, antidepressants, or alcohol). It is essential to discuss risk-avoidance strategies with the patient, both for work (i.e., dangerous machinery, heights) and leisure (i.e., swimming or bathing unsupervised). Issues such as: driving, oral contraceptives, pregnancy, education, and management of tonic-clonic seizures must be discussed. Relatives must be informed about first aid measures. The legislation regarding work and driving will vary from country to country and in the US, from state to state. UK regulations can be found on www.dvla.gov.uk.[16]

Tonic-clonic seizures are most likely to become completely controlled with medication, whereas focal seizures are only completely controlled by a single anticonvulsant in 30% to 40%, with an additional 30% to 40% achieving a 50% reduction in seizure frequency. Any of several anticonvulsants can be used to control seizures. Anticonvulsants have not been compared head to head in tumor-associated epilepsy. The anticonvulsant used will depend on the urgency for treatment (e.g., status epilepticus), possible interactions with other drugs likely to be used in management of the tumor and cost-effectiveness issues. Carbamazepine, phenytoin, and phenobarbital are enzyme-inducing agents whereas valproate, lamotrigine, levetiracetam, and topiramate are not. The newer anticonvulsants may be better tolerated, have fewer drug interactions, and may have fewer cognitive side effects, but they are more expensive.[17,18] Guidelines are available on the efficacy and tolerability of the newer antiepileptic drugs.[19] These recommend initial use of the older agents unless there is a satisfactory reason for not using them. Certain antiepileptic agents may alter the bioavailability of chemotherapy (see later). Whether this has any significant effect on survival or outcome is still uncertain. Acute seizure management is crucial, because prolonged seizures cause neurochemical changes occur that lead to neuronal damage. Evidence from a trial comparing four treatment regimes for the management of status epilepticus has demonstrated that intravenous injection of lorazepam 0.1 mg/kg, at a rate of less than 2 mg/min, is effective in the initial treatment in 65% of patients. Phenobarbital (15 mg/kg) was effective in 58%, diazepam (0.15 mg/kg) followed by phenytoin 18 mg/kg was effective in 56%, and phenytoin alone in 44% of cases. The American Academy of Neurology Guidelines for the management ofstatus epilepticus have been summarized in Table 12-1.

Surgical resection of some low-grade neoplasms (gangliogliomas, pilocytic astrocytomas, dysembryoplastic neuroepithelial tumors) can cure epilepsy or reduce seizure frequency, particularly if the epileptogenic area, as determined by noninvasive recordings, is resected in addition to the tumor.[20] Fractionated radiotherapy and radiosurgery can reduce seizure frequency to Engel classification I or II in 54% of patients with brain tumors and intractable epilepsy.[21] As with

TABLE 12-1 Management of Status Epilepticus

- **0 minute**: Make the diagnosis by observing one additional seizure in a patient with a history of recent seizures or impaired consciousness, or by observing continuous seizure activity for more than 10 minutes.
- **5 minutes**: Ensure that the airway is maintained, sufficient oxygen is being received, circulation is adequate. Insert an intravenous cannula and start an infusion with normal saline after drawing blood for serum chemistry, hematology, anticonvulsant levels, and toxic drug screen, if appropriate. If hypoglycemia is suspected, confirm by a fingerstick, then administer 100 mg thiamine followed by 50 ml of 50% glucose by direct push.
- **10 minutes**: Administer lorazepam 0.1 mg/kg by intravenous push (<2 mg/min).
- **25 minutes**: If status epilepticus does not stop, start phenytoin 15 to 20 mg/kg by slow intravenous infusion at a rate of no more than 50 mg/min directly into the intravenous port nearest the patient. Monitor the blood pressure and electrocardiogram during and after the infusion. If it does not stop after 20 mg/kg of phenytoin, a further 5 mg/kg, repeated if necessary up to a maximum of 30 mg/kg, should be tried.
- **60 minutes**: If status persists, consider intubation. Also consider giving intravenous propofol or barbiturates (e.g., phenobarbital 20 mg/kg by intravenous push [<100 mg/min]).
- **90 minutes**: If status persists, intubate, ventilate, and start barbiturate coma, or give intravenous propofol to suppress all epileptiform activity on EEG. Monitor BP, ECG, and respiratory function closely.

tumor-associated epilepsy surgery, temporal lobe tumors had a better success rate than extratemporal tumors. Temozolomide may reduce the seizure frequency in intractable epilepsy.[22]

There does not seem to be a difference in how patients with brain tumors cope with their illness as compared to patients with other brain diseases such as stroke and Parkinson disease.[23] Anxiety or depression may occur due to uncertainty about symptoms, likelihood of control of symptoms, and worries about the immediate future, including death, or family and financial matters. All of these affect quality of life. Psychological morbidity is related to physical and neuropsychological functioning. Psychological morbidity is associated with high levels of physical disability and also with cognitive dysfunction, but is not related to the grade of tumor or the extent to which the patient was aware of the nature of his or her disease. In one prospective study, 5% had clinically significant levels of anxiety, and six (15%) had clinically significant levels of depression, yet 92% felt they had full or intermediate knowledge about their prognosis.

A variety of psychological approaches have been used, but cognitive-behavior therapy (CBT) has been most researched in people with cancer. Treatment with antidepressants has been shown to be more effective than either placebo or no treatment in patients with physical illness.[24] However, there are no randomized controlled trials of the use of antidepressants in patients with brain tumors. Management guidelines for the treatment of depression in those who are also physically ill have been published.[25] Short-term, highly focused forms of psychotherapy such as cognitive-behavioral, supportive, and group therapies are helpful but time-consuming. They may be the only forms of treatment available in patients disinclined to accept antidepressants or who are intolerant of them. CBT is as effective as antidepressants. By 3 to 8 months, 50% to 60% of patients are in remission, compared with only 27% treated with placebo.[26,27]

Depression should be and can be successfully treated.[28] The importance of this is supported by the observation that the presence of depression impacts negatively on both psychological and physical quality-of-life outcomes in patients with brain tumors.[29] Neuropsychiatrists may be able to help identify whether sedation, confusion, and possible lowered seizure threshold are related to the disease or to antidepressant or antipsychotic medication.[30] There are no randomized controlled trials of different treatment approaches in the neuropsychiatric management of patients with brain or CNS tumors. The advice, therefore, is at the level of recommendations for best practice from a consensus group of experts. In the "Glioma Outcome" study (2004) that included 598 patients diagnosed with a glioma,[31] concordance between physician recognition of depression and treatment of depression was initially low (33%), but increased at 3 and 6 months (51%and 60%, respectively). Antidepressants may have an adverse effect on seizure control, although this is rarely a serious complication in my experience, and it has not been found in recent prospective studies.[32] Antidepressants should be prescribed when necessary, as depression is a major cause of poor quality of life in patients with epilepsy.[33] Selective serotonin-reuptake inhibitors have largely replaced tricyclic antidepressants in the management of somatic psychiatric conditions, but good comparative treatment studies in patients with brain tumors are not available.

Prophylactic Perioperative Care

PROPHYLACTIC ANTICONVULSANTS

Although it has been common practice in the USA and parts of Europe to prescribe prophylactic anticonvulsants prior to neurosurgery for malignant brain tumors, there is now evidence from a meta-analysis of randomized controlled trials showing that anticonvulsant prophylaxis does not reduce the seizure incidence (OR 1.09; 95% CI, 0.63 to 1.89; p=0.8), seizure-free survival (OR 1.03; 95% CI, 0.74 to 1.44; p=0.9), or overall survival (OR 0.93; 95% CI, 0.65 to 1.32; p=0.7) in patients with brain tumors who have not had an epileptic seizure.[34] More recent studies, in which patients were randomized either to no treatment or to treatment with carbamazepine or phenytoin for 6 or 24 months, showed no significant differences in any group. A high incidence of drug-related side effects was found in this and other studies.[35–37] Anticonvulsant prophylaxis in patients with newly diagnosed brain tumors is therefore not justified.

PROPHYLACTIC ANTICOAGULATION

Cancer, immobility, hemiplegia, and surgery are all risk factors for deep vein thrombosis and pulmonary embolus. Risk of DVT and/or pulmonary embolus is age-related, with an annual incidence of less than 1:3000 in patients under the age of 40 and 1:500 in those over the age of 80.[38] The frequency of DVT in malignant glioma is between 19% and 28%, and the risk that a patient with a brain tumor will display a DVT in follow-up studies is between 22% and 45%.[39] The frequency of DVT is highest in meningioma (72%), followed by glioma (60%) and metastasis (20%).[40,41] Despite the very high likelihood of thrombotic complications in patients with malignant glioma, there is no consensus about DVT prophylaxis.[42] The risk of DVT is reduced by use of compression stockings, pneumatic intermittent compression boots, early mobilization, low-dose heparin or fractionated heparin. A meta-analysis of four randomized controlled trials of heparin prophylaxis in neurosurgical patients has shown that with placebo, 29% of people develop DVT, compared with 16% of those receiving low molecular weight heparin or unfractionated heparin.[43] A critical appraisal of the literature on prophylactic anticoagulation therapy in neurosurgery concluded that treatment with heparin resulted in a 45% relative risk reduction of venous thromboembolism (OR 0.48; 95% CI 0.35-0.66; p<0.001).[44] Major bleeding complications were infrequent, but heparin (both UFH and LMWH) resulted in a 71% increased relative risk of major bleeding events (OR 1.71; 95% CI 0.69-4.27; p=0.24). A randomized controlled trial of heparin 5000 U subcutaneously, starting 2 hours before surgery and continuing every 12 hours thereafter until full ambulation or for 7 days, in 103 patients undergoing surgery for removal of a supratentorial tumor, showed no increase in bleeding tendency in any of the parameters examined compared with the placebo arm.[45] There is no evidence to suggest that enoxaparin 40 mg/day is superior to unfractionated heparin. In the randomized controlled trial comparing these agents as prophylaxis, none of the 150 participants in the study suffered symptomatic DVT and less than 10% had asymptomatic DVT (mostly calf) using the combination of graduated compression stockings, intermittent pneumatic compression, and either enoxaparin or subcutaneous heparin 5000 U twice daily.[46] A multimodality approach to prophylaxis, using compression stockings, pneumatic intermittent compression boots, and prophylactic perioperative minidose heparin during surgery is safe and is recommended.

Complications Indirectly Related to the Tumor and Its Effects

DEEP VEIN THROMBOSIS AND PULMONARY EMBOLUS

Deep vein thrombosis (DVT) may be difficult to diagnose. Although DVT may cause unilateral calf or thigh swelling, pain and tenderness along the line of the deep veins, low-grade pyrexia, distension of superficial veins, or color change, many cases are asymptomatic. Homan sign is poorly predictive. There is a 10% rate of symptomatic pulmonary embolus in untreated proximal DVT, and 18% to 30% mortality if this is left untreated.[47] Pulmonary embolus is rare if the DVT is treated by anticoagulation therapy.[48] DVT can be complicated by critical limb ischemia (less than 5%), recurrent DVT (20% in 5 years), or postthrombotic syndrome (50% to 75%). If clinically suspected, intravenous heparin should be started until the diagnosis is excluded by diagnostic imaging.[49] as the benefits of anticoagulation outweigh the risks of tumor hemorrhage. Compression ultrasound will reliably identify proximal DVT, but contrast venography is the gold standard if ultrasound is negative.

Unfractionated heparin is the initial treatment of choice followed by oral anticoagulation.[49,50] Low molecular weight heparin is an effective alternative to unfractionated heparin and may reduce both the occurrence of major bleeding during initial treatment and overall mortality.[51] Low molecular weight heparin is more costly, but it can be given once per day by subcutaneous injection and there is no need to monitor blood tests. If DVT is confirmed, heparin should be continued for 4 to 6 days while oral anticoagulation is being introduced. An international normalized ratio (INR) of greater than 2.0 on 2 consecutive days should be obtained before heparin is stopped. The optimal INR after a first DVT is 2.5. Anticoagulation should be continued for at least 3 months, although 6 months is commonly recommended. Aspirin and nonsteroidal antiinflammatory drugs should be avoided when on heparin or warfarin. Hypersensitivity (drug-induced thrombocytopenia), local injection site bruising, and bleeding are common complications of heparin. Graduated elastic compression stockings worn on the affected leg for at least 2 years after a DVT reduces the incidence of postthrombotic syndrome from 23% to 11%.[52,53]

Effort dyspnea, syncope, and tiredness may herald small pulmonary emboli, while medium-sized emboli usually cause pleuritic chest pain, cough, and hemoptysis. Large pulmonary emboli cause central chest pain, collapse, shock, tachypnea, and tachycardia. A spiral computed tomogram of the chest usually demonstrates emboli well, but occasionally a pulmonary angiogram is required. Alternatively, a ventilation-perfusion scan using technecium-99m may show mismatch. Blood gases, electrocardiogram, chest x-ray, erythrocyte sedimentation rate, and full blood count may be supportive where pulmonary angiogram or spiral CT are not readily available. Medical management of pulmonary embolism consists of 100% oxygen, intravenous fluids to increase the right ventricular filling pressure, heparin, and oral anticoagulation. Venous thrombectomy and pulmonary embolectomy may be indicated for massive pulmonary emboli. If there is a clear contraindication to anticoagulation (e.g., known hypersensitivity to heparin or pork products, major active bleeding, thrombocytopenia <50,000 platelets/μl, or a history of heparin-induced thrombocytopenia), inferior vena caval filters can be used. Filters often do not prevent pulmonary emboli, and some studies suggest a 40% recurrence rate and a high complication rate (62%).[54,55]

Complications from Medical Treatment

STEROIDS

Common gastrointestinal complications of dexamethasone include dyspepsia, candidiasis, and abdominal distention, and less commonly peptic or esophageal ulceration or acute pancreatitis. These can be minimized by keeping the steroid dose as low as possible and giving an H2 receptor antagonist (e.g., cimetidine or ranitidine) or a proton pump inhibitor (e.g., omeprazole or lansoprazole). Musculoskeletal effects, particularly proximal myopathy, osteoporosis with vertebral fractures, avascular necrosis of the hip, and tendon rupture are generally the result of long-term high-dose usage, but proximal myopathy can start after a few weeks of high-dose dexamethasone. Endocrine effects such as increased appetite, weight gain, unmasked diabetes, and increased susceptibility to infection (e.g., *Candida*) appear early. Adrenal suppression is a late feature. Neuropsychiatric side effects such as insomnia are very common early symptoms, ever at lower doses whereas euphoria, anxiety, or acute confusional state and psychosis are, usually, early dose-related effects. Psychological dependence and depression may occur with long-term usage. Worsening of glaucoma is a rare but serious early complication, while other ophthalmological complications such as cataract and scleral thinning occur with prolonged use. Ankle edema, skin atrophy, bruising, striae, telangectasia, and acne can occur after a few weeks at high dosage.

Cautions for usage include advanced age, past history of tuberculosis, heart, liver or renal failure, diabetes, hypertension, glaucoma, or a past history of severe psychosis. With long-term usage, elevation in blood sugar occur in 47% to 72%, peripheral edema in 11%, anxiety or psychiatric disorders in 10%, oropharyngeal candidiasis in 6% to 8%, Cushing syndrome in 15%, and muscular weakness in 60%. Rarely, an acute myopathy can come on within a week of starting high-dose corticosteroids and can involve respiratory muscles. Myopathy is more common with 9-alpha-fluorinated corticosteroids, such as dexamethasone; classical steroid myopathy is painless, with a slow onset, and affects proximal lower limb muscles and occasionally proximal upper limbs.[56] The mechanism of this steroid myopathy is felt to be due to inhibition of messenger RNA synthesis of muscle-specific proteins. Withdrawal of dexamethasone after usage for some months must be done fairly slowly, and may be associated with changes in mood, myalgia, arthropathy, headaches, or loss of appetite. Dexamethasone-withdrawal headache is nonspecific and may lead to the reinstatement of higher doses due to concerns of raised intracranial pressure. Evidence of reduced tumor mass effect and reassurance that withdrawal can cause headache may aid eventual withdrawal and limit psychological dependence.

ANTIEPILEPTIC DRUGS (AEDs)

AEDs should be prescribed after discussions with the patient about the benefits and side effect profiles. Ideally, epilepsy should be treated with a single anticonvulsant agent at the lowest effective dose. Combination therapy may be necessary, but is commonly associated with complex drug interactions and increased frequency of side effects. A careful watch must be kept in the early stages of drug introduction, especially for early hematological, hypersensitivity, or central nervous system side effects. Early allergic responses necessitate withdrawal. AED hypersensitivity syndrome is characterized by multisystem involvement, fever, lymphadenopathy, mucocutaneous rash, hypertransaminasemia, and peripheral eosinophilia. This potentially lethal complication is a feature of aromatic enzyme-inducing antiepileptics (phenytoin, phenobarbital, carbamazepine) through the hepatic cytochrome P450 (CYP) isoenzyme mechanism.[57] There is cross-reactivity between these antiepileptics. The risk of allergic rash or blood dyscrasias is approximately 5% to 10% with carbamazepine, phenytoin, and lamotrigine. This generally occurs within the first 2 months of starting therapy. Stevens-Johnson syndrome, toxic epidermal necrolysis, and hepatic complications are rare but serious complications. In patients with drug-induced skin rash, valproate, gabapentin, topiramate, tiagabine, and levetiracetam are moderately safe choices.

The enzyme-inducing AEDs will commonly increase the gamma GT by up to three times the upper limit, but this usually only requires monitoring rather than drug alteration. However, all drugs (especially valproate) can cause serious hepatic toxicity and liver failure; therefore, although these complications are rare, it is advisable to monitor liver function during the introduction and the following 6 months. The incidence of hematological toxicity from valproate is low and mainly consists of dose-dependent thrombocytopenia. Interactions are usually due to hepatic enzyme induction or inhibition, and are variable and often unpredictable. AED interactions are summarized in Table 12-2.

Metabolism of phenytoin may be altered by drugs influencing CYP2C9 or CYP2C19, such as diazepam, leading to phenytoin toxicity. Tricyclic antidepressants inhibit CYP2C19. P450 enzyme-inducing anticonvulsants reduce serum levels of chemotherapeutic agents metabolized by CYP3A4 and CYP2A6. This could have a beneficial effect on reducing the toxicity of chemotherapeutic agents, but may also reduce the effectiveness of these agents. Whether this has any significant effect on survival or outcome is still uncertain. When survival was studied in chemotherapy trials of patients with glioblastoma who were or were not on enzyme-inducing AEDs, enzyme-inducing AEDs were associated with better overall survival and progression-free survival (HR=0.75, p=0.0029 and HR 0.81, p=0.024, respectively).[58] Enzyme-inhibiting AEDs (e.g., valproic acid) can increase the concentration of chemotherapy. The newer generation of AEDs (e.g., lamotrigine, gabapentin, and levetiracetam) are not metabolized by CYP, and may be as effective in managing seizures.[59] Procarbazine oxidation is enhanced by enzyme-inducing AEDs and may increase the likelihood of hypersensitivity reactions to procarbazine.[60] The risk of thrombocytopenia with valproate may be worsened if patients are receiving fotomustine-cisplatinum chemotherapy, but it responds to valproate dose reduction.[61]

In the context of management of patients with brain tumors, AEDs may cause central nervous system side effects that may be difficult to distinguish from tumor

TABLE 12-2 Antiepileptic Drug Addiction and the Effect on Existing Drugs

Carbamazepine	Often lowers concentration	Clonazepam, clobazam, lamotrigine, phenytoin, valproate, topirimate, oxcarbazepine, tiagabine
	May increase concentration	Phenytoin, phenobarbital
Gabapentin	No interactions	
Lamotrigine	May increase	Active metabolite carbamazepine
Levetiracetam	No interactions	
Oxcarbazepine	May lower concentration	Carbamazepine
	May raise concentration	Carbamazepine
Phenobarbital	Often lowers concentration	Clonazepam, carbamazepine Lamotrigine, phenytoin, valproate, topirimate, oxcarbazepine,tiagabine
	May increase concentration	Phenytoin
Phenytoin	Often lowers concentration	Clonazepam, carbamazepine Lamotrigine, valproate, topirimate, oxcarbazepine, tiagabine
	Often increases concentration	Phenobarbital
Topiramate	May raises concentration	Phenytoin
Valproate	May lower concentration	Active metabolite oxcarbazepine
	Often raises concentration	Active metabolite carbamazepine Lamotrigine, Phenobarbital, Phenytoin

progression or may influence management in other ways. These are summarized in Table 12-3. Carbamazepine can cause a mild neutropenia and hyponatremia that may influence the later use of chemotherapy. Valproate is often associated with weight gain that can be a problem if the patient also requires steroids. Valproate can also inhibit platelet aggregation and the coagulation cascade which may lead to a higher tendency to hemorrhage when used with heparins, warfarin, or nonsteroidal antiinflammatory drugs. Valproate can cause a fine tremor, which is often more noticeable in the hemiparetic limb in patients with an existing hemiparesis. Toxicity, with AEDs inducing dysarthria, ataxia, lethargy, and weakness, can be easily mistaken for tumor progression, although the presence of nystagmus and intermittent diplopia and the absence of papilledema or focal neurological deficit are helpful pointers to the likely diagnosis of AED toxicity. Many AEDs are associated with headache, cognitive, speech or memory problems, or psychiatric symptoms that may be mistaken for tumor progression. Some suggest that patients with cognitive problems may be best suited to treatment with newer agents such as lamotrigine, gabapentin, tiagabine, levetiracetam or oxcarbazepine, although this is only by extrapolation from studies in patients with nontumor-associated epilepsy. Obese patients may benefit from topiramate or zonisamide, as these have a tendancy to produce weight loss. Acute angle closure glaucoma has been associated with topiramate and reverses when the

TABLE 12-3 Important, Common, or CNS Side Effects of Anticonvulsants

Carbamazepine	Cautions:	Hepatic, renal, cardiac disease. Glaucoma. Beware of early severe blood and skin disorders
Oxcarbazepine	Toxicity:	Diplopia, dizziness; confusion, ataxia, tremor
	Side effects:	Rash, agitation; leukopenia and other blood disorders, jaundice, renal failure, hypersensitivity reaction, depression, psychosis, alopecia, hyponatremia, edema, osteomalacia
Gabapentin	Cautions:	Psychotic illness, renal impairment, diabetes
	Toxicity:	Tiredness, diplopia, dizziness, ataxia, tremor
	Side effects:	Rash, leukopenia and other blood disorders, myalgia, headache, memory problems, hypersensitivity reaction, cough, paresthesia
Lamotrigine	Cautions:	Hepatic, renal. Beware of early severe blood and skin disorders and aplastic anemia
	Toxicity:	Diplopia, dizziness; confusion and ataxia
	Side effects:	Rash, hypersensitivity reaction, flu-like illness, worsening seizures, agitation; leukopenia and other blood disorders, dizziness, drowsiness, insomnia, headache, agitation
Levetiracetam	Cautions:	Hepatic, renal disease
	Toxicity:	Drowsiness, fatigue, and dizziness
	Side effects:	Drowsiness, fatigue, and dizziness. Rarely amnesia, psychiatric symptoms, insomnia, headache, rash
Phenobarbital	Cautions:	Hepatic, renal disease; careful in elderly
	Toxicity:	Drowsiness, fatigue, and dizziness
	Side effects:	Drowsiness, fatigue, and dizziness, psychiatric symptoms(depression or agitation), insomnia, megaloblastic anemia (folate deficiency)
Phenytoin	Cautions:	Hepatic disease. Beware of early severe blood and skin disorders.
	Toxicity:	Diplopia, dizziness; confusion, ataxia, tremor
	Side effects:	Rash, agitation; leukopenia and other blood disorders, jaundice, SLE, hypersensitivity reaction, depression, psychosis, gum hypertrophy, peripheral neuropathy, megaloblastic anemia, osteomalacia
Topiramate	Cautions:	Hepatic disease and renal disease. May cause secondary acute angle closure glaucoma in myopes in first month.
	Toxicity:	Diplopia, dizziness; confusion, ataxia, tremor
	Side effects:	Rash, agitation; leukopenia and other blood disorders, jaundice, weight loss, paresthesia, memory problems, fatigue, speech problems, depression, psychosis
Valproate	Cautions:	Hepatic disease, clotting disorders. Pancreatitis
	Toxicity:	Tremor. Diplopia, dizziness; confusion, ataxia
	Side effects:	Leukopenia and other blood disorders, alopecia, weight gain, gastrointestinal side effects, memory problems, dementia, gynecomastia

drug is withdrawn. Vigabatrin is not commonly used now because of its association with irreversible visual field loss and the requirement for visual fields to be checked regularly.[62]

H2 RECEPTOR ANTAGONISTS AND PROTON PUMP INHIBITORS

These drugs are commonly started around the same time as dexamethasone in order to prevent gastric symptoms, particularly if there is concomitant use of aspirin or nonsteroidal antiinflammatory agents, or because of gastric symptoms caused by dexamethasone. These agents can cause headache, dizziness, rash, and tiredness, and rarely confusion, depression, and hallucinations. Leukopenia, thrombocytopenia, rash, and disturbance of hepatic enzymes may mimic either anticonvulsant allergy or side effects of chemotherapy. Cimetidine binds to microsomal cytochrome P450 and should be avoided in patients on warfarin and phenytoin. Ranitidine does not inhibit drug metabolism. Proton pump inhibitors may also cause headache, hypersensitivity reactions, peripheral edema, muscle and joint pains, alopecia, and blurring of vision. Omeprazole and lansoprazole can rarely be associated with hyponatremia and with acute confusional states, agitation, and hallucinations.

ANTIDEPRESSANTS AND ANXIOLYTICS

As mentioned earlier, not all patients with anxiety or depression require medication. Anxiolytic and antidepressant use should not be embarked upon lightly. Tricyclic antidepressants are contraindicated in patients with urinary outflow obstruction, narrow-angle glaucoma, cardiac arrhythmias, or postural hypotension. Fluoxetine, paroxetine, and high dose sertraline are contraindicated in patients receiving codeine compounds. Antidepressants in general are associated with new-onset seizures in 0.2% of otherwise healthy patients; the frequency is likely to be higher in those with an underlying brain tumor. Worsening of seizures is always a risk, although not as commonly seen as one might expect in patients already on antiepileptic drugs.

Tricyclic antidepressants can be divided into sedative and less sedative drugs. The sedating agents are drugs such as amitripyline, clomipramine, dothiepin, doxepin, mianserin, and trazodone. The less sedating drugs are imipramine, lofepramine, and nortriptyline. Imipramine and amitriptyline have more muscarinic and cardiac side effects. Lofepramine has fewer muscarinic side effects and is less dangerous in overdose, but may be associated with hepatic toxicity. Gradual introduction is important in the elderly because of hypotensive effects with dizziness or syncope. Tricyclic agents may be associated with hyponatremia.

Selective serotonin-reuptake inhibitors (SSRIs) have fewer muscarinic side effects and are less cardiotoxic than tricyclic agents. Gastric side effects of nausea and vomiting are common. Hyponatremia is more common with SSRIs than with tricyclics and may cause confusion, tiredness, and worsening of seizures. Anxiolytics are helpful in acute panic disorders and for the short-term relief of severe anxiety, but cautious use in advised in patients with respiratory disease or muscle weakness and in the elderly. Side effects include drowsiness, confusion, ataxia, memory problems, paradoxical increase in aggression, muscle weakness, and occasionally headache, vertigo, hypotension, and visual disturbance.

Antipsychotic agents such as chlorpromazine and haloperidol have sedative, antimuscarinic, and extrapyramidal side effects; they are contraindicated in patients with epilepsy, as they are pro-convulsant.

Neurological and Psychiatric Postoperative Complications

POSTOPERATIVE HEADACHES

Postoperative headache is frequently a source of concern for patients, and sometimes for their doctors. As in all cases of headache, a full history of the headache should be taken. The timing of onset, site, character, frequency, severity, temporal development, relieving and aggravating factors, and associated features (nausea, vomiting, focal signs, papilledema, fever) should be sought. After craniotomy, it is common for patients to complain of local tenderness at the craniotomy site, which may persist for weeks, months, or years. These headaches generally do not require more than simple analgesia (e.g., acetaminophen). In addition, there may be an intermittent sharp, stabbing pain that is momentary but frequently recurrent. There can sometimes be a sensation of water running down that side of the scalp, or another unusual sensation. There is scalp and skull tenderness, but usually no clearly discernible sensory loss. Generally, reassurance, local massage (when the wound has healed), or heat and simple analgesia may be all that is required. The sharp, stabbing pains are usually so brief that analgesia is not helpful. Frequent or particularly severe neuralgic pains may, rarely, require analgesia with carbamazepine or amitriptyline. Postsurgical migraines are not uncommon, particularly in previous migraineurs.

NEUROLOGICAL IMPAIRMENTS

In a prospective database, 788 patients who underwent their first or second craniotomy for malignant glioma were analyzed for perioperative complications.[63] Perioperative complications occurred in 24% of patients after a first operation and 33% of patients after a second ($p = 0.1$). Most patients were the same or better neurologically after surgery, but 8% displayed significant worsening after the first operation and 18% after the second ($p = 0.007$). Regional complications occurred at similar rates in both groups, but systemic infections occurred more frequently in the second surgery group (4.4% compared with 0%; $p < 0.0001$), as did depression (20% compared with 11%; $p = 0.02$). The perioperative mortality rate was 1.5% following a first operation and 2.2% after a second. Nevertheless, most selected patients are neurologically stable or improved after either their first or second craniotomy.[64] Studies using intraoperative image guidance and functional mapping in patients with low-grade glioma identified a high percentage of postoperative cognitive deficits, but these often resolve within 3 months.[65,66] In one study of neurocognitive dysfunction in patients with insular tumors undergoing surgery, neurosurgeons presurgically identified altered mental status in 13%; however, neuropsychological testing demonstrated cognitive problems in 73%. Postsurgical decline (median 16 days postoperatively) was identified in all patients in at least one cognitive domain.[67] See Table 12-4.

TABLE 12-4 Postoperative Change in Neurological Impairment (Edinburgh Functional Impairment Tests [EFIT]), Disability (Barthel Disability Index), and Performance (Karnofsky Performance Scale) in Patients with Single Intracerebral Tumors

(n=193)	Improved	Stable	Worse
EFIT (Resection + steroids)	31 (24%)	59 (46%)	39 (36%)
EFIT (Biopsy + steroids)	10 (16%)	31 (48%)	23 (36%)
Barthel Disability Index	10 (10%)	59 (61%)	26 (27%)
Karnofsky Performance Scale	11 (11%)	59 (61%)	26 (27%)

ACUTE CONFUSIONAL STATES/ACUTE PANIC ATTACKS

In patients who are confused or demented or who have receptive dysphasia, all forms of treatment should be discussed with the next of kin. In patients with postsurgical acute confusional states, it is essential to consider infection, hypoxia, endocrine or metabolic derangement, drug-related side effects, and underlying psychiatric conditions. Psychiatrists are skilled in assessments of mental capacity and consent, and if the psychiatric disturbance is severe, the patient may require to be detained and treated under section. Patients with acute confusional states in the early postsurgical phase are almost always being treated with steroids. The management of these patients generally follows the usual principles of management of an acute delirium in a medically sick patient. Some advice concerning psychiatric complications in cancer patients has been published in the literature.[68] A study from Memorial Sloan-Kettering Cancer Center found that 41% of inpatient psychiatric referrals were diagnosed with organic mental disorders.[30]

Acute panic attacks are uncommon and must be differentiated from epileptic panic attacks. They usually occur in patients with a past history of anxiety or depression and are more common in younger patients (under 50 years of age). Early identification of patients with anxiety and appropriate counseling (information clearly given, reassurance, message of hope, advice about side effects of medication, a contact telephone number to call if anxious, e.g., neuro-oncology nurse), may be highly effective in reducing the likelihood of panic attacks. Epileptic panic attacks are usually short-lived, stereotyped, and nonsituational; also, the patient is well between attacks. An electroencephalogram may show a discharging seizure focus. The treatment is appropriate antiepileptic drugs. The recognized treatments for severe acute (nonepileptic) panic attacks include cognitive behavior therapy and, particularly in the USA, alprazolam treatment.[28,30] In general, short-acting drugs with a good side-effect profile (less potent anticholinergic effects) should be prescribed at low doses.

Conclusions

The management of patients with intrinsic brain tumors in the early perioperative and postoperative period can be challenging. As can be seen from this chapter, there are important diagnostic and management roles that have historically been the remit of neurologists or psychiatrists, and others that involve the neurosurgeon's skills. Neuro-oncology specialist nurses are in an ideal position to bridge the gap between primary care physician, neurologist, and neurosurgeon as well as to act as a initial point of contact for the patient or primary care physician following diagnosis. Increasingly, it is perceived that a multidisciplinary team approach to care is superior to the single clinician approach. It is hoped that this chapter has highlighted areas in the management of brain tumors where this multidisciplinary paradigm will improve care.

I would like to thank Dr Alasdair Rooney, Neuro-Oncology Psychiatry Fellow, Edinburgh Centre for Neuro-Oncology for his input into the psychiatric management of people with brain tumors.

REFERENCES

1. Grant R. Overview: Brain tumour diagnosis and management/Royal College of Physician Guidelines. J Neurol Neurosurg Psychiat 2004;75(Suppl. 2):18–23.
2. Forsyth PA, Posner JB. Headaches in patients with brain tumors. Neurology 1993;43:1678–83.
3. Fisher CM. Brain herniation: a revision of classical concepts. Can J Neurol Sci 1995;22(2):83–91.
4. Schaller B, Ruegg SJ. Brain tumor and seizures: pathophysiology and its implications for treatment revisited. Epilepsia 2003;44(9):1223–32.
5. Clyde Z, Chataway J, Signorini D, Gregor A, Grant R. Significant change in tests of neurological impairment in patients with brain tumours. J Neurooncol 1998;39:81–90.
6. Tucha O, Smely C, Preier M, Lange KW. Cognitive deficits before treatment among patients with brain tumors. Neurosurgery 2000;47:324–33.
7. Pringle A, Taylor R, Whittle IR. Anxiety and depression in patients with intracranial neoplasm before and after tumour surgery. Br J Neurosurg 1999;13(1):46–51.
8. Mainio A, Hakko H, Niemela A, Tuurinkoski T, Koivukangas J, Rasanen P. The effect of brain tumour laterality on anxiety levels among neurosurgical patients. J Neurol Neurosurg Psychiat 2003;74:1278–82.
9. Gupta RK, Kumar R. Benign brain tumours and psychiatric morbidity: a 5 years retrospective data analysis. Austral New Zealand J Psychiat 2004;38:316–9.
10. Pelletier G, Verhoef M, Khatri N, Hagen N. Quality of life in brain tumor patients: the relative contributions of depression, fatigue, emotional distress and existential issues. J Neurooncol 2002;57(1):41–9.
11. Wellisch D, Kaleita T, Freeman D, Cloughesy T, Goldman J. Predicting major depression in brain tumor patients. Psychooncol 2002;11(3):230–8.
12. Hahn CA, Dunn RH, Logue PE, King JH, Edwards CL, Halperin EC. Prospective study of neuropsychologic testing and quality-of-life assessment of adults with primary malignant brain tumors. Int J Radiat Oncol Biol Phys 2003;55(4):992–9.
13. Hemper C, Weiss E, Hess CF. Dexamethasone treatment in patients with brain metastases and primary brain tumors: do the benefits outweigh the side effects? Sup Care Cancer 2002;10:322–8.
14. Vecht CJ, Hovestadt A, Verbiest HB, van Vliet JJ, van Puten. Dose effect relationship of dexamethasone on Karnofsky performance in metastatic brain tumors: a randomized study of doses of 4, 8, and 16mg per day. Neurology 1994;44(4):675–80.
15. Watling CJ, Cairncross JG. Acetazolamide therapy for symptomatic plateau waves in patients with brain tumors. Report of three cases. J Neurosurg 2002;97(1):224–6.
16. www.dvla.gov.uk.
17. Bergey GK. Initial treatment of epilepsy: special issues in treating the elderly. Neurology 2004;63(10 Suppl. 4):S40–8.
18. Wagner GL, Wilms EB, van Donselaar CA, Vecht ChJ. Levetiracetam: preliminary experience in patients with primary tumours. Seizure 2003;12(8):585–6.
19. Beghi E. efficacy and tolerability of the newer anti-epileptic drugs: comparison of two recent guidelines. Lancet Neurol 2004;3(10):618–21.
20. Zenter J, Hufnagel A, Wolf HK, Ostertun B, Behrens E, Campos M, et al. Surgical treatment of neoplasms associated with medically intractable epilepsy. Neurosurgery 1997;41(2):378–86.

21. Schrottner O, Eder HG, Unger F, Feichtinger K, Pendl G. Radiosurgery in lesional epilepsy: brain tumors. Stereotact Funct Neurosurg 1998;70(Suppl. 1):50–6.
22. Hoang-Xuan K, Capelle L, Kujas M, et al. Temozolomide as initial treatment for adults with low-grade oligodendroglioma or oligoastrocytomas and correlation with chromosome 1p deletions. J Clin Oncol 2004;22(15):3133–8.
23. Herrmann M, Curio N, Petz T, Synowitz H, Wagner S, Bartels C, et al. Coping with illness after brain diseases—a comparison between patients with malignant brain tumors, stroke, Parkinson's disease and traumatic brain injury. Disabil Rehab 2000 Aug 15;22(12):539–46.
24. Gill D, Hatcher S. A systematic review of the treatment of depression with antidepressant drugs in patients who also have physical illness. J Psychosomat Res 1999;47(2):131–43.
25. Voellinger R, Berney A, Bauman P, Annoni J-M, Bryois C, Buclin T, et al. Major depressive disorder in the general hospital: adaptation of the practice guidelines. Gen Hosp Psychiat 2003;25(3):185–93.
26. Mynors-Wallis L, et al. Problem-solving treatment: evidence for effectiveness and feasibility in primary care. Int J Psychiat Med 1996;26:249–62.
27. Schulberg HC, Block MR, Madonia MJ, Scott CP, Rodriguez E, Imber SD, et al. Treating major depression in primary care practice: eight month clinical outcomes. Arch Gen Psychiat 1996;58:112–8.
28. Wein S. Cancer. In: Robinson R, Yates W, editors. Psychiatric Treatment of the Mentally Ill. New York: Marcel Dekker, Inc; 1999. p. 229–51.
29. Huang ME, Wartella J, Kreutzer J, Broaddus W, Lyckholm L. Functional outcomes and quality of life in patients with brain tumours: a review of the literature. Brain Inj 2001;15:843–56.
30. Passik S, Ricketts P. Central Nervous System Tumors. Psycho-oncology 1998. JC Holland. Oxford: Oxford University Press; p. 303–13.
31. Litofsky NS, Farace E, Anderson Jr F, Meyers CA, Huang W, Laws Jr ER. Glioma Outcomes Project Investigators. Depression in patients with high-grade glioma: results of the Glioma Outcomes Project. Neurosurgery 2004;54(2):358–66 Feb (discussion 366–7).
32. Kuhn KU, Quednow BB, Thiel M, Falkai P, Maier W, Elger CE. Anti-depressive treatment in patients with temporal lobe epilepsy and major depression: a prospective study with three different antidepressants. Epilepsy Behav 2003;4(6):674–9.
33. Boylan LS, Flint LA, Labovitz DL, Jackson SC, Starner K, Devinsky O. Depression but not seizure frequency predicts quality of life in treatment-resistant epilepsy. Neurology 2004;62(2):258–61.
34. Glantz MJ, Cole BF, Forsyth PA, Recht LD, Wen PY, Chamberlain MC, et al. Practice Parameter: Anticonvulsant prophylaxis in patients with newly diagnosed brain tumours. Report of the Quality Standards Subcommittee of the American Academy of Neurology 2000. http://www.aan.com/professionals/practice/index.
35. Foy PM, Chadwick DW, Rajgopalan N, Johnson AL, Shaw MD. Do prophylactic anticonvulsant drugs alter the pattern of seizures after craniotomy? J Neurol Neurosurg Psychiat 1992 Sep;55(9): 753–7.
36. De Santis A, Villani R, Sinisi M, Stocchetti N, Perucca E. Add-on phenytoin fails to prevent early seizures after surgery for supratentorial brain tumors: a randomized controlled study. Epilepsia 2002;43(2):175–82.
37. Pace A, Bove L, Innocenti P, et al. Epilepsy in gliomas: incidence and treatment in 119 patients. J Exp Clin Cancer Res 1998;17(4):479–82.
38. DH. Advice on travel related deep vein thrombosis. London Department of Health 2002. www.doh.gov.uk/dvt/index.htm.
39. Sawaya RE, Ligon BL. Thromboembolic complications associated with brain tumors. J Neurooncol 1994;22:173–81.
40. Sawaya R, Zuccarello M, Elkalliny M, Nishiyama H. Post-operative venous thromboembolism and brain tumors: part 1. Clinical profile. J Neurooncol 1992;14:119–25.
41. Levi AD, Wallace MC, Bernstein M, Walters BC. Venous thromboembolism after brain tumor surgery: a retrospective review. Neurosurgery 1991;28:859–63.
42. Danish SF, Burnett MG, Stein SC. Prophylaxis for deep venous thrombosis in patients with craniotomies: a review. Neurosurg Focus 2004;17:1–8.
43. Iorio A, Agnelli G. Low *molecular* weight and unfractionated heparin for prevention of venous thromboembolism in neurosurgery—a meta-analysis. Arch Int Med 2000;160(15):2327–32.
44. Abdulwadud O. Anticoagulation therapy as prophylaxis for prevention of DVT or pulmonary embolism in neurosurgery. [Online]. Available from http://www.med.monash.edu.au/healthservices/cce/ 2002.
45. Constantini S, Kanner A, Friedman A, Shoshan Y, Israel Z, Ashkenazi E, et al. Safety of perioperative minidose heparin in patients undergoing brain tumor surgery: a prospective, randomized, double blind study. J Neurosurg 2001;94(6):918–21.

46. Goldhaber SZ, Dunn K, Gerhard-Herman M, Park JK, Black PMcL. Low rate of venous thromboembolism after craniotomy for brain tumor using multimodality prophylaxis. Chest 2002;122:1933–7.
47. Hull RD, Pineo GF. Prophylaxis of deep venous thrombosis and pulmonary embolism. Current recommendations. Med Clin North Am 1998;82(3):477–93.
48. Hutten BA, Prins MH. Duration of oral anticoagulant treatment for symptomatic venous thromboembolism (Cochrane Review). The Cochrane Library 2002;(4). Oxford. Update Software.
49. SIGN Anti-thrombotic therapy. Report Number 36. Scottish Intercollegiate Guidelines Network www.sign.ac.uk; 1999.
50. Brandjes DP, Heijboer H, Butler HR, de Rijk M, Jagt H, ten Cate JW. Acenocoumerol and heparin compared with acenocoumerol alone in the initial treatment of proximal vein thrombosis. N Engl J Med 1992;327(21):1485–9.
51. van den Belt AGM, Prins MH, Lensing AW, et al. Fixed dose subcutaneous low molecular weight heparin for the long term treatment of symptomatic venous thromboembolism. (Cochrane Review). The Cochrane Library 2002;(4) Oxford. Update software.
52. Brandes AA, Scelzi E, Salmistraro G, Ermani M, Carollo C, Berti F, et al. Incidence of risk of thromboembolism during treatment of high grade gliomas: a prospective study. Eur J Cancer 1997;33:1592–6.
53. McCollum C. Avoiding the consequences of deep vein thrombosis. Elevation and compression are important and too often forgotten. Brit Med J 1998;317:696.
54. Levin JM, Schiff D, Loeffler JS, Fine HA, Black PM, Wen PY. Complications of therapy for venous thromboembolic disease in patients with brain tumors. Neurology 1993;43:1111–4.
55. Schiff D, DeAngelis L. Therapy for venous thromboembolism in patients with brain metastases. Cancer 1994;73:493–8.
56. Batchelor TT, Taylor LP, Thaler HT, Posner JB, DeAngelis LM. Steroid myopathy in cancer patients. Neurology 1997;48:1234–8.
57. Maldonado RN, Tello SJ, Garcia-Baquero RE, Castano HA. Anticonvulsant hypersensitivity syndrome with fatal outcome. Eur J Dermatol 2002;12(5):503–5.
58. Jaekle KA, Ballman K, Uhm J, O'Fallon J, Schomberg P, Scheithauer C, et al. Comparison of survival endpoints in glioblastoma patients receiving or not receiving enzyme-inducing anticonvulsants in NCCTG Trails. 113s ASCO 2004. Abstract No 1525 J Clini Oncol 2004;22(Suppl. 14):113s.
59. Vecht CJ, Wagner GL, Wilms EB. Treating seizures in patients with brain tumors: Drug interactions between antiepileptic and chemotherapeutic agents. Semin Oncol 2003;30(6 Suppl. 19):49–52.
60. Lehmann DF, Hurteau TE, Newman N, Coyle TE. Anticonvulsant usage is associated with an increased risk of procarbazine hypersensitivity reactions in patients with brain tumors. Clin Pharmacol Ther 1997;62(2):225–9.
61. Bourg V, Lebrun C, Chichmanian RM, Thomas P, Frenay M. Nitroso-urea-cisplatin-based chemotherapy associated with valproate: increase of haematological toxicity. Ann Oncol 2001;12(2):217–9.
62. Asconape JJ. Some common issues in the use of antiepileptic drugs. Semin Neurol 2002;22(1):27–39.
63. Chang SM, Parney IF, McDermott M, Barker 2nd FG, Schmidt MH, Huang W, et al. Glioma Outcomes Investigators. Perioperative complications and neurological outcomes of first and second craniotomies among patients enrolled in the Glioma Outcome Project. J Neurosurg 2003;Jun 98(6):1175–81.
64. Grant R, Slattery J, Gregor A, Whittle IR. Recording neurological impairment in clinical trials of glioma. J Neuro-Oncol 1994;19:37–49.
65. Duffau H, Capelle L, Denvil D, et al. Functional recovery after surgical resection of low grade gliomas in eloquent brain: hypothesis of brain compensation. J Neurol Neurosurg Psychiat 2003;74:901–7.
66. Duffau H, Capelle L, Denvil D, et al. Usefulness of intra-operative electrical subcortical mapping during surgery for low grade gliomas located within eloquent brain regions: functional results in a consecutive series of 103 patients. J Neurosurg 2003;98:764–85.
67. Wefel JS, Lang FF, Nadar R, Meyers CA. Neurocognitive sequelae of surgical resection for previously untreated intrinsic insular region tumor. Neurooncol 2003;3350.
68. Olofsson S, Weitzner M, Valentine A, Baile W, Meyers C. A retrospective study of the psychiatric management of delirium in the cancer patient. Support Care Cancer 1996;4(5):351–7.

13 Brain Metastases

SILVIA HOFER • MICHAEL BRADA

Introduction

Brain metastases are a common manifestation of malignancy, affecting approximately 10% of patients with solid tumors. The majority develop in the context of known primary or metastatic disease, although a small proportion of patients present with intracranial lesions as the first feature of malignancy. The approach to management has, for many years, consisted of corticosteroids, brain irradiation, and surgery for solitary lesions. With developments in high precision radiotherapy and advances in systemic treatment, the range of treatment options has increased, even though the evidence base for management alternatives is limited and in only few instances supported by randomized trials. This chapter deals with the management of patients with metastatic disease in the brain parenchyma and does not address the issue of meningeal dissemination.

Incidence

The frequency of brain metastases reflects the incidence of primary malignancy as well as the propensity for CNS dissemination. Lung, breast, melanoma, renal, and colorectal cancers account for the majority of cases of brain metastases. The overall risk of developing brain metastases in patients with solid tumors is in the region of 10%. The reported incidence for patients with lung cancer is 20%, melanoma 7%, renal carcinoma 7%, breast cancer 5%, and colorectal cancer 2%. Patients with breast cancer aged 20 to 39 years have the highest proportional risk of brain metastases.[1]

Presentation and Diagnosis

Patients with brain metastases may present with the classical features of a brain tumor. In the presence of multiple lesions, the presentation may be with a nonspecific global deficit and confusional state or epilepsy. Although cognitive impairment is common, detected in up to 65% of patients,[2] it requires detailed neuropsychological testing. Any patient with known malignant disease presenting with any features indicating an intracranial problem requires imaging with CT, or preferably MRI, with and without contrast.

Brain metastases are typically isodense or hyperdense on CT and isointense or hyperintense on MRI, usually with surrounding low density assumed to represent edema. Most brain metastases enhance with intravenous contrast. The difficulty in differential diagnosis arises in the presence of hemorrhage into the lesion, which does not allow for visualization of the underlying tumor. While the majority of brain metastases lie within the brain parenchyma, they may occasionally mimic tumors such as meningioma or acoustic neuroma. It may not be possible to distinguish the two diagnoses on imaging alone, particularly as patients with disseminated malignancy may have coexisting benign tumors. The imaging diagnosis is also difficult in patients presenting with a single intracranial lesion in the absence of systemic disease; the differential diagnosis includes other enhancing single lesions, such as high-grade gliomas.

The need for a histological confirmation of metastatic disease in the brain is summarized in an algorithm (Figure 13-1). In the presence of known systemic malignancy and metastatic disease, there is no indication for biopsy of intracranial lesions unless there is a high index of suspicion for an alternative diagnosis such as an atypical infection. In patients presenting with lesions in the brain, without previous history of primary malignancy, histological confirmation of diagnosis is generally required, preferably from an extracranial site.

The management of brain metastases is influenced by the extent and activity of systemic disease; this information would be part of the routine workup of a patient with known malignant disease and should be available prior to a decision on treatment. In patients with presumed solitary brain metastases, any decision on local treatment should only be made after confirmation of the solitary nature of the tumor by MRI.

Prognosis

Patients with brain metastases have a limited prognosis, with few or no long-term survivors. Median survival in patients with multiple brain metastases is in the region of 3 to 4 months, and 1 year survival is in the region of 12%.[3]

Prognostic factors for survival are performance status, age, and the presence and activity of systemic disease. Patients with all four favorable prognostic factors

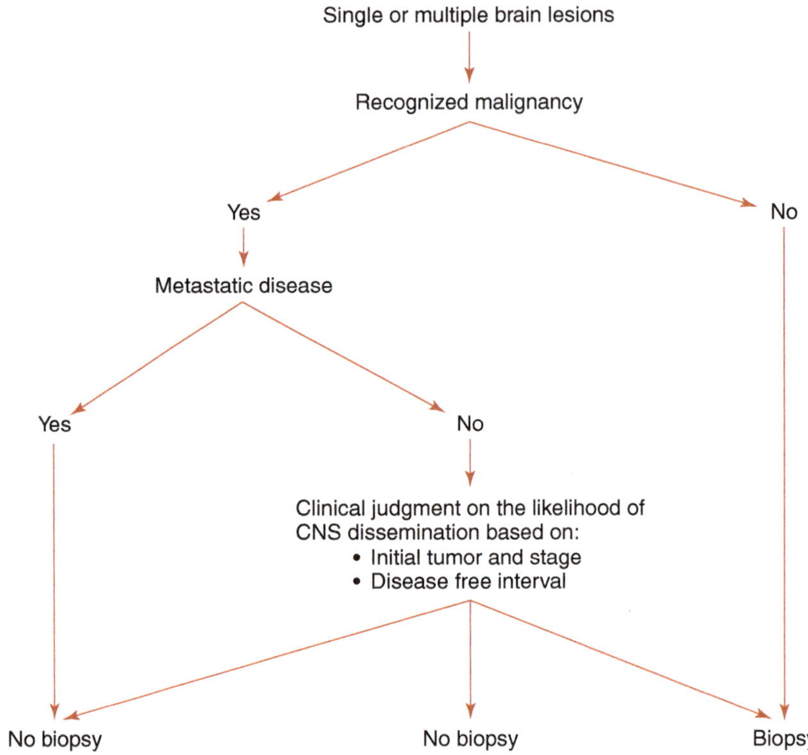

Figure 13-1 Need for histological confirmation of presumed brain metastases.

(Karnofsky Performance Status [KPS] >70, no extracranial metastases, controlled primary tumor, age under 65 years) have a median survival in the region of 7 months. In the presence of one adverse prognostic factor, the median survival drops to 4 months, and, if KPS score is below 70, the median survival is just over 2 months (Table 13-1).[4] More recent prognostic indices also include the number of metastases, distinguishing between solitary lesions and the presence of two or three lesions or more than three.

TABLE 13-1 RPA Classes I-III[4]

Class	Age	Karnofsky PS	Primary		Extracranial metastases	Median survival
I	<65	≥ 70%	Controlled	and	absent	6 to 7 months
II	Any	≥ 70%	Uncontrolled	and/or	present	4 to 5 months
III	Any	<70%	Uncontrolled	and/or	present	2 to 3 months

RPA, recursive partitioning analysis
PS, Performance Status

Medical Management

The aim of treatment of brain metastases is palliation, to improve neurological deficit and quality of life and to prolong survival. Mass effect and neurological deficit assumed to be due to surrounding edema are appropriately treated with corticosteroids. Oral dexamethasone is generally employed as the drug of choice and can be administered in a single daily dose. The tendency has been to recommend a large loading dose followed by reduced daily doses, although it is not clear whether this approach leads to a faster improvement in function. The only regimen subject to a randomized trial is the administration of low-dose dexamethasone (4 mg daily) in comparison to high-dose dexamethasone (12 mg daily). The improvement in function at one week was the same regardless of dose. Patients receiving higher doses experienced more severe side effects,[5] which suggests that 4 mg dexamethasone given in a single daily dose is sufficient and should only be increased in the absence of response after 2 or 3 days. In patients with clinical features of increased intracranial pressure, higher loading doses are recommended. After a clinical benefit has been achieved, the dose should be gradually titrated down to the lowest necessary to maintain improvement in symptoms. It is also important to reduce and discontinue corticosteroids after definitive treatment, to avoid cushingoid side effects.

In patients presenting with brain metastases detected on routine imaging who have no or minimal symptoms, corticosteroids should not be automatically administered. Corticosteroids are also not recommended as a prophylactic treatment prior to cranial irradiation or chemotherapy. Prolonged use may, theoretically, alter the uptake of water-soluble chemotherapeutic agents due to alteration in the blood brain barrier (BBB), although the clinical relevance is not clear. The principal reason for withholding corticosteroids in patients with minimal or no symptoms is to avoid disabling proximal myopathy and other steroid-induced side effects.

The management of seizures in patients with brain metastases should be along the lines of management of epilepsy in patients with any brain tumor. There is no evidence for benefit of prophylactic anticonvulsants.[6] If chemotherapy is part of the management (see below), it is preferable to avoid enzyme-inducing anticonvulsants that increase the metabolism of taxanes, anthracyclines, vinca alkaloids and small molecular tyrosine kinase inhibitors, leading to lower effective doses. Lamotrigine is a reasonable first choice as it does not induce liver enzymes.

Specific Treatment Modalities

SURGERY

Surgery is the appropriate treatment for accessible solitary brain metastases in noneloquent areas. The aim is complete tumor removal to obtain symptomatic relief of increased intracranial pressure or focal deficit from the tumor mass and to achieve local disease control. In patients with multiple brain metastases, surgical excision is generally not indicated, unless one large and easily accessible lesion is responsible for the majority of symptoms. Although resection of multiple brain

TABLE 13-2 WBRT vs. Surgery/WBRT in Patients with Solitary Brain Metastases (Randomized Studies)

Reference	Number of patients	WBRT dose (Gy)	Median survival (months)	
			WBRT alone	*Surgery + WBRT*
Patchell et al., 1990[9]	48	36	3.8	10
Vecht et al., 1993[10]	63	40	6	10
Mintz et al., 1996[11]	84	30	6.3	5.6

WBRT, whole brain radiotherapy

metastases has been recommended by some authors, the apparent favorable survival seen in the reported cohorts is most likely due to patient selection rather than the efficacy of surgery.[7,8]

The survival benefit of surgical resection of solitary brain metastases has been tested in three small randomized trials comparing surgery and whole brain radiotherapy (WBRT) with WBRT alone. Two studies had shown prolongation in survival, but this was not confirmed in the third study (Table 13-2).[9,10,11] The consensus of opinion is that surgery is the appropriate treatment for patients with solitary brain metastases, with the aim being to prolong survival and improve quality of life (QoL). However, radical excision should be reserved for patients with favorable prognostic factors, particularly those without progressive systemic disease.

RADIOTHERAPY

Whole brain irradiation has been the mainstay of treatment of patients with brain metastases. Only one randomized trial compared supportive care (corticosteroids alone) with whole brain radiotherapy (WBRT); it showed a small improvement in median survival in patients receiving WBRT.[12] Subsequent randomized studies examining the role of WBRT compared different dose fractionation schedules to identify the most effective regimen. None have shown benefit for more intensive treatment employing higher doses, given either as daily fractionation or as accelerated radiotherapy using multiple treatments per day. A UK study comparing 30 Gy in 10 fractions with 12 Gy in two fractions had shown a survival benefit for longer fractionation in favorable-prognosis patients,[13] and one or two fraction regimens are rarely employed. The preferred WBRT for patients with multiple brain metastases is 20 Gy in 5 fractions, or 30 Gy in 10 fractions. WBRT improves neurological function in over half of patients with a deficit, although part of the improvement may be due to corticosteroids.

It is generally accepted that patients with good performance status and reasonable prognosis may benefit from WBRT both in terms of survival and neurological function/QoL. However, the value of radiotherapy in patients with marked disability and poor performance status is questioned,[14] and at present it is not clear whether WBRT is appropriate. Randomized trials currently underway examine survival and quality of life benefits of WBRT in patients with multiple brain metastases and poor prognosis.

Patients with brain metastases from chemosensitive tumors are appropriately treated with primary chemotherapy, as discussed later in this chapter. Because of presumed residual microscopic disease following the completion of chemotherapy, patients are usually offered consolidation WBRT, although randomized studies assessing the additional value of irradiation are not available.

In diseases with a high incidence of intracranial dissemination of disease, brain irradiation may be used as prophylaxis, similar to the use of craniospinal irradiation in acute lymphatic leukemia in childhood. Prophylactic cranial irradiation (PCI) improves intracranial tumor control and survival in patients with limited and advanced-stage small cell lung cancer who achieve good remission with chemotherapy[15,16]; however, the magnitude of gain in life expectancy is not large and neurocognitive deficits in long-term survivors are of concern. So far there is not enough evidence to support PCI in patients with other solid tumors.

RADIOTHERAPY AND RADIOSENSITIZERS

A number of radiation sensitizers have been tested in addition to radiotherapy with the aim of improving disease control in the brain as well as survival. Electron-affinic sensitizers (metronidazole, misonidazole)[17,18] and sensitizers of proliferating cells (BUdr)[19] have not demonstrated benefit in randomized studies. The addition of radiation sensitizers motexafin gadolinium, which is preferentially taken up by enhancing lesions,[20] and efaproxiral do not improve survival or disease control.

RADIOSURGERY

Radiosurgery (stereotactic radiotherapy) is a high-precision localized radiation which can be delivered with a linear accelerator (using multiple fixed fields or multiple arcs of rotation) or with a multiheaded cobalt unit (gamma knife). Stereotactic radiotherapy delivers more localized radiation than would be achieved with conventional irradiation for lesions less than 4 cm in diameter.[21]

Radiosurgery has been considered as a noninvasive equivalent of surgical excision, although the apparent equivalence of tumor control and survival is based on reported data from largely retrospective phase II studies.[22]

Following a single radiation dose (radiosurgery) of 15 to 25 Gy, the "response rate," measured as a reduction in the size of solitary metastases, is in the range of 80% to 90%, although complete disappearance is uncommon. In patients with MRI-proven solitary brain metastases the addition of radiosurgery to whole brain radiotherapy (WBRT) improves survival and tumor control.[23] Radiosurgery does not prolong survival in patients with multiple (two or more) brain metastases.[23]

The prognostic factors for survival in patients with solitary brain metastases are the same as in patients with multiple brain metastases.[24] The dominant adverse prognostic factor for survival is performance status.[25] Patients with poor performance status and marked disability have survival similar to patients with multiple brain metastases, and radiosurgery is not appropriate as first-line palliative treatment.

The present recommendation is to offer radiosurgery to patients with solitary brain metastases and good performance status. While it is generally reserved for patients with surgically inaccessible lesions, it can be considered as an alternative

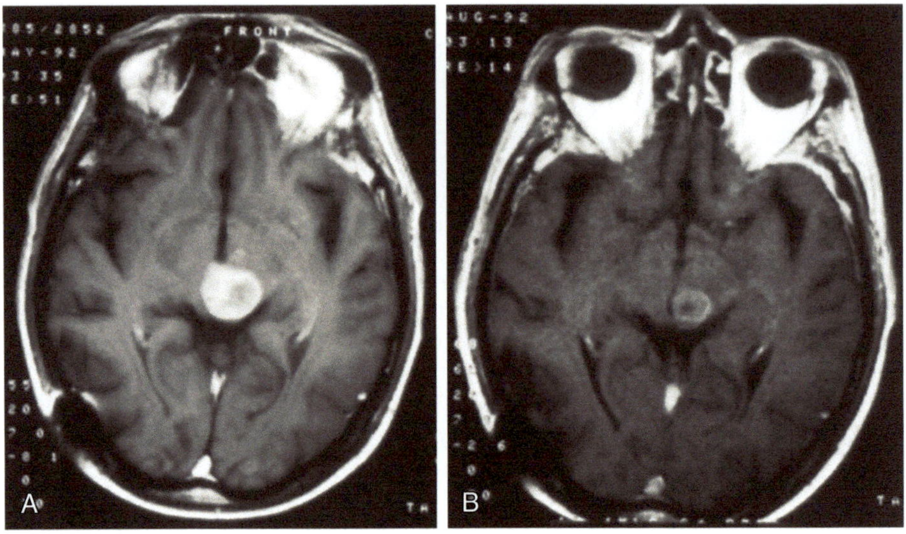

Figure 13-2 MRI of a patient with a solitary brain metastasis from renal cell carcinoma before **(A)** and 1 month after **(B)** linear accelerator radiosurgery.

to surgery and therefore can be offered as an alternative to surgical excision even in operable lesions. It is a less invasive, less costly, and largely outpatient procedure (Figure 13-2). Radiosurgery can occasionally be offered to selected patients with two (or rarely three) metastases, good performance status, and absent or controlled systemic disease.

The role of WBRT following surgery or radiosurgery is currently debated. One small randomized study has shown that the addition of WBRT prolongs intracranial disease control. This was not translated into survival benefit and the overall value of adding WBRT is not clear.[26] A large prospective randomized trial addressing this question is underway. Our institutional policy is not to offer WBRT to patients following successful local treatment, and to continue close monitoring with repeat imaging (e.g., every 3 months). Routine addition of WBRT is an alternative approach. Patients considered for radiosurgery as primary treatment often have initial WBRT as rapid initial therapy, allowing time for more technologically-intensive radiosurgery.

SYSTEMIC TREATMENT

The blood-brain barrier (BBB) has been considered a bar to effective delivery of systemic agents that are not lipid-soluble. Nevertheless, the administration even of water-soluble drugs, which cannot cross an intact BBB, results in regression of brain metastases, and the concept of BBB should not, therefore, be considered the reason for withholding potentially effective chemotherapy, particularly as enhancing brain metastases are likely to have impaired BBB. In addition, the expression of P-glycoprotein (P-gp), a major protein constituent in the intact BBB, which pumps drugs and toxins out of the brain, is low in tumors with metastatic potential to the brain (e.g., lung, melanoma, breast) and in the neovasculature of metastatic tumors. This further suggests that the choice of chemotherapy should be based on histology of the primary tumor rather than the perceived ability of agents to get into the intact brain.

Chemotherapy does not prevent the development of brain metastases, as adjuvant chemotherapy in lung and breast cancer[27,28] does not reduce the incidence of brain metastases. The response rate of brain metastases to chemotherapy tends to reflect the responsiveness of the malignancy outside the brain.[29,30,31] Decision on the use of systemic agents should therefore be based on the assessment of chemosensitivity of the disease. In patients with brain metastases from untreated chemosensitive tumors such as non-Hodgkin lymphoma, small cell lung cancer (SCLC), and germ cell tumors, the appropriate first-line treatment is chemotherapy. In other solid tumors, clinical data on the efficacy of chemotherapy as the sole treatment for brain metastases are mostly limited to small phase II studies, often in heavily pretreated patients, which provide limited information on the choice of agents.

Chemotherapy has been considered as an additional treatment to WBRT in patients with established brain metastases. Randomized phase II studies of concomitant and adjuvant temozolomide, teniposide or other drugs with radiation show no survival benefit and at best a small difference in response rate and progression-free survival.[32]

Management in Common Solid Tumors

NON–SMALL CELL LUNG CANCER (NSCLC)

The actuarial 2-year cumulative risk of developing brain metastases in patients with locally advanced stage III adenocarcinoma and squamous cell carcinoma following combined modality treatment is 22% and 10% respectively, and nearly half present within 4 months of completion of treatment.[27] While the use of chemotherapy reduces the risk of extracranial failure, it has no effect on the incidence of CNS relapse. PCI has been suggested in patients with locally advanced NSCLC. It may reduce the risk of developing disease in the brain, but the overall benefit is yet to be defined.[33]

Patients with brain metastases from NSCLC tend to be heavily pretreated and have less chance of responding to second-line or third-line agents; they should, therefore, receive short palliative WBRT. The response rates to platinum-based chemotherapy as a preferred first-line regimen are similar to those in systemic NSCLC. In asymptomatic chemonaïve patients not in need of immediate radiotherapy, chemotherapy can therefore be considered as an alternative, particularly in the presence of disseminated or locally advanced and progressive disease, with radiotherapy reserved for progressive intracranial disease.[34] Temozolomide, an alkylating agent with good CNS penetration, has no single agent activity in NSCLC[35] and has little role in patients with NSCLC brain metastases.

Tyrosine kinase (TK) inhibitors of the epidermal growth factor receptor (EGFR), have activity in patients with brain metastases,[36,37] similar to that seen with extracranial disease. Vascular endothelial growth factor (VEGF) inhibitors such as bevacizumab and small-molecule TK receptor-inhibitors such as sorafenib and sunitinib are currently under investigation. Additional benefit from antiangiogenesis agents is postulated by their ability to reduce peritumoral edema, with the hope of reducing steroid dependence.

SMALL CELL LUNG CANCER (SCLC)

The incidence of brain metastases is particularly high in SCLC. In patients with limited disease who achieve complete or good remission, PCI has become part of the initial treatment. It decreases the incidence of brain metastases and has a modest survival benefit.[15] Even in responding patients with extensive disease, PCI reduces the incidence of brain metastases and improves survival, albeit at the cost of some toxicity.[16] Although there is concern regarding the impact of PCI on QoL and cognitive function, there are no consistent differences between patients with or without PCI, and no major impairment attributable solely to PCI.[33,38,39]

Intracranial metastases from SCLC respond to chemotherapy as disease at other sites. In newly diagnosed (chemonaïve) patients with SCLC, the response of brain metastases to chemotherapy (without irradiation) is 70% to 80%, while at relapse (pretreated group) it is 40% to 50%.[29] The use of additional WBRT does not translate into improved survival, suggesting that extracranial disease is the major determinant of outcome[40] in this group of patients.

BREAST CANCER

Because of the high incidence of the disease, nearly a quarter of patients presenting with brain metastases have underlying breast cancer. The risk of developing brain metastases is higher in younger patients who have negative estrogen receptor status, grade 3 disease, large tumors and HER-2 overexpression, and is also more common in the presence of visceral metastases, especially lung.[41,42] Patients with HER-2–overexpressing tumors are more prone to developing brain metastases, and the incidence is not reduced by the HER-2 monoclonal antibody trastuzumab. Dual EGFR and HER-2 tyrosine kinase inhibitor lapatinib, which penetrates the BBB, has not, so far, shown improved efficacy.

Breast cancer is both chemoresponsive and radioresponsive. There are no randomized trials comparing the two treatment modalities. WBRT remains the standard of care in the majority of symptomatic patients. Patients with brain metastases who have chemosensitive tumors, particularly with metastatic disease at other sites, can be considered for systemic chemotherapy, and, if they have hormone responsive disease, for hormone therapy. Capecitabine, an oral fluoropyrimidine has shown activity in the brain,[43,44] while temozolomide has minimal activity and is unlikely to be effective for brain metastases.

MALIGNANT MELANOMA

Malignant melanoma is a relatively chemoresistant and radioresistant tumor. Although radiotherapy is perceived to be poorly effective, patients with melanoma brain metastases have not been identified as having significantly worse survival, and WBRT remains the treatment of choice.

While response rates to single agent dacarbazine (DTIC), temozolomide (TMZ), and fotemustine are 5% to 15%, in the brain they are only around 7%.[45,46]

Although a more aggressive approach with platinum and DTIC combined with IL-2 and interferon may result in marginally better response rates (and occasional complete response) outside the brain, it does not prevent the development of brain metastases. A phase III randomized trial comparing fotemustine with DTIC in patients with disseminated melanoma suggested a longer median time to developing brain metastases (22.7 vs. 7.2 months), although this did not reach statistical significance (p= .059).[47] Replacing DTIC with temozolomide has been claimed to reduce the incidence of CNS progression, but did not result in improved survival.[48] The addition of thalidomide to temozolomide in metastatic melanoma has also not altered the incidence of brain metastases, but has added to toxicity.[49]

GERM CELL TUMORS

Approximately 10% of all patients with advanced gonadal germ cell tumors present with brain metastases. CNS disease may also appear as part of systemic relapse. The primary treatment in patients with brain metastases is chemotherapy, as in advanced nonseminoma germ cell tumors. Despite a high response rate to chemotherapy, radiotherapy (WBRT) is recommended as adjuvant treatment.[50,51]

Conclusions

Brain metastases during the course of a malignant disease are generally a hallmark of incurable disseminated disease. In this context, the primary aim of management is palliative; this can be achieved with symptomatic management and a range of oncological treatments, of which WBRT remains the most effective. More aggressive treatment approaches with surgery, radiosurgery, and combined therapies are best reserved for a subset of patients with solitary brain metastases, who have minimal neurological deficit and absent or static systemic disease. Intensive local treatments are inappropriate for patients with multiple brain metastases, particularly in the context of other metastatic disease.

Palliative care services have an important and often primary role in the care of patients affected by brain metastases, as well as their families. The aim in all patients with brain metastases should be to allow symptom-free independent life at home or in a palliative care setting; the focus must be on support and not oncological treatment alone.

REFERENCES

1. Barnholtz-Sloan JS, Sloan AE, Davis FG, Vigneau FD, Lai P, Sawaya RE. Incidence proportions of brain metastases in patients diagnosed (1973 to 2001) in the Metropolitan Detroit Cancer Surveillance System. J Clin Oncol 2004;22(14):2865–72.
2. Chang EL, Wefel JS, Maor MH, Hassenbusch SJ, Mahajan A, Lang FF, et al. A pilot study of neurocognitive function in patients with one to three new brain metastases initially treated with stereotactic radiosurgery alone. Neurosurgery 2007;60:277–83.
3. Lagerwaard FJ, Levendag PC, Nowak PJ, Eijkenboom WM, Hanssens PE, Schmitz PI. Identification of prognostic factors in patients with brain metastases: a review of 1292 patients. Int J Radiat Oncol Biol Phys 1999;43(4):795–803.
4. Gaspar LE, Scott C, Murray K, Curran W. Validation of the RTOG recursive partitioning analysis (RPA) classification for brain metastases. Int J Radiat Oncol Biol Phys 2000;47(4):1001–6.

5. Vecht CJ, Wagner GL, Wilms EB. Interactions between antiepileptic and chemotherapeutic drugs. Lancet Neurol 2003;2(7):404–9.
6. Glantz MJ, Cole BF, Forsyth PA, Recht LD, Wen PY, Chamberlain MC, et al. Practice parameter: anticonvulsant prophylaxis in patients with newly diagnosed brain tumors. Report of the Quality Standards Subcommittee of the American Academy of Neurology. Neurology 2000;54(10):1886–93.
7. Bindal RK, Sawaya R, Leavens ME, Lee JJ. Surgical treatment of multiple brain metastases. J Neurosurg 1993;79(2):210–6.
8. Wronski M, Arbit E, Burt M, Galicich JH. Survival after surgical treatment of brain metastases from lung cancer: a follow-up study of 231 patients treated between 1976 and 1991. J Neurosurg 1995;83(4):605–16.
9. Patchell RA, Tibbs PA, Walsh JW, Dempsey RJ, Maruyama Y, Kryscio RJ, et al. A randomized trial of surgery in the treatment of single metastases to the brain. N Engl J Med 1990;322(8):494–500.
10. Vecht CJ, Haaxma Reiche H, Noordijk EM, Padberg GW, Voormolen JHC, Hoekstra FH, et al. Treatment of single brain metastasis: Radiotherapy alone or combined with neurosurgery? Ann Neurol 1993;33:583–90.
11. Mintz AH, Kestle J, Rathbone MP, Gaspar L, Hugenholtz H, Fisher B, et al. A randomised trial to assess the efficacy of surgery in addtion to radiotherapy in patients with a single cerebral metastasis. Cancer 1996;78:1470–6.
12. Horton J, Baxter DH, Olson KB. The management of metastases to the brain by irradiation and corticosteroids. Am J Roentgenol Radium Ther Nucl Med 1971;111(2):334–6.
13. Priestman TJ, Dunn J, Brada M, Rampling R, Baker PG. Final results of the Royal College of Radiologists' trial comparing two different radiotherapy schedules in the treatment of cerebral metastases. Clin Oncol R Coll Radiol 1996;8(5):308–15.
14. Tsao MN, Sultanem K, Chiu D, Copps F, Dixon P, Easton D, et al. Supportive care management of brain metastases: what is known and what we need to know. Conference proceedings of the National Cancer Institute of Canada (NCIC) Workshop on Symptom Control in Radiation Oncology. Clin Oncol (R Coll Radiol) 2003;15(7):429–34.
15. Auperin A, Arriagada R, Pignon JP, Le Pechoux C, Gregor A, Stephens RJ, et al. Prophylactic cranial irradiation for patients with small-cell lung cancer in complete remission. Prophylactic Cranial Irradiation Overview Collaborative Group [see comments]. N Engl J Med 1999;341(7):476–84.
16. Slotman B, Faivre-Finn C, Kramer G, Rankin E, Snee M, Hatton M, et al. Prophylactic cranial irradiation in extensive small-cell lung cancer. N Engl J Med 2007;357(7):664–72.
17. Eyre HJ, Ohlsen JD, Frank J, LoBuglio AF, McCracken JD, Weatherall TJ, et al. Randomized trial of radiotherapy versus radiotherapy plus metronidazole for the treatment metastatic cancer to brain. A Southwest Oncology Group study. J Neurooncol 1984;2(4):325–30.
18. Komarnicky LT, Phillips TL, Martz K, Asbell S, Isaacson S, Urtasun RA, et al. protocol for the evaluation of misonidazole combined with radiation in the treatment of patients with brain metastases (RTOG-7916). Int J Radiat Oncol Biol Phys 1991;20(1):53–8.
19. Phillips TL, Scott CB, Leibel SA, Rotman M, Weigensberg IJ. Results of a randomized comparison of radiotherapy and bromodeoxyuridine with radiotherapy alone for brain metastases: report of RTOG trial 89–05. Int J Radiat Oncol Biol Phys 1995;33(2):339–48.
20. Mehta MP, Rodrigus P, Terhaard CH, Rao A, Suh J, Roa W, et al. Survival and neurologic outcomes in a randomized trial of motexafin gadolinium and whole-brain radiation therapy in brain metastases. J Clin Oncol 2003;21(13):2529–36.
21. Brada M, Foord T. Radiosurgery for brain metastases. Clin Oncol (R Coll Radiol) 2002;14(1):28–30.
22. Pirzkall A, Debus J, Lohr F, Fuss M, Rhein B, Engenhart Cabillic R, et al. Radiosurgery alone or in combination with whole-brain radiotherapy for brain metastases. J Clin Oncol 1998;16(11):3563–9.
23. Andrews DW, Scott CB, Sperduto PW, Flanders AE, Gaspar LE, Schell MC, et al. Whole brain radiation therapy with or without stereotactic radiosurgery boost for patients with one to three brain metastases: phase III results of the RTOG 9508 randomised trial. Lancet 2004;363(9422):1665–72.
24. Milker-Zabel S, Debus J, Thilmann C, Schlegel W, Wannenmacher M. Fractionated stereotactically guided radiotherapy and radiosurgery in the treatment of functional and nonfunctional adenomas of the pituitary gland. Int J Radiat Oncol Biol Phys 2001;50(5):1279–86.
25. Jyothirmayi R, Saran FH, Jalali R, Perks J, Warrington A, Ashley S, et al. Stereotactic radiotherapy for solitary brain metastases. Clin Oncol 2001;13:228–34.

26. Patchell RA, Tibbs PA, Regine WF, Dempsey RJ, Mohiuddin M, Kryscio RJ, et al. Postoperative radiotherapy in the treatment of single metastases to the brain: a randomized trial. JAMA 1998;280(17):1485–9.
27. Gaspar LE, Chansky K, Albain KS, Vallieres E, Rusch V, Crowley JJ, et al. Time from treatment to subsequent diagnosis of brain metastases in stage III non-small-cell lung cancer: a retrospective review by the Southwest Oncology Group. J Clin Oncol 2005;23(13):2955–61.
28. Crivellari D, Pagani O, Veronesi A, Lombardi D, Nole F, Thurlimann B, et al. High incidence of central nervous system involvement in patients with metastatic or locally advanced breast cancer treated with epirubicin and docetaxel. Ann Oncol 2001;12(3):353–6.
29. Kristensen CA, Kristjansen PEG, Hansen HH. Systemic chemotherapy of brain metastases from small cell lung cancer. J Clin Oncol 1992;10:1498–502.
30. Bernardo G, Cuzzoni Q, Strada MR, Bernardo A, Brunetti G, Jedrychowska I, et al. First-line chemotherapy with vinorelbine, gemcitabine, and carboplatin in the treatment of brain metastases from non-small-cell lung cancer: a phase II study. Cancer Invest 2002;20(3):293–302.
31. Boogerd W, Dalesio O, Bais EM, Sade JJ. Response of brain metastases from breast cancer to systemic chemotherapy. Cancer 1992;927–80.
32. Verger E, Gil M, Yaya R, Vinolas N, Villa S, Pujol T, et al. Temozolomide and concomitant whole brain radiotherapy in patients with brain metastases: a phase II randomized trial. Int J Radiat Oncol Biol Phys 2005;61(1):185–91.
33. Pöttgen C, Eberhardt W, Grannass A, Korfee S, Stüben G, Teschler H, et al. Prophylactic cranial irradiation in operable stage IIIA non-small-cell lung cancer treated with neoadjuvant chemoradiotherapy: Results from a german multicenter randomized trial. J Clin Oncol 2007;25:4987–92.
34. Robinet G, Thomas P, Breton JL, Lena H, Gouva S, Dabouis G, et al. Results of a phase III study of early versus delayed whole brain radiotherapy with concurrent cisplatin and vinorelbine combination in inoperable brain metastasis of non-small-cell lung cancer: Groupe Francais de Pneumo-Cancerologie (GFPC) Protocol 95-1. Ann Oncol 2001;12(1):59–67.
35. Dziadziuszko R, Ardizzoni A, Postmus PE, Smit EF, Price A, Debruyne C, et al. Temozolomide in patients with advanced non-small cell lung cancer with and without brain metastases. a phase II study of the EORTC Lung Cancer Group (08965). Eur J Cancer 2003;39(9):1271–6.
36. Ceresoli GL, Cappuzzo F, Gregorc V, Bartolini S, Crino L, Villa E. Gefitinib in patients with brain metastases from non-small-cell lung cancer: a prospective trial. Ann Oncol 2004;15(7):1042–7.
37. Hotta K, Kiura K, Ueoka H, Tabata M, Fujiwara K, Kozuki T, et al. Effect of gefitinib ('Iressa', ZD1839) on brain metastases in patients with advanced non-small-cell lung cancer. Lung Cancer 2004;46(2):255–61.
38. Gregor A, Cull A, Stephens RJ, Kirkpatrick JA, Yarnold JR, Girling DJ, et al. Prophylactic cranial irradiation is indicated following complete response to induction therapy in small cell lung cancer: results of a multicentre randomised trial. United Kingdom Coordinating Committee for Cancer Research (UKCCCR) and the European Organization for Research and Treatment of Cancer (EORTC) [see comments]. Eur J Cancer 1997;33(11):1752–8.
39. Arriagada R, Le Chevalier T, Borie F, et al. Prophylactic cranial irradiation for patients with small-cell lung cancer in complete remission. J Natl Cancer Inst 1995;87:183–90.
40. Postmus PE, Haaxma-Reiche H, Smit EF, Groen HJ, Karnicka H, Lewinski T, et al. Treatment of brain metastases of small-cell lung cancer: comparing teniposide and teniposide with whole-brain radiotherapy—a phase III study of the European Organization for the Research and Treatment of Cancer Lung Cancer Cooperative Group. J Clin Oncol 2000;18(19):3400–8.
41. Gonzalez-Angulo AM, Cristofanilli M, Strom EA, Buzdar AU, Kau SW, Broglio KR, et al. Central nervous system metastases in patients with high-risk breast carcinoma after multimodality treatment. Cancer 2004;101(8):1760–6.
42. Slimane K, Andre F, Delaloge S, Dunant A, Perez A, Grenier J, et al. Risk factors for brain relapse in patients with metastatic breast cancer. Ann Oncol 2004;15(11):1640–4.
43. Wang ML, Yung WK, Royce ME, Schomer DF, Theriault RL. Capecitabine for 5-fluorouracil-resistant brain metastases from breast cancer. Am J Clin Oncol 2001;24(4):421–4.
44. Siegelmann-Danieli N, Stein M, Bar-Ziv J. Complete response of brain metastases originating in breast cancer to capecitabine therapy. Isr Med Assoc J 2003;5(11):833–4.
45. Middleton MR, Grob JJ, Aaronson N, Fierlbeck G, Tilgen W, Seiter S, et al. Randomized phase III study of temozolomide versus dacarbazine in the treatment of patients with advanced metastatic malignant melanoma. J Clin Oncol 2000;18(1):158–66.
46. Agarwala SS, Kirkwood JM, Gore M, Dreno B, Thatcher N, Czarnetski B, et al. Temozolomide for the treatment of brain metastases associated with metastatic melanoma: a phase II study. J Clin Oncol 2004;22(11):2101–7.

47. Avril MF, Aamdal S, Grob JJ, Hauschild A, Mohr P, Bonerandi JJ, et al. Fotemustine compared with dacarbazine in patients with disseminated malignant melanoma: A phase III study. J Clin Oncol 2004;22:1118–25.
48. Atkins MB, Gollob JA, Sosman JA, McDermott DF, Tutin L, Sorokin P, et al. A phase II pilot trial of concurrent biochemotherapy with cisplatin, vinblastine, temozolomide, interleukin 2, and IFN-alpha 2B in patients with metastatic melanoma. Clin Cancer Res 2002;8(10):3075–81.
49. Hwu WJ, Krown SE, Menell JH, Panageas KS, Merrell J, Lamb LA, et al. Phase II study of temozolomide plus thalidomide for the treatment of metastatic melanoma. J Clin Oncol 2003;21(17):3351–6.
50. Schmoll HJ, Souchon R, Krege S, Albers P, Beyer J, Kollmannsberger C, et al. European consensus on diagnosis and treatment of germ cell cancer: a report of the European Germ Cell Cancer Consensus Group (EGCCCG). Ann Oncol 2004;15(9):1377–99.
51. Spears W. Brain metastases and testicular tumors: long term survival. Int J Radiat Oncol Biol Phys 1991;22:17–22.

14 Spinal Metastases

TALI SIEGAL • TZONY SIEGAL

Introduction

Spinal metastases may affect different components of the spine, and the approach to treatment depends on correct localization of the affected compartment. Metastases to the spine most frequently involve the vertebral elements and the epidural space.[1–4] In a small proportion of patients, symptoms and signs may arise from metastases that spread to the intradural spinal compartment, either extramedullary or intramedullary (Table 14-1).[5–7] The approach to treatment varies according to the affected site, and ideally requires the shared decision of a multidisciplinary team. The specific treatment may include various combinations of steroids, irradiation, surgery, chemotherapy, hormonotherapy, and bisphosphonates, as appropriate for the underlying neoplasm.

Vertebral Metastases

Metastases most commonly affect the lungs, liver, and skeletal system. Bone metastases are a significant cause of morbidity, due to pain, pathologic fractures, hypercalcemia, and spinal cord compression.[3,4,8,9] The vertebral column is the most common site for skeletal metastases,[10] and in autopsy series, 60% of patients dying of cancer were found to have spinal and epidural metastases.[11] Destructive vertebral lesions are a common source of morbidity, with pain the presenting complaint in the majority of cases.

All patients with vertebral metastases are at potential risk of developing spinal instability and neurological impairment. Therefore, it is useful to classify vertebral

TABLE 14-1 Spinal Metastases

Vertebral metastases
- Biomechanically stable
- Potentially unstable
  - Without compression fracture
  - With compression fracture
- Biomechanically unstable
  - Without compression fracture
  - With compression fracture

Vertebral metastases with epidural extension
- Without root/neural elements displacement ± instability
- With nerve roots displacement/encasement ± instability
- With spinal cord displacement/compression ± instability
- With cauda equina displacement ± instability

Epidural metastases without vertebral lesion
- Paravertebral mass with an epidural extension
- Epidural mass without a paravertebral tumor

Intradural metastases
- Intradural extramedullary mass
- Intramedullary spinal mass

metastases according to biomechanical stability and the presence or absence of dural sac displacement or neural element compression (Table 14-1). This classification allows for early recognition of potential complications. Treatment can be adjusted to meet the potential risks and preserve or restore normal function.

Assessment of the extent of vertebral metastases is based on imaging findings that range from spine radiography and bone scintigraphy to positron emission tomography (PET) using F-18 2-fluoro-2-deoxy-D-glucose (FDG),[12] computerized tomography (CT), and magnetic resonance imaging (MRI). MRI is sensitive to both focal vertebral lesions and bone marrow involvement, in both hematologic malignancies and in solid tumors.[13]

Even in patients with diffuse marrow involvement, the spine may not be defined as mechanically unstable. The criteria for determining spinal stability in neoplastic disease are complex, and differ from those established for trauma. Unfortunately, no validated system exists for making this determination.

CLINICAL AND IMAGING CRITERIA FOR SPINAL STABILITY IN NEOPLASTIC DISEASE

Determining spinal stability is of paramount importance in choosing the appropriate form of management for patients with spinal metastases, since a major goal of treatment is restoration or maintenance of spinal stability. In trauma, the accepted biomechanical model for thoracolumbar stability after fractures is the three-column concept of the spine (Figure 14-1).[14]

- The anterior column consists of the anterior half of the vertebral body, the anterior longitudinal ligament, and the anterior annulus fibrosus.
- The middle column includes the posterior longitudinal ligament, the posterior half of the vertebral body, and the posterior annulus.

The posterior column consists of the neural arch (laminae and pedicles), facets, the ligamentum flavum, and the supraspinous and interspinous ligaments.

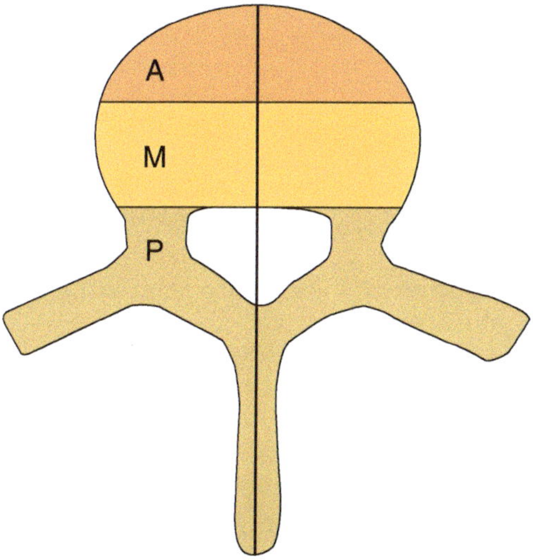

Figure 14-1 Classification system for the evaluation of spinal stability. The three-column system of Denis[14] was devised for assessment of spinal column stability in trauma. The system divides the spine into the anterior (A), middle (M), and posterior (P) columns. The spine is considered unstable if two of the three columns are disrupted. The six-column system of Kostuik and Errico[15] was devised for evaluating stability in spine tumors. Here the three columns, as defined by Denis, are subdivided into left (L) and right (R) halves. The spine is unstable if three to four of the columns are destroyed.

The spine is considered unstable if two of the three columns are disrupted. Spinal fractures are also classified according to the mechanism of injury.

In neoplastic destruction of the spine these concepts may not always be applicable, because trauma and tumors are quite different conditions in terms of the disruption of bone, disc, and ligament; the quality of surrounding bone stock; and the ability of the spine to heal. A set of criteria, which requires validation, has been developed for spinal tumors.[15] The spine is divided into six columns: the three columns defined above[14] subdivided into left and right halves (Figure 14-1). The spine is considered to be unstable if three to four of the columns are destroyed, and markedly unstable if five to six of the columns are involved. Angulation of 20 degrees or more adds to the consideration of instability.

Instability does not usually develop when involvement is limited to the vertebral spongy bone core or to the anterior column. When the posterior half (middle column) of the vertebral body is also involved (cortical bone included), pathologic compression fracture can occur, producing kyphosis and extrusion of bone, tumor, or disc into the spinal canal, with resulting neural compromise. Tumor involvement of the middle and posterior column may produce forward shearing deformity. In addition, segmental instability is probably present when the clinical syndrome is characterized by pain that is aggravated by movement (in the absence of significant neural encroachment), and associated with progressive collapse of vertebral bodies or localized kyphosis on imaging studies. The MRI appearance of acute vertebral fractures was studied in a series of 100 patients evaluated for suspected spinal cord compression (SCC).[16] Pathological fracture of the vertebral body was present in 51% of compressive levels. Of these, 68% had loss of height greater than 50%; vertebral bodies in the lower thoracic region were more likely to have pathological fractures.

A systematic approach to determining clinical instability of the spine should include anatomic, biomechanical, symptomatic, and therapeutic considerations.[17,18] Apart from imaging studies that define anatomic details used in the three-column spinal model (Figure 14-1),[16] the concept of clinical instability should be taken into account. Clinical instability is defined as "loss of the ability of the spine under physiologic loads to maintain relationships between vertebrae in such a way that there is either damage or subsequent irritation to the spinal cord or nerve roots, and in addition there is development of incapacitating deformity or pain due to structural changes."[18]

TREATMENT OF VERTEBRAL METASTASES

Biomechanically Stable Vertebral Metastases

Although some vertebral metastases are painless, many cause significant and debilitating pain. Besides pain, vertebral metastases can also give rise to pathological fracture and SCC, which are two important complications that result in significant morbidity. Treatment of vertebral metastases often requires a multimodality approach, with the main aims of alleviating pain and preventing future complications. It is important to base the treatment plan on the overall clinical situation, since vertebral metastases represent only one aspect of the disease process. Treatment of biomechanically-stable vertebral metastases usually includes analgesic medication and focal radiotherapy as the immediate modalities to alleviate pain. In certain tumor types, hormone therapy, cytotoxic drugs, and bisphosphonates are added, in view of the likelihood of further skeletal involvement.

Radiation Therapy

Radiotherapy is effective in reducing metastatic bone pain and, in some instances, causing tumor shrinkage or growth inhibition.[8,19–21] There is, as yet, no consensus regarding the most appropriate way of delivering radiotherapy for metastatic bone pain. The practice differs significantly between countries and, indeed, between treatment centers within the same country.

One of the controversies is whether single fraction radiotherapy is as effective as multifraction radiotherapy. Single fraction radiotherapy is more convenient for the patient, and it is also less costly compared with multifraction radiotherapy. However, there are some important concerns relating to single fraction therapy. The equivalent biological dose of single fraction treatment is usually smaller than the total multifraction treatment dose. As a result, the pain response to a single dose may be inferior to the multifraction radiotherapy response. Even if the initial pain response is similar, it may not be durable enough to ensure that the patient remains asymptomatic. In addition, with a potentially reduced tumoricidal effect, single fraction radiotherapy may not be as effective in preventing complications such as pathological fractures and SCC. Systematic reviews of randomized studies examining the effectiveness of single fraction radiotherapy versus multiple fraction radiotherapy pooled the results and used meta-analysis to estimate the effect of treatment on pain response, retreatment rate, and complications.[8,19] There was no difference between the two radiotherapy schedules for both overall and complete pain response rates; however, patients treated by single fraction radiotherapy had a higher retreatment rate and a higher rate of pathological fractures compared with patients treated by multifraction schedule. The SCC rates were similar for both arms of the treatment schedules, although there was a trend of increasing SCC rates for patients treated by single fraction radiotherapy. Based on the above analysis of the two treatment schedules, we recommend multifraction radiotherapy for most vertebral metastases except in those patients whose life expectancy is considered to be extremely short, in which case a single fraction schedule may be appropriate for immediate pain control. The treatment schedule should be tailored for each patient based on the type of palliative therapy required and the complications that may yet develop.

Bisphosphonates

These agents work by several different mechanisms to reduce both bone resorption and bone formation.[22,23] Bisphosphonates can be divided into two groups: those resembling pyrophosphate (for example, clodronate and etidronate), and the aminobisphosphonates (for example, pamidronate and zoledronic acid). The latter group inhibits enzymes of the mevalonate pathway, disrupting the signaling function of key regulatory proteins. The net effect in both groups is inhibition of osteoclast function, which leads to a decrease in bone resorption. Systematic review showed that bisphosphonates significantly decreased skeletal morbidity, and reduced the probability of vertebral fracture.[3,4,9] However, the incidence of SCC was not reduced. This may be related to the fact that studies examining skeletal events were insufficiently powered to show a difference between bisphosphonates and controls for SCC, which is a relatively rare skeletal event. Based on the systematic review, recommendations are that treatment with bisphosphonate medications should start when bone metastases are diagnosed and continue until no longer clinically relevant.[3]

Vertebral Metastases with Biomechanical Potential or Overt Instability

Vertebral metastases that lead to biomechanical spine instability, or potential instability, produce a range of symptoms and signs that should direct therapeutic consideration. Patients with localized kyphosis, collapsed vertebra, fracture-dislocation, retropulsion of a bone fragment, or segmental instability may require various surgical procedures tailored to meet decompression, stabilization, or pain relief requirements, depending on symptomatology (Figure 14-2). However, not

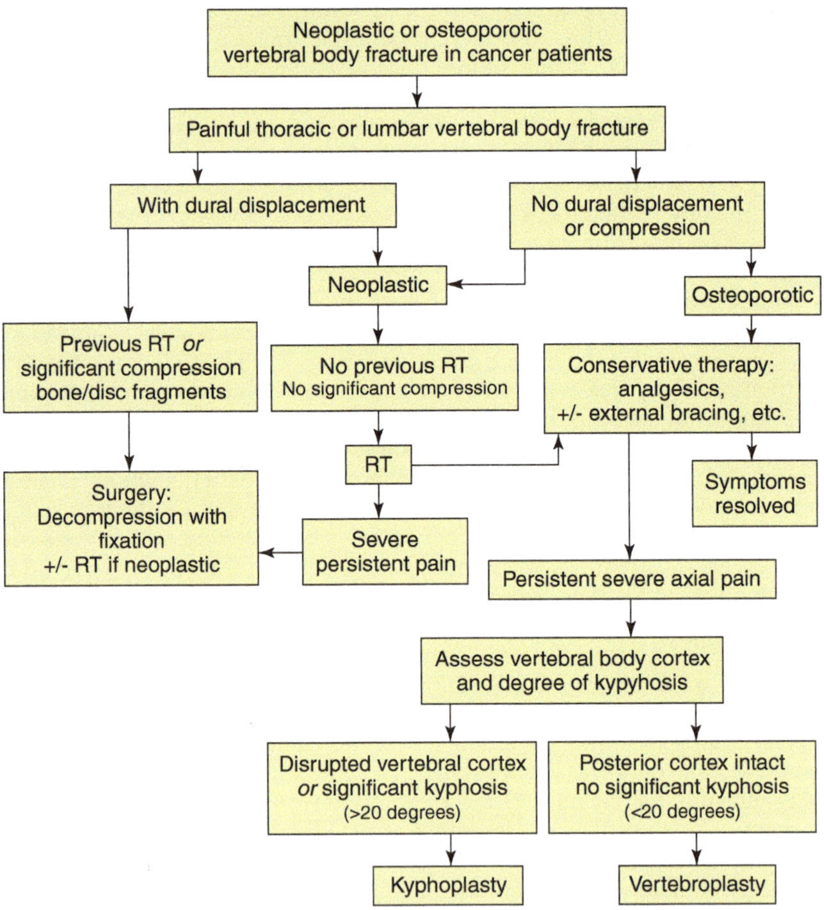

Figure 14-2 Treatment algorithm for painful thoracic or lumbar vertebral body fractures. The fracture can be either osteoporotic or secondary to disruption of the vertebral cortical shell by metastatic tumor.

every case defined by the criteria for unstable spine requires surgical intervention. If the tumor is relatively radiosensitive, radiotherapy may result in satisfactory axial settling and pain relief over a period of weeks or months (Figure 14-2). These patients should be carefully followed because they are still potentially unstable. Surgical procedures are reserved for symptomatic cases, because preventive surgery is probably unjustified in the management of metastatic disease of the spine.

When the anterior and middle columns are destroyed by tumor, treatment considerations should include decompression as well as restoration of stability by instrumentation and vertebral replacement constructs. If the posterior column structures are involved, then the treatment plan is to replace or substitute for the support role of these structures by posterior decompression combined with posterior instrumentation to maintain stability.

Recommendations for patient selection and optimal methods of decompression and stabilization are constantly evolving. The criteria for spinal instability that should lead to consideration of spinal stabilization are summarized in Table 14-2.

VERTEBRAL COMPRESSION FRACTURE IN CANCER PATIENTS

Acute vertebral compression fractures are common and may occur because of osteoporosis, neoplastic infiltration of the vertebral body, or trauma (Figure 14-3). Patients may present with osteoporotic fracture secondary to various precipitating factors such as age, steroid therapy, immobility, and prolonged use of low molecular weight heparin. Neoplastic vertebral compression is a common occurrence in both hematological malignancies and solid tumors.[13,24–26]

The differential diagnosis may be difficult. Imaging findings are suggestive, but often inconclusive. It has been reported, for example, that osteoporotic fractures may accumulate FDG to varying degrees, and false-positive findings may occur when FDG-PET imaging is performed to assess whether metastases are present.[12,27] Accurate differentiation of simple osteoporotic fracture from pathological fracture often requires the integration of imaging findings (PET/CT combined technique and MRI) with clinical assessment. MRI findings may be useful (Figure 14-3). A convex posterior border of the vertebral body, abnormal signal intensity of the

TABLE 14-2 Categories of Spinal Instability in Metastatic Disease that Require Consideration for Spinal Fixation*

- Anterior + middle column involvement or >50% collapse of vertebral body height
- Middle + posterior column involvement or shearing deformity
- Three–column involvement
- Involvement of same column in two or more adjacent vertebrae
- Iatrogenic
  - Laminectomy in face of anterior and/or middle column disease
  - Prospective resection of >50% of cut surface of the vertebral body

*Definition of potential instability relies on imaging studies and is valid only if the vertebral cortical shell is involved.

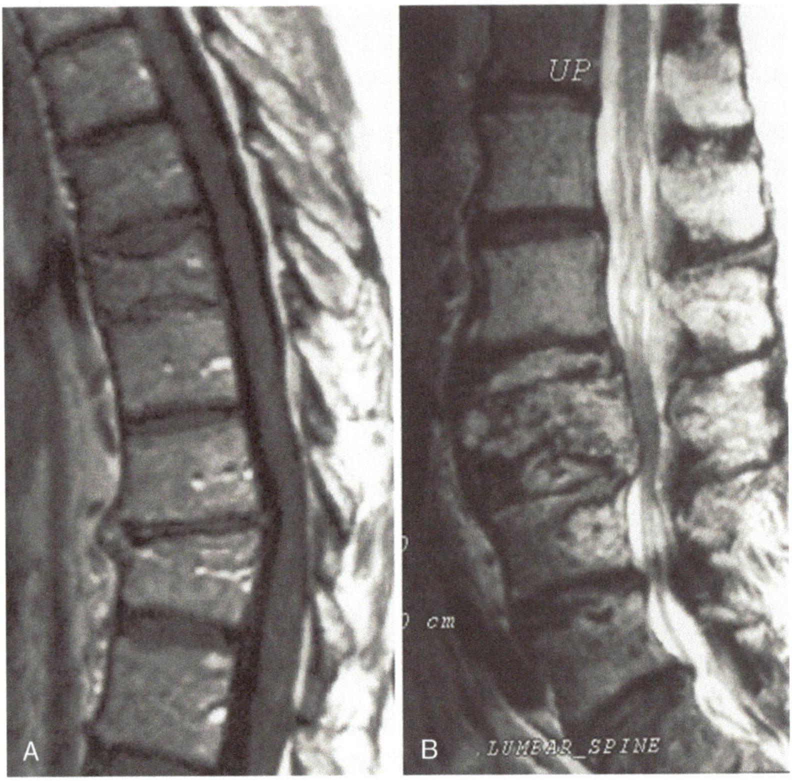

Figure 14-3 MRI of vertebral fractures in cancer patients. (**A**) Osteoporotic collapse of thoracic vertebra in a female patient with primary CNS lymphoma. The patient had been treated with dexamethasone for several months to control increased intracranial pressure induced by the brain tumor, and subsequently received additional steroids as part of the treatment schedule. She presented with a new incapacitating back pain. MRI reveals central collapse of the 6th thoracic vertebra. (**B**) Neoplastic collapse of the third lumbar vertebra associated with compression of the thecal sac. Note that the tumor (prostatic carcinoma) also involves the 4th and 5th lumbar vertebrae.

pedicle or posterior elements, epidural mass, focal paraspinal mass, and other spinal metastases are suggestive of metastatic compression fractures. In contrast, findings suggestive of osteoporotic compression fractures are: a low signal-intensity band on T_1-weighted and T_2-weighted images, spared normal bone marrow signal intensity of the vertebral body, retropulsion of a posterior bone fragment, multiple compression fractures, and fluid collection (the fluid sign) that results from bone marrow edema.[24,25]

Treatment Options for Vertebral Compression Fracture (Figure 14-2)

Vertebral compression fracture is associated with severe pain and is frequently the cause of immobility. A multidisciplinary approach to patient selection and management is essential (Figure 14-2).Once vertebral body fracture is diagnosed, it is important to evaluate whether dural displacement or significant neural compression is present. In cases with significant compression of neural elements secondary to impingement of bone, disc fragments, or tumor mass, early consideration of surgical decompression combined with stabilization should take place. In neoplastic vertebral fractures where dural displacement is present but compression is not significant, radiotherapy followed by conservative therapy can form the initial approach. Conservative treatment of thoracic or lumbar vertebral fracture includes analgesic medications with or without external bracing and encouragement to maintain weight-bearing activities. Radiotherapy is also added to metastatic vertebral fractures that are not associated with dural displacement. None of these latter modalities is uniformly effective in relieving pain or improving ambulatory status.

For patients who fail to improve with conservative management and have no evidence of cord or thecal sac compression, a minimally-invasive procedure that involves percutaneous injection of polymethylmethacrylate (PMMA), a surgical bone cement, under imaging guidance can be offered.[28,29] Precise indications for these techniques are still evolving.

The goal of vertebroplasty is to provide pain relief and bone strengthening in painful vertebral body compression fracture. Selected patients with focal, intense, and intractable midline spinal pain at the level of the fracture, or within two vertebral levels below it, and who failed conservative management, are candidates for this minimally-invasive procedure. Vertebroplasty does not re-expand a collapsed vertebra, but it provides a certain degree of reinforcement and stabilization of the fracture, which alleviates pain. The procedure is relatively contraindicated for patients with evidence of dural displacement or compression,[30] and suitable for patients with no radicular signs. Contraindications to the procedure include bleeding disorder and unstable fracture due to posterior element involvement. Procedural complications are relatively rare; most are related to PMMA leakage through cortical defects.[29–32] Cement leakage rates range from 9% to 88%, and, in most cases, leakage is asymptomatic. Neural element compression resulting from cement extravasation remains a rare event.

Percutaneous balloon kyphoplasty, a recent modification of vertebroplasty, involves inflation of a balloon within a collapsed vertebral body to restore height and reduce kyphotic deformity prior to stabilization with PMMA. The risk of cement extravasation is reduced because inflation of the balloon creates a void within the vertebral body into which the cement can be injected under relatively low pressure. Therefore, this procedure is indicated once there is evidence for disrupted posterior cortex of the collapsed vertebra, and in cases where significant kyphotic deformity contributes to the pathophysiology of spinal pain.

Current experience with vertebroplasty and kyphoplasty for painful vertebral fractures in cancer patients remains limited, but favorable results can be obtained with careful selection of appropriate patients.[28–30,33,34] Marked or complete pain relief is reported in 70% to 84% of procedures performed in neoplastic vertebral fractures, and the rate exceeds 90% in osteoporotic fractures. No change in the level of pain is reported in about 9% of neoplastic fractures. Pain relief and increased mobility are expected within 24 hours postprocedure, but occasionally these responses occur after a few days. As a result, analgesic consumption is also significantly reduced in the majority of treated patients.[29] Based on current knowledge, these procedures can be applied with a good safety profile in well-selected patients with osteoporotic fractures and in patients with multiple myeloma or metastatic cancer who have refractory spinal pain.

Vertebral Metastases with Epidural Extension

Sixty percent of vertebral metastases associated with epidural extension in adults are related to breast, lung, and prostate cancer.[1,35–38] Other common neoplasms include lymphoma, renal cancer, sarcoma, and multiple myeloma. The origin of metastases cannot be identified in 7% to 12% of cases.[13,37,39,40] All patients with vertebral metastases are at potential risk of developing compression of the neural roots, cauda equina, and/or the spinal cord. Epidural metastases are the most common cause of spinal cord and cauda equina dysfunction in cancer patients. The term SCC is used in this chapter to include cauda equina compression, unless otherwise noted.

FREQUENCY

The incidence of SCC is unknown. Retrospective clinical studies suggest that 2% to 20% of patients with vertebral metastases develop myelopathy secondary to SCC.[10,37,41] A recent population-based study of neoplastic SCC in Ontario found that the cumulative probability of experiencing at least one episode of SCC in the last five years preceding death from cancer was 2.5% and ranged from 0.2% in cancer of the pancreas to 7.9% in myeloma.[37] An autopsy study estimated that 5% of cancer patients develop spinal epidural tumor deposits,[42] but a proportion may remain clinically silent. SCC may present as the initial manifestation of malignancy in about 8% to 20% of patients with symptomatic epidural deposits.[43,44] Carcinoma of the lung, cancer of unknown primary site, multiple myeloma, and non-Hodgkin lymphoma are disproportionately represented (accounting for 78% of episodes) in a series of SCC occurring as initial manifestation of malignancy. These primary tumors account for only 26% of SCC in patients with a previously-established diagnosis of malignancy.

The incidence of SCC secondary to lymphoma, breast, and prostate cancer has decreased over the years.[45] This declining incidence probably reflects a shift in oncological treatment policies towards the early use of radiotherapy, or more effective and earlier treatment of the primary tumor reducing the rate of metastatic complications. The routine use of advanced imaging techniques (CT, PET/CT, and MRI) also contributes to early detection and treatment of clinically silent spinal metastases.[1,2,12,16,39,40] Imaging of the whole spine is feasible with these techniques. When performed, for example, in patients with clinical symptomatology suggestive of SCC, whole spine images often reveal that two or more levels of compression are present, affecting more than one region of the spine. Multiple levels of neural element compression are detected in 25% to 43% of suspected SCC.[2,16,39,40,46]

LOCATION OF EPIDURAL TUMOR IN RELATION TO THE SPINAL CORD AND THE YIELD OF DIAGNOSTIC IMAGING

Epidural SCC usually results from metastases to one of three sites: the vertebrae, the paravertebral tissue, or the epidural space itself. Extension of the tumor into the spinal canal may produce variable involvement of the anterior (ventral) compartment, lateral gutters, posterior compartment, or any combination of these sites (Figure 14-4).

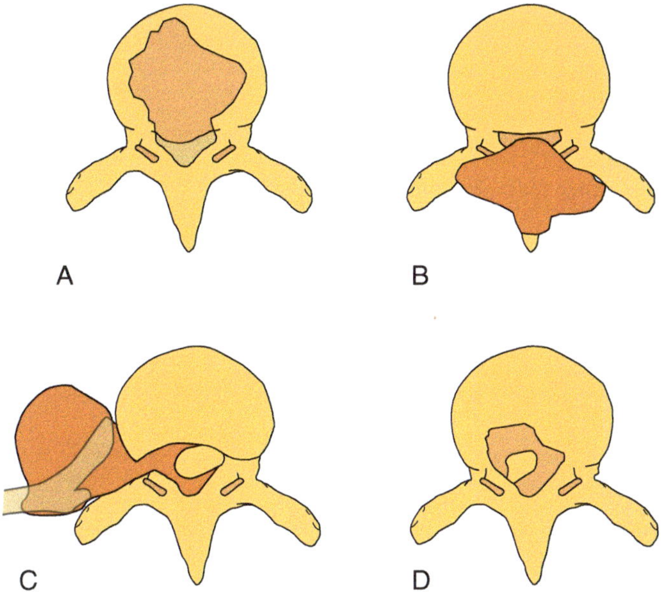

Figure 14-4 Modes of invasion into the spinal canal by metastatic tumors. Epidural metastases usually arise from extension of metastases located in the adjacent vertebral column into the spinal canal (**A** and **B**), or from paravertebral masses penetrating through the intervertebral foramina (**C**). The extension of the tumor into the spinal canal produces variable involvement of (**A**) the anterior (ventral) compartment, (**B**) the posterior compartment, (**C**) the lateral gutter, or (**D**) any combination of these conditions.

Spinal radiography is predictive of epidural disease,[47] and an epidural mass is identified at 86% of symptomatic spinal segments. However, radiographic results require 30% to 70% bony destruction before they become positive. An MRI study demonstrated that, although an absent pedicle is often the first radiographic sign of metastatic disease, the pedicle is involved by direct extension from either the vertebral body or the posterior elements, and is therefore a late occurrence in the disease process.[48] The region of the vertebral column that is most often involved is the vertebral body, probably because of its extensive vascular supply; thus, most epidural tumors arise in a vertebral body and invade the epidural space anteriorly.[16,49] MRI evaluation of neoplastic SCC showed that metastatic disease was present in the bodies of all 160 vertebral levels that were studied.[16] Assessment of vertebral quadrants' (one anterior, two laterals and one posterior column) involvement showed that 97% of the vertebrae had more than 50% involvement. Four columns were affected in 52% and three columns in 30%. Single column involvement was seen only in the anterior column, and accounted for 3% of affected vertebrae. Coexisting anterior and posterior column disease was observed in 75%. The extensive vertebral involvement associated with SCC suggests that any attempt to perform decompressive surgery should always be combined with measures to stabilize the spine.

Normal spinal roentgenograms, seen in 6% of SCC, do not exclude epidural metastases. Normal radiographs are found in 89% of lymphoma patients with epidural compression,[45] in whom a paravertebral tumor mass invades the epidural space through the intervertebral foramina, rather than via vertebral extension (Figure 14-4). This mode of epidural invasion is seen in lymphomas, renal cell cancer, superior sulcus tumors (Pancoast syndrome), and neuroblastoma, and accounts for approximately 10% of all SCC.[45] Up to 36% of patients with paraspinal tumor have epidural metastases on myelography.[50] With the advent of CT scanning and MRI, which adequately demonstrate paravertebral soft tissues, these lesions are being more frequently recognized. A paraspinal mass is detected by MRI at the site of SCC in 28% of patients, and only one third of the masses were detected on plain radiography.[40] Pure, exclusively epidural lesions are rare, and their incidence is not known. In a consecutive series of 100 patients with SCC evaluated by MRI, no isolated epidural lesion was noted.[16]

The location of the extradural metastases within the vertebral canal has important surgical implications. Accurate definition of the epidural mass as posterior, lateral, cuff, or anterior (Figure 14-4) requires CT-myelography or a noninvasive MRI study. MRI is the procedure of choice to evaluate the vertebral column, spinal cord, and soft tissue parts, and usually eliminates the need for other imaging studies.[39,51–53] It is the imaging method of choice both for screening and for ultimate diagnosis of SCC whenever it is readily available.[2,16,39,40,54,55] Still, spinal CT is an excellent screening method to diagnose patients at risk, and to verify presence of an epidural mass in an emergency setting.[1]

In a study of 342 episodes of suspected neoplastic SCC evaluated with spinal CT, additional MRI assessment was required due to diagnostic uncertainty in only 5%.[1] However, MRI has a broader impact on management. It detects unexpected vertebral and epidural lesions that lead to a change in treatment in up to 50% of patients.[2,16,39,54,55] Thus, when SCC is suspected, a complete spine evaluation is indicated, and MRI provides significant economic benefits compared with other imaging modalities used for evaluation.[56]

Myelography combined with CT should be performed only when there is inability to perform MRI, either because patients are unable to undergo MRI (because of pacemakers or claustrophobia), or when a technically adequate MRI cannot be obtained (e.g., presence of spinal instrumentation at the investigated level or extreme obesity).

SYMPTOMS AND SIGNS

Onset of SCC symptoms may be acute or insidious, and symptom duration varies widely. Pain is the initial symptom in 96% of cases, preceding other symptoms by approximately 2 to 3 months.[35,57] Pain can be localized close to the site of the lesion or can be radicular. Pain generally results from nerve root compression or infiltration, compression fractures, segmental instability, displacement of the dura, or dural invasion. Therefore, all patients with symptomatic spinal metastases must be considered at risk for SCC. The site of pain may not correspond to the site of epidural compression on imaging,[35] and it may be nonspecific or referred to other sites, frequently leading to a delay in diagnosis.[35,57] This is especially true in patients without a previous history of cancer.

At the time of diagnosis, neurological signs are common,[35,45,51,57] and include various degrees of muscle weakness in 76%, bladder and bowel dysfunction in over 50%, and sensory deficit in about 50% of patients with SCC. However, weakness and sensory abnormalities are often reported late and identified even later, despite patients having reported pain for a considerable time. Nearly half of severely affected patients develop a complete deficit (no residual spinal cord function) after diagnosis and before undergoing any treatment. Of the paraparetic patients, 28% become paraplegic in less than 24 hours and before initiation of treatment.[58] SCC should therefore be treated as soon as possible, and early diagnosis is crucial, as functional outcome largely depends on the neurological function before treatment.[45,58–60]

Apart from the typical manifestations of SCC, unusual clinical presentations may be seen. These includes atypical facial pain and numbness, Brown-Séquard syndrome, ataxia secondary to posterior column dysfunction, or herpetic rash along the affected dermatomes.[45,51,61]

PATHOPHYSIOLOGY

The mechanisms that determine the degree of irreversible tissue damage are poorly understood, but appear to be associated with a neurochemical cascade activated by the initial event of compressive injury. Comprehension of the secondary autodestructive processes has increased with the use of well-characterized animal models.[62–76] These laboratory studies demonstrate that pharmacologic treatments modify neurochemical changes, attenuate spinal cord edema, ameliorate structural destruction, and significantly delay neurologic deterioration, even if the compressing tumor is not removed. Figure 14-5 summarizes the paradigm of secondary events in neoplastic SCC, and the pharmacological strategies used to ameliorate them in experimental animal models.

The mechanism of injury induced by the expanding extradural tumors is complex and multifactorial. The extradural tumor causes early obstruction of the epidural venous plexus, and also induces arteriolar dilatation via local spinal autoregulatory mechanisms such as activation of endothelial NO synthase.[64,65,77] These changes in vascular tone and drainage enhance production of a vasogenic type of edema. With increase of edema and mechanical pressure, a decrease in spinal cord blood flow at the site of compression eventually follows. Ischemia may then play the final deleterious role, leading to cell death if compression is not promptly alleviated. In animal models, development of conduction block and neurologic signs of myelopathy were related to myelin destruction,[76] which was probably caused by both mechanical compression and ischemia, and by activation of death receptor pathways associated with oligodendroglial apoptosis.[78] Although demyelination can occur at sites of spinal compression,[79,80] remyelination may take place after transient compression,[81] possibly correlating with recovery of function after prompt decompression.

Local production of cytokines such as prostaglandins, interleukin (IL)-1 and IL-6, may promote an inflammatory response with associated physiological changes of vasodilation, plasma exudation, and edema formation.[75,82] In keeping with this concept, a rapid antiedema effect is achieved by steroidal or nonsteroidal antiinflammatory drugs (e.g., indomethacin),[67,69,70] or by inhibitors of phagocytic activity.[75,82] It was found that IL-1 induces upregulation of adhesion molecules,

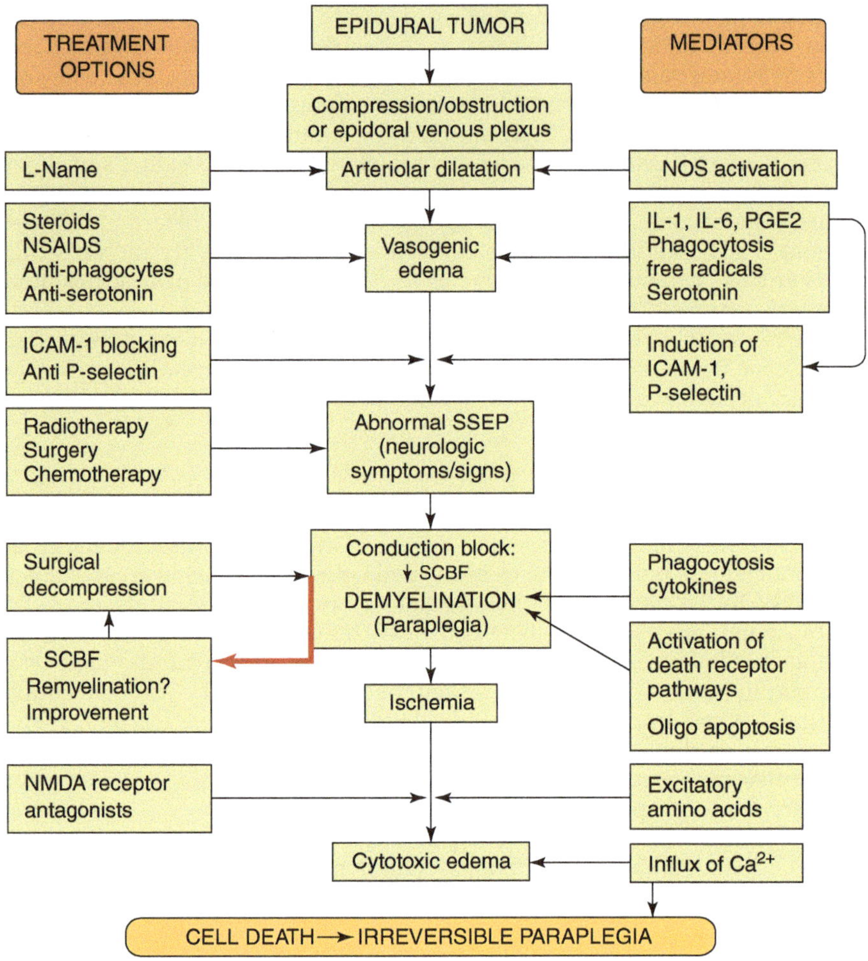

Figure 14-5 An algorithm of the recognized mechanisms involved in the pathophysiology of spinal cord compression. Pharmacological treatment options may reduce neural tissue damage. Data related to pharmacologic manipulations are derived from investigation of animal models of neoplastic SCC. The relationship of the currently used therapeutic modalities in humans (corticosteroids, radiotherapy, surgery, and chemotherapy) to the specific stage of spinal cord injury is also shown.

such as P-selectin and ICAM-1. Blockage of this process resulted in white matter preservation and improved neurological outcome.[83,84]

Other studies looked at the microglia and phagocytic activity. Immunohistochemical studies showed that in tumor-bearing paraplegic rats, the normal population of resting microglia was replaced by activated amoeboid cells, probably engaged in phagocytosis.[75] At onset of paraplegia, marked disruption of normal neurofilament cytoarchitecture was evident. In vivo pharmacological inhibition of phagocytosis (using chloroquine and colchicines) was associated with a reduced ratio of amoeboid microglia, marked preservation of neurofilament structure, diminished synthesis of cytokines (PGE_2, IL-1, IL-6), and significant attenuation in spinal cord edema. Initiating this treatment at first sign of neurologic dysfunction significantly delayed the onset of paraplegia, and protracted the course of neurological deterioration toward paraplegia.

These results suggest that inhibition of phagocytosis may delay structural damage, and thus enhance the chance of recovery following antitumor therapy. It provides the scientific background for the clinical use of steroids, and it also explains the favorable neurological outcome in patients with SCC who are treated by radiotherapy and receive high-dose dexamethasone.[85] Although dexamethasone is incapable of blocking phagocytosis, it does inhibit inflammatory responses and production of some cytokines that play a role in the phagocytic cascade.

A marked increase in serotonin utilization is present in the compressed cord segments. Inhibition of serotonin receptors results in attenuated vascular permeability and a protracted clinical course toward paraplegia, similar to the favorable effect produced by antiinflammatory agents.[73–75,82] Receptor-activated serotonergic mechanisms that are distinct from the mechanism associated with the inflammatory response probably participate in the disruption of the blood-spinal cord barrier in the subacutely developing compression injury. These mechanisms can be separately manipulated pharmacologically to yield measurable effects in experimental models. Finally, in the end stage, when conduction block and ischemia set in, excitotoxins (such as glutamate) mediate the evolution of cytotoxic edema that adds its deleterious role.[71,72]

These experimental findings indicate that early pharmacological intervention may offer the potential to delay neurological deterioration, and may attenuate neuronal damage. Given the complexity of pathophysiological mechanisms, such manipulations should be carefully assessed before their extrapolation to human clinical studies.

SURVIVAL AND SPINAL CORD COMPRESSION

The magnitude of the clinical problem of SCC is usually underestimated. The best evidence suggests that approximately 5% of patients dying of cancer have suffered from epidural metastases.[37,42] This calculated incidence exceeds the annual rate of traumatic spinal cord injury. However, because of the high mortality among these patients (50% to 70% at one year), the socioeconomic impact of neoplastic SCC is less than traumatic injury. The overall median survival following the first episode of SCC is short, ranging from 3 to 4 months.[36,37,86] As a result, neoplastic SCC accounts for only 10% to 14% of all spinal cord injury admissions to rehabilitation units.[87] It was demonstrated that pretreatment ambulatory function is the main determinant for posttreatment gait function, and the survival of nonambulatory patients can only be improved with restoration of gait function by immediate treatment.[36,38,88,89]

In spite of the poor prognosis of the disease, most patients should receive active treatment[36,51,90] to preserve or restore mobility and continence, and to alleviate intractable pain. SCC in itself is usually not the direct cause of death, except when it occurs in the upper portion of the cervical spine. Survival in SCC is related to the natural history of the systemic malignancy. Only about 30% of patients are expected to survive beyond 1 year, and rarely as long as 4 to 9 years.[43,91–93]

FACTORS INFLUENCING RECOVERY OF FUNCTION

Tumor Biology and Cell Type

The biological activity of the primary neoplasm determines the aggressiveness of both local and systemic disease, the success of therapy, and the posttreatment survival rate.[37,58,94] Patients with myeloma, lymphoma, Ewing sarcoma, neuroblastoma, or carcinoma of the breast have a favorable prognosis for recovery of function, and they survive longer after the first episode of SCC.[37] The outlook for patients with metastatic bronchogenic carcinoma or metastatic disease of an unknown primary site is generally poor. Overall, radiosensitivity and chemosensitivity is associated with a more favorable prognosis and functional outcome, while radioresistant tumors tend to have worse results.[37,58,95]

Pretreatment Neurological Status

SCC outcome depends in good part on the patient's neurological status at the time of treatment. A positive correlation exists between the pretreatment mobility and functional outcome.[51,58,94,96–100] From 80% to 90% of patients who can walk at the time of diagnosis remain ambulant after treatment, 35% to 45% of those who are initially paraparetic become ambulatory, and only 5% to 7% of paraplegic patients regain the ability to walk. The success of therapy in paraplegic patients depends on whether the patient has complete functional cord transection, or whether there is preservation of some neurological function, with motor function the most significant. Only 2% of patients with complete transection recover ambulation, compared to 20% of patients with residual neurological function. Regardless of the mode of therapy, complete paraplegia carries a bad functional prognosis.

The value of early diagnosis is clear, and with the advent of modern imaging techniques the percentage of patients diagnosed while still able to walk is steadily increasing. Series in which modern imaging techniques were used to diagnose SCC contain 42% to 56% ambulatory patients,[85,99–101] unlike previous reports in which only 25% of patients were ambulatory at diagnosis.[59,95,102,103] Nevertheless, an unacceptable delay in diagnosis, investigation, and referral occurs in many patients with neoplastic SCC, with a median delay of 14 days from the onset of symptoms. This delay results in preventable loss of function before treatment.[35,104,105]

Progression Rate of Symptoms

It has been suggested that a rapid onset and progression of neurological symptoms is associated with a worse prognosis as compared to a gradual onset and slow progression of neurological deficit.[58,88,106–108] The importance of the rate of symptom progression was emphasized in a study of 15 paraplegic patients treated with radiation therapy.[109] Five of the 15 patients regained ambulation after a delay of 3 months or more. The median time from the initial motor symptoms to total paralysis was longer (45 days) in patients who recovered than in those who remained paralyzed (9 days). The progression rate of motor deficit was found to be an independent prognostic factor for posttreatment functional outcome in a study that analyzed variables by multiple logistic regression analysis.[88,107,108] A slower development of motor dysfunction predicted a better outcome, and was found to be a stronger predictor than other prognostic factors such as the type of tumor or the pretreatment ambulatory status. However, if the degree of spinal cord damage is taken into account, the neurological grade still has a great influence on prognosis in patients with rapidly developing symptoms (less than 24 hours).[58] In patients with rapidly evolving deficit, 20% of paraparetic patients recover, compared with none of the paraplegic patients.

Therefore, residual cord function should also be taken into account as an important prognostic variable in the rapidly evolving deficit. Once paraplegia has set in, the duration of paralysis does have prognostic significance, although anecdotal recovery has been reported even after periods of 4 to 8 weeks.[109]

Treatment with Corticosteroids

The use of steroids in the treatment of SCC is widely accepted.[58,60,85,95,103,110] The scientific basis for steroid use stems from animal models of SCC, in which reduction of spinal cord edema and delayed onset of paraplegia were observed after treatment with dexamethasone.[62,64,66,67,69,75] The clinical basis for use of high-dose steroids is the rapid symptom relief noted in some patients receiving initial doses of 100 mg of dexamethasone, although the outcome was not superior compared to historical controls who received lower doses of steroids.[95] In a prospective study, 37 patients with SCC were randomly assigned to receive initial treatment with either high-dose dexamethasone (100 mg) or a conventional intravenous bolus dose (10 mg) of dexamethasone followed by 16 mg/day orally.[110] No dose effect was observed on neurological outcome, but a substantial effect on pain was noted within 24 hours after high-dose treatment. There is only one well-designed, randomized, controlled trial that compared high-dose dexamethasone to no steroids in 57 patients with metastatic SCC treated with radiotherapy alone.[85] There was a statistically and clinically significant difference between the steroid-treated and control arms. Of patients receiving steroids, 81% were ambulatory after treatment, compared to only 63% of patients in the control arm. However, steroid treatment was associated with significant side effects in 11%.

Several investigators observed a dramatic resolution of symptoms after treatment with steroids alone.[45,111,112] Such steroid-related improvement probably results from a direct oncolytic effect observed in lymphomas and leukemias. This response differs from the pharmacologic effect of steroids that protracts the cascade of deleterious events leading to irreversible spinal cord damage, which are demonstrated in Figure 14-5.

PRINCIPLES OF MANAGEMENT

The management of metastatic SCC is controversial.[58–60,94,99,100,113,114] Controversy stems from the lack of prospective, well-designed, controlled clinical studies directly comparing various treatment modalities, and from an absence of standard criteria for evaluation of response. Patients with metastatic SCC have, by definition, tumors that have spread from a primary site and thus are no longer curable by local measures. The therapeutic modalities of surgery and radiotherapy are palliative, and preservation or restoration of ambulation and bladder control are

TABLE 14-3 Therapeutic Modalities in Spinal Epidural Metastases

Pharmacotherapy
- Specific (antineoplastic; combination chemotherapy)
- Nonspecific (antiedema, analgesia)

Radiation Therapy
- External beam radiotherapy—conventional fields
- Image-guided intensity-modulated radiosurgery
- Fractionated stereotactic conformal radiotherapy

Surgery
- Laminectomy (posterior decompression) ± spinal fixation
- Vertebral body resection (anterior decompression) + spinal fixation
- Combined anterior and posterior decompression + spinal fixation (may be staged as sequential procedures)

the criteria for successful therapy. Pain relief is also an important, but secondary goal.

Because the treatment is not curative, its effect on the quality of further survival is particularly important. The therapeutic modalities currently available for the treatment of patients with epidural SCC are listed in Table 14-3. An algorithm for treatment selection in the various categories of SCC is shown in Figure 14-6.

Pharmacotherapy

Specific Chemotherapy

Epidural metastases arising from chemoresponsive primary tumors are likely to respond to chemotherapy, particularly early in the course of the disease. The response of lymphomas affecting the spine to corticosteroids[45] may serve as an example. Several reports suggest that good recovery of neurological function can be obtained by chemotherapy alone in chemosensitive neoplasms such as lymphoma, myeloma, Ewing sarcoma, germ cell tumors, and neuroblastoma.[114–119] The published experience of chemotherapy alone is limited and large-scaled studies are not available.

Chemotherapy should be considered for treating spinal metastases with epidural components in the following settings:

1. In some patients with lymphoma, neuroblastoma, germ cell tumors, or Ewing sarcoma with SCC as the presenting manifestation of malignancy, or when SCC is recognized during evaluation of the extent of disease. The best approach to treatment in these settings is still unclear. We believe that in SCC diagnosed in the above setting, with mild neurological dysfunction and no sign of rapid deterioration, chemotherapy can be used first.
2. Patients with SCC whose level of neural compression was previously irradiated, and who are not candidates for further radiation or surgical therapy. These patients should be considered for chemotherapy.
3. Chemotherapy can be used in chemosensitive tumors in conjunction with either surgery or radiotherapy in the acute treatment of symptomatic SCC.

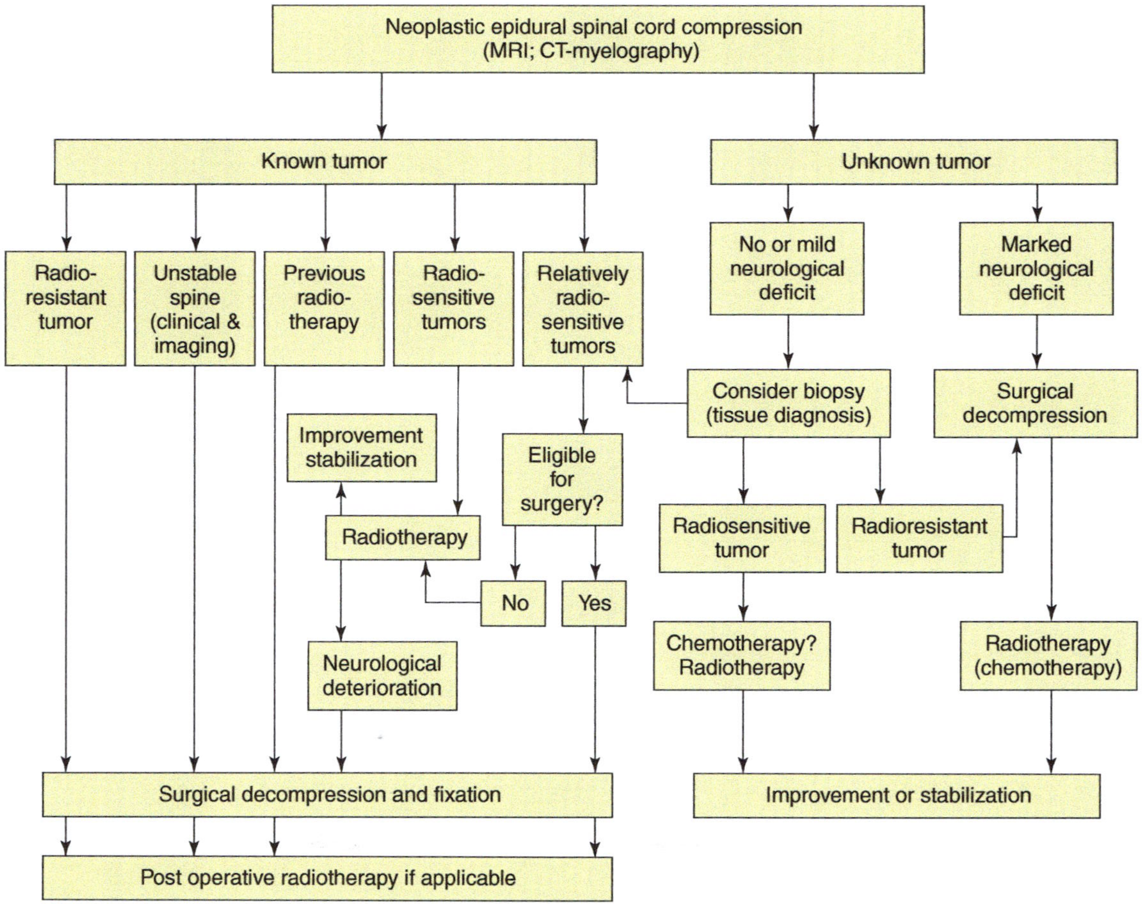

Figure 14-6 An algorithm for evaluating and selecting the preferred therapeutic approach in patients with neoplastic SCC.

Nonspecific pharmacotherapy

- ***Corticosteroids:*** Glucocorticoids rarely achieve the dramatic relief from neurological disability that is seen in patients with brain metastases. However, when high doses of corticosteroids are used to treat SCC, most patients experience dramatic relief from pain.[95,110] Some experience an arrest of progressively-deteriorating neurological function, and a few may improve from corticosteroids alone. High doses of steroids are frequently used in SCC as specified above.[60,95,110] The associated side effects that can arise with the use of corticosteroids should be an important consideration. The incidence of serious steroid-related complications in neuro-oncology patients has been the subject of several studies.[120–122] At least one steroid-related side effect was observed in 51% of treated patients, and 19% required hospital admission. Both the duration and the total dose of steroid therapy predicted toxicity. A significant increase in severe complications, including fatal sepsis, was noted when dexamethasone was used for more than 40 days to treat SCC.[123] In addition, patients with SCC treated with steroids present fewer signs and symptoms of peritonitis when they develop intestinal perforation. Because major complications occur in patients who receive steroids for more than 1 month, they must be used judiciously, and should be discontinued as rapidly as possible, or tapered down to the lowest possible level that is compatible with clinical benefit.

  The following recommendations apply for the use of steroids:
  1. For patients with imaging evidence of SCC, but without signs of myelopathy, dexamethasone does not need to be given during treatment by radiotherapy.[60,124]
  2. Patients with SCC and moderate pain, but without myelopathy, may be treated with a standard dose (16 mg/day) of dexamethasone for pain relief. Nonsteroidal antiinflammatory agents may serve as substitutes.
  3. Patients with SCC and signs of myelopathy should be treated initially with high doses of dexamethasone to increase their chance for posttreatment ambulation.[85] This comes with a moderate risk of serious toxicity, which has to be accepted in view of the expected benefit. The drug should be tapered off as soon as definitive treatment has been initiated.
- ***Analgesia:*** Because pain is the presenting symptom in over 95% of patients with epidural SCC,[35,45,90,95] the principles of good analgesic management must be applied. In most patients, treatment with either radiotherapy alone or resection of tumor and restoration of stability frequently results in pain relief.[45,49,51]

Radiation Therapy

The results of radiation therapy in 1211 patients with a variety of metastatic tu mors[36,43,45,85,95,96,99,101,125–129] can be summarized as follows: Between 28% and 50% of patients either regain or maintain ambulation at the end of therapy, and, of those who survive one year, 50% maintain that improvement.[45,95] The proportion of patients who are ambulatory at diagnosis is increasing, and they comprise 42% to 64% of patients diagnosed with SCC.[36,45,85,99,101] Up to 96% of patients who are ambulatory at diagnosis are likely to maintain mobility. However, 4% to 20% of patients who can walk at the start of treatment will deteriorate to nonambulatory status during or soon after completion of radiotherapy. Radiation therapy also results in pain relief in 50% to 80% of patients.[36,45,49,51,94,98,99]

The efficacy of radiation therapy depends on the radiosensitivity of the tumor, the neurological status at time of treatment, and maintenance of spinal stability. Patients with highly radiosensitive tumors (such as lymphoma, Ewing sarcoma, seminoma, neuroblastoma, and myeloma) are more likely to regain or maintain ambulation than those with less radiosensitive tumors (overall, 60% to 80% versus 40%).[49,58,103,112,114] Improvement after the initiation of radiation therapy may be delayed for a few days before it becomes evident, even in patients with radiosensitive tumors.

Radiotherapy should also be considered as primary therapy for moderately radiosensitive neoplasms, such as breast carcinoma. However, the need for surgical intervention should be critically reviewed for each patient. Radiotherapy is considered as the treatment of first choice for patients who are ambulatory at presentation, and whose spinal stability is maintained. However, in nonambulatory patients, surgical decompression should be considered as the primary avenue of therapy because radiotherapy requires a time interval that may cause an irreversible delay in the reduction of spinal cord damage. A randomized study assigned patients with SCC to primary treatment with either radiotherapy alone or to surgical decompression with stabilization followed by postoperative radiotherapy.[130] Patients treated by immediate direct surgical decompressive surgery plus radiotherapy retained the ability to walk longer and regained the ability to walk more often than patients treated by radiotherapy alone. Radiotherapy alone should be employed if surgery is contraindicated because of the patient's poor general medical status, multiple compression levels, or long-standing paraplegia.

The indication for primary radiotherapy is less clear for tumors generally regarded as poorly radioresponsive. Nevertheless, radiotherapy should be tried as a primary modality if the patient's neurological deficit is not severe, and if the rate of progression of the deficit is such that there would be time to resort to surgical decompression should radiotherapy fail. Still, if the odds are that surgery will be required, the increased rate of postoperative complications observed in previously irradiated patients should be carefully weighed against the benefit of early surgical intervention. Where surgery is the primary therapy, postoperative radiation is employed to prevent local recurrence of tumor and to contribute to pain relief.

No controlled studies have compared the various dose and fractionation schedules of radiation therapy given to patients with SCC.[60] Single-arm studies and retrospective reviews of nonrandomized studies[108,127,131–133] suggest that neither the dose nor the fractionation schedule has a major impact on outcome. The chosen treatment schedule should be a short palliative regimen at doses below spinal cord tolerance. The frequently used schedules are 20 Gy in five fractions, 28 Gy in seven fractions, and 30 Gy in ten fractions.

Surgery

Surgical treatment of SCC has been a subject of debate for a long time. A recent randomized trial compared direct decompressive surgical resection plus radiotherapy to treatment with radiotherapy alone.[130] This trial proved that primary treatment with surgical decompression and stabilization yields a better outcome than treatment with radiotherapy alone. Prior to this study, surgical series suggested that a high proportion of patients regain or maintain ambulation (approximately 75%).[45,97,100,103,134–147] However, the risk associated with operative morbidity (average rate 14%) and mortality (4.5%) should be carefully weighed against the expected gain from surgery. Surgery is usually indicated for patients with SCC who have an expected survival that exceeds 3 to 6 months. This expected survival is longer than the overall median survival of patients with SCC, which ranges between 3 and 4 months.[36,37,86]

The traditional approach to the treatment of neoplastic SCC has been decompressive laminectomy, with or without postoperative radiation therapy.[41,43,45,85,95,96,99,101,102,112,125–127,141] Ambulation following laminectomy is maintained or regained in 35% to 50% of treated patients, a result similar to that achieved by radiation therapy alone. Pain is improved in 50% to 70% of patients, a rate which is also similar to that for radiation therapy. Approximately 14% of patients treated by radiotherapy can deteriorate,[36,43,45,85,95,96,125–129] compared to approximately 15% of the patients reported to have worse neurological outcome after laminectomy. Thus, results of laminectomy used as a decompressive surgery are similar to those reported for radiation therapy alone. Therefore, oncology literature favored initial radiotherapy in the majority of the patients, reserving surgery for salvage or diagnosis.

Laminectomy via the midline posterior approach is technically easy and safe, and allows for tissue diagnosis, but provides adequate decompression only when the tumor mass lies dorsolateral to the dura. Laminectomy also destabilizes the spine if the vertebral body and the pedicles are destroyed by tumor, and only allows a limited access to tumor lying ventral to the cord. The reasons for surgical failures in the past were: (1) nonselective use of one surgical approach (laminectomy), (2) inadequate tumor resection, (3) ineffective stabilization, and (4) poor patient selection. To obtain an effective decompression, the surgical approach should be selected according to the location of the main compressing mass within the spinal canal. Spinal fixation should follow as an integral part of the decompressive procedure in order to establish spinal stability and restore ambulation.

Indications for Surgical Intervention

Figure 14-6 specifies the circumstances in which surgery should be considered.

Diagnosis in Doubt

In 8% of patients with neoplastic SCC, spinal involvement is the initial presentation of cancer.[44,102] When the etiology of the spinal lesion is in doubt, surgical decompression should be considered to obtain a tissue diagnosis and to achieve rapid decompression. Current image-assisted (CT-guided) percutaneous needle biopsy of vertebral lesions is diagnostic in 95% of patients[44,148] and has a reported complication rate of less than 1%. Therefore, surgery is rarely needed simply to establish the diagnosis of malignancy. If the biopsy shows a chemosensitive tumor (e.g., lymphoma) the patient can immediately proceed to treatment without the delay imposed by surgery. If the biopsy results are not diagnostic, or if the patient's ability to walk is already impaired and neurological status is unstable, decompression is advisable to achieve an accurate diagnosis and to initiate treatment without delay.

Spinal Instability or Bone Compression:

A major goal of treatment is the restoration or maintenance of spinal stability; therefore, it is essential to diagnose spinal instability. The criteria for spinal stability in neoplastic disease of the spine are specified in section 2.1 of this chapter. Apart from the neuroimaging studies that define anatomic details used in the three-column spinal model (Figure 14-1), the concept of clinical instability should be taken into account.[18] Clinical instability should be suspected whenever an incapacitating pain develops under physiologic loads and is associated with structural changes identified on imaging. Thus symptoms and signs should direct therapeutic consideration. Patients with fracture-dislocation, localized kyphosis, collapsed vertebra with retropulsion of a bone fragment, or segmental instability, may require surgical decompression and stabilization if either pain or neurological symptomatology is present. Not every case defined by the criteria for unstable spine requires surgical intervention. If the tumor is relatively radiosensitive, and no neurological deficit is present, radiotherapy may result in satisfactory axial settling and pain relief over a period of weeks or months. These patients should be carefully followed, because they are potentially unstable.

When the anterior and middle columns are destroyed by tumor, treatment considerations should include decompression by the anterior approach to the spine as well as restoration of stability by vertebral body replacement constructs. If the posterior column structures are involved, then the treatment plan is to replace (or substitute) for the support role of these structures by posterior decompression combined with posterior instrumentation for maintenance of stability.

The criteria of spinal instability that should bring about consideration for spinal stabilization are summarized in Table 14-2. The criteria for patient selection, the surgical approach for decompression, and the methods of stabilization vary. Recommendations for patient selection and optimal methods of decompression and stabilization are undergoing constant development.

Previous Radiation Exposure:

When radiotherapy cannot be used because of previous irradiation, surgical decompression is indicated as the primary therapeutic modality because of the risk of exceeding spinal cord tolerance by further irradiation. Surgery is warranted for relapse occurring months or even years after a successful previous treatment, in the hope of preserving neurological function. In many patients, however, life expectancy at the time of relapse of SCC is short. Retreatment with radiotherapy often preserves ambulation with a low risk of radiation myelopathy during the remaining lifespan.[131,149–151]

Radioresistant Tumors:

In radioresistant tumors, e.g., renal cell carcinoma, decompressive surgery might be considered as the primary mode of therapy. Postoperative radiotherapy is administered with the hope of retarding tumor regrowth. However, this indication is not generally accepted, and sometimes, especially in neurologically-stable patients, radiotherapy may be tried first.

Neurological Deterioration During Radiotherapy:

Neurological deterioration occurring during radiotherapy of a relatively radiosensitive tumor should prompt an early consideration for surgical decompression. The decline in neurological function may reflect radioresistance, progressive spinal instability, or bone compression secondary to vertebral collapse, all of which may be most effectively treated by spinal decompression and stabilization.

Selection of Surgical Approach

The goal of surgery is the optimal removal of the compressing epidural mass and restoration of spinal stability. Therefore, the selection of the surgical approach should be determined by variables such as the location of the tumor inside and outside the spinal canal, the main cause of the instability, and feasible options for stabilization. Table 14-4 details the preoperative assessment required for determining the surgical approach. The location of the epidural mass should dictate the approach for decompression. Primary spinal tumors are classified based on tumor location and according to the zones of involvement (McLain and Weinstein classification),[152] and this information is used to determine the optimal surgical approach (Figure 14-7). These guidelines are also applicable to metastatic lesions.

In patients with metastatic spine disease and limited life expectancy, radical excision of the vertebral tumor is not always the main goal; therefore, selection of surgical approach also requires other considerations. In patients with progressive kyphosis without anterior cord compression, or in patients with thoracic

TABLE 14-4 Pretreatment or Preoperative Assessment of Tumor Location and Extent of Pathology in Tumors of the Spine

Bone involvement (CT, MRI)
- Vertebral body and pedicles, posterior elements, or a combination of both
- Number of vertebrae involved
- Percentage of bone mass loss of the vertebral cut surface

Epidural mass (CT myelography, MRI)
- Epidural mass related or unrelated to the bone lesion
- Number of spinal levels involved
- Position of the epidural mass: anterior, lateral, posterior, and/or encircling

Spinal stability (spinal radiography, CT and MRI)
- Involvement of two or more adjacent vertebrae
- Involvement of two or more spinal columns as well as the vertebral cortical shell
- Loss of more than 50% of the vertebral width
- Shearing deformity
- Any combination of the above

Retroperitoneal and/or paravertebral mass (CT, MRI)
- Location
- Extent
- Involvement of adjacent structures or organs (kidneys, uterus, large vessels)
- Involvement of posterior chest or abdominal wall

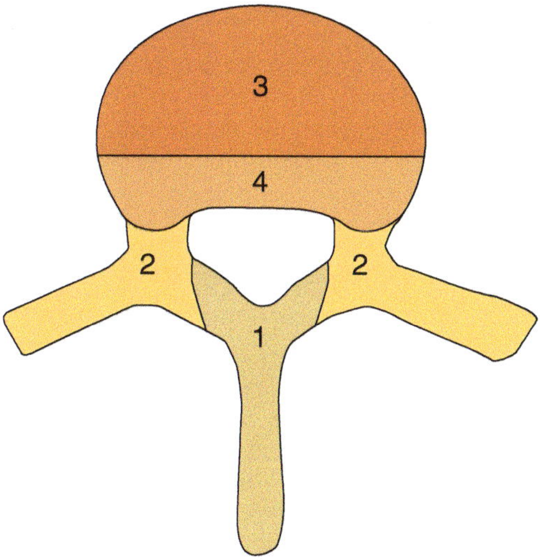

Figure 14-7 Classification system of McLain and Weinstein[152] suggested for determining the optimal surgical approach for resection of spinal tumors. The spine is divided into four zones of possible tumor involvement. Zone 1 is best approached posteriorly. Zone 2 tumors may be resected via a posterior or posterolateral approach. Zone 3 tumors are best approached anteriorly. Zone 4 is the most inaccessible region, hence a combined anterior and posterior approach may be recommended.

or lumbar pathological fracture or dislocation without significant soft tissue or bony neural compromise, posterior realignment and stabilization may relieve pain and most cord impingement. In patients for whom the anterior approach is not feasible due to technical reasons, poor medical status, or widespread disease, partial decompression and stabilization via a posterior approach may be a useful palliative procedure.[153]

COMPLICATIONS

Radiotherapy

Most papers dealing with radiotherapy alone do not comment on complications of therapy or mortality. Death in the first month after radiotherapy is most likely the result of active primary or metastatic disease. The main determinants of survival are performance status and tumor burden; 70% of patients considered severely ill at the time of SCC diagnosis were reported to die within 30 days after diagnosis.[103] The risk of radiation myelopathy is related to dose/fractionation parameters, which, in palliative treatment, are below the level of spinal cord tolerance. The proportion of patients with neoplastic SCC surviving for more than 2 years is less than 3%, and these patients are at risk of developing radiation myelopathy.[131] Of patients who survive for more than 18 months, 5% may develop symptomatic myelopathy.[131]

Surgical Complications

Mortality

The incidence of death within the first month after decompressive laminectomy is approximately 8%.[45,154–157] The surgical mortality rate after vertebral body resection of 4% to 8% falls within the same range.[45,97,100,103,134–137,142,144,145]

Morbidity

The risk of neurological deterioration as a result of surgery is a major concern in patients who present while they are still able to walk. Its average rate following laminectomy is 15% (range: 5% to 30%).[45,93,158,159] Neurological deterioration is rare after vertebral body resection, and occurs in only 2% to 6% of patients.[97,103,134,160]

Nonneurological complications in patients undergoing laminectomy combined with radiotherapy include wound infection, wound dehiscence, spinal epidural hematoma, cerebrospinal fluid leak, and spinal instability. The frequency of these complications ranges from 8% to 54%, with a mean of 12%.[45,59] Only a few authors mentioned the problem of instability,[45,102] which amounts to about 9% of cases.

As the use of instrumentation increases, nonneurological complications, especially instrumentation-related complications such as dislodgment and infections, are increasing (Table 14-5). Preoperative protein depletion and perioperative administration of corticosteroids are risk factors for wound infection.[144,161] The likelihood of postoperative complications is significantly increased in patients with poor neurological outcome, and in patients who develop severe motor deficit prior to surgery.[144] Spinal radiation before surgical decompression is associated with a significantly higher rate of major wound complications.[162,163] Patients with preoperative irradiation had a 32% major wound complication rate, which was threefold higher than the 12% rate observed in patients who underwent de novo surgery.[163] It should be noted that a tailored, patient-specific approach, including vertebral body resection and spinal instrumentation techniques, requires considerable expertise. These procedures should be undertaken only by a surgeon familiar with the specific techniques for posterior and anterior spinal instrumentation, including the different options to suit specific levels along the spine.

RECURRENT EPIDURAL SCC

About 10% of patients will eventually develop local recurrence of spinal metastasis. Most of these patients have received radiotherapy and some have had previous surgery. Little attention has been paid to this subgroup of patients. For the majority, no reliably effective chemotherapy option remains at this stage. Spinal surgery should be considered in these patients, although many have advanced visceral disease limiting their life expectancy to a few months, or widespread

TABLE 14-5 Surgery-related Nonneurological Morbidity in Neoplastic Spinal Cord Compression

Surgical Procedure	Morbidity (%)	
	Range	Average
Laminectomy	8-54	15
Laminectomy and fixation	1-21	11
Vertebral body resection and fixation	8-41	23
Patient-specific approach (anterior, posterior or both) and fixation	25-48	37

spinal metastases, which limit surgical feasibility. Surgical decompression after previous radiotherapy is associated with an increased rate of morbidity.[162,163] A retrospective study of 51 patients undergoing a second course of spinal radiation found that reirradiation was highly successful in preserving neurologic function and rarely resulted in radiation myelopathy.[149]

CONCLUSIONS FOR EPIDURAL METASTASES

Early diagnosis and treatment of neoplastic SCC improve outcome. A high index of suspicion is essential, especially in patients known to harbor a neoplastic process. Wider acceptance and judicious use of modern and novel surgical techniques for spinal decompression and stabilization may improve the quality of life of subgroups of patients too often denied such treatment. Early consideration of surgery in patients with life expectancy greater than 6 months may bring about improved mobility, better quality of life, fewer surgical complications, and longer survival. More trials are needed to identify patients who would benefit from advanced surgical techniques.

Intradural Metastases

Metastatic disease within the confines of the dura constitutes less than 5% of all spinal metastases. Intradural metastases that affect the spinal cord are categorized into those located in the subarachnoid space, causing intradural SCC (Figure 14-8a), and intramedullary metastases that invade the cord substance (Figure 14-8b).

INTRADURAL EXTRAMEDULLARY METASTASES

Metastatic tumors involving the subarachnoid space are by definition leptomeningeal metastases. Unlike the multifocal manifestations produced by diffuse seeding of the subarachnoid space, a metastatic spread may present as a single intradural extramedullary mass lesion compressing the spinal cord.[164–166] The clinical features of these metastases are essentially identical to those of patients with epidural SCC. Primary tumors in a series of ten patients included breast, lung, melanoma, and uterine neoplasm in a descending order of frequency.[165] Of the ten tumors, nine appeared to have spread from brain metastases via the cerebrospinal fluid pathway; in another series brain metastases anteceded the spinal spread in 80% of cases.[164]

The intradural location of the tumor can be identified by MRI evaluation. The treatment of choice is probably radiotherapy. However, if neurological deterioration is relentless and there is no evidence for diffuse spread of metastatic disease in the subarachnoid space, then surgical intervention may be justified.

INTRAMEDULLARY METASTASES

Intramedullary spinal metastases arise either from hematogenous spread to the spinal parenchyma, or by growth of subarachnoid tumor along nerve roots directly into the spinal cord.[167] Intramedullary metastases comprise 8.5% of all CNS metastases, and were found in 2% of cancer patients who had autopsy.

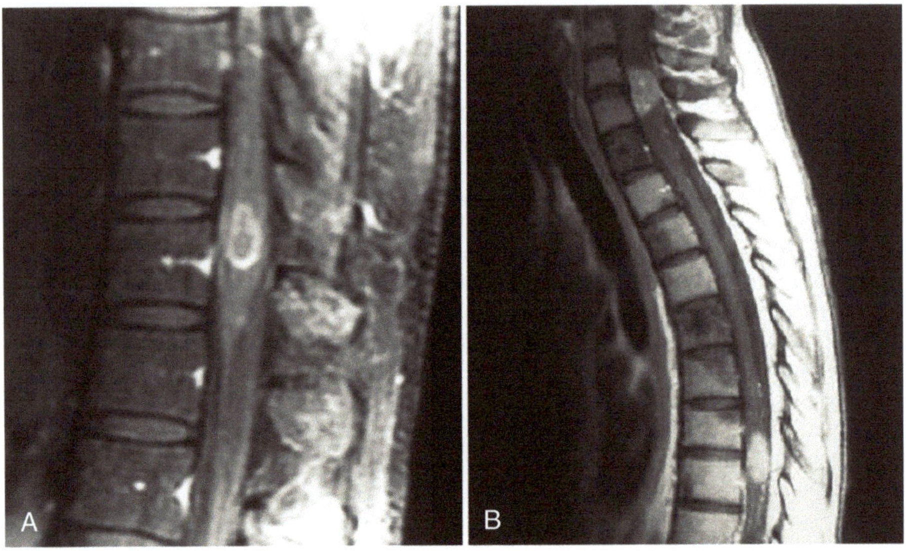

Figure 14-8 **Intramedullary metastases: A,** MRI (enhanced T_1-weighted) shows an enhancing intramedullary metastasis at the T11 vertebral level. The patient had a known metastatic breast carcinoma. Note the associated spinal cord swelling. **B,** A patient with a metastatic non-small cell lung carcinoma with a previous history of brain metastases presented with back pain and myelopathy. MRI (enhanced T_1-weighted) reveals two enhancing intradural lesions. The lesion at the level of C7-T1 is located intradurally, but it is an extramedullary metastasis. The second lesion at the T8-T9 vertebral level is an intramedullary metastasis with an oval-shaped enhancement. Note the vertebral body metastases at multiple levels.

Lung cancer is a common primary tumor, accounting for approximately 50% of these metastases,[5,7,45,167,168] breast cancer contributes about 15%, and lymphoma and melanoma each account for another 10% of cases.[5,45,167,168] In two series, intramedullary metastases were the initial manifestation of cancer in 30% of cases.[5,169]

Disease at other levels of the neuroaxis is common in patients with intramedullary metastases;[5,6,168] approximately 50% of patients have brain metastases and 30% have multiple spinal cord metastases. Brain metastases are almost invariably diagnosed prior to the intramedullary lesion, although sometimes the diagnosis is simultaneous. Leptomeningeal seeding coexists in 15% to 44% of patients, and one autopsy study showed that seeding was associated with focal or multifocal direct extension of the leptomeningeal tumor across the pia into the parenchyma of the spinal cord.[167]

The clinical features of intramedullary metastases include pain in approximately 50% of patients, sensory deficit in more than 80%, weakness in 90%, and urinary incontinence in more than 60%.[5,45,168] None of these features reliably differentiates intramedullary metastases from epidural SCC. However, markedly asymmetric neurologic findings (Brown-Séquard or pseudo–Brown-Séquard syndrome), reported in approximately 30% of cases, are suggestive of an intramedullary rather than extramedullary lesion.

Contrast-enhanced MRI is the ultimate diagnostic examination, but when MRI is contraindicated a CT-myelography should be performed.[5,6] Myelography is less sensitive than MRI and yields a positive diagnosis in only 50% to 80% of symptomatic cases.[5,45] MRI shows that intramedullary metastases are most commonly isolated, small, oval-shaped lesions, without or with slight deformation of the spinal profile. The lesions are enhancing with contrast, and on T_2-weighted sequences pencil-shaped hyperintensity frequently extends cranial to the lesion.[6] Lumbosacral myelomeres are the most frequently affected segments, but involvement of the thoracic and cervical myelomeres is often encountered. Because multiple spinal lesions are found in approximately one third of patients, the MRI study should encompass the entire spine or the whole neuroaxis. Differential diagnoses include primary intramedullary tumors (e.g., glioma or ependymoma), radiation myelopathy in previously irradiated patients, spinal cord infarction from embolus or vascular occlusion, and paraneoplastic necrotic myelopathy. In patients with no history of malignancy, the differential diagnosis also includes myelitis or acute demyelinating plaque. Imaging evaluation of the whole neuroaxis combined with a careful history and neurological examination may aid in the differential diagnosis.

Intramedullary metastases commonly develop late in the course of malignancy. The median survival from diagnosis of the intramedullary lesion is approximately 4 months.[5] Patients with radiosensitive or relatively radiosensitive neoplasms may respond to radiotherapy. Most patients who are ambulatory when diagnosed will experience durable stabilization of function following radiotherapy.

In a small subset of patients surgical resection of an intramedullary lesion should be considered. This is frequently the case when the intramedullary lesion is the first manifestation of malignancy. As with brain metastases, intramedullary deposits are frequently circumscribed, with little invasion of the surrounding spinal medulla, and are thus amenable for gross total resection. In patients with a known diagnosis of cancer, radiation may be considered when the metastasis is isolated, and when the mode of spread is likely to be hematogenous rather than via the subarachnoid space. A few patients who underwent surgical removal of intramedullary metastases are reported to have long-term survival with good neurologic function after treatment.[170–173]

REFERENCES

1. Talcott JA, Stomper PC, Drislane FW, Wen PY, Block CC, Humphrey CC, et al. Assessing suspected spinal cord compression: a multidisciplinary outcomes analysis of 342 episodes. Support Care Cancer 1999;7(1):31–8.
2. Cook AM, Lau TN, Tomlinson MJ, Vaidya M, Wakeley CJ, Goddard P. Magnetic resonance imaging of the whole spine in suspected malignant spinal cord compression: impact on management. Clin Oncol (R Coll Radiol) 1998;10(1):39–43.
3. Ross JR, Saunders Y, Edmonds PM, Patel S, Broadley KE, Johnston SR. Systematic review of role of bisphosphonates on skeletal morbidity in metastatic cancer. BMJ 2003;327(7413):469.
4. Pavlakis N, Stockler M. Bisphosphonates for breast cancer. Cochrane Database Syst Rev 2002;(1) CD003474.
5. Schiff D, O'Neill BP. Intramedullary spinal cord metastases: clinical features and treatment outcome. Neurology 1996;47(4):906–12.
6. Crasto S, Duca S, Davini O, Rizzo L, Pavanello IG, Avataneo T, et al. MRI diagnosis of intramedullary metastases from extra-CNS tumors. Eur Radiol 1997;7(5):732–6.
7. Potti A, Abdel-Raheem M, Levitt R, Schell DA, Mehdi SA. Intramedullary spinal cord metastases (ISCM) and non-small cell lung carcinoma (NSCLC): clinical patterns, diagnosis and therapeutic considerations. Lung Cancer 2001;31(2–3):319–23.
8. Wai MS, Mike S, Ines H, Malcolm M. Palliation of Metastatic Bone Pain: Single Fraction versus Multifraction Radiotherapy–A Systematic Review of the Randomised Trials. Cochrane Database Syst Rev 2004;(2) CD004721.

9. Rosen LS, Gordon D, Tchekmedyian S, Yanagihara R, Hirsh V, Krzakowski M, et al. Zoledronic acid versus placebo in the treatment of skeletal metastases in patients with lung cancer and other solid tumors: a phase III, double-blind, randomized trial—the Zoledronic Acid Lung Cancer and Other Solid Tumors Study Group. J Clin Oncol 2003;21(16):3150–7.
10. Schaberg J, Gainor BJ. A profile of metastatic carcinoma of the spine. Spine 1985;10(1):19–20.
11. Abrams HL, Spiro R, Goldstein N. Metastases in carcinoma. Analysis of 1000 autopsied cases. Cancer 1950;3:74–85.
12. Metser U, Lerman H, Blank A, Lievshitz G, Bokstein F, Even-Sapir E. Malignant involvement of the spine: assessment by 18F-FDG PET/CT. J Nucl Med 2004;45(2):279–84.
13. Vande Berg BC, Lecouvet FE, Michaux L, Ferrant A, Maldague B, Malghem J. Magnetic resonance imaging of the bone marrow in hematological malignancies. Eur Radiol 1998;8(8):1335–44.
14. Denis F. Spinal instability as defined by the three-column spine concept in acute spinal trauma. Clin Orthop 1984;(189)65–76.
15. Kostuik JP, Errico JN. Differential diagnosis and surgical treatment of metastatic spine tumors. In: Frymoyer JW, editor. New York: Raven Press; 1991. p. 861–88.
16. Khaw FM, Worthy SA, Gibson MJ, Gholkar A. The appearance on MRI of vertebrae in acute compression of the spinal cord due to metastases. J Bone Joint Surg Br 1999;81(5):830–4.
17. Bradford DS. Spinal instability: orthopedic perspective and prevention. Clin Neurosurg 1980;27:591–610.
18. White AAI, Panjabi MM. Clinical biomechanics of the spine. Philadelphia: Lippincott J. B; 1987. p. 191–276.
19. Sze WM, Shelley MD, Held I, Wilt TJ, Mason MD. Palliation of metastatic bone pain: single fraction versus multifraction radiotherapy—a systematic review of randomised trials. Clin Oncol (R Coll Radiol) 2003;15(6):345–52.
20. Saarto T, Janes R, Tenhunen M, Kouri M. Palliative radiotherapy in the treatment of skeletal metastases. Eur J Pain 2002;6(5):323–30.
21. Jeremic B. Single fraction external beam radiation therapy in the treatment of localized metastatic bone pain. A review. J Pain Symptom Manage 2001;22(6):1048–58.
22. Fleisch H. Development of bisphosphonates. Breast Cancer Res 2002;4(1):30–4.
23. Fleisch H. Bisphosphonates in osteoporosis. Eur Spine J 2003.
24. Baur A, Stabler A, Arbogast S, Duerr HR, Bartl R, Reiser M. Acute osteoporotic and neoplastic vertebral compression fractures: fluid sign at MR imaging. Radiology 2002;225(3):730–5.
25. Jung HS, Jee WH, McCauley TR, Ha KY, Choi KH. Discrimination of metastatic from acute osteoporotic compression spinal fractures with MR imaging. Radiographics 2003;23(1):179–87.
26. Kim JK, Learch TJ, Colletti PM, Lee JW, Tran SD, Terk MR. Diagnosis of vertebral metastasis, epidural metastasis, and malignant spinal cord compression: are T(1)-weighted sagittal images sufficient? Magn Reson Imaging 2000;18(7):819–24.
27. Shon IH, Fogelman I. F-18 FDG positron emission tomography and benign fractures. Clin Nucl Med 2003;28(3):171–5.
28. Peh WC, Gilula LA. Percutaneous vertebroplasty: indications, contraindications, and technique. Br J Radiol 2003;76(901):69–75.
29. Fourney DR, Schomer DF, Nader R, Chlan-Fourney J, Suki D, Ahrar K, et al. Percutaneous vertebroplasty and kyphoplasty for painful vertebral body fractures in cancer patients. J Neurosurg 2003;98(1 Suppl):21–30.
30. Appel NB, Gilula LA. Percutaneous vertebroplasty in patients with spinal canal compromise. AJR Am J Roentgenol 2004;182(4):947–51.
31. Yeom JS, Kim WJ, Choy WS, Lee CK, Chang BS, Kang JW. Leakage of cement in percutaneous transpedicular vertebroplasty for painful osteoporotic compression fractures. J Bone Joint Surg Br 2003;85(1):83–9.
32. Mousavi P, Roth S, Finkelstein J, Cheung G, Whyne C. Volumetric quantification of cement leakage following percutaneous vertebroplasty in metastatic and osteoporotic vertebrae. J Neurosurg 2003;99(1 Suppl):56–9.
33. Alvarez L, Perez-Higueras A, Quinones D, Calvo E, Rossi RE. Vertebroplasty in the treatment of vertebral tumors: postprocedural outcome and quality of life. Eur Spine J 2003;12(4):356–60.
34. Coumans JV, Reinhardt MK, Lieberman IH. Kyphoplasty for vertebral compression fractures: 1-year clinical outcomes from a prospective study. J Neurosurg 2003;99(1 Suppl):44–50.
35. Levack P, Graham J, Collie D, Grant R, Kidd J, Kunkler I, et al. Don't wait for a sensory level—listen to the symptoms: a prospective audit of the delays in diagnosis of malignant cord compression. Clin Oncol (R Coll Radiol) 2002;14(6):472–80.

36. Zaidat OO, Ruff RL. Treatment of spinal epidural metastasis improves patient survival and functional state. Neurology 2002;58(9):1360–6.
37. Loblaw DA, Laperriere NJ, Mackillop WJ. A population-based study of malignant spinal cord compression in Ontario. Clin Oncol (R Coll Radiol) 2003;15(4):211–7.
38. Helweg-Larsen S, Sorensen PS, Kreiner S. Prognostic factors in metastatic spinal cord compression: a prospective study using multivariate analysis of variables influencing survival and gait function in 153 patients. Int J Radiat Oncol Biol Phys 2000;46(5):1163–9.
39. Schiff D, O'Neill BP, Wang CH, O'Fallon JR. Neuroimaging and treatment implications of patients with multiple epidural spinal metastases. Cancer 1998;83(8):1593–16601.
40. Husband DJ, Grant KA, Romaniuk CS. MRI in the diagnosis and treatment of suspected malignant spinal cord compression. Br J Radiol 2001;74(877):15–23.
41. Cobb 3rd CA, Leavens ME, Eckles N. Indications for nonoperative treatment of spinal cord compression due to breast cancer. J Neurosurg 1977;47(5):653–8.
42. Barron KD, Hirano A, Araki S, Terry RD. Experiences with metastatic neoplasms involving the spinal cord. Neurology 1959;9(2):91–106.
43. Bach F, Larsen BH, Rohde K, Borgesen SE, Gjerris F, Boge-Rasmussen T, et al. Metastatic spinal cord compression. Occurrence, symptoms, clinical presentations and prognosis in 398 patients with spinal cord compression. Acta Neurochir 1990;107(1–2):37–43.
44. Schiff D, O'Neill BP, Suman VJ. Spinal epidural metastasis as the initial manifestation of malignancy: clinical features and diagnostic approach. Neurology 1997;49(2):452–6.
45. Posner JB. Spinal metastases In: Posner JB, editor. . Philadelphia: Davis, F. A. Company; 1995. p. 111–42.
46. Chamberlain MC, Kormanik PA. Epidural spinal cord compression: a single institution's retrospective experience. Neuro-oncol 1999;1(2):120–3.
47. Portenoy RK, Galer BS, Salamon O, Freilich M, Finkel JE, Milstein D, et al. Identification of epidural neoplasm. Radiography and bone scintigraphy in the symptomatic and asymptomatic spine. Cancer 1989;64(11):2207–13.
48. Asdourian PL, Weidenbaum M, DeWald RL, Hammerberg KW, Ramsey RG. The pattern of vertebral involvement in metastatic vertebral breast cancer. Clin Orthop 1990;(250)164–70.
49. Siegal T,. Spinal epidural metastases from solid tumors. Clinical diagnosis and management. In: Twijnstra A, Keyser A, Ongerboer de Visser BW, editors. The Netherlands: Elsevier Science Publications; 1993. p. 283–305.
50. Graus F, Krol G, FK M. Early diagnosis of spinal epidural metastases: correlation with clinical and radiological findings (abstr). Conference, 1985.
51. Byrne TN. Spinal cord compression from epidural metastases. N Engl J Med 1992; 327(9):614–9.
52. Carmody RF, Yang PJ, Seeley GW, Seeger JF, Unger EC, Johnson JE. Spinal cord compression due to metastatic disease: diagnosis with MR imaging versus myelography. Radiology 1989;173(1):225–9.
53. Colletti PM, Dang HT, Deseran MW, Kerr RM, Boswell WD, Ralls PW. Spinal MR imaging in suspected metastases: correlation with skeletal scintigraphy. Magn Reson Imaging 1991;9(3):349–55.
54. Heldmann U, Myschetzky PS, Thomsen HS. Frequency of unexpected multifocal metastasis in patients with acute spinal cord compression. Evaluation by low-field MR imaging in cancer patients. Acta Radiol 1997;38(3):372–5.
55. Colletti PM, Siegel HJ, Woo MY, Young HY, Terk MR. The impact on treatment planning of MRI of the spine in patients suspected of vertebral metastasis: an efficacy study. Comput Med Imaging Graph 1996;20(3):159–62.
56. Jordan JE, Donaldson SS, Enzmann DR. Cost effectiveness and outcome assessment of magnetic resonance imaging in diagnosing cord compression. Cancer 1995;75(10):2579–86.
57. Solberg A, Bremnes RM. Metastatic spinal cord compression: diagnostic delay, treatment, and outcome. Anticancer Res 1999;19(1B):677–84.
58. Barcena A, Lobato RD, Rivas JJ, Cordobes F, de Castro S, Cabrera A, et al. Spinal metastatic disease: analysis of factors determining functional prognosis and the choice of treatment. Neurosurgery 1984;15(6):820–7.
59. Findlay GF. Adverse effects of the management of malignant spinal cord compression. J Neurol Neurosurg Psychiatry 1984;47(8):761–8.
60. Loblaw DA, Laperriere NJ. Emergency treatment of malignant extradural spinal cord compression: an evidence-based guideline. J Clin Oncol 1998;16(4):1613–24.

61. Hainline B, Tuszynski MH, Posner JB. Ataxia in epidural spinal cord compression. Neurology 1992;42(11):2193–5.
62. Ushio Y, Posner R, Kim JH, Shapiro WR, Posner JB. Treatment of experimental spinal cord compression caused by extradural neoplasms. J Neurosurg 1977;47(3):380–90.
63. Ushio Y, Posner R, Posner JB, Shapiro WR. Experimental spinal cord compression by epidural neoplasm. Neurology 1977;27(5):422–9.
64. Ikeda H, Ushio Y, Hayakawa T, Mogami H. Edema and circulatory disturbance in the spinal cord compressed by epidural neoplasms in rabbits. J Neurosurg 1980;52(2):203–9.
65. Kato A, Ushio Y, Hayakawa T, Yamada K, Ikeda H, Mogami H. Circulatory disturbance of the spinal cord with epidural neoplasm in rats. J Neurosurg 1985;63(2):260–5.
66. Delattre JY, Arbit E, Thaler HT, Rosenblum MK, Posner JB. A dose-response study of dexamethasone in a model of spinal cord compression caused by epidural tumor. J Neurosurg 1989;70(6):920–5.
67. Siegal T, Shapira Y, Sandbank U, Catane R. Indomethacin and dexamethasone treatment in experimental neoplastic spinal cord compression: Part 1. Effect on water content and specific gravity. Neurosurgery 1988;22(2):328–33.
68. Siegal T, Shohami E, Shapira Y. Indomethacin and dexamethasone treatment in experimental neoplastic spinal cord compression: Part 2. Effect on edema and prostaglandin synthesis. Neurosurgery 1988;22(2):334–9.
69. Siegal T, Shohami E, Shapira Y. Comparison of soluble dexamethasone sodium phosphate with free dexamethasone and indomethacin in treatment of experimental neoplastic spinal cord compression. Spine 1988;13(10):1171–6.
70. Siegal T, Siegal T, Shapira Y, Shohami E. The early effect of steroidal and non-steroidal anti-inflammatory agents on neoplastic epidural cord copmpression. Ann NY Acad Sci 1989;559:488–90.
71. Siegal T, Lossos F. Experimental neoplastic spinal cord compression: effect of anti-inflammatory agents and glutamate receptor antagonists on vascular permeability. Neurosurgery 1990;26(6):967–70.
72. Siegal T, Shohami E, Lossos F. Experimental neoplastic spinal cord compression: effect of ketamine and MK-801 on edema and prostaglandins. Neurosurgery 1990;26(6):963–6.
73. Siegal T. Participation of serotonergic mechanisms in the pathophysiology of experimental neoplastic spinal cord compression. Neurology 1991;41(4):574–80.
74. Siegal T. Serotonergic manipulations in experimental neoplastic spinal cord compression. J Neurosurg 1993;78(6):929–37.
75. Siegal T. Spinal cord compression: from laboratory to clinic. Eur J Cancer 1995;31A(11): 1748–53.
76. Siegal T, Siegal TZ, Sandbank U, Shohami E, Shapira J, Gomori JM, et al. Experimental neoplastic spinal cord compression: evoked potentials, edema, prostaglandins, and light and electron microscopy. Spine 1987;12(5):440–8.
77. Ishikawa M, Sekizuka E, Krischek B, Sure U, Becker R, Bertalanffy H. Role of nitric oxide in the regulation of spinal arteriolar tone. Neurosurgery 2002;50(2):371–7; discussion 377–8.
78. Casha S, Yu WR, Fehlings MG. Oligodendroglial apoptosis occurs along degenerating axons and is associated with FAS and p75 expression following spinal cord injury in the rat. Neuroscience 2001;103(1):203–18.
79. Blight AR, Decrescito V. Morphometric analysis of experimental spinal cord injury in the cat: the relation of injury intensity to survival of myelinated axons. Neuroscience 1986;19(1):321–41.
80. Waxman SG. Demyelination in spinal cord injury. J Neurol Sci 1989;91(1–2):1–14.
81. Gledhill RF, McDonald WI. Morphological characteristics of central demyelination and remyelination: a single-fiber study. Ann Neurol 1977;1(6):552–60.
82. Siegal T, Shezen E, Siegal T. The effect of in-vivo inhibition of phagocytic activity in experimental neoplastic spinal cord compression: Immunohistochemistry, vascular permeability and neurologic function. J Neuro-Oncol 1994;21:68 (Abst P269).
83. Farooque M, Isaksson J, Olsson Y. Improved recovery after spinal cord injury in neuronal nitric oxide synthase-deficient mice but not in TNF-alpha-deficient mice. J Neurotrauma 2001;18(1):105–14.
84. Farooque M, Isaksson J, Olsson Y. White matter preservation after spinal cord injury in ICAM-1/P-selectin-deficient mice. Acta Neuropathol (Berl) 2001;102(2):132–40.
85. Sorensen S, Helweg-Larsen S, Mouridsen H, Hansen HH. Effect of high-dose dexamethasone in carcinomatous metastatic spinal cord compression treated with radiotherapy: a randomised trial. Eur J Cancer 1994;30A(1):22–7.

86. Guo Y, Young B, Palmer JL, Mun Y, Bruera E. Prognostic factors for survival in metastatic spinal cord compression: a retrospective study in a rehabilitation setting. Am J Phys Med Rehabil 2003;82(9):665–8.
87. McKinley WO, Huang ME, Tewksbury MA. Neoplastic vs. traumatic spinal cord injury: an inpatient rehabilitation comparison. Am J Phys Med Rehabil 2000;79(2):138–44.
88. Rades D, Heidenreich F, Bremer M, Karstens JH. Time of developing motor deficits before radiotherapy as a new and relevant prognostic factor in metastatic spinal cord compression: final results of a retrospective analysis. Eur Neurol 2001;45(4):266–9.
89. Eriks IE, Angenot EL, Lankhorst GJ. Epidural metastatic spinal cord compression: functional outcome and survival after inpatient rehabilitation. Spinal Cord 2004;42(4):235–9.
90. Schiff D. Spinal cord compression. Neurol Clin 2003;21(1):67–86 viii.
91. Podd TJ, Carpenter DS, Baughan CA, Percival D, Dyson P. Spinal cord compression: prognosis and implications for treatment fractionation. Clin Oncol (R Coll Radiol) 1992;4(6):341–4.
92. Tatsui H, Onomura T, Morishita S, Oketa M, Inoue T. Survival rates of patients with metastatic spinal cancer after scintigraphic detection of abnormal radioactive accumulation. Spine 1996;21(18):2143–8.
93. Bauer HC, Wedin R. Survival after surgery for spinal and extremity metastases. Prognostication in 241 patients. Acta Orthop Scand 1995;66(2):143–6.
94. Maranzano E, Latini P. Effectiveness of radiation therapy without surgery in metastatic spinal cord compression: final results from a prospective trial. Int J Radiat Oncol Biol Phys 1995;32(4):959–67.
95. Greenberg HS, Kim JH, Posner JB. Epidural spinal cord compression from metastatic tumor: results with a new treatment protocol. Ann Neurol 1980;8(4):361–6.
96. Constans JP, de Divitiis E, Donzelli R, Spaziante R, Meder JF, Haye C. Spinal metastases with neurological manifestations. Review of 600 cases. J Neurosurg 1983;59(1):111–8.
97. Sundaresan N, Galicich JH, Lane JM, Bains MS, McCormack P. Treatment of neoplastic epidural cord compression by vertebral body resection and stabilization. J Neurosurg 1985;63(5):676–84.
98. Turner S, Marosszeky B, Timms I, Boyages J. Malignant spinal cord compression: a prospective evaluation. Int J Radiat Oncol Biol Phys 1993;26(1):141–6.
99. Helweg-Larsen S. Clinical outcome in metastatic spinal cord compression. A prospective study of 153 patients. Acta Neurol Scand 1996;94(4):269–75.
100. Sundaresan N, Sachdev VP, Holland JF, Moore F, Sung M, Paciucci PA, et al. Surgical treatment of spinal cord compression from epidural metastasis. J Clin Oncol 1995;13(9):2330–5.
101. Huddart RA, Rajan B, Law M, Meyer L, Dearnaley DP. Spinal cord compression in prostate cancer: treatment outcome and prognostic factors. Radiother Oncol 1997;44(3):229–36.
102. Gilbert RW, Kim JH, Posner JB. Epidural spinal cord compression from metastatic tumor: diagnosis and treatment. Ann Neurol 1978;3(1):40–51.
103. Siegal T. Surgical decompression of anterior and posterior malignant epidural tumors compressing the spinal cord: a prospective study. Neurosurgery 1985;17(3):424–32.
104. Husband DJ. Malignant spinal cord compression: prospective study of delays in referral and treatment. Bmj 1998;317(7150):18–21.
105. Helweg-Larsen S, Sorensen PS. Symptoms and signs in metastatic spinal cord compression: a study of progression from first symptom until diagnosis in 153 patients. Eur J Cancer 1994;30A(3):396–8.
106. Rades D, Blach M, Bremer M, Wildfang I, Karstens JH, Heidenreich F. Prognostic significance of the time of developing motor deficits before radiation therapy in metastatic spinal cord compression: one-year results of a prospective trial. Int J Radiat Oncol Biol Phys 2000;48(5):1403–8.
107. Rades D, Heidenreich F, Karstens JH. Final results of a prospective study of the prognostic value of the time to develop motor deficits before irradiation in metastatic spinal cord compression. Int J Radiat Oncol Biol Phys 2002;53(4):975–9.
108. Rades D, Karstens JH, Alberti W. Role of radiotherapy in the treatment of motor dysfunction due to metastatic spinal cord compression: comparison of three different fractionation schedules. Int J Radiat Oncol Biol Phys 2002;54(4):1160–4.
109. Helweg-Larsen S, Rasmusson B, Sorensen PS. Recovery of gait after radiotherapy in paralytic patients with metastatic epidural spinal cord compression. Neurology 1990;40(8):1234–6.
110. Vecht CJ, Haaxma-Reiche H, van Putten WL, de Visser M, Vries EP, Twijnstra A. Initial bolus of conventional versus high-dose dexamethasone in metastatic spinal cord compression. Neurology 1989;39(9):1255–7.
111. Clarke PR, Saunders M. Steroid-induced remission in spinal canal reticulum cell sarcoma. Report of two cases. J Neurosurg 1975;42(3):346–8.

112. Marshall LF, Langfitt TW. Combined therapy for metastatic extradural tumors of the spine. Cancer 1977;40(5):2067–70.
113. Siegal T. Current considerations in the management of neoplastic spinal cord compression. Spine 1989;14(2):223–8.
114. Siegal T. Spinal epidural involvement in haematological tumors: clinical featuresand therapeutic options. Leuk Lymphoma 1991;5:101–10.
115. Wong ET, Portlock CS, O'Brien JP, DeAngelis LM. Chemosensitive epidural spinal cord disease in non-Hodgkins lymphoma. Neurology 1996;46(6):1543–7.
116. Cooper K, Bajorin D, Shapiro W, Krol G, Sze G, Bosl GJ. Decompression of epidural metastases from germ cell tumors with chemotherapy. J Neurooncol 1990;8(3):275–80.
117. Gale GB, O'Connor DM, Chu JY, Tantana S, Weber TR. Successful chemotherapeutic decompression of epidural malignant germ cell tumor. Med Pediatr Oncol 1986;14(2):97–9.
118. Gale J, Mead GM, Simmonds PD. Management of spinal cord and cauda equina compression secondary to epidural metastatic disease in adults with malignant germ cell tumours. Clin Oncol (R Coll Radiol) 2002;14(6):481–90.
119. Hayes FA, Thompson EI, Hvizdala E, O'Connor D, Green AA. Chemotherapy as an alternative to laminectomy and radiation in the management of epidural tumor. J Pediatr 1984;104(2):221–4.
120. Fadul CE, Lemann W, Thaler HT, Posner JB. Perforation of the gastrointestinal tract in patients receiving steroids for neurologic disease. Neurology 1988;38(3):348–52.
121. Weissman DE. Glucocorticoid treatment for brain metastases and epidural spinal cord compression: a review. J Clin Oncol 1988;6(3):543–51.
122. Weiner HL, Rezai AR, Cooper PR. Sigmoid diverticular perforation in neurosurgical patients receiving high-dose corticosteroids. Neurosurgery 1993;33(1):40–3.
123. Martenson Jr JA, Evans RG, Lie MR, Ilstrup DM, Dinapoli RP, Ebersold MJ, et al. Treatment outcome and complications in patients treated for malignant epidural spinal cord compression (SCC). J Neurooncol 1985;3(1):77–84.
124. Maranzano E, Latini P, Beneventi S, Perruci E, Panizza BM, Aristei C, et al. Radiotherapy without steroids in selected metastatic spinal cord compression patients. A phase II trial. Am J Clin Oncol 1996;19(2):179–83.
125. Obbens EA, Kim JH, Thaler H, Deck MD, Posner JB. Metronidazole as a radiation enhancer in the treatment of metastatic epidural spinal cord compression. J Neurooncol 1984;2(2):99–104.
126. Harrison KM, Muss HB, Ball MR, McWhorter M, Case D. Spinal cord compression in breast cancer. Cancer 1985;55(12):2839–44.
127. Maranzano E, Latini P, Perrucci E, Beneventi S, Lupattelli M, Corgna E. Short-course radiotherapy (8 Gy x 2) in metastatic spinal cord compression: an effective and feasible treatment. Int J Radiat Oncol Biol Phys 1997;38(5):1037–44.
128. Kovner F, Spigel S, Rider I, Otremsky I, Ron I, Shohat E, et al. Radiation therapy of metastatic spinal cord compression. Multidisciplinary team diagnosis and treatment. J Neurooncol 1999;42(1):85–92.
129. Brown PD, Stafford SL, Schild SE, Martenson JA, Schiff D. Metastatic spinal cord compression in patients with colorectal cancer. J Neurooncol 1999;44(2):175–80.
130. Regine WF, Tibbs PA, Young A, Payne R, Saris S, Kryscio RJ, et al. Metastatic spinal cord compression: a randomized trial of direct decompressive surgical resection plus radiotherapy vs. radiotherapy alone. Int J Radiat Oncol Biol Phys 2003;57(Suppl. 2):S125.
131. Maranzano E, Bellavita R, Floridi P, Celani G, Righetti E, Lupattelli M, et al. Radiation-induced myelopathy in long-term surviving metastatic spinal cord compression patients after hypofractionated radiotherapy: a clinical and magnetic resonance imaging analysis. Radiother Oncol 2001;60(3):281–8.
132. Hoskin PJ, Grover A, Bhana R. Metastatic spinal cord compression: radiotherapy outcome and dose fractionation. Radiother Oncol 2003;68(2):175–80.
133. Rades D, Karstens JH. A comparison of two different radiation schedules for metastatic spinal cord compression considering a new prognostic factor. Strahlenther Onkol 2002;178(10):556–61.
134. Harrington KD. Anterior cord decompression and spinal stabilization for patients with metastatic lesions of the spine. J Neurosurg 1984;61(1):107–17.
135. Siegal T, Tiqva P. Vertebral body resection for epidural compression by malignant tumors. Results of forty-seven consecutive operative procedures. J Bone Joint Surg Am 1985;67(3):375–82.
136. Cooper PR, Errico TJ, Martin R, Crawford B, DiBartolo T. A systematic approach to spinal reconstruction after anterior decompression for neoplastic disease of the thoracic and lumbar spine. Neurosurgery 1993;32(1):1–8.

137. Onimus M, Schraub S, Bertin D, Bosset JF, Guidet M. Surgical treatment of vertebral metastasis. Spine 1986;11(9):883–91.
138. Onimus M, Papin P, Gangloff S. Results of surgical treatment of spinal thoracic and lumbar metastases. Eur Spine J 1996;5(6):407–11.
139. Tomita K, Kawahara N, Kobayashi T, Yoshida A, Murakami H, Akamaru T. Surgical strategy for spinal metastases. Spine 2001;26(3):298–306.
140. Durr HR, Wegener B, Krodel A, Muller PE, Jansson V, Refior HJ. Multiple myeloma: surgery of the spine: retrospective analysis of 27 patients. Spine 2002;27(3):320–4; discussion 325–6.
141. Schoeggl A, Reddy M, Matula C. Neurological outcome following laminectomy in spinal metastases. Spinal Cord 2002;40(7):363–6.
142. Hirabayashi H, Ebara S, Kinoshita T, Yuzawa Y, Nakamura I, Takahashi J, et al. Clinical outcome and survival after palliative surgery for spinal metastases: palliative surgery in spinal metastases. Cancer 2003;97(2):476–84.
143. Hatrick NC, Lucas JD, Timothy AR, Smith MA. The surgical treatment of metastatic disease of the spine. Radiother Oncol 2000;56(3):335–9.
144. Wise JJ, Fischgrund JS, Herkowitz HN, Montgomery D, Kurz LT. Complication, survival rates, and risk factors of surgery for metastatic disease of the spine. Spine 1999;24(18):1943–51.
145. Walsh GL, Gokaslan ZL, McCutcheon IE, Mineo MT, Yasko AW, Swisher SG, et al. Anterior approaches to the thoracic spine in patients with cancer: indications and results. Ann Thorac Surg 1997;64(6):1611–8.
146. Sapkas G, Kyratzoulis J, Papaioannou N, Babis G, Rologis D, Tzanis S. Spinal cord decompression and stabilization in malignant lesions of the spine. Acta Orthop Scand Suppl 1997;275:97–100.
147. Gokaslan ZL, York JE, Walsh GL, McCutcheon IE, Lang FF, Putnam Jr JB, et al. Transthoracic vertebrectomy for metastatic spinal tumors. J Neurosurg 1998;89(4):599–609.
148. Fyfe IS, Henry AP, Mulholland RC. Closed vertebral biopsy. J Bone Joint Surg Br 1983; 65(2):140–3.
149. Schiff D, Shaw EG, Cascino TL. Outcome after spinal reirradiation for malignant epidural spinal cord compression. Ann Neurol 1995;37(5):583–9.
150. Grosu AL, Andratschke N, Nieder C, Molls M. Retreatment of the spinal cord with palliative radiotherapy. Int J Radiat Oncol Biol Phys 2002;52(5):1288–92.
151. Milker-Zabel S, Zabel A, Thilmann C, Schlegel W, Wannenmacher M, Debus J. Clinical results of retreatment of vertebral bone metastases by stereotactic conformal radiotherapy and intensity-modulated radiotherapy. Int J Radiat Oncol Biol Phys 2003;55(1):162–7.
152. McLain RF, Weinstein JN. Tumors of the spine. Semin Spine Surgery 1990;2:157–80.
153. Shimizu K, Shikata J, Iida H, Iwasaki R, Yoshikawa J, Yamamuro T. Posterior decompression and stabilization for multiple metastatic tumors of the spine. Spine 1992;17(11):1400–4.
154. Levy WJ, Latchaw Jr JP, Hardy RW, Hahn JP. Encouraging surgical results in walking patients with epidural metastases. Neurosurgery 1982;11(2):229–33.
155. Dunn Jr RC, Kelly WA, Wohns RN, Howe JF. Spinal epidural neoplasia. A 15-year review of the results of surgical therapy. J Neurosurg 1980;52(1):47–51.
156. DeWald RL, Bridwell KH, Prodromas C, Rodts MF. Reconstructive spinal surgery as palliation for metastatic malignancies of the spine. Spine 1985;10(1):21–6.
157. Perrin RG, McBroom RJ. Anterior versus posterior decompression for symptomatic spinal metastasis. Can J Neurol Sci 1987;14(1):75–80.
158. Heller M, McBroom RJ, MacNab T, Perfin R. Treatment of metastatic disease of the spine with posterolateral decompression and Luque instrumentation. Neuroorthopedics 1986;2:70–4.
159. Sherman RM, Waddell JP. Laminectomy for metastatic epidural spinal cord tumors. Posterior stabilization, radiotherapy, and preoperative assessment. Clin Orthop 1986;(207)55–63.
160. Slatkin NE, Posner JB. Management of spinal epidural metastases. Clin Neurosurg 1983;30:698–716.
161. McPhee IB, Williams RP, Swanson CE. Factors influencing wound healing after surgery for metastatic disease of the spine. Spine 1998;23(6):726–32 discussion 732–3.
162. Sundaresan N, Rothman A, Manhart K, Kelliher K. Surgery for solitary metastases of the spine: rationale and results of treatment. Spine 2002;27(16):1802–6.
163. Ghogawala Z, Mansfield FL, Borges LF. Spinal radiation before surgical decompression adversely affects outcomes of surgery for symptomatic metastatic spinal cord compression. Spine 2001;26(7):818–24.
164. Chow TS, McCutcheon IE. The surgical treatment of metastatic spinal tumors within the intradural extramedullary compartment. J Neurosurg 1996;85(2):225–30.

165. Perrin RG, Livingston KE, Aarabi B. Intradural extramedullary spinal metastasis. A report of 10 cases. J Neurosurg 1982;56(6):835–7.
166. Mirimanoff RO, Choi NC. Intradural spinal metastases in patients with posterior fossa brain metastases from various primary cancers. Oncology 1987;44(4):232–6.
167. Costigan DA, Winkelman MD. Intramedullary spinal cord metastasis. A clinicopathological study of 13 cases. J Neurosurg 1985;62(2):227–33.
168. Grem JL, Burgess J, Trump DL. Clinical features and natural history of intramedullary spinal cord metastasis. Cancer 1985;56(9):2305–14.
169. Dunne JW, Harper CG, Pamphlett R. Intramedullary spinal cord metastases: a clinical and pathological study of nine cases. Q J Med 1986;61(235):1003–20.
170. Schijns OE, Kurt E, Wessels P, Luijckx GJ, Beuls EA. Intramedullary spinal cord metastasis as a first manifestation of a renal cell carcinoma: report of a case and review of the literature. Clin Neurol Neurosurg 2000;102(4):249–54.
171. Gasser TG, Pospiech J, Stolke D, Schwechheimer K. Spinal intramedullary metastases. Report of two cases and review of the literature. Neurosurg Rev 2001;24(2–3):88–92.
172. Ogino M, Ueda R, Nakatsukasa M, Murase I. Successful removal of solitary intramedullary spinal cord metastasis from colon cancer. Clin Neurol Neurosurg 2002;104(2):152–6.
173. Findlay JM, Bernstein M, Vanderlinden RG, Resch L. Microsurgical resection of solitary intramedullary spinal cord metastases. Neurosurgery 1987;21(6):911–5.

15 Neoplastic Meningitis

MARC C. CHAMBERLAIN

Introduction

Neoplastic meningitis (NM) is the result of seeding of the leptomeninges by malignant cells. NM is not infrequent, and is becoming more common as cancer patients live longer.[1–5] NM results in significant morbidity, and median survival is short despite therapy. However, treatment can result in significant palliation of the CNS and is best approached by a multidisciplinary team.

Epidemiology

Neoplastic meningitis is diagnosed in 1% to 5% of patients with solid tumors (in which case it is termed carcinomatous meningitis), 5% to 15% of patients with leukemia (termed leukemic meningitis) and lymphoma (termed lymphomatous meningitis), and 1% to 2% of patients with primary brain tumors.[5] Autopsy studies show that 19% of patients with cancer and neurologic signs and symptoms have evidence of meningeal involvement.[6] Adenocarcinoma is the most frequent histology, and breast, lung, and melanoma are the most common primary sites to metastasize to the leptomeninges.[3,7,8] Although small cell lung cancer and melanoma have the highest rates of spread to the leptomeninges (11% and 20%, respectively), because of the higher incidence of breast cancer (with a 5% rate of spread), the later accounts for most cases in large series of the disorder.[1,7,9–11] Carcinomas of unknown primary constitute 1% to 7% of all cases of NM.[7]

NM usually presents in patients with widely disseminated and progressive systemic cancer (>70%) but it can present after a disease-free interval (20%) and may even be the first manifestation of cancer (5% to 10%), occasionally in the absence of other evidence of systemic disease.[7,12–14]

Pathogenesis

Cancer cells reach the meninges by various routes: (1) hematogenous spread, either through the venous plexus of Batson or by arterial dissemination; (2) direct extension from contiguous tumor deposits; (3) and through centripetal migration from systemic tumors along perineural or perivascular spaces.[15–18]

Once cancer cells have entered the subarachnoid space, cancer cells are transported by CSF flow, resulting in disseminated and multifocal neuraxis seeding of the leptomeninges. Tumor infiltration is most prominent at the base of the brain, the dorsal surface of the spinal cord, and, in particular, the cauda equina.[5,18] Hydrocephalus or impairment of CSF flow may occur at any level of the neuraxis and is due to ependymal nodules or tumor deposits obstructing CSF outflow.

Clinical Features

NM classically presents with pleomorphic clinical manifestations encompassing symptoms and signs in three domains of neurological function: (1) the cerebral hemispheres; (2) the cranial nerves; and (3) the spinal cord and roots. Signs on examination generally exceed the symptoms reported by the patient.

The most common manifestations of cerebral hemisphere dysfunction are headache and mental status changes. Other signs include confusion, cognitive impairment, seizures and hemiparesis. Diplopia is the most common symptom of cranial nerve dysfunction with cranial nerve VI being the most frequently affected, followed by cranial nerves III and IV. Trigeminal sensory or motor loss, cochlear dysfunction and optic neuropathy are also common findings. Spinal signs and symptoms include weakness (lower extremities more often than upper), dermatomal or segmental sensory loss, and pain in the neck, back, or following radicular patterns. Nuchal rigidity is only present in 15% of cases.[3,7,8,13,19]

A high index of suspicion needs to be entertained in order to make the diagnosis of NM. The finding of multifocal neuraxis disease in a patient with known malignancy is strongly suggestive of NM, but it is also common for patients with NM to present with isolated syndromes such as symptoms of raised intracranial pressure, cauda equina syndrome, or cranial neuropathy.

New neurological signs and symptoms may represent progression of NM but must be distinguished from the manifestations of parenchymal disease (30% to 40% of patients with NM will have coexistent parenchymal brain metastases), from side effects of chemotherapy or radiation used for treatment, and, rarely, from paraneoplastic syndromes. At presentation, NM must also be differentiated from chronic meningitis due to tuberculosis, fungal infection or sarcoidosis, as well as from metabolic and toxic encephalopathies in the appropriate clinical setting.[7,20]

Diagnosis

CSF EXAMINATION

The most useful laboratory test in the diagnosis of NM is the CSF examination. Abnormalities include increased opening pressure (>200 mm H_2O), increased leukocytes (>4/mm^3), elevated protein (>50 mg/dl) or decreased glucose (<60 mg/dl), which though suggestive of NM are not diagnostic. The presence of malignant cells in the CSF is diagnostic of NM, but in general, as is true for most cytological analysis, assignment to a particular tumor is not possible.[21]

In patients with positive CSF cytology (discussed later), up to 45% will be cytologically negative on initial examination.[6] The yield is increased to 80% with a second CSF examination, but little benefit is obtained from repeat lumbar punctures after the second.[7] Of note, a series by Kaplan, including lymphomatous and leukemic meningitis, observed the frequent dissociation between CSF cell count and malignant cytology (29% of cytologically-positive CSF had concurrent CSF counts of less than 4/mm^3).[3] Murray showed that CSF levels of protein, glucose, and malignant cells vary at different levels of the neuraxis, even if there is no obstruction of the CSF flow.[22,23] This finding reflects the multifocal nature of neoplastic meningitis and explains that CSF obtained from a site distant to that of the pathologically-involved meninges may yield a negative cytology.

Of the 90 patients reported by Wasserstrom, 5% had positive CSF cytology only from either the ventricles or cisterna magna.[7] In a series of 60 patients with NM, positive lumbar CSF cytology at diagnosis, and no evidence of CSF flow obstruction, ventricular and lumbar cytologies obtained simultaneously were discordant in 30% of cases.[24] The authors observed that in the presence of spinal signs or symptoms, the lumbar CSF was more likely to be positive and, conversely, in the presence of cranial signs or symptoms, the ventricular CSF was more likely to be positive. Not obtaining CSF from a site of symptomatic or radiographically demonstrated disease was found, in a prospective evaluation of 39 patients, to correlate with false-negative cytology results, as did withdrawing small CSF volumes (<10.5 ml), delaying processing of specimens, and obtaining less than two samples.[25] Even after correcting for these factors, there remains a substantial group of patients with NM who have persistently negative CSF cytology. Glass reported on a postmortem study of the value of premortem CSF cytology,[6] and demonstrated that up to 40% of patients with clinically suspected NM proven at the time of autopsy are cytologically negative. This figure increased to over 50% in patients with focal NM.

The low sensitivity of CSF cytology not only makes it difficult to diagnose NM, but also to assess the response to treatment. Biochemical markers, immunohistochemistry, and molecular biology techniques applied to CSF have been explored in an attempt to find a reliable biological marker of disease.

Numerous biochemical markers have been evaluated but, in general, their use has been limited by poor sensitivity and specificity. Particular tumor markers, such as CEA (carcinoembryogenic antigen) from adenocarcinomas, and AFP (α-fetoprotein) and β-HCG (β-human chorionic gonadotropin) from testicular cancers and primary extragonadal CNS tumors, can be relatively specific for NM when elevated in CSF in the absence of markedly elevated serum levels.[16,26] Nonspecific tumor markers such as CK-BB (creatine-kinase BB isoenzyme),

TPA (tissue polypeptide antigen, $\beta_2$microglobulin, β-glucoronidase, LDH isoenzyme-5 and more recently VEGF (vascular endothelial growth factor) can be strong indirect indicators of NM, but none are sensitive enough to improve the cytological diagnosis.[27–31] The use of these biochemical markers can be helpful as adjunctive diagnostic tests and, when followed serially, to assess response to treatment. Occasionally, in patients with clinically suspected NM and negative CSF cytology, they may support the diagnosis of NM.[32]

Use of monoclonal antibodies for immunohistochemical analysis in NM does not significantly increase the sensitivity of cytology alone.[33–35] However, in the case of leukemia and lymphoma, antibodies against surface markers can be used to distinguish between reactive and neoplastic lymphocytes in the CSF.[36]

Cytogenetic studies have also been evaluated in an attempt to improve the diagnostic accuracy of NM. Flow cytometry and DNA single cell cytometry, techniques that measure the chromosomal content of cells, and fluorescent in situ hybridization (FISH), that detects numerical and structural genetic aberrations as a sign of malignancy, can give additional diagnostic information, but still have a low sensitivity.[37–39] Polymerase-chain reaction (PCR) can establish a correct diagnosis when cytology is inconclusive, but the genetic alteration of the neoplasia must be known for it to be amplified with this technique, and this is generally not the case, particularly in solid tumors.[40]

In cases where there is no manifestation of systemic cancer and CSF examinations remain inconclusive, a meningeal biopsy may be diagnostic. The yield of this test increases if the biopsy is taken from an enhancing region on MRI (see below).[41]

NEURORADIOGRAPHIC STUDIES

Magnetic resonance imaging with gadolinium enhancement (MR-Gd) is the technique of choice to evaluate patients with suspected NM (Figures 15-1 through 15-4).[42–44] Because NM involves the entire neuraxis, imaging of the entire CNS is required in patients considered for further treatment. T1-weighted sequences, with and without contrast, combined with fat-suppression T2-weighted sequences constitute the standard examination.[42–45] MRI has been shown to have a higher sensitivity than cranial contrast-enhanced computed tomography (CE-CT) in several series, and is similar to computerized tomographic myelography (CT-M) for the evaluation of the spine, but significantly better tolerated.[42,44–46]

Any irritation of the leptomeninges (i.e., subarachnoid blood) will result in their enhancement on MRI, which is seen as a fine signal-intense layer that follows the gyri and superficial sulci. Subependymal involvement of the ventricles often results in ventricular enhancement. Some changes, such as cranial nerve enhancement on cranial imaging and intradural extramedullary enhancing nodules on spinal MR (most frequently seen in the cauda equina), can be considered diagnostic of NM in patients with cancer.[47] Lumbar puncture itself can rarely cause a meningeal reaction leading to dural-arachnoidal enhancement, so imaging should, preferably, be obtained prior to the procedure.[48] MR-Gd still has a ≥30% incidence of false-negative results, so a normal study does not exclude the diagnosis of NM. On the other hand, in cases with a typical clinical presentation, abnormal MR-Gd alone is adequate to establish the diagnosis of NM.[32,42,46,47]

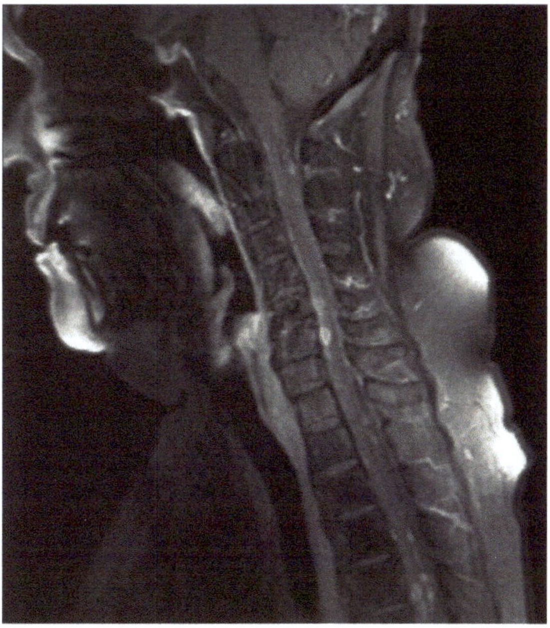

Figure 15-1 Fat-suppressed sagittal postcontrast MRI of cervical/thoracic spine demonstrating subarachnoid nodules anterior and posterior to the spinal cord in a patient with non–small cell lymphoma.

Radionuclide studies, using either ^{111}Indium-diethylenetriamine pentaacetic acid or ^{99}Tc macro-aggregated albumin, constitute the technique of choice to evaluate CSF flow dynamics.[17,49] Abnormal CSF circulation has been demonstrated in 30% to 70% of patients with NM, with blocks commonly occurring at the skull base, the spinal canal, and over the cerebral convexities.[46,49,50] Patients with interruption of CSF flow demonstrated by radionuclide ventriculography have

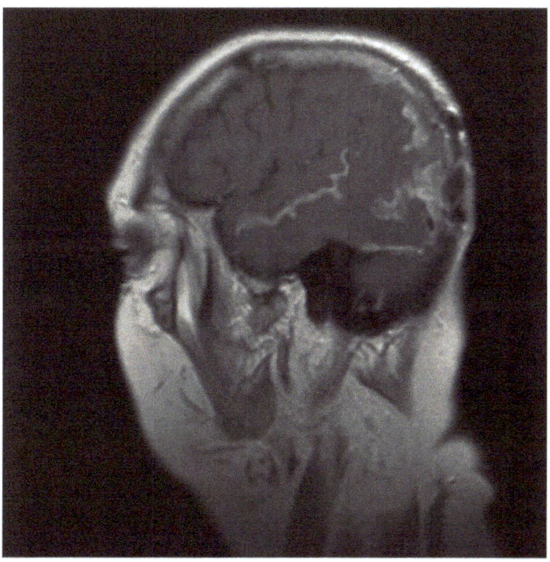

Figure 15-2 Sagittal T1-weighted postcontrast brain MRI demonstrating leptomeningeal enhancement of the Sylvian cistern and occipital lobe in a patient with non–small cell lung cancer.

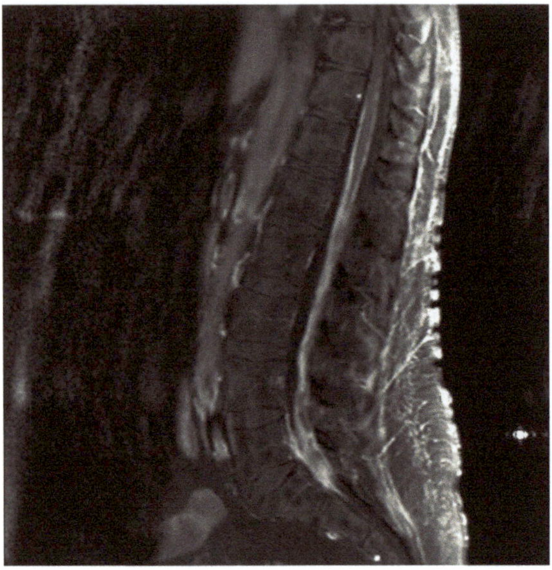

Figure 15-3 Sagittal T2-weighted lumbar spine MRI revealing nodules in the lumbar cistern in a patient with breast cancer.

been shown, in three clinical series, to have decreased survival when compared to those with normal CSF flow.[49,51,52] Involved-field radiotherapy to the site of CSF flow obstruction restores flow in 30% of patients with spinal disease and 50% of patients with intracranial disease.[53,54] Reestablishment of CSF flow with involved-field radiotherapy followed by intrathecal chemotherapy led to longer survival, lower rates of treatment-related morbidity, and a lower rate of death from progressive NM, compared to the group that had persistent CSF blocks.[49,51]

Staging

In summary, patients with suspected NM should undergo one or two lumbar punctures, cranial MR-Gd, spinal MR-Gd, and a radioisotope CSF flow study to rule out sites of CSF block. If cytology remains negative and radiological studies are not definitive, consideration may be given to ventricular or lateral cervical spine CSF analysis based on the suspected site of predominant disease. If the clinical scenario or radiological studies are highly suggestive of NM, treatment is warranted despite persistently negative CSF cytologies.

Prognosis

The median survival of untreated patients with NM is 4 to 6 weeks; death generally occurs due to progressive neurological dysfunction.[7] Treatment is intended to improve or stabilize the neurological status, maintain neurological quality of life, and prolong survival. Fixed neurological defects are rarely improved with

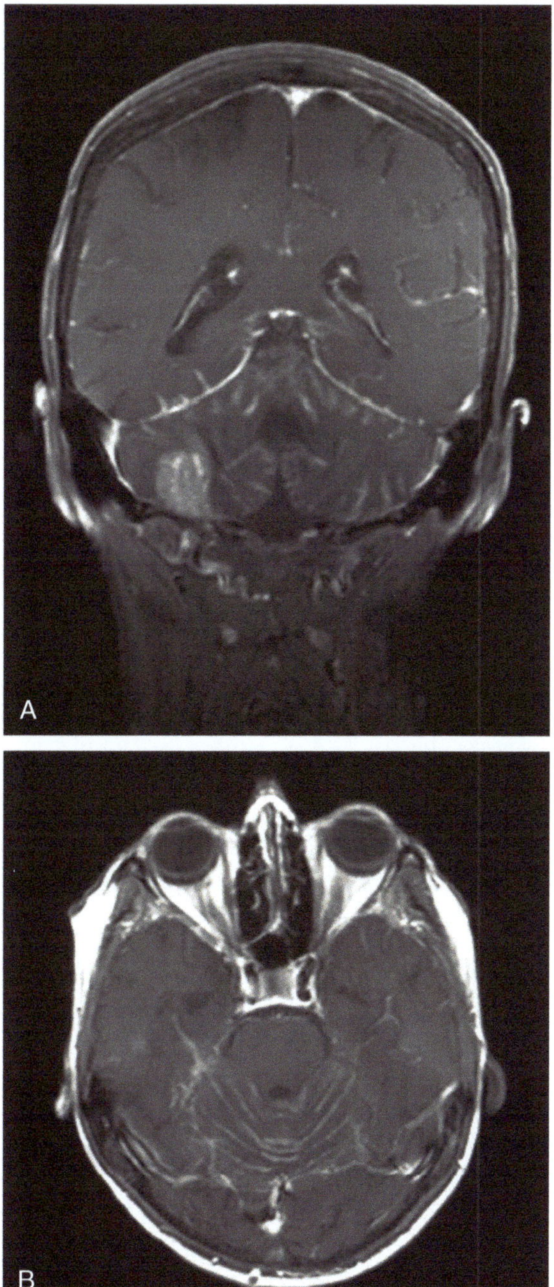

Figure 15-4 Coronal and axial T1-weighted postcontrast brain MRI demonstrating interfolial enhancement of the cerebellum and a right inferior cerebellar brain metastasis in a patient with breast cancer.

treatment, but progression of neurological deterioration may be halted in some patients and median survival can be increased to 4 to 6 months.[16] Of the solid tumors, breast cancer responds best, with median survivals of 6 months and 11% to 25% 1-year survivals.[26,55] Numerous prognostic factors for survival and response have been studied (age, gender, duration of signs of NM, increased protein or low glucose in CSF, ratio of lumbar/ventricular CEA, etc.), but many remain controversial.[55] It is commonly accepted, however, that patients will do poorly with intensive treatment of NM if they have poor performance status, multiple fixed neurologic deficits, bulky CNS disease, coexistent carcinomatous encephalopathy, and CSF flow abnormalities demonstrated by radionuclide ventriculography. In general, patients with widely metastatic aggressive cancers that do not respond well to systemic chemotherapies are also less likely to benefit from intensive therapy.[56,57] What appears clear is that, optimally, NM should be diagnosed in the early stages of disease to prevent progression of disabling neurological deficits, analogous to the clinical situation of epidural spinal cord compression.

Treatment

The evaluation of treatment of NM is complicated by the lack of standard treatments, the difficulty of determining response to treatment given the suboptimal sensitivity of the diagnostic procedures and that most patients will die of systemic disease, and the fact that most studies are small, nonrandomized, and retrospective. However, it is clear that treatment of NM can provide effective palliation and, in some cases, result in prolonged survival. Treatment in most cases requires the combination of surgery, radiation, and chemotherapy (Box 15-1). Figure 15-5 outlines a treatment algorithm for NM.

BOX 15-1 STANDARD TREATMENT MODALITIES FOR NEOPLASTIC MENINGITIS

CHEMOTHERAPY

Regional

- Methotrexate
- Cytarabine or Ara-C
- DepoCyt®
- Thio-TEPA

Systemic: High-dose intravenous:

- Methotrexate
- Cytarabine or Ara-C
- ThioTEPA

RADIOTHERAPY

Limited-field
Craniospinal

SURGERY

CSF reservoir and intra-CSF catheter
CSF diversion

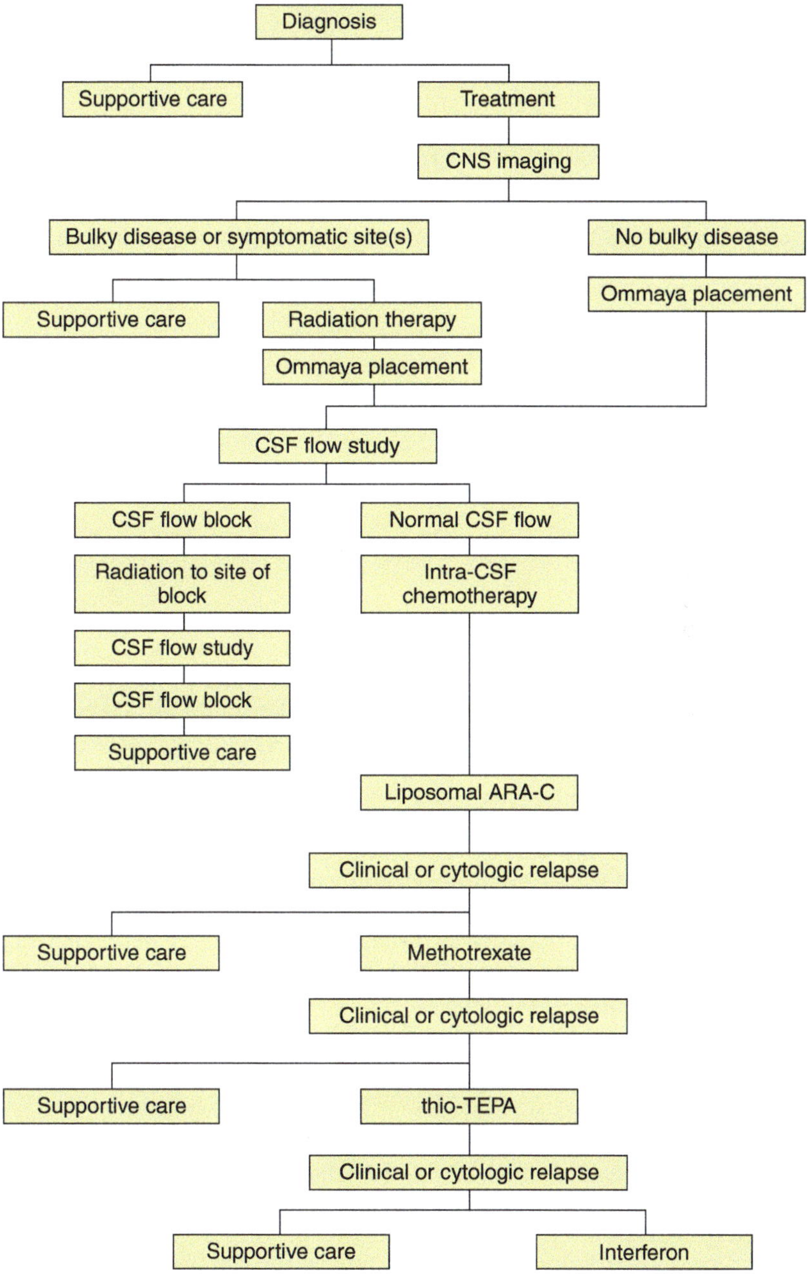

Figure 15-5 Treatment algorithm for neoplastic meningitis.

SURGERY

Surgery is used in the treatment of NM for the placement of (1) intraventricular catheter and subgaleal reservoir for administration of cytotoxic drugs and (2) ventriculoperitoneal shunt in patients with symptomatic hydrocephalus.

Drugs can be instilled into the subarachnoid space by lumbar puncture or via an intraventricular reservoir system. The latter is the preferred approach because it is simpler, more comfortable for the patient, and safer than repeated lumbar punctures. It also results in a more uniform distribution of the drug in the CSF space and produces the most consistent CSF levels. In up to 10% of lumbar punctures, the drug is delivered to the epidural space (even if there is CSF return after placement of the needle), and drug distribution has been shown to be better after drug delivery through a reservoir.[58–60]

NM often causes communicating hydrocephalus leading to symptoms of raised intracranial pressure. Relief of sites of CSF flow obstruction with involved-field radiation should be attempted to avoid the need for CSF shunting. If hydrocephalus persists, a ventriculoperitoneal shunt should be placed to relieve the pressure, as relief of pressure often results in clinical improvement.

RADIOTHERAPY

Radiotherapy is used in the treatment of NM for (1) palliation of symptoms, such as a cauda equina syndrome, (2) to decrease bulky disease such as coexistent parenchymal brain metastases, and (3) to correct CSF flow abnormalities demonstrated by radionuclide ventriculography. Patients may have significant symptoms without radiographic evidence of bulky disease and still benefit from radiation. For example, patients with low back pain and leg weakness should be considered for radiation to the cauda equina, and those with cranial neuropathies should be offered whole-brain or base-of-skull radiotherapy.[26]

Radiotherapy of bulky disease is indicated as intra-CSF chemotherapy is limited by diffusion to 2 to 3 mm penetration into tumor nodules. In addition, involved-field radiation can correct CSF flow abnormalities, and this has been shown to improve patient outcome as discussed above. Whole neuraxis radiation is rarely indicated in the treatment of NM from solid tumors because it is associated with significant systemic toxicity (severe myelosuppression and mucositis among other complications) and is not curative.

CHEMOTHERAPY

Chemotherapy is the only treatment modality that can treat the entire neuraxis, and may be administered systemically or intrathecally.

Intrathecal chemotherapy is the mainstay of treatment for NM (Table 15-1). Retrospective analysis or comparison to historical series suggest that the administration of chemotherapy to the CSF improves the outcome of patients with NM.[1,20,51,61,62] However, it is noted that most series will exclude patients that are too sick to receive any treatment, which may be up to one third of patients with NM.[63] Three agents are routinely used: methotrexate, cytarabine (including liposomal cytarabine or DepoCyt®), and thioTEPA. No difference in response has been seen when comparing single agent methotrexate with thioTEPA or when

TABLE 15-1 Regional Chemotherapy for Neoplastic Meningitis

Drugs	*Induction Regimens*		*Consolidation Regimen*		*Maintenance regimen*	
	Bolus Regimen	**CxT Regimen**	**Bolus Regimen**	**CxT Regimen**	**Bolus Regimen**	**CxT Regimen**
Methotrexate[65,66,67,84,85]	10–15 mg twice weekly (total 4 weeks)	2 mg/day for 5 days every other week (total 8 weeks)	10–15 mg once weekly (total 4 weeks)	2 mg/day for 5 days every other week (total 4 weeks)	10–15 mg once a month	2 mg/day for 5 days once a month
Cytarabine[68,84]	25–100 mg 2 times weekly (total 4 weeks)	25 mg/day for 3 days weekly (total 4 weeks)	25–100 mg once weekly (total 4 weeks)	25 mg/day for 3 days every other week (total 4 weeks)	25–100 mg once a month	25 mg/day for 3 days once a month
DepoCyt®[67,68,84]	50 mg every 2 weeks (total 8 weeks)		50 mg every 4 weeks (total 24 weeks)			
Thiotepa[66]	10 mg 2 times weekly (total 4 weeks)	10 mg/day for 3 days weekly (total 4 weeks)	10 mg once weekly (total 4 weeks)	10 mg/day for 3 days every other week (total 4 weeks)	10 mg once a month	10 mg/day for 3 days once a month
α-Interferon[83]	$1{\times}10^6$ U 2 times weekly (total 4 weeks)		$1{\times}10^6$ U 3 times weekly every other week (total 4 weeks)		$1{\times}10^6$ U 3 times weekly 1 week per month)	
Etoposide[82]		0.5 mg/day for 5 days every other week (total 8 weeks)		0.5 mg/day for 5 days every other week (total 4 weeks)		0.5 mg/day for 5 days once a month
Topotecan[76]	0.4 mg 2 times weekly (total 4 weeks)		0.4 mg 2 times weekly every other week (total 4 weeks)		0.4 mg 2 times weekly once a month	
Rituximab[81]	25 mg 2 times weekly (total 4 weeks)		25 mg 2 times weekly every other week (total 4 weeks)		25 mg 2 times weekly once a month	

using multiple agent (methotrexate, thioTEPA and cytarabine, or methotrexate and cytarabine) versus single agent methotrexate treatment.[64–66] Table 15-2 outlines the randomized clinical trials conducted for NM while Table 15-1 is an outline of the common treatment regimens for intra-CSF chemotherapy. A sustained-release form of cytarabine (DepoCyt®) results in cytotoxic cytarabine levels in the CSF for greater than or equal to 10 days, and when given bimonthly and compared to biweekly methotrexate, resulted in longer time to neurological progression in patients with NM.[67,68] Furthermore, quality of life and cause of death favored DepoCyt® over methotrexate. These findings were confirmed in a study of lymphomatous meningitis and in an open label study, suggesting that DepoCyt® should be considered the drug of first choice in the treatment of NM.[68,69]

Complications of intrathecal chemotherapy include those related to the ventricular reservoir and those related to the chemotherapy administered (Box 15-2). The most frequent complications of ventricular reservoir placement are malposition (rates reported 3% to 12%), obstruction, and infection (usually skin flora). CSF infection occurs in 2% to 13% of patients receiving intrathecal chemotherapy. It commonly presents with headache, changes in neurologic status, fever, and malfunction of the reservoir. CSF pleocytosis is commonly encountered. The most frequently isolated organism is *Staphylococcus epidermidis*. Treatment requires intravenous antibiotics, with or without oral and intraventricular antibiotics. Some authors advocate the routine removal of the ventricular reservoir, whilst others reserve device removal for those that do not clear with antibiotic therapy.

Myelosuppression may occur after administration of intrathecal chemotherapies, and some recommend that folinic acid rescue (10 mg every 6 hours for 24 hours) be given orally after the administration of methotrexate to mitigate this complication. Chemical aseptic meningitis occurs in nearly half of patients treated by intrathecal administration and is manifested by fever, headache, nausea, vomiting, meningismus, and photophobia. In the majority of patients, this inflammatory reaction can be treated in the outpatient setting with oral antipyretics, antiemetics, and corticosteroids. Rarely, treatment-related neurotoxicity occurs and may result in a symptomatic subacute leukoencephalopathy or myelopathy. However, in patients with NM and prolonged survival, the combination of radiotherapy and chemotherapy frequently results in a late leukoencephalopathy evident on neuroradiographic studies, which is occasionally symptomatic.[1,5,70–72]

The rationale to give intrathecal chemotherapy is based on the presumption that most chemotherapeutic agents, when given systemically, have poor CSF penetration and do not reach therapeutic levels. Exceptions to this would be systemic high-dose methotrexate, cytarabine, and thioTEPA, all of which result in cytotoxic CSF levels. Their systemic administration, however, is limited by systemic toxicity and the difficulty to integrate these regimens into other chemotherapeutic programs being used to manage systemic disease. Some authors argue that intrathecal chemotherapy does not add to improved outcome in the treatment of NM, since systemic therapy can obtain access to the subarachnoid deposits through their own vascular supply.[63] In a retrospective comparison of patients treated with systemic chemotherapy and radiation to involved areas, plus or minus intrathecal chemotherapy, Bokstein did not find significant differences in response rates, median survival, or proportion of long-term survivors between the two groups

TABLE 15-2 Randomized Clinical Trials

Study	Design	Response	Toxicity
Shapiro[84]	Solid tumors (n=103) DepoCyt vs. MTX Lymphoma (n=25) DepoCyt vs. Ara-C	DepoCyt vs. MTX/Ara-C: PFS*: 35 vs. 43 d DepoCyt vs. MTX: PFS: 35 vs. 37.5 DepoCyt vs. Ara-C: CR*: 33.3% vs. 16.7% PFS: 34 vs. 50 d	DepoCyt vs. MTX/Ara-C: Drug-related AEs: 48% vs. 60% Serious AEs: 86% vs. 77%
Boogerd[85]	N=35 Breast cancer IT vs. no IT †	IT vs. no IT: Improvement or stabilization: 59% vs. 67% TTP: 23 vs. 24 wk Median survival: 18.3 vs. 30.3 wk	IT vs. no IT: Neurological complications: 47% vs. 6%
Glantz[68]	N=28 Lymphoma DepoCyt vs. Ara-C	DepoCyt vs. Ara-C: TTP*: 78.5 vs. 42 d OS*: 99.5 vs. 63 d RR: 71% vs. 15%	DepoCyt vs. Ara-C: Headache: 27% vs. 2%; nausea: 9% vs. 2%; fever: 8% vs. 4%; pain: 5% vs. 4%; confusion: 7% vs. 0%; somnolence: 8% vs. 4%
Glantz[67]	N=61 Solid tumors DepoCyt vs. MTX	DepoCyt vs. MTX: RR* 26% vs. 20% OS* 105 vs. 78 d TTP 58 vs. 30 d	DepoCyt vs. MTX: Sensory/motor: 4% vs. 10%; altered mental status: 5% vs. 2%; headache: 4% vs. 2%
Grossman[66]	N=59 Solid tumors and lymphoma (in 90%) IT MTX vs. thiotepa	IT MTX vs. thiotepa: Neurological improvements: none Median survival: 15.9 vs. 14.1 wk	IT MTX vs. thiotepa: Serious toxicities similar between groups Mucositis and neurological complications more common in MTX group
Hitchins[65]	N=44 Solid tumors and lymphomas IT MTX vs. MTX + Ara-C	IT MTX vs. MTX + Ara-C: RR*: 61% vs. 45% Median survival*: 12 vs. 7 wk	IT MTX vs. MTX + Ara-C: N/V: 36% vs. 50%; septicemia, neutropenia: 9% vs. 15%; mucositis: 14% vs. 10%; pancytopenia: 9% vs. 10%. AEs related to reservoir: blocked Ommaya: 17% vs. 0%; intracranial hemorrhage: 11% vs. 0%

*No significant differences between groups.
†Appropriate systemic chemotherapy and/or radiotherapy given in both arms.
AEs = adverse events; CR = complete response; MTX = methotrexate; N/V = nausea/vomiting; OS = overall survival; PFS = progression-free survival; RR = response rate; TTP = time to progression

BOX 15-2 COMMON COMPLICATIONS OF INTRAVENTRICULAR CHEMOTHERAPY[86]

1. Related to the Ventricular Reservoir
   Catheter Malposition
   Catheter Obstruction
   Bacterial Infection (*Staphylococcus epidermidis*)
2. Related to Chemotherapy
   Systemic Toxicity:
   Myelosuppression
   Regional Toxicity:
   Aseptic Chemical Meningitis
   Direct Neurotoxicity
   Late Leukoencephalopathy

but, of course, the group that did not receive the intrathecal treatment was spared the complications of this modality.[73] Glantz treated 16 patients with high-dose intravenous methotrexate and compared their outcome with a reference group of 15 patients treated with intrathecal methotrexate.[74] They found response rates and survival were significantly better in the group treated with intravenous therapy. Finally, a recent report describes two patients with breast cancer in whom NM was controlled with systemic hormonal treatment.[75]

Nonetheless, intrathecal chemotherapy remains the preferred treatment route for NM at this time. New drugs are being explored to try to improve the efficacy of treatment. These include mafosphamide, diaziquone, topotecan, interferon-α, and temozolomide. Immunotherapy, using IL-2 and IFN-α, ^{131}I-radiolabelled monoclonal antibodies, gene therapy, and retuximab are other modalities that are being explored in clinical trials.[76–81]

SUPPORTIVE CARE

Not all patients with NM are candidates for the aggressive treatment outlined above (Box 15-3). Most authors agree that combined-modality therapy should be offered to patients with life expectancy greater than 3 months and a Karnofsky performance status of greater than 60%.

Supportive care should be offered to every patient, regardless of whether they receive NM-directed therapy. These therapies include anticonvulsants for

BOX 15-3 PROGNOSTIC FACTORS IN NEOPLASTIC MENINGITIS[17,20,42,47,49–52,56,57]

- Performance status (function of neurologic disability)
- Tumor histology
- Status of systemic disease
- CSF compartmentalization
- Coexistent bulky metastatic CNS disease
- Presence of carcinomatous encephalopathy

seizure control (seen in 10% to 15% of patients with NM), adequate analgesia with opioid drugs as needed, as well as antidepressants and anxiolytics if necessary. Corticosteroids have a limited use in NM-related neurological symptoms, but can be useful to treat vasogenic edema associated with intraparenchymal or epidural metastases, or for the symptomatic treatment of nausea and vomiting together with routine antiemetics. Decreased attention and somnolence secondary to whole brain radiation can be treated with psychostimulants.[5]

Conclusions

NM is a complicated disease, for a variety of reasons. First, most reports concerning NM treat all subtypes as equivalent with respect to CNS staging, treatment, and outcome. However, clinical trials in oncology are based on specific tumor histology. Comparing responses in patients with carcinomatous meningitis due to breast cancer to patients with non-small cell lung cancer outside of investigational new drug trials may be misleading. A general consensus is that breast cancer is inherently more chemosensitive than non–small cell lung cancer or melanoma and therefore, survival following chemotherapy is likely to be different. This observation has been substantiated in patients with systemic metastases, although comparable data regarding CNS metastases, and in particular NM, is meager.

A second feature of NM, which complicates therapy, is deciding whom to treat (Box 15-3). Not all patients necessarily warrant aggressive CNS-directed therapy, however, few guidelines exist directing appropriate choice of therapy. Based on the prognostic variables determined clinically and by evaluation of extent of disease, a sizable minority of patients will not be candidates for aggressive NM-directed therapy. Therefore, supportive comfort care (radiotherapy to symptomatic disease, antiemetics, and narcotics) is reasonably offered to patients with NM considered poor candidates for aggressive therapy, as seen in Figure 15-1.

Third, optimal treatment of NM remains poorly defined. Given these constraints, the treatment of NM today is palliative and rarely curative, with a median patient survival of 2 to 3 months, based on data of the four prospective randomized trials in this disease. However, palliative therapy of NM often affords the patient protection from further neurological deterioration and consequently an improved neurologic quality of life. No studies to date have attempted an economic assessment of the treatment of NM and therefore no information is available regarding a cost-benefit analysis, as has been performed for other cancer-directed therapies.

Finally, in patients with NM, the response to treatment is primarily a function of CSF cytology and, secondarily, of clinical improvement of neurologic signs and symptoms. Aside from CSF cytology and perhaps biochemical markers, no other CSF parameters predict response. Furthermore, because CSF cytology may manifest a rostral-caudal disassociation, consecutive negative cytologies (defined as a complete response to treatment) require confirmation by both ventricular and lumbar CSF cytologies. In general, only pain-related neurologic symptoms improve significantly with treatment. Neurologic signs such as confusion, cranial nerve deficit(s), ataxia, and segmental weakness show only minimal improvement or stabilize with successful treatment.

REFERENCES

1. Shapiro WR, Posner JB, Ushio Y, et al. Treatment of meningeal neoplasms. Cancer Treat Rep 1977;61:733–43.
2. Nugent JL, Bunn Jr PA, Matthews MJ, et al. CNS metastases in small cell bronchogenic carcinoma: increasing frequency and changing pattern with lengthening survival. Cancer 1979;44:1885–93.
3. Kaplan JG, DeSouza TG, Farkash A, et al. Leptomeningeal metastases: comparison of clinical features and laboratory data of solid tumors, lymphomas and leukemia's. J Neuro Oncol 1990;9:225–9.
4. Siegal T, Lossos A, Pfeffer MR. Leptomeningeal metastases: analysis of 31 patients with sustained off- therapy response following combined-modality therapy. Neurology 1994;44:1463–9.
5. Chamberlain MC. Carcinomatous meningitis. Arch Neurol 1997;54(1):16–7.
6. Glass JP, Melamed M, Chernik NL, et al. Malignant cells in cerebrospinal fluid (CSF): the meaning of a positive CSF cytology. Neurology 1979;29(10):1369–75.
7. Wasserstrom WR, Glass JP, Posner JB. Diagnosis and treatment of leptomeningeal metastases from solid tumors: experience with 90 patients. Cancer 1982;49(4):759–72.
8. Little JR, Dale AJ, Okazaki H. Meningeal carcinomatosis. Clinical manifestations. Arch Neurol 1974;30(2):138–43.
9. Rosen ST, Aisner J, Makuch RW, et al. Carcinomatous leptomeningitis in small cell lung cancer: a clinicopathologic review of the National Cancer Institute experience. Medicine (Baltimore) 1982;61(1):45–53.
10. Amer MH, Al Sarraf M, Baker LH, et al. Malignant melanoma and central nervous system metastases: incidence, diagnosis, treatment and survival. Cancer 1978;42(2):660–8.
11. Yap HY, Yap BS, Tashima CK, et al. Meningeal carcinomatosis in breast cancer. Cancer 1978;42(1):283–6.
12. van Oostenbrugge RJ, Twijnstra A. Presenting features and value of diagnostic procedures in leptomeningeal metastases. Neurology 1999;53(2):382–5.
13. Balm M, Hammack J. Leptomeningeal carcinomatosis. Presenting features and prognostic factors. Arch Neurol 1996;53(7):626–32.
14. Sorensen SC, Eagan RT, Scott M. Meningeal carcinomatosis in patients with primary breast or lung cancer. Mayo Clin Proc 1984;59(2):91–4.
15. Gonzalez-Vitale JC, Garcia-Bunuel R. Meningeal carcinomatosis. Cancer 1976;37(6):2906–11.
16. Grossman SA, Krabak MJ. Leptomeningeal carcinomatosis. Cancer Treat Rev 1999;25(2):103–19.
17. Chamberlain MC. Radioisotope CSF flow studies in leptomeningeal metastases. J Neuro Oncol 1998;38(2–3):135–40.
18. Boyle R, Thomas M, Adams JH. Diffuse involvement of the leptomeninges by tumour—a clinical and pathological study of 63 cases. Postgrad Med J 1980;56(653):149–58.
19. Wolfgang G, Marcus D, Ulrike S. Leptomeningeal Carcinomatosis; Clinical syndrome in different primaries. J Neuro Oncol 1998;38:103–10.
20. Chamberlain MC, Kormanik PR. Carcinomatous meningitis secondary to breast cancer: predictors of response to combined modality therapy. J Neuro Oncol 1997;35(1):55–64.
21. Kolmel HW. Cytology of neoplastic meningosis. J Neuro Oncol 1998;38(2–3):121–5.
22. Murray JJ, Greco FA, Wolff SN, et al. Neoplastic meningitis. Marked variations of cerebrospinal fluid composition in the absence of extradural block. Am J Med. 1983;75(2):289–94.
23. Rogers LR, Duchesneau PM, Nunez C, et al. Comparison of cisternal and lumbar CSF examination in leptomeningeal metastasis. Neurology 1992;42(6):1239–41.
24. Chamberlain MC, Kormanik PA, Glantz MJ. A comparison between ventricular and lumbar cerebrospinal fluid cytology in adult patients with leptomeningeal metastases. Neuro-Oncol 2001;3(1):42–5.
25. Glantz MJ, Cole BF, Glantz LK, et al. Cerebrospinal fluid cytology in patients with cancer: minimizing false-negative results. Cancer 1998;82(4):733–9.
26. DeAngelis LM. Current diagnosis and treatment of leptomeningeal metastasis. J Neuro Oncol 1998;38(2–3):245–52.
27. Wasserstrom WR, Schwartz MK, Fleisher M, et al. Cerebrospinal fluid biochemical markers in central nervous system tumors: a review. Ann Clin Lab Sci 1981;11(3):239–51.
28. Van Zanten AP, Twijnstra A, Hart AA, et al. Cerebrospinal fluid lactate dehydrogenase activities in patients with central nervous system metastases. Clin Chim Acta 1986;161(3):259–68.
29. Klee GG, Tallman RD, Goellner JR, et al. Elevation of carcinoembryonic antigen in cerebrospinal fluid among patients with meningeal carcinomatosis. Mayo Clin Proc 1986;61(1):9–13.

30. Twijnstra A, van Zanten AP, Hart AA, et al. Serial lumbar and ventricle cerebrospinal fluid lactate dehydrogenase activities in patients with leptomeningeal metastases from solid and haematological tumours. J Neurol Neurosurg Psychiatry 1987;50(3):313–20.
31. Stockhammer G, Poewe W, Burgstaller S, et al. Vascular endothelial growth factor in CSF: a biological marker for carcinomatous meningitis. Neurology 2000;54(8):1670–6.
32. Chamberlain MC. Cytologically negative carcinomatous meningitis: usefulness of CSF biochemical markers. Neurology 1998;50(4):1173–5.
33. Garson JA, Coakham HB, Kemshead JT, et al. The role of monoclonal antibodies in brain tumour diagnosis and cerebrospinal fluid (CSF) cytology. J Neuro Oncol 1985;3(2):165–71.
34. Hovestadt A, Henzen-Logmans SC, Vecht CJ. Immunohistochemical analysis of the cerebrospinal fluid for carcinomatous and lymphomatous leptomeningitis. Br J Cancer 1990;62(4):653–4.
35. Boogerd W, Vroom TM, van Heerde P, et al. CSF cytology versus immunocytochemistry in meningeal carcinomatosis. J Neurol Neurosurg Psychiatry 1988;51(1):142–5.
36. Van Oostenbrugge RJ, Hopman AH, Ramaekers FC, et al. In situ hybridization: a possible diagnostic aid in leptomeningeal metastasis. J Neuro Oncol 1998;38(2–3):127–33.
37. Cibas ES, Malkin MG, Posner JB, et al. Detection of DNA abnormalities by flow cytometry in cells from cerebrospinal fluid. Am J Clin Pathol 1987;88(5):570–7.
38. Biesterfeld S, Bernhard B, Bamborschke S, et al. DNA single cell cytometry in lymphocytic pleocytosis of the cerebrospinal fluid. Acta Neuropathol (Berl) 1993;86(5):428–32.
39. Van Oostenbrugge RJ, Hopman AH, Arends JW, et al. The value of interphase cytogenetics in cytology for the diagnosis of leptomeningeal metastases. Neurology 1998;51(3):906–8.
40. Rhodes CH, Glantz MJ, Glantz L, et al. A comparison of polymerase chain reaction examination of cerebrospinal fluid and conventional cytology in the diagnosis of lymphomatous meningitis. Cancer 1996;77(3):543–8.
41. Cheng TM, O'Neill BP, Scheithauer BW, et al. Chronic meningitis: the role of meningeal or cortical biopsy. Neurosurgery 1994;34(4):590–5.
42. Chamberlain MC, Sandy AD, Press GA. Leptomeningeal metastasis: a comparison of gadolinium-enhanced MR and contrast-enhanced CT of the brain. Neurology 1990;40(3 Pt 1):435–8.
43. Schumacher M, Orszagh M. Imaging techniques in neoplastic meningiosis. J Neuro Oncol 1998;38(2–3):111–20.
44. Sze G, Soletsky S, Bronen R, et al. MR imaging of the cranial meninges with emphasis on contrast enhancement and meningeal carcinomatosis. AJR Am J Roentgenol 1989;153(5):1039–49.
45. Schuknecht B, Huber P, Buller B, et al. Spinal leptomeningeal neoplastic disease. Evaluation by MR, myelography and CT myelography. Eur Neurol. 1992;32(1):11–6.
46. Chamberlain MC. Comparative spine imaging in leptomeningeal metastases. J Neuro Oncol 1995;23(3):233–8.
47. Freilich RJ, Krol G, DeAngelis LM. Neuroimaging and cerebrospinal fluid cytology in the diagnosis of leptomeningeal metastasis. Ann Neurol 1995;38(1):51–7.
48. Mittl Jr RL, Yousem DM. Frequency of unexplained meningeal enhancement in the brain after lumbar puncture. AJNR Am J Neuroradiol 1994;15(4):633–8.
49. Glantz MJ, Hall WA, Cole BF, et al. Diagnosis, management, and survival of patients with leptomeningeal cancer based on cerebrospinal fluid-flow status. Cancer 1995;75(12):2919–31.
50. Grossman SA, Trump CL, Chen DCP, Thompson G, Camargo E. Cerebrospinal flow abnormalities in patients with neoplastic meningitis. Am J Med 1982;73:641–7.
51. Chamberlain MC, Kormanik PA. Prognostic significance of 111indium-DTPA CSF flow studies in leptomeningeal metastases. Neurology 1996;46(6):1674–7.
52. Mason WP, Yeh SD, DeAngelis LM. 111Indium-diethylenetriamine pentaacetic acid cerebrospinal fluid flow studies predict distribution of intrathecally administered chemotherapy and outcome in patients with leptomeningeal metastases. Neurology 1998;50(2):438–44.
53. Chamberlain MC, Corey-Bloom J. Leptomeningeal metastases: 111indium-DTPA CSF flow studies. Neurology 1991;41(11):1765–9.
54. Chamberlain MC, Kormanik P, Jaeckle KA, et al. 111Indium-diethylenetriamine pentaacetic acid CSF flow studies predict distribution of intrathecally administered chemotherapy and outcome in patients with leptomeningeal metastases. Neurology 1999;52(1):216–7.
55. Hildebrand J. Prophylaxis and treatment of leptomeningeal carcinomatosis in solid tumors of adulthood. J Neuro Oncol 1998;38(2–3):193–8.
56. Chamberlain MC, Kormanik PA. Prognostic significance of coexistent bulky metastatic central nervous system disease in patients with leptomeningeal metastases. Arch Neurol 1997;54(11):1364–8.

57. Chamberlain MC. Neoplastic meningitis-related encephalopathy: prognostic significance. Neurology 2003;60(5):A17–8.
58. Shapiro WR, Young DF, Mehta BM. Methotrexate: distribution in cerebrospinal fluid after intravenous, ventricular and lumbar injections. N Engl J Med 1975;293(4):161–6.
59. Berweiler U, Krone A, Tonn JC. Reservoir systems for intraventricular chemotherapy. J Neuro Oncol 1998;38(2–3):141–3.
60. Sandberg DI, Bilsky MH, Souweidane MM, et al. Ommaya reservoirs for the treatment of leptomeningeal metastases. Neurosurgery 2000;47(1):49–54.
61. Sause WT, Crowley J, Eyre HJ, et al. Whole brain irradiation and intrathecal methotrexate in the treatment of solid tumor leptomeningeal metastases--a Southwest Oncology Group study. J Neuro Oncol 1988;6(2):107–12.
62. Chamberlain MC, Kormanik P. Carcinoma meningitis secondary to non-small cell lung cancer: combined modality therapy. Arch Neurol 1998;55(4):506–12.
63. Siegal T. Leptomeningeal metastases: rationale for systemic chemotherapy or what is the role of intra-CSF-chemotherapy?. J Neuro Oncol 1998;38(2–3):151–7.
64. Giannone L, Greco FA, Hainsworth JD. Combination intraventricular chemotherapy for meningeal neoplasia. J Clin Oncol 1986;4(1):68–73.
65. Hitchins RN, Bell DR, Woods RL, et al. A prospective randomized trial of single-agent versus combination chemotherapy in meningeal carcinomatosis. J Clin Oncol 1987;5(10):1655–62.
66. Grossman SA, Finkelstein DM, Ruckdeschel JC, et al. Randomized prospective comparison of intraventricular methotrexate and thiotepa in patients with previously untreated neoplastic meningitis. J Clin Oncol 1993;11:561–9.
67. Glantz MJ, Jaeckle KA, Chamberlain MC, et al. A randomized controlled trial comparing intrathecal sustained-release cytarabine (DepoCyt) to intrathecal methotrexate in patients with neoplastic meningitis from solid tumors. Clin Cancer Res 1999;5(11):3394–402.
68. Glantz MJ, LaFollette S, Jaeckle KA, Shapiro W, Swinnen L, Rozental JR, et al. Randomized Trial of a Slow Release Versus a Standard Formulation of Cytarabine for the Intrathecal Treatment of Lymphomatous Meningitis. J Clin Oncol 1999;17:3110–6.
69. Jaeckle KA, Batchelor T, O'Day SJ, Phuphanich S, New P, Lesser G, et al. An open trial of sustained-release cytarabine (Depocyt) for the intrathecal treatment of solid tumor neoplastic meningitis. J Neuro Oncol 2002;57(3):231–9.
70. Siegal T, Pfeffer MR, Steiner I. Antibiotic therapy for infected Ommaya reservoir systems. Neurosurgery 1988;22(1 Pt 1):97–100.
71. Kerr JZ, Berg S, Blaney SM. Intrathecal chemotherapy. Crypt Rev Oncol Hematol 2001;37(3):227–36.
72. Bleyer WA, Drake JC, Chabner BA. Neurotoxicity and elevated cerebrospinal-fluid methotrexate concentration in meningeal leukemia. N Engl J Med 1973;289(15):770–773.
73. Bokstein F, Lossos A, Siegal T. Leptomeningeal metastases from solid tumors: a comparison of two prospective series treated with and without intra-cerebrospinal fluid chemotherapy. Cancer 1998;82(9):1756–63.
74. Glantz MJ, Cole BF, Recht L, et al. High-Dose Intravenous Methotrexate for Patients with Nonelukemic Leptomeningeal Cancer: Is Intrathecal Chemotherapy Necessary? J Clin Oncol 1998;16(4):1561–7.
75. Boogerd W, Dorresteijn LDA, van der Sande JJ, et al. Response of leptomeningeal metastases from breast cancer to hormonal therapy. Neurology 2000;55(1):117–9.
76. Blaney SM, Poplack DG. New cytotoxic drugs for intrathecal administration. J Neuro Oncol 1998;38:219–23.
77. Sampson JH, Archer GE, Villavicencio AT, et al. Treatment of Neoplastic Meningitis with Intrathecal Temozolomide. Clin Cancer Res 1999;5:1183–8.
78. Herrlinger U, Weller M, Schabet M. New aspects of immunotherapy of leptomeningeal metastasis. J Neuro Oncol 1998;38:233–9.
79. Coakham HB, Kemshead JT. Treatment of neoplastic meningitis by targeted radiation using ^{131}I-radiolabelled monoclonal antibodies. J Neuro Oncol 1998;38:225–32.
80. Vrionis FD. Gene Therapy of Neoplastic Meningiosis. J Neuro Oncol 1998;38:241–4.
81. Rubenstein JI, Fridlyand J, Abrey L, et al. Phase 1 study of intraventricular administration of rituximab in patients with recurrent CNS and intraocular lymphoma. J Clin Oncol 2007;25(11):1350–6.
82. Chamberlain MC, Wei-Tao DD, Groshen S. A Phase 2 trial of intra-CSF etoposide in the treatment of neoplastic meningitis. Cancer 2006;31(9):2021–7.

83. Chamberlain MC. Alpha-Interferon in the Treatment of Neoplastic Meningitis. Cancer 2002;94:2675–80.
84. Shapiro WR, Schmid M, Glantz M, Miller JJ. A randomized phase III/IV study to determine benefit and safety of cytarabine liposome injection for treatment of neoplastic meningitis. J Clin Oncol 2006;24(June 6 Suppl):1528 (abstract).
85. Boogerd W, van den Bent MJ, Koehler PJ, Heimans JJ, Van der Sande JJ, et al. The relevance of intraventricular chemotherapy for leptomeningeal metastasis in breast cancer: a randomized study. Eur J Cancer 2004;40:2726–33.
86. Chamberlain MC, Kormanik PA, Barba D. Complications associated with intraventricular chemotherapy in patients with leptomeningeal metastases. J Neurosurg 1997;87:694–9.

16 Neurotoxicity of Chemotherapy

KATE SCATCHARD • SIOW MING LEE

Introduction

Neurological side effects are a common complication following chemotherapy, and can adversely affect clinical management of the cancer patient. The overall incidence of these toxicities is unknown, but they are becoming more common with the escalations in cytotoxic dose that are now possible with modern hydration regimens, and the use of growth factor support and/or peripheral blood stem cells rescue to prevent myelosuppression. Additionally, as more patients survive long term, late neurological side effects are becoming increasingly recognized, such as impaired cognitive function and/or dementia.

Types of Neurological Damage

COGNITIVE DYSFUNCTION

Cancer patients have frequently recognized decreased cognitive function ("chemobrain") during chemotherapy, which, in the past, was attributed by their physicians to stress or depression. Patients report problems with memory retrieval, learning, and concentration, which may persist after treatment has finished or never fully resolve.[1] The incidence of acute problems during treatment ranges from 15% to 70%, with 50% of patients in one study identifying persistent problems a year after treatment.[2] Cross-sectional studies also suggest persistent cognitive dysfunction in 20% to 30% of patients 2 to 10 years posttreatment.[3,4]

Mechanisms for this functional decline are not fully understood, but recent work by Han et al.[5] on 5-fluorouracil neurotoxicity in mice suggest extensive myelin damage and persistent suppression of both oligodendrocyte and progenitor cell proliferation in the subventricular zone, hippocampus, and corpus callosum.

ACUTE ENCEPHALOPATHY

Acute encephalopathy is a common problem in oncology patients; it has a wide range of precipitating factors including metabolic derangements, hypoxia, brain metastases, meningeal carcinomatosis, infection, paraneoplastic phenomena, and drugs.[6] Presenting symptoms typically include lethargy, confusion, somnolence, seizures, or coma. The diagnosis of drug-induced encephalopathy is typically one of exclusion. A careful drug history should be taken, including recent administration of narcotic analgesia and antiemetic cover, used frequently for cancer patients undergoing chemotherapy and/or for symptom control. CNS infections should also be excluded, particularly in immunocompromised and neutropenic patients. Investigations should include urea/electrolytes, liver function, serum glucose, calcium magnesium, viral serology, and CSF examination. If focal neurological deficit is present, CT or MRI imaging may be helpful and, in any case, should be undertaken prior to a lumbar puncture. EEG is particularly helpful if seizures occur, and will typically show generalized slowing with delta wave activity.[7] Encephalopathy due to cytotoxic drug exposure is generally self-limiting and recovers spontaneously. The only specific therapy is the use of methylene blue in ifosfamide-induced encephalopathy, which should be considered in any patients undergoing ifosfamide chemotherapy. Risk factors include extremes of age, dose/ schedule, previous cranial radiotherapy, and renal or hepatic dysfunction.[8,9]

LEUKOENCEPHALOPATHY

Leukoencephalopathy may follow on from acute encephalopathy, but may also be the first indication of neurotoxicity several months to years after administration of cytotoxic drugs. Patients present with cognitive deficits, which may progress to dementia, coma, and death.[10–14] MRI imaging shows widespread changes throughout the white matter,[15–18] and histologically, there is axonal swelling, demyelination, and neuronal death.[19] Those most at risk are patients treated with methotrexate or cytarabine, particularly if given intrathecally or if cranial radiotherapy preceded cytotoxic administration.[9] Elderly patients with primary central nervous system lymphoma undergoing treatment with high-dose methotrexate and whole-brain radiotherapy (WBRT) are at particularly high risk of developing this complication.[20] There is no specific therapy that can halt the progressive decline, and overall the prognosis is poor. Elderly patients with primary CNS lymphoma should be informed about these risks;

it should also be considered by the treating oncologists whether these patients can be treated with reduced-dose WBRT or avoid WBRT altogether after-high dose methotrexate.

CEREBELLAR DYSFUNCTION

Cerebellar signs in an oncology patient are usually due to direct spread of cancer, particularly if it is asymmetric. In rarer situations, this can be due to paraneoplastic syndromes, which tend to have a subacute onset and may be associated with the presence of antineuronal antibodies.[6] Care should also be taken to distinguish cerebellar ataxia from sensory ataxia due to a severe sensory neuropathy. Cytarabine and 5-fluorouracil are the cytotoxics most likely to cause cerebellar dysfunction including truncal ataxia, gait disturbance, and ataxia.[8,14,21,22] Acutely, the MRI tends to be normal, but subsequent scans may show chronic atrophy due to irreversible Purkinje cell loss.[15–18]

SPINAL CORD TOXICITY

Spinal cord toxicity can occur following intrathecal administration of certain cytotoxics in acute leukemias, lymphomas, and brain tumors. Intrathecal chemotherapy is administered either as part of a lumbar puncture procedure or into the ventricles, via an Ommaya reservoir.[6] The drugs most commonly used are cytarabine, methotrexate, and hydrocortisone; they may be given singly, sequentially, or together as "triple therapy." Symptoms usually arise after multiple cycles of therapy and include both spinal cord and nerve root signs. Loss of neurological function may progress upwards.[23] Histologically, there are focal areas of necrosis, particularly at the periphery of the spinal cord, associated with axonal swelling and demyelination. Myelin basic protein levels in the CSF may be elevated.[24] Typically, only half of those affected will show any sign of recovery.

PERIPHERAL NEUROPATHY

Peripheral neuropathies are the most common neurological complications in patients receiving chemotherapy, especially with regimens containing taxanes (taxol, docataxel), platinum (cisplatin, carboplatin, oxaliplatin), and vinca alkaloids (vincristine). The neuropathy tends to be predominantly sensory in nature, with a glove and stocking distribution. Generally, symptoms are self-limiting, but in some patients the symptoms persist. The effect is cumulative,[6] and patients frequently complain of acute subjective paresthesia of the extremities 2 to 3 days after chemotherapy. With subsequent treatment cycles, symptoms may progress to permanent paresthesia, with decreased sensation to pinprick, light touch, and vibration on formal testing.[9,25–29] At this stage, chemotherapy should be stopped or the dose reduced, as continuing can lead to difficulty with activities of daily living. The neuropathy is largely reversible over several months but many patients may be left with some degree of paresthesia. In rare instances, neuropathy may be paraneoplastic in origin. Oxaliplatin is unusual in that it causes acute cold dysesthesias, as well as pharyngolaryngospasm, which usually starts shortly after administration of chemotherapy and then resolves.

Grading Toxicity

There is no universal grading system for the evaluation of patients with neurological toxicity although two neurotoxicity scoring systems are frequently used: NCI-CTC 3 (National Cancer Institute Common Toxicity Criteria version 3) and ECOG (Eastern Cooperative Oncology Group).[30] The NCI-CTCAE scores a variety of symptoms from ataxia to motor neuropathy on a scale of 0 to 5, with 0 being normal, 1 mild self-limiting, 2 moderate, 3 severe undesirable, 4 life-threatening, and 5 death induced by adverse event. The full version can be downloaded from www.fda.gov. The ECOG criteria are organized in a similar manner with a scale from 0 to 4 and can be viewed at www.ecog.org. Generally patients with a toxicity score of 1 to 2 can continue with their treatment unmodified, while those with a score of 3 or 4 require dose modification or cessation of treatment.

Prevention

Neurotoxicity is a frequent and dose-limiting side effect of chemotherapy, particularly as supportive measures aimed at overcoming bone marrow suppression have led to the use of higher doses of a number of cytotoxic agents.

The patients most at risk are those receiving a high cumulative dose or intensive schedule, particularly if there is a preexisting condition such as diabetes mellitus, hereditary neuropathy, or multiple sclerosis.[31] Previous radiotherapy may also increase the risk of developing neurotoxicity if patients are subsequently treated with cisplatin or methotrexate.[32,33]

Patients with HIV-related malignancies are also at increased risk of cytotoxic-induced neuropathy, since both HIV and the drugs used to treat it (highly active antiretroviral therapy, or HAART) can cause neurological damage independently.[34] Distal sensory neuropathy is the commonest form of HIV-associated neuropathy and can be difficult to distinguish from that caused by specific nucleoside antiretrovirals. In addition, compounded neurological toxicities frequently occur because of reduced clearance of vincristine, vinblastine, and taxane; these complications can be reduced by changing these patients' antiretroviral medications. More rarely, patients can develop inflammatory demyelinating polyneuropathy, mononeuritis multiplex, or neuronal damage due to opportunistic infections such as CMV and HZV.

Currently there are few therapies able to prevent neurological toxicity preemptively. Infusions of methylene blue are used prophylatically in patients receiving ifosfamide who have previously developed acute encephalopathy. A number of trials have investigated the benefits of agents such as calcium-magnesium infusions, carbamazepine, gabapentin, amifostine, and glutathione.[7,35–52] However, the trials are small studies and no specific prophylaxis can be routinely recommended.

Treatment of Neurotoxicity

Apart from dose reduction or discontinuing the drugs implicated in the development of neurotoxicity, there is very little in the way of specific pharmacological management to reverse their side effects. Methylene blue is used for ifosfamide-induced encephalopathy and infusional calcium with magnesium may lessen the severity of established peripheral neuropathy due to oxaliplatin. However, considerable input from the multidisciplinary team is required in the holistic care of the patient,[53] including analgesia for neuropathic pain, maximization of mobility (with occupational and physiotherapist involvement where there is loss of balance, sensory loss, or muscle weakness), and good nursing care to manage bowel or bladder dysfunction, protection of pressure areas in immobilized patients, and maintenance of a safe environment if patients are confused.

Cytotoxic Agents and Their Neurological Toxicities (See Table 16-1)

5-FLUOROURACIL

5-fluorouracil (5-FU), a pyrimidine analogue, is widely used in the treatment of gastrointestinal malignancies; it is administered either as a short intravenous bolus or as a prolonged continuous infusion. Neurotoxicity is rare, but may include acute cerebellar dysfunction in 3% to 7% of patients, causing gait ataxia, nystagmus, and scanning speech.[54,55] Symptoms tend to resolve spontaneously within a few days of treatment cessation although administration of thiamine may be helpful.[22] Patients may also develop acute confusion in the absence of cerebellar signs, which may recur on reexposure to 5-FU.[56] The main risk factor for development of neurotoxicity is deficiency of the enzyme dihydropyrimidine dehydrogenase which metabolizes 5-FU.[57–59]

A subacute form of leukoencephalopathy occurs in approximately 2% of patients receiving 5-FU in combination with levamisole (an immunomodulatory agent).[60–64] Presentation is with focal neurological abnormalities and cognitive impairment that may be mistaken for metastatic disease. MRI shows patchy abnormalities within the white matter that enhance with gadolinium. Histologically, these patches contain an intense inflammatory infiltration with demyelination but axonal sparing. It is thought that the levamisole disrupts the blood-brain barrier potentiating 5-FU's access to the CNS. Although treatment with steroids has been advocated, this syndrome is frequently self-limiting and patients usually recover completely over the course of several weeks without specific therapy. In some patients, thymidine has also been used successfully.[58] Rarely, a peripheral sensory neuropathy has also been reported.[65] Because many patients received adjuvant 5-FU based treatments for a variety of cancers, including breast, gastrointestinal, and bowel cancers, patients should be monitored for possible long-term neurocognitive damage.[5]

ASPARAGINASE

Asparaginase (either as the L- or pegylated formulation) is a component of remission-induction therapy used to treat acute lymphoblastic leukemia (ALL). It may cause cerebrovascular accidents during the first few weeks of its administration.[66] This is due to depletion of plasma proteins involved in coagulation, such as fibrinogen and antithrombin III. Thrombosis typically occurs within the

TABLE 16-1 List of Cytotoxic Agents

Cytotoxic Agent	Use	Neurological Toxicity	Specific Therapy
5-Fluorouracil	GI malignancy	Acute cerebellar dysfunction Leukoencephalopathy	
Busulfan	Hodgkin lymphoma Dysgeminoma Testicular cancer	Tonic-clonic seizures	Prophylactic anticonvulsants
Cisplatin	Gynecological Head and neck Urological	Peripheral neuropathy Ototoxicity Encephalopathy	
Cytarabine	Leukemia and Lymphoma	Acute cerebellar dysfunction Spinal cord toxicity Peripheral neuropathy Acute encephalopathy	
Fludarabine	Lymphoma	Peripheral neuropathy Somnolence Encephalopathy	
Ifosfamide	Sarcoma Neuroblastoma Wilm tumor Lymphoma	Acute encephalopathy	Methylene blue 50 mg IV × 6/day
L-asparaginase	ALL	Cerebrovascular events Psychiatric disturbance	Anticoagulation for venous thrombosis
Methotrexate		Acute encephalitis Leukoencephalopathy Spinal cord toxicity	
Nitrosoureas		Encephalopathy	
Oxaliplatin	GI malignancy	Transient acute dysesthesia Distal sensory peripheral neuropathy	Symptoms triggered by cold
Procarbazine	Lymphoma	Peripheral neuropathy Somnolence	
Taxanes	Breast and ovarian cancers	Peripheral neuropathy	
Vinca alkaloids Vincristine Vinblastine Vindesine Vinorelbine	Hematologic malignancy Sarcoma Breast Lung	Peripheral neuropathy Autonomic neuropathy Fatal myeloencephalopathy with intrathecal administration	CSF lavage for inadvertent IT administration

dural sinuses and cerebral veins, leading to secondary hemorrhage or infarction.[67] Patients present with a range of symptoms from mild headache to coma and death, which are caused by rapid increases in intracranial pressure. Once diagnosed, the asparaginase should be stopped and the patient anticoagulated unless hemorrhage is present.

Asparaginase acts to cleave asparagine, an essential amino acid required by rapidly proliferating cells (hence its antimitotic action) and also as a neurotransmitter. Therefore depletion of asparagine during treatment has also been associated with the development of neuropsychiatric symptoms such as depression and hallucinations.[68]

CYCLOPHOSPHAMIDE

Cyclophosphamide is a prodrug, which alkylates DNA after hepatic activation.[69] It is used in a wide range of malignancies, including lymphoma, breast cancer, and testicular cancer. When given in high doses, it may lead to inappropriate secretion of ADH (SIADH), and hence a secondary metabolic encephalopathy may occur, with confusion, seizures, or coma.[70–72] There have been a few case reports of cyclophosphamide also being associated with blurred vision, dizziness, and confusion in the absence of SIADH.[73,74]

CYTARABINE

Cytarabine is an analogue of adenosine, causing chain termination during DNA synthesis; it is one of the most effective cytotoxic drugs in the treatment of acute leukemia. It is used either at a conventional dose of 100 to 200 mg/m^2/day or at high doses of 2 to 6 g/m^2/day.[69] Neurotoxicity is particularly common at the higher dose levels, affecting 16% to 50% of patients;[8] it predominantly affects the central nervous system. The risk of neurotoxicity is increased by age, dose/ schedule (particularly cumulative dose), renal or hepatic impairment, and the concurrent use of neurotropic antiemetics such as phenothiazines.[8,75,76]

The mechanism of toxicity is not well-understood, but it appears that cytarabine directly causes neuronal death, possibly by the inhibition of cytidine-dependent neurotropic signal transduction,[77] although it has also been shown to stimulate the production of reactive oxygen species that may also damage DNA directly by inducing strand breaks.[78]

Acute cerebellar dysfunction is the commonest central neurotoxicity, occurring in approximately 14% of patients; they typically present with dysarthria, nystagmus, gait ataxia, and confusion. Onset usually occurs during administration of a multiday regimen, particularly above a cumulative dose of 36 g/m^2 and generally resolves rapidly once cytarabine is withdrawn.[8,9,14] However, toxicity may be permanent once more than 8% to 20% of Purkinje cells have been lost.[8] Acute encephalopathy is also common, presenting with somnolence or seizures. MRI scanning reveals diffuse high-intensity lesions within the central matter on T2-weighting that may be reversible.[18] The encephalopathy should rapidly resolve entirely on stopping cytarabine; however, damage may be permanent and progress to leukoencephalopathy in a minority of patients, usually those with preexisting organ dysfunction or neurological problems.[8] Less commonly, optic neuropathy, anosmia, and an incompletely reversible myelopathy have been reported.[14] As with methotrexate, the intrathecal administration of cytarabine may cause ascending myelitis.[8,79–81] There have also been case reports of sensory peripheral neuropathy following cytarabine exposure.[82]

ETOPOSIDE

Etoposide, a topoisomerase II inhibitor used in treatment of hematological, lung, ovarian, and testicular cancers,[69] causes very little neurotoxicity, although at very high doses there have been reports of peripheral neuropathy, headache, seizures, and somnolence, in bone marrow transplant recipients and patients with malignant gliomas.[83,84]

FLUDARABINE

Neurotoxicity with the antimetabolite fludarabine is uncommon, but somnolence, acute encephalopathy, and chronic leukoencephalopathy progressing to coma and death have all been reported.[85]

IFOSFAMIDE

Central nervous system toxicity occurs in approximately 10% to 20% of patients receiving ifosfamide, who present with personality changes, confusion, hallucinations, stupor, and coma.[9] More unusually, patients may experience seizures, myoclonus, cranial nerve palsies, or extrapyramidal symptoms.[86,87] Symptoms usually begin 12 to14 hours after initiation of an ifosfamide infusion and spontaneously resolve 2 to 3 days after its cessation, although rarely symptoms may persist or even be fatal. EEG tends to show severe slowing with delta wave activity with or without seizure activity. Patients most at risk are those with impaired renal function, low serum albumin, pelvic tumors, and previous exposure to cisplatin.[88] The risk of encephalopathy varies with route of administration. It is more common after oral administration, and is also more frequent with short intravenous infusion durations.[89–91] The mechanism of toxicity is unclear but may be related to accumulation of metabolites such as chloracetaldehyde and chloroethylamine, which deplete intracellular glutathione and NAD and impair mitochondrial electron transport.[92] Methylene blue, 300 mg IV in 6 divided doses, is used in the treatment of ifosfamide-induced encephalopathy and 50 mg IV qds may be given prophylatically.[93–96] It is thought to act primarily as an alternative electron acceptor restoring mitochondrial respiratory chain function, but may also oxidate NADH and inhibits plasma monoamine oxidases.

METHOTREXATE

Methotrexate is one of the most widely used cytotoxic antimetabolites in the treatment of hematological, breast, and head/ neck cancers.[9] In addition, prophylactic intrathecal use in ALL and high grade non-Hodgkin lymphomas has reduced the incidence of CNS relapse in high risk patients.[97] Methotrexate acts by inhibiting dihydrofolate reductase, thus blocking purine and thymidine biosynthesis. Its neurotoxicity is thought to stem from widespread disruption of various metabolic pathways in the brain and can be acute or chronic.

Acute encephalopathy is associated with the administration of high-dose methotrexate ($>3\,mg/m^2$) and is characterized by somnolence, confusion, and seizures.[98] Other symptoms include emotional lability and alternating hemiparesis, giving rise to the misdiagnosis of a functional disorder. The imaging appearances are characteristic and show symmetrical restricted diffusion on diffusion-weighted imaging, even when the T2-weighted sequences appear normal (Figure 16-1). Patients most at risk are children, those who have received previous cranial radiotherapy, or those receiving concomitant intravenous and intrathecal therapy. Metabolic abnormalities associated with the development

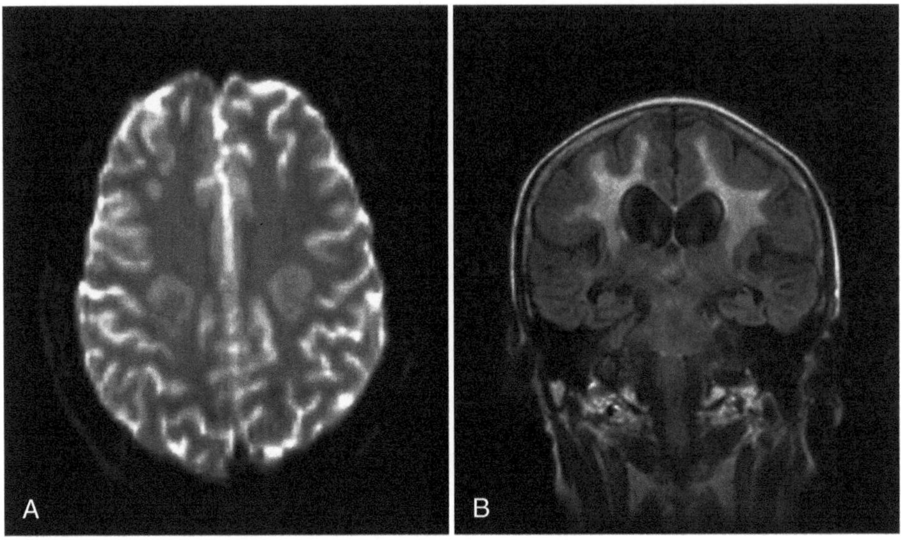

Figure 16-1 Acute methotrexate encephalopathy. 18-year-old girl with T-cell lymphoblastic lymphoma who presented with first left-sided, then right-sided weakness (alternating hemiparesis) and dysphasia following high-dose intrathecal MTX. The MRI shows symmetric circular areas of restricted diffusion in the centrum semiovale, which appear bright on the diffusion-weighted imaging **(A)** and dark on the ADC map **(B)**. Her recovery was slow and incomplete. She has been left with severe balance difficulties, orofacial apraxia, and dysphasia.

of encephalopathy include widespread reduction in glucose utilization and protein synthesis,[99] which are reversible by replacing depleted folate stores with the administration of leucovorin.[100] Leucovorin is now given routinely following high-dose methotrexate (folinic acid rescue). Other studies have also postulated that changes in adenosine,[101] homocysteine,[102,103] or biopterin[104] levels may also contribute to development of encephalopathy. In one study, aminophylline (2.5 mg/kg IV over 1 hour), given to six encephalopathic patients, caused immediate resolution of symptoms in four and improved symptoms in the remaining two patients.[101]

Administration of intrathecal methotrexate alone may result in an aseptic meningitis, with headache, neck stiffness, vomiting, and fever developing 2 to 4 hours after injection and lasting 12 to 72 hours.[105] Transverse myelopathy has also been associated with intrathecal methotrexate, but usually in patients who have received repeated administrations. Patients develop progressive back pain, sensory loss, paraplegia, and sphincter disturbance over several days or weeks. Myelin basic protein may be raised in the CSF prior to the development of neurological signs.[106] Approximately half the patients recover some function. Histologically, there are areas of focal necrosis associated with axonal swelling and demyelination. Pathogenesis is due to transient inhibition of myelin formation by S-adenosylmethionine[107] and choline[16] depletion secondary to methotrexate-induced folate deficiency.

Leukoencephalopathy may develop several months to years after both intravenous and intrathecal methotrexate administration. Patients present with cognitive impairment, gait abnormalities, focal neurologic deficits, and/or seizures, and

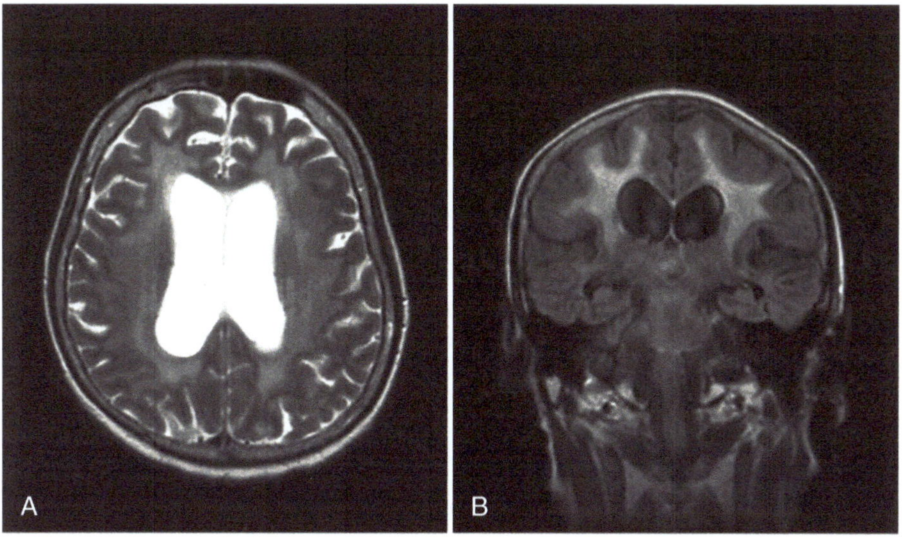

Figure 16-2 Methotrexate leukoencephalopathy. 62-year-old woman with primary CNS lymphoma affecting the posterior fossa, treated with high-dose intravenous methotrexate followed by RT in 2003. She presented in 2006 with increasing gait ataxia and memory loss. Her condition progressed rapidly in the final months of 2008. MRI shows generalized volume loss and extensive confluent high-signal white matter change and enlarged ventricles on axial T2-weighted **(A)** and coronal FLAIR **(B)**, typical of methotrexate leukoencephalopathy.

may progress to coma and death. MRI reveals diffuse atrophy, ventricular dilation, and cortical calcification (Figure 16-2).[108] Histologically, there are areas of axonal necrosis with associated myelin loss as well as microangiopathic calcification within the vasculature.[19] As with the development of acute encephalopathy, those most at risk appear to be children and recipients of cranial radiotherapy prior to chemotherapy.[20] The neurological damage is not reversible, and there is no available treatment. Neurocognitive complications are significantly increased in older patients with primary CNS lymphoma treated with high-dose methotrexate and whole brain radiotherapy.

NITROSOUREAS

The nitrosureas, carmustine (BCNU) and lomustine (CCNU) are DNA-alkylating agents that cross the blood-brain barrier and are therefore commonly used in the treatment of brain tumors, melanoma, and CNS lymphomas.[69] At conventional doses neurotoxicity is unusual; however, when used at high doses, particularly in association with intraarterial injection or previous radiotherapy, blindness due to optic neuropathy, encephalopathy, and seizures have been reported.[109–112]

PLATINUM COMPOUNDS

Platinum-containing compounds such as cisplatin, carboplatin, and oxaliplatin all act by alkylating DNA to produce interstrand and intrastrand breaks, which result in lethal DNA strand breakage during replication.[69]

The commonest neurological toxicity is a painful sensory peripheral neuropathy, which is dose-related and cumulative. Patients typically present with dysesthesia and decreased proprioception and vibration sense, and may have absent deep tendon reflexes.[27,113–125] If treatment is halted at this stage, these symptoms generally resolve completely over several months.[126] However, if treatment continues, mild motor neuropathy and severe sensory ataxia may develop, affecting ambulation in some patients. The pathogenesis of the peripheral neuropathy is unknown, but histologically there is axonal swelling and myelin sheath breakdown, predominantly affecting large sensory fibers within the dorsal column.[127]

Oxaliplatin also causes an acute sensory disturbance in 80% to 90% of patients, characterized by transient distal or perioral paresthesia that starts during drug administration, is frequently triggered by cold and touching cold objects, and resolves completely over several hours to days. It is thought to be caused by disruption of voltage-gated ion channels within neurons. Symptoms can, therefore, be dramatically reduced if patients are advised to keep warm and avoid cold food or drinks.[115]

Irreversible high-frequency hearing loss associated with tinnitus also occurs frequently with cisplatin exposure and may progress to affect lower frequency ranges if treatment is not terminated.[116,128–131] Cisplatin appears to be toxic to the outer hair cells of the cochlea, while the vestibular apparatus is unaffected. Young age and previous cranial radiotherapy increase risk, as does peak plasma cisplatin concentration and cumulative dose. Despite the frequent occurrence of hearing loss, most patients remain asymptomatic, although small losses can be a significant problem for professional singers and musicians.

More rarely, patients may develop Lhermitte sign, optic neuropathy, or cortical blindness secondary to cisplatin-induced nerve demyelination, all of which are capable of total spontaneous recovery if treatment is stopped.[9]

Cisplatin is the most neurotoxic of the platinum compounds, with 23% of patients developing peripheral neuropathy[27,132,133] and up to 81% developing high frequency hearing loss on audiometry,[134] while carboplatin is the least with only 1% of patients developing peripheral neuropathy and 19%, asymptomatic hearing loss.[27,131,133]

There have been many small trials looking at prophylaxis of neuropathy in platinum-treated patients, predominantly with compounds containing thiol groups or heavy metal chelators such as glutathione, antiepileptics, and amifostine. Some of these trials reported some benefit.[35–39,41–52] However, study numbers are small and no definite conclusion can be drawn from these studies. Infusional calcium gluconate with magnesium sulfate (1g of each in 250 ml 5% dextrose IV over 20 minutes, pre- and post-chemotherapy) may lessen the severity of established peripheral neuropathy due to oxaliplatin.[135]

PROCARBAZINE

Procarbazine is a DNA alkylator commonly used in the treatment of Hodgkin lymphoma; it readily crosses the blood brain barrier.[69] It causes an acute encephalopathy with confusion and somnolence in 14% to 33% of patients, which is probably secondary to its ability to inhibit monoamine oxidase.[109,136,137] Symptoms are therefore worsened by concurrent administration of phenothiazines such as chlorpromazine, which is used frequently as antiemetic prophylaxis. Peripheral neuropathy has also been reported in 2% to 20% of patients receiving procarbazine. Patients typically present with a subjective paresthesia, which usually resolves completely on cessation of treatment.[136,137]

TAXANES

The taxanes paclitaxol and docetaxol both act by stabilizing microtubule polymerization, thus preventing the completion of successful mitosis. They are widely used in the treatment of breast, lung, and ovarian cancers. Unfortunately, their mechanism of action also leads to microtubule accumulation within axons, interfering with axonal transport and causing neurotoxicity. This is predominantly in the form of a distal peripheral polyneuropathy; patients typically present with painful paresthesia in a glove-and-stocking distribution, associated with reduced vibration sense, absent deep tendon reflexes, and difficulty with activities of daily living.[138] Infrequently, there may also be a mild motor neuropathy, proximal muscle weakness, or autonomic neuropathy. Histologically, there is axonal atrophy, lack of axonal sprouting, and secondary demyelination predominantly involving small pain and temperature fibers, although motor and large sensory fibers may also be affected to a lesser extent. Risk of neuropathy is greater with paclitaxol than docetaxol[139] and increases with dose, cumulative exposure, diabetes, or other preexisting neuropathy, and multiple sclerosis. Once peripheral neuropathy has developed, the taxane should be stopped and spontaneous recovery will usually occur over several months. Pyridoxine may speed recovery in the case of docetaxol, and amitryptiline or gabapentin may be useful if neuropathic pain is significant. Although no neuroprotective agents can be recommended at present, laboratory studies with nerve growth factor,[140] ACTH analogues,[141] and phase I clinical trials of glutamate and amifostine[25] have produced some encouraging results.

CNS toxicity is rare, reflecting poor penetrance of the blood-brain barrier, although there have been occasional case reports of paclitaxol precipitating a mild encephalopathy. Presentation was with confusion, dysphasia, and nonspecific diffuse slowing on EEG, and recurred on reexposure.[142] Transient visual disturbances have also been documented during taxane infusions, which may respond to a slowing of the rate of infusion.

VINCA ALKALOIDS

The vinca alkaloids vincristine, vinblastine, vindesine, and vinorelbine are widely used in the treatment of hematological malignancies, sarcomas, breast cancer, and lung cancer. They act by binding tubulin and thus inhibit microtubule polymerization during mitosis.[9] Neurotoxicity, in the form of peripheral or autonomic neuropathy, occurs with all of these drugs, especially with vincristine. It is less frequently reported with vinblastine, vindesine, or vinorelbine. The neuropathy is probably caused by impairment of axonal flow due to inhibition of axonal microtubules, leading to axonal atrophy and adjacent myelin sheath damage. Patients usually present with a predominantly sensory peripheral neuropathy, which may be accompanied by the loss of deep tendon reflexes or, in the severest forms, distal muscle weakness. Constipation also occurs frequently due to reduced bowel motility, requiring treatment with stimulant laxatives. More rarely ocular palsies, voice hoarseness, and autonomic neuropathy (with postural hypotension and bladder atony) may occur. There have been several case reports of vincristine administration unmasking previously undiagnosed Charcot-Marie-Tooth syndrome, and therefore vinca alkaloids are not recommended for patients with hereditary polyneuropathies.[143–148] Because of the fact that this toxicity is dose related and cumulative, the dose of vincristine is always capped at 2 mg. Concurrent administration of itraconazole or nifedipine has also been reported to enhance neurotoxicity by inhibiting vincristine degradation within the liver. Following development of significant neuropathy, vinca alkaloid treatment should either be reduced in dose or stopped. Symptomatic recovery usually occurs spontaneously, although this can take several months. There has been one case report of lithium (600 mg od PO) administration[149] successfully reversing vincristine-induced peripheral neuropathy, allowing vincristine therapy to continue.

When administered intrathecally, vincristine is usually fatal due an ascending myeloencephalopathy causing ascending paralysis, coma, and death. At postmortem, there is widespread necrosis within the central nervous system, particularly the periventricular regions. Even so, there are several cases worldwide each year of inadvertent intrathecal administration,[150–153] usually as a result of a series of procedural errors including mistaking vincristine for an intended intrathecal drug, not checking physician orders, mistaking the route of administration and mislabeling of syringes.[154] Stringent regulations have now been introduced in the UK regarding who can administer intrathecal chemotherapy, and where and how this takes place. Once this mistake has been discovered, cerebrospinal fluid exchange should be initiated immediately and continued until as much of the vincristine as possible has been recovered.[151,154] Unfortunately, most patients still suffer extensive neurological damage resulting in death despite aggressive cerebrospinal lavage.

Biological Agents

Since the late 1990s, the search for new anticancer agents has switched away from classical cytotoxics that kill cancer cells by inducing DNA damage to agents that modify growth signaling pathways. There are two main types of agents, the -mabs, which are monoclonal antibodies that target either cell surface receptors (e.g., trastuzumab against Her 2 receptors) or circulating ligand (e.g., bevacizumab against VEGF), and the -ibs, which are small drug molecules that target intracellular stages of signaling pathways (e.g., erlotinib which inhibits the tyrosine kinase complexed to the intracellular portion of the epidermal growth factor (EGF) receptor). In general, these drugs have a much gentler side effect profile compared with cytotoxic agents and very little in the way of neurotoxicity has been reported in the literature to date, although there have been isolated case reports of reversible posterior leukoencephalopathy (RPLE) with bevacizumab and sorafenib.[155–157] This condition typically presents with headache, cortical blindness, and seizures. MRI imaging reveals vasogenic edema in the posterior cerebral white matter. Although the exact etiology is unknown, RPLE is frequently associated with hypertension, which is a commonly reported side effect of this group of drugs. Concomitant cytotoxic chemotherapy may also be an additional influence on the development of RPLE by causing endothelial damage or vasospasm.

Bortezomib, a proteosome inhibitor used in patients with multiple myeloma, causes a peripheral sensory neuropathy in one third of patients.[158] On examination, affected patients typically have reduced ankle reflexes, decreased vibration sensation, and impaired heel-toe gait. Symptoms generally improve with dose reduction or discontinuation of therapy. More rarely, it has been associated with life-threatening motor neuropathy.[159]

Thalidomide is also currently widely used in myeloma because of its immunomodulatory and antiangiogenic effects. Unfortunately, up to 50% of patients develop a distal sensory peripheral neuropathy and a smaller number, a motor neuropathy. Patients may benefit from dose reductions when these complications occur. Newer thalidomide analogues such as lenalidomide seem to have a more favorable toxicity profile with reduced incidences of neuropathy (<5%).[160]

REFERENCES

1. Meyers CA. How chemotherapy damages the central nervous system. J Biol 2008;7:11.
2. Wefel JS, et al. The cognitive sequelae of standard dose adjuvant chemotherapy in women with breast cancer: results of a prospective, randomised longitudinal trial. Cancer 2004;100:2292–9.
3. Ahles TA, et al. Neuropsychological impact of standard dose chemotherapy in long-term survivors of breast cancer and lymphoma. J Clin Oncol 2002;20:485–93.
4. Schagen SB, et al. Cognitive deficits after post-operative chemotherapy for breast cancer. Cancer 1999;85:640–50.
5. Han R, et al. Systemmic 5-fluorouracil treatment causes a syndrome of delayed myelin destruction in the central nervous system. J Biol 2008;7:12.
6. Gilbert M. Neurologic complications. In: Abeloff MD, editor. Clinical Oncology. Philadelphia: Churchill Livingstone; 2000.
7. Korinthenberg R, et al. On the origin of EEG-slowing and encephalopathy during induction treatment of acute lymphoblastic leukemia. Med Pediatr Oncol 2002;39(6):566–72.
8. Baker WJ, Royer Jr GL, Weiss RB. Cytarabine and neurologic toxicity. J Clin Oncol 1991;9(4):679–93.
9. Verstappen CC, et al. Neurotoxic complications of chemotherapy in patients with cancer: clinical signs and optimal management. Drugs 2003;63(15):1549–63.
10. Saumoy M, et al. Progressive multifocal leukoencephalopathy in chronic lymphocytic leukemia after treatment with fludarabine. Leuk Lymphoma 2002;43(2):433–6.
11. Choi SM, et al. 5-fluorouracil-induced leukoencephalopathy in patients with breast cancer. J Korean Med Sci 2001;16(3):328–34.
12. Honkaniemi J, et al. Reversible posterior leukoencephalopathy after combination chemotherapy. Neuroradiology 2000;42(12):895–9.
13. Gonzalez H, et al. Progressive multifocal leukoencephalitis (PML) in three patients treated with standard-dose fludarabine (FAMP). Hematol Cell Ther 1999;41(4):183–6.
14. Hoffman DL, et al. Encephalopathy, myelopathy, optic neuropathy, and anosmia associated with intravenous cytosine arabinoside. Clin Neuropharmacol 1993;16(3):258–62.
15. Leung LH, et al. White-matter diffusion anisotropy after chemo-irradiation: a statistical parametric mapping study and histogram analysis. Neuroimage 2004;21(1):261–8.
16. Davidson A, et al. Proton magnetic resonance spectroscopy ((1)H-MRS) of the brain following high-dose methotrexate treatment for childhood cancer. Med Pediatr Oncol 2000;35(1):28–34.
17. Rao RD, et al. Methotrexate induced seizures associated with acute reversible magnetic resonance imaging (MRI) changes in a patient with acute lymphoblastic leukemia. Leuk Lymphoma 2002;43(6):1333–6.

18. Vaughn DJ, et al. High-dose cytarabine neurotoxicity: MR findings during the acute phase. AJNR Am J Neuroradiol 1993;14(4):1014–6.
19. Liu HM, et al. Methotrexate encephalopathy. A neuropathologic study. Hum Pathol 1978;9(6):635–48.
20. Blay JY, et al. High-dose methotrexate for the treatment of primary cerebral lymphomas: analysis of survival and late neurologic toxicity in a retrospective series. J Clin Oncol 1998;16(3):864–71.
21. Barbieux C, et al. (Acute cerebellar syndrome after treatment with 5-fluorouracil). Bull Cancer 1996;83(1):77–80.
22. Pirzada NA, Ali II, Dafer RM. Fluorouracil-induced neurotoxicity. Ann Pharmacother 2000;34(1):35–8.
23. Hodgson PS, et al. The neurotoxicity of drugs given intrathecally (spinal). Anesth Analg 1999;88(4):797–809.
24. Clark AW, et al. Paraplegia following intrathecal chemotherapy: neuropathologic findings and elevation of myelin basic protein. Cancer 1982;50(1):42–7.
25. Makino H. Treatment and care of neurotoxicity from taxane anticancer agents. Breast Cancer 2004;11(1):100–4.
26. Othieno-Abinya NA, Nyabola LO. Experience with vincristine—associated neurotoxicity. East Afr Med J 2001;78(7):376–8.
27. Hilkens PH, et al. Peripheral neuropathy induced by combination chemotherapy of docetaxel and cisplatin. Br J Cancer 1997;75(3):417–22.
28. Cella D, et al. Measuring the side effects of taxane therapy in oncology: the functional assesment of cancer therapy-taxane (FACT-taxane). Cancer 2003;98(4):822–31.
29. Uhm JH, Yung WK. Neurologic Complications of Cancer Therapy. Curr Treat Options Neurol 1999;1(5):428–37.
30. Cavaletti G, et al. Grading of chemotherapy-induced peripheral neurotoxicity using the Total Neuropathy Scale. Neurology 2003;61(9):1297–300.
31. Quasthoff S, Hartung HP. Chemotherapy-induced peripheral neuropathy. J Neurol 2002;249(1):9–17.
32. Schlegel U, et al. Neurologic sequelae of treatment of primary CNS lymphomas. J Neurooncol 1999;43(3):277–86.
33. Taphoorn MJ. Neurocognitive sequelae in the treatment of low-grade gliomas. Semin Oncol 2003;30(6 Suppl. 19):45–8.
34. Pardo CA, McArthur JC, Griffin JW. HIV neuropathy: insights in the pathology of HIV peripheral nerve disease. J Peripher Nerv Syst 2001;6(1):21–7.
35. Aloe L, et al. Evidence that nerve growth factor promotes the recovery of peripheral neuropathy induced in mice by cisplatin: behavioral, structural and biochemical analysis. Auton Neurosci 2000;86(1–2):84–93.
36. Bokemeyer C, et al. Silibinin protects against cisplatin-induced nephrotoxicity without compromising cisplatin or ifosfamide anti-tumour activity. Br J Cancer 1996;74(12):2036–41.
37. Capizzi RL. Protection of normal tissues from the cytotoxic effects of chemotherapy by amifostine (Ethyol): clinical experiences. Semin Oncol 1994;21(5 Suppl. 11):8–15.
38. Cavaletti G, et al. Neuroprotectant drugs in cisplatin neurotoxicity. Anticancer Res 1996; 16(5B):3149–59.
39. Cascinu S, et al. Neuroprotective effect of reduced glutathione on oxaliplatin-based chemotherapy in advanced colorectal cancer: a randomized, double-blind, placebo-controlled trial. J Clin Oncol 2002;20(16):3478–83.
40. Cassidy J, et al. Clinical trials of nimodipine as a potential neuroprotector in ovarian cancer patients treated with cisplatin. Cancer Chemother Pharmacol 1998;41(2):161–6.
41. Eckel F, et al. (Prevention of oxaliplatin-induced neuropathy by carbamazepine. A pilot study). Dtsch Med Wochenschr 2002;127(3):78–82.
42. Foster-Nora JA, Siden R. Amifostine for protection from antineoplastic drug toxicity. Am J Health Syst Pharm 1997;54(7):787–800.
43. Kanat O, et al. Protective effect of amifostine against toxicity of paclitaxel and carboplatin in non-small cell lung cancer: a single center randomized study. Med Oncol 2003;20(3):237–45.
44. Lersch C, et al. Prevention of oxaliplatin-induced peripheral sensory neuropathy by carbamazepine in patients with advanced colorectal cancer. Clin Colorectal Cancer 2002;2(1):54–8.
45. Links M, Lewis C. Chemoprotectants: a review of their clinical pharmacology and therapeutic efficacy. Drugs 1999;57(3):293–308.
46. Orditura M, et al. Amifostine: A selective cytoprotective agent of normal tissues from chemo-radiotherapy induced toxicity (Review). Oncol Rep 1999;6(6):1357–62.

47. Pace A, et al. Neuroprotective effect of vitamin E supplementation in patients treated with cisplatin chemotherapy. J Clin Oncol 2003;21(5):927–31.
48. Rick O, et al. Assessment of amifostine as protection from chemotherapy-induced toxicities after conventional-dose and high-dose chemotherapy in patients with germ cell tumor. Ann Oncol 2001;12(8):1151–5.
49. Smyth JF, et al. Glutathione reduces the toxicity and improves quality of life of women diagnosed with ovarian cancer treated with cisplatin: results of a double-blind, randomised trial. Ann Oncol 1997;8(6):569–73.
50. Spencer CM, Goa KL. Amifostine. A review of its pharmacodynamic and pharmacokinetic properties, and therapeutic potential as a radioprotector and cytotoxic chemoprotector. Drugs 1995;50(6):1001–31.
51. Sumiyoshi Y, et al. (Glutathione chemoprotection therapy against CDDP-induced neurotoxicity in patients with invasive bladder cancer). Gan To Kagaku Ryoho 1996;23(11):1506–8.
52. Viele CS, Holmes BC. Amifostine: drug profile and nursing implications of the first pancytoprotectant. Oncol Nurs Forum 1998;25(3):515–23.
53. Hildebrand J. Neurological complications of cancer chemotherapy. Curr Opin Oncol 2006;18(4):321–4.
54. Bygrave HA, et al. Neurological complications of 5-fluorouracil chemotherapy: case report and review of the literature. Clin Oncol (R Coll Radiol) 1998;10(5):334–6.
55. Moore DH, Fowler Jr WC, Crumpler LS. 5-Fluorouracil neurotoxicity. Gynecol Oncol 1990;36(1):152–4.
56. Ki SS, et al. A case of neurotoxicity following 5-fluorouracil-based chemotherapy. Korean J Intern Med 2002;17(1):73–7.
57. Shehata N, Pater A, Tang SC. Prolonged severe 5-fluorouracil-associated neurotoxicity in a patient with dihydropyrimidine dehydrogenase deficiency. Cancer Invest 1999;17(3):201–5.
58. Takimoto CH, et al. Severe neurotoxicity following 5-fluorouracil-based chemotherapy in a patient with dihydropyrimidine dehydrogenase deficiency. Clin Cancer Res 1996;2(3):477–81.
59. Morrison GB. Dihydropyrimidine dehydrogenase deficiency: a pharmacogenetic defect causing severe adverse reactions to 5-fluorouracil-based chemotherapy. Oncol Nurs Forum 1997;24(1):83–8.
60. Hsu CH, et al. Weekly 24-hour infusion of high-dose 5-fluorouracil and leucovorin in the treatment of advanced gastric cancers. An effective and low-toxic regimen for patients with poor general condition. Oncology 1997;54(4):275–80.
61. Figueredo AT, et al. Disabling encephalopathy during 5-fluorouracil and levamisole adjuvant therapy for resected colorectal cancer: a report of two cases. Cancer Invest 1995;13(6):608–11.
62. Murray CL, et al. Multifocal inflammatory leukoencephalopathy after fluorouracil and levamisole therapy for colon cancer. AJNR Am J Neuroradiol 1997;18(8):1591–2.
63. Saletti P, et al. Two cases of neurotoxicity possibly related to 5-fluorouracil and FA administration. Ann Oncol 1996;7(2):213–4.
64. Wang WS, et al. Weekly 24-hour infusion of high-dose 5-fluorouracil and leucovorin in patients with advanced colorectal cancer: Taiwan experience. Jpn J Clin Oncol 1998;28(1):16–9.
65. van Laarhoven HW, et al. 5-FU-induced peripheral neuropathy: a rare complication of a well-known drug. Anticancer Res 2003;23(1B):647–8.
66. Ray M, Marwaha RK, Trehan A. Chemotherapy related fatal neurotoxicity during induction in acute lymphoblastic leukemia. Indian J Pediatr 2002;69(2):185–7.
67. Feinberg WM, Swenson MR. Cerebrovascular complications of L-asparaginase therapy. Neurology 1988;38(1):127–33.
68. Holland JC. Psychiatric symptoms assocated with L-asparaginase therapy. J Psychiatr Res 1974;10:174.
69. Perry MC, Anderson CM, Donehower RC. Chemotherapy. In: Abeloff MD, editor. Clinical Oncology. Philadelphia: Churchill Livingstone; 2000.
70. Webberley MJ, Murray JA. Life-threatening acute hyponatraemia induced by low dose cyclophosphamide and indomethacin. Postgrad Med J 1989;65(770):950–2.
71. Tsujita Y, et al. (Syndrome of inappropriate secretion of antidiuretic hormone and neurotoxicity induced by vincristine and alkylating agents during chemotherapy for malignant lymphoma of thyroid gland). Gan To Kagaku Ryoho 1998;25(5):757–60.
72. DeFronzo RA, et al. Proceedings: Cyclophosphamide and the kidney. Cancer 1974;33(2):483–91.
73. Kende G, et al. Blurring of vision: a previously undescribed complication of cyclophosphamide therapy. Cancer 1979;44(1):69–71.

74. Tashima CK. Immediate cerebral symptoms during rapid intravenous administration of cyclophosphamide (NSC-26271). Cancer Chemother Rep 1975;59(2 Pt 1):441–2.
75. Schiller G, Lee M. Long-term outcome of high-dose cytarabine-based consolidation chemotherapy for older patients with acute myelogenous leukemia. Leuk Lymphoma 1997; 25(1–2):111–9.
76. Smith GA, et al. High-dose cytarabine dose modification reduces the incidence of neurotoxicity in patients with renal insufficiency. J Clin Oncol 1997;15(2):833–9.
77. Martin DP, Wallace TL, Johnson Jr EM. Cytosine arabinoside kills postmitotic neurons in a fashion resembling trophic factor deprivation: evidence that a deoxycytidine-dependent process may be required for nerve growth factor signal transduction. J Neurosci 1990;10(1):184–93.
78. Geller HM, et al. Oxidative stress mediates neuronal DNA damage and apoptosis in response to cytosine arabinoside. J Neurochem 2001;78(2):265–75.
79. Garcia-Tena J, et al. Intrathecal chemotherapy-related myeloencephalopathy in a young child with acute lymphoblastic leukemia. Pediatr Hematol Oncol 1995;12(4):377–85.
80. Ozon A, et al. Acute ascending myelitis and encephalopathy after intrathecal cytosine arabinoside and methotrexate in an adolescent boy with acute lymphoblastic leukemia. Brain and Development 1994;16(3):246–8.
81. Ruggiero A, et al. Intrathecal chemotherapy with antineoplastic agents in children. Paediatr Drugs 2001;3(4):237–46.
82. Borgeat A, De Muralt B, Stalder M. Peripheral neuropathy associated with high-dose Ara-C therapy. Cancer 1986;58(4):852–4.
83. Imrie KR, et al. Peripheral neuropathy following high-dose etoposide and autologous bone marrow transplantation. Bone Marrow Transplant 1994;13(1):77–9.
84. Leff RS, et al. Acute neurologic dysfunction after high-dose etoposide therapy for malignant glioma. Cancer 1988;62(1):32–5.
85. Chun HG, et al. Central nervous system toxicity of fludarabine phosphate. Cancer Treat Rep 1986;70(10):1225–8.
86. Meyer T, Ludolph AC, Munch C. Ifosfamide encephalopathy presenting with asterixis. J Neurol Sci 2002;199(1–2):85–8.
87. Primavera A, Audenino D, Cocito L. Ifosfamide encephalopathy and nonconvulsive status epilepticus. Can J Neurol Sci 2002;29(2):180–3.
88. Curtin JP, et al. Ifosfamide-induced neurotoxicity. Gynecol Oncol 1991;42(3):193–6 discussion 191–2.
89. Comandone A, et al. Two episodes of ifosfamide-related neurotoxicity in the same patient following different schedules and doses of the drug. A case report. Tumori 2000;86(6):483–6.
90. Carlson L, et al. Toxicity, pharmacokinetics, and in vitro hemodialysis clearance of ifosfamide and metabolites in an anephric pediatric patient with Wilms' tumor. Cancer Chemother Pharmacol 1998;41(2):140–6.
91. Keizer HJ, et al. Ifosfamide treatment as a 10-day continuous intravenous infusion. J Cancer Res Clin Oncol 1995;121(5):297–302.
92. Sood C, O'Brien PJ. 2-Chloroacetaldehyde-induced cerebral glutathione depletion and neurotoxicity. Br J Cancer Suppl 1996;27:S287–93.
93. Turner AR, Duong CD, Good DJ. Methylene blue for the treatment and prophylaxis of ifosfamide-induced encephalopathy. Clin Oncol (R Coll Radiol) 2003;15(7):435–9.
94. Raj AB, Bertolone SJ, Jaffe N. Methylene blue reversal of ifosfamide-related encephalopathy. J Pediatr Hematol Oncol 2004;26(2):116.
95. Kupfer A, Aeschlimann C, Cerny T. Methylene blue and the neurotoxic mechanisms of ifosfamide encephalopathy. Eur J Clin Pharmacol 1996;50(4):249–52.
96. Kupfer A, et al. Prophylaxis and reversal of ifosfamide encephalopathy with methylene-blue. Lancet 1994;343(8900):763–4.
97. Hill JM, et al. A comparative study of the long term psychosocial functioning of childhood acute lymphoblastic leukemia survivors treated by intrathecal methotrexate with or without cranial radiation. Cancer 1998;82(1):208–18.
98. Walker RW, et al. Transient cerebral dysfunction secondary to high-dose methotrexate. J Clin Oncol 1986;4(12):1845–50.
99. Phillips PC, et al. Acute high-dose methotrexate neurotoxicity in the rat. Ann Neurol 1986;20(5):583–9.
100. Phillips PC, et al. High-dose leucovorin reverses acute high-dose methotrexate neurotoxicity in the rat. Ann Neurol 1989;25(4):365–72.

101. Bernini JC, et al. Aminophylline for methotrexate-induced neurotoxicity. Lancet 1995; 345(8949):544–7.
102. Kishi S, et al. Homocysteine, pharmacogenetics, and neurotoxicity in children with leukemia. J Clin Oncol 2003;21(16):3084–91.
103. Quinn CT, et al. Elevation of homocysteine and excitatory amino acid neurotransmitters in the CSF of children who receive methotrexate for the treatment of cancer. J Clin Oncol 1997;15(8):2800–6.
104. Millot F, et al. Changes of cerebral biopterin and biogenic amine metabolism in leukemic children receiving 5 g/m2 intravenous methotrexate. Pediatr Res 1995;37(2):151–4.
105. Mott MG, Stevenson P, Wood CB. Methotrexate meningitis. Lancet 1972;2(7778):656.
106. Bates SE, et al. Ascending myelopathy after chemotherapy for central nervous system acute lymphoblastic leukemia: correlation with cerebrospinal fluid myelin basic protein. Med Pediatr Oncol 1985;13(1):4–8.
107. Surtees R, Clelland J, Hann I. Demyelination and single-carbon transfer pathway metabolites during the treatment of acute lymphoblastic leukemia: CSF studies. J Clin Oncol 1998;16(4):1505–11.
108. Lien HH, et al. Osteogenic sarcoma: MR signal abnormalities of the brain in asymptomatic patients treated with high-dose methotrexate. Radiology 1991;179(2):547–50.
109. Postma TJ, et al. Neurotoxicity of combination chemotherapy with procarbazine, CCNU and vincristine (PCV) for recurrent glioma. J Neurooncol 1998;38(1):69–75.
110. Shingleton BJ, et al. Ocular toxicity associated with high-dose carmustine. Arch Ophthalmol 1982;100(11):1766–72.
111. Rosenblum MK, et al. Fatal necrotizing encephalopathy complicating treatment of malignant gliomas with intra-arterial BCNU and irradiation: a pathological study. J Neurooncol 1989;7(3):269–81.
112. Wilson WB, Perez GM, Kleinschmidt-Demasters BK. Sudden onset of blindness in patients treated with oral CCNU and low-dose cranial irradiation. Cancer 1987;59(5):901–7.
113. Donzelli E, et al. Neurotoxicity of platinum compounds: comparison of the effects of cisplatin and oxaliplatin on the human neuroblastoma cell line SH-SY5Y. J Neurooncol 2004; 67(1–2):65–73.
114. Gent P, Massey K. An overview of chemotherapy-induced peripheral sensory neuropathy, focusing on oxaliplatin. Int J Palliat Nurs 2001;7(7):354–9.
115. Grothey A. Oxaliplatin-safety profile: neurotoxicity. Semin Oncol 2003;30(4 Suppl. 15):5–13.
116. Cavaletti G, et al. Neurotoxicity and ototoxicity of cisplatin plus paclitaxel in comparison to cisplatin plus cyclophosphamide in patients with epithelial ovarian cancer. J Clin Oncol 1997;15(1):199–206.
117. Fossa SD, et al. Clinical and biochemical long-term toxicity after postoperative cisplatin-based chemotherapy in patients with low-stage testicular cancer. Oncology 1995;52(4):300–5.
118. Higa GM, Wise TC, Crowell EB. Severe, disabling neurologic toxicity following cisplatin retreatment. Ann Pharmacother 1995;29(2):134–7.
119. Keime-Guibert F, Napolitano M, Delattre JY. Neurological complications of radiotherapy and chemotherapy. J Neurol 1998;245(11):695–708.
120. Lorusso V, et al. Carboplatin plus ifosfamide as salvage treatment of epithelial ovarian cancer: a pilot study. J Clin Oncol 1993;11(10):1952–6.
121. Neijt JP, Lund B. Paclitaxel with carboplatin for the treatment of ovarian cancer. Semin Oncol 1996;23(6 Suppl. 15):2–4.
122. Petersen PM, Hansen SW. The course of long-term toxicity in patients treated with cisplatin-based chemotherapy for non-seminomatous germ-cell cancer. Ann Oncol 1999;10(12):1475–83.
123. Fu KK, Kai EF, Leung CK. Cisplatin neuropathy: a prospective clinical and electrophysiological study in Chinese patients with ovarian carcinoma. J Clin Pharm Ther 1995;20(3):167–72.
124. Troy L, et al. Cisplatin-based therapy: a neurological and neuropsychological review. Psychooncology 2000;9(1):29–39.
125. von Schlippe M, Fowler CJ, Harland SJ. Cisplatin neurotoxicity in the treatment of metastatic germ cell tumour: time course and prognosis. Br J Cancer 2001;85(6):823–6.
126. Cassidy J, Misset JL. Oxaliplatin-related side effects: characteristics and management. Semin Oncol 2002;29(5 Suppl. 15):11–20.
127. Gregg RW, et al. Cisplatin neurotoxicity: the relationship between dosage, time, and platinum concentration in neurologic tissues, and morphologic evidence of toxicity. J Clin Oncol 1992;10(5):795–803.

128. Salvinelli F, et al. Bilateral irreversible hearing loss associated with the combination of carboplatin and paclitaxel chemotherapy: a unusual side effect. J Exp Clin Cancer Res 2003;22(1):155–8.
129. Kollmannsberger C, et al. Late toxicity following curative treatment of testicular cancer. Semin Surg Oncol 1999;17(4):275–81.
130. Calhoun EA, et al. Perceptions of cisplatin-related toxicity among ovarian cancer patients and gynecologic oncologists. Gynecol Oncol 1998;71(3):369–75.
131. Bokemeyer C, et al. Evaluation of long-term toxicity after chemotherapy for testicular cancer. J Clin Oncol 1996;14(11):2923–32.
132. Chaudhary UB, Haldas JR. Long-term complications of chemotherapy for germ cell tumours. Drugs 2003;63(15):1565–77.
133. Perol M, et al. Multicenter randomized trial comparing cisplatin-mitomycin-vinorelbine versus cisplatin-mitomycin-vindesine in advanced non-small cell lung cancer. 'Groupe Francais de Pneumo-Cancerologie'. Lung Cancer 1996;14(1):119–34.
134. van der Hulst RJ, Dreschler WA, Urbanus NA. High frequency audiometry in prospective clinical research of ototoxicity due to platinum derivatives. Ann Otol Rhinol Laryngol 1988;97(2 Pt 1):133–7.
135. Gamelin L, Boisdron-Celle M, Delva R. Prevention of oxaliplatin related neurotoxicity by calcium and magnesium infusions: A retrospective study of 161 patints receiving oxaliplatin combined with 5-fluorouracil and leucovorin for advanced colorectal cancer. Clin Cancer Res 2004;10:4055–61.
136. Spivack SD. Drugs 5 years later: procarbazine. Ann Int Med 1974;81(6):795–800.
137. Stolinsky DC, et al. Clinical experience with procarbazine in Hodgkin's disease, reticulum cell sarcoma, and lymphosarcoma. Cancer 1970;26(5):984–90.
138. Kuroi K, Shimozuma K. Neurotoxicity of taxanes: symptoms and quality of life assessment. Breast Cancer 2004;11(1):92–9.
139. Guastalla 3rd JP, Dieras V. The taxanes: toxicity and quality of life considerations in advanced ovarian cancer. Br J Cancer 2003;89(Suppl. 3):S16–22.
140. Apfel SC, et al. Nerve growth factor prevents toxic neuropathy in mice. Ann Neurol 1991;29(1):87–90.
141. Hamers FP, et al. The ACTH-(4–9) analog, ORG 2766, prevents taxol-induced neuropathy in rats. Eur J Pharmacol 1993;233(1):177–8.
142. Perry JR, Warner E. Transient encephalopathy after paclitaxel (Taxol) infusion. Neurology 1996;46(6):1596–9.
143. Naumann R, et al. Early recognition of hereditary motor and sensory neuropathy type 1 can avoid life-threatening vincristine neurotoxicity. Br J Haematol 2001;115(2):323–5.
144. Chauvenet AR, et al. Vincristine-induced neuropathy as the initial presentation of charcot-marie-tooth disease in acute lymphoblastic leukemia: a Pediatric Oncology Group study. J Pediatr Hematol Oncol 2003;25(4):316–20.
145. Trobaugh-Lotrario AD, Smith AA, Odom LF. Vincristine neurotoxicity in the presence of hereditary neuropathy. Med Pediatr Oncol 2003;40(1):39–43.
146. Uno S, et al. (Acute vincristine neurotoxicity in a non-Hodgkin's lymphoma patient with Charcot-Marie-Tooth disease). Rinsho Ketsueki 1999;40(5):414–9.
147. Neumann Y, et al. Vincristine treatment triggering the expression of asymptomatic Charcot-Marie-Tooth disease. Med Pediatr Oncol 1996;26(4):280–3.
148. Orejana-Garcia AM, Pascual-Huerta J, Perez-Melero A. Charcot-Marie-Tooth disease and vincristine. J Am Podiatr Med Assoc 2003;93(3):229–33.
149. Petrini M, et al. Is lithium able to reverse neurological damage induced by vinca alkaloids? (Short communication). J Neural Transm 1999;106(5–6):569–75.
150. Al Ferayan A, et al. Cerebrospinal fluid lavage in the treatment of inadvertent intrathecal vincristine injection. Childs Nerv Syst 1999;15(2–3):87–9.
151. Alcaraz A, et al. Intrathecal vincristine: fatal myeloencephalopathy despite cerebrospinal fluid perfusion. J Toxicol Clin Toxicol 2002;40(5):557–61.
152. Kwack EK, et al. Neural toxicity induced by accidental intrathecal vincristine administration. J Korean Med Sci 1999;14(6):688–92.
153. Meggs WJ, Hoffman RS. Fatality resulting from intraventricular vincristine administration. J Toxicol Clin Toxicol 1998;36(3):243–6.
154. Fernandez CV, et al. Intrathecal vincristine: an analysis of reasons for recurrent fatal chemotherapeutic error with recommendations for prevention. J Pediatr Hematol Oncol 1998;20(6):587–90.

155. Glusker P, Recht L, Lane B. Reversible posterior leukoencephalopathy syndrome and bevacizumab. N Engl J Med 2006;354(9):980–2; discussion 980–2.
156. Peter S, et al. Reversible posterior leukoencephalopathy syndrome and intravenous bevacizumab. Clin Experiment Ophthalmol 2008;36(1):94–6.
157. Vaughn C, Zhang L, Schiff D. Reversible posterior leukoencephalopathy syndrome in cancer. Curr Oncol Rep 2008;10(1):86–91.
158. Badros A, et al. Neurotoxicity of bortezomib therapy in multiple myeloma: a single-center experience and review of the literature. Cancer 2007;110(5):1042–9.
159. Gupta S, et al. Life-threatening motor neurotoxicity in association with bortezomib. Haematologica 2006;91(7):1001.
160. Kannarkat G, Lasher EE, Schiff D. Neurologic complications of chemotherapy agents. Curr Opin Neurol 2007;20(6):719–25.

17 Neurological Complications of Radiation Therapy

DAMIEN RICARD • CAROLE SOUSSAIN • ANTHONY BÉHIN • DAYSI CHI

Introduction

Radiation therapy (RT) plays a key role in neuro-oncology but is associated with significant, sometimes life-threatening, neurotoxicity. The development of new techniques (such as radiosurgery or brachytherapy) has widened the indications of RT to include more benign conditions (e.g., trigeminal neuralgia or vascular malformations), and has increased rates of long-term survivors who may develop late toxicity. Thus, complications of RT have gained increasing interest. Nervous tissue tolerance depends on several currently well-defined factors such as volume, total dose, dose per fraction, and duration of irradiation. In addition, other factors that may increase the risk of radiation-induced toxicity are older age, concurrent diseases (such as diabetes, hypertension), vascular disease, adjuvant chemotherapy, and probably genetic predisposition.[1,2] The adverse neurological effects of radiotherapy are usually classified according to the time course in relation to irradiation and include acute disorders (days to weeks), early-delayed complications (1 to 6 months) and late-delayed complications (more than 6 months) (Table 17-1). Radiation damage may be direct to the central or peripheral nervous system, or secondary to vascular or endocrine lesions or to the development of a radiation-induced tumor (Figure 17-1).

HISTOPATHOLOGY

Due to the difficulty in obtaining irradiated human tissue, histopathological studies of irradiated brains in human are scarce. However, a few autopsy studies in adults and children are available and show similar features of vascular and demyelinating lesions at light microscopic level. Lai et al.[3] studied the brains of five adult patients with primary CNS lymphoma who were in complete remission, but who died after combined modality therapy with WBRT and chemotherapy. The MRIs showed cerebral atrophy, ventricular dilatation, and white matter hyperintensity on FLAIR and T2 images. Occasional enhancing lesions were observed. The corresponding histopathological lesions were myelin and axonal loss, spongiosis, gliosis in white matter, fibrotic thickening of small blood vessels in the deep white matter, and atherosclerosis of the large vessels in the circle of Willis. All patients but one were older than 60, and symptoms of neurotoxicity developed within 3 months of completion of treatment. An autopsy study was performed in 34 children with gliomas, 22 of whom had undergone CNS radiation therapy.[4] Causes of death were not detailed in this study and the cognitive status of the children before they died was unknown. Lesions such as demyelination, focal necrosis, cortical atrophy, endothelial proliferation, vascular thrombosis, and vascular

TABLE 17-1 Main Neurological Complications of Radiotherapy

SITE	ACUTE COMPLICATIONS <4 weeks after RT	EARLY-DELAYED COMPLICATIONS 1 to 6 months after RT	LATE-DELAYED COMPLICATIONS > 6 months after RT
Brain	Acute encephalopathy	Somnolence syndrome Worsening of preexisting symptoms Transient cognitive impairment Subacute rhombencephalitis	Focal brain radionecrosis Cognitive impairment and leukoencephalopathy Secondary brain tumors
Spinal cord		Lhermitte sign	Focal spinal radionecrosis Progressive myelopathy Spinal hemorrhage
Cranial nerves		Transient hearing loss Anosmia Ageusia	Hearing loss Visual loss Lower cranial nerve palsies
Peripheral nerves	Paresthesias	Brachial or lumbosacral plexopathy (transient)	Brachial or lumbosacral plexopathy Malignant nerve sheath tumors Lower motor neuron syndrome

thickening were more frequently observed in irradiated brains, whereas neuronal degeneration, cerebral edema, and gliosis were common in irradiated and nonirradiated brains. Demyelination was observed at all time points from 6 months but was more frequent 9 months after radiotherapy. Vascular changes appeared as a late effect of radiation injury. Panagiotakos et al.[5] performed an original and extensive study on human normal and irradiated white matter brain samples from surgical biopsies of glial tissue around tumor. Histological assessments of human tissue were completed by ultrastructural analysis and immunohistochemistry. Samples from irradiated patients exhibited persistent loss of oligoprogenitors starting as early as 2 months after radiation, whereas the decline of more mature oligodendrocytes only started beyond a year after irradiation. Early and transitory endothelial cell loss was noted. Myelin sheaths showed signs of degradation. Signs suggesting axonal damage were only seen late after irradiation. Neuronal cell bodies seemed to be spared from radiation injury.

Radiation-induced histolopathological lesions in brain were studied in rats in a few prospective studies, using either only light microscopy analysis or more sophisticated methods such as immunocytochemical and ultrastructural analysis. Kamiryo et al.[6] studied histological changes in the rat brain within 1 year of radiation at doses of 50, 75, and 120 Gy, mimicking therapeutic radiosurgery. The authors observed time-dependent and dose-dependent changes. The first lesions to appear were morphological changes in astrocytes, followed by vasodilation and fibrin deposition in capillary walls for all the studied doses. BBB leakage (Evans blue permeability assay) was observed only after 75 and

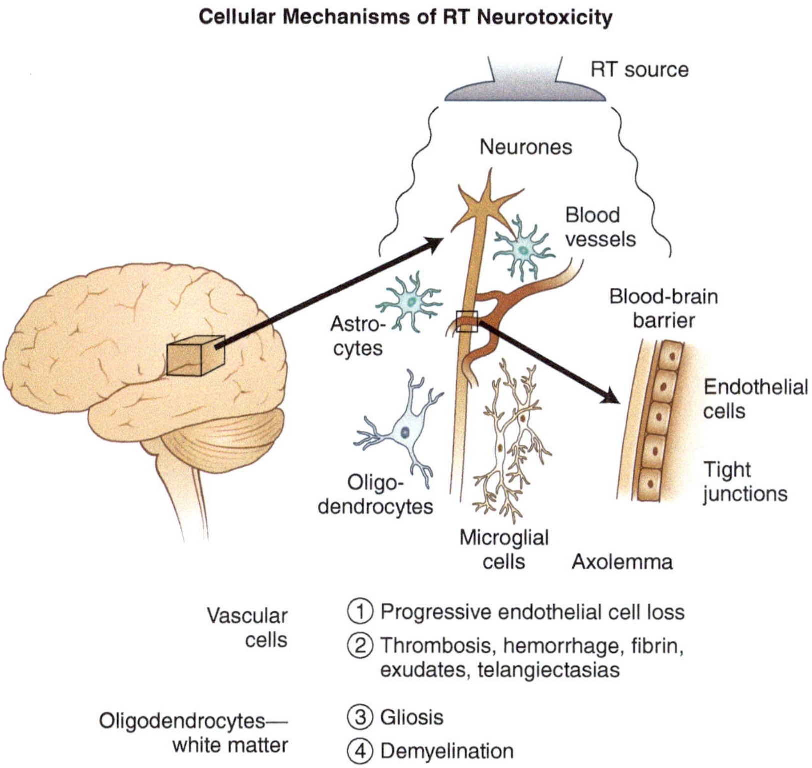

Figure 17-1 Pathophysiology of RT-induced neurotoxicity. The mechanism of RT-induced damage to the CNS is complex and likely to include a combination of vascular injury, demyelination and neuronal damage. The vascular injury is thought to be partly responsible for the abnormal vasculature, thrombosis, and fibrinoid necrosis seen in radiation necrosis. RT also causes depletion of oligodendrocytes, which in turn leads to demyelination and white matter necrosis. Other targets of RT damage include neurons, astrocytes, and microglia.

120 Gy, and necrosis only after 120 Gy. The time course of these lesions varied dramatically with radiation dose: after 120 Gy, the first lesions were observed only 3 days after irradiation and the whole set of lesions occurred within 4 weeks, whereas after 50 Gy, first lesions were only seen at 3 months and developed over 12 months.

An earlier study by Calvo et al.[7] focused on radiation-induced damage in the choroid plexus of the rat brain after a single dose of 17.5 to 25 Gy. They observed early morphological changes in the epithelial cells, followed by interstitial fibrosis associated with degenerative changes of arterioles and thrombi. Severity of lesions was dose and time dependent. The same authors later showed that necrosis was more frequent and occurred earlier in the fimbria than in the internal capsule and corpus callosum. They found a correlation between the incidence of necrosis in the white matter, seen after a latent interval of 26 weeks, and earlier changes in the vasculature such as blood vessel dilatation, blood vessel wall thickening, endothelial cell nuclear enlargement, and hypertrophy of perivascular astrocytes.

Fractionated (eight fractions) WBRT (40 Gy) was delivered to adult rats by Yoneoka et al.,[8] more closely modeling therapeutic irradiation in humans. Though rats showed radiation-induced cognitive dysfunction, no histological abnormalities were found in irradiated brains over 12 months after irradiation. This study suggested that cognitive dysfunction can either precede morphological changes in the brain, or even arise without them. It is worthy of note that only light microscopic examination was performed. Vascular permeability was not assessed.

Iradiation of the spinal cord led to progressive abnormalities in the white matter, beginning at 19 weeks, for doses greater than 17 Gy. The spinal cord of paralyzed animals showed areas of necrosis and demyelination, but neither gross vascular lesion nor inflammatory infiltrate was found.[9] Occasional vessel dilation was observed.

PATHOPHYSIOLOGY

The pathophysiology of white matter abnormalities potentially leading to necrosis are not fully understood, but several hypotheses have been proposed. Because histological examination usually shows vascular lesions and demyelination, vessels and glial cells have often been considered as the primary target of radiation injury (Figure 17-1). However, the situation is probably more complicated: recently, the interactions between radiation and other cell types have been studied more closely, as well as the regenerative abilities of the CNS.[10] A short discussion of the main aspects of the pathophysiology of RT-related injuries is described in the following sections.

Vascular Damage

Transient disruption of the blood-brain barrier, possibly initiated by sphingomyelinase-mediated endothelial apoptosis, is thought to be responsible for the *acute or early-delayed*, steroid-responsive forms of radiation toxicity.[11–13] A vascular theory has also been advocated to explain radiation necrosis. Necrosis would be a consequence of ischemia secondary to blood vessel damage. Vascular damage is indeed prominent during radionecrosis, including thrombosis, hemorrhage, fibrinous exudates, telangiectasias, vascular fibrosis/hyalinization with luminal stenosis, and fibrinoid vascular necrosis. Furthermore, a progressive endothelial cell loss and vessel rarefaction seems to precede white matter necrosis.[12] Thus, a cascade (involving signaling molecules among others) could be initiated at the time of irradiation, producing gradual cell loss throughout the clinically silent period.[3] At the molecular level, VEGF seems to play a pivotal role in the endothelial cell loss.[9] This progressive loss would eventually lead to overt necrosis.[14] Despite these findings, several points argue against a purely ischemic model: first, neurons are very sensitive to ischemia and should be prominently damaged if the lesion was primarily vascular, whereas neurons are in fact largely spared during radionecrosis.[15] Second, vascular damage is not always present in radionecrosis.[16] Other cellular mechanisms may be involved and perpetuate vascular damage or contribute to edema, gliosis, and demyelination in the brain, such as upregulation of diverse adhesion molecules,[17] production of cytokines,[18,19] or cumulative oxidative stress in endothelial cells.

Oligodendrocytes

The demyelinating lesions observed after RT underscore the putative role of oligodendrocytes as a target of radiation damage. Oligodendrocytes are responsible for the production of the myelin sheath in the CNS and derive from progenitor cells such as O-2A. CNS radiation induces depletion of oligodendrocytes and suppresses, at least transiently, the production of oligodendrocyte progenitors,[20–22] possibly through a p53-dependent pathway.[23–25] However, the contribution of demyelination in tissue destruction remains questionable since severely demyelinating conditions such as multiple sclerosis do not lead to overt necrosis.[15]

Other CNS Cell Types

Several studies over the past few years have focused on the potential role of neurons, astrocytes, and microglia in the development of radiation-induced lesions, either as primary targets or through alterations of their regulatory capacity.[26–28] Particularly noteworthy is the possible role of microglia[29] that may enhance radiation injury through persistent oxidative stress.[30,31] Radiation damage to the subventricular zone, a tissue containing glial and neural stem cells, was reported more than 25 years ago.[32] Recent studies have found a dose-dependent reduction of neural stem cells of the subependyma after irradiation in this region.[33,34] Their implication in radiation injury thus seems probable but remains to be elucidated.

As a whole, the development of radiation injury is complex, and results from interactions between vascular cells and oligodendrocytes, as well as neural stem cells and the physiological responses of these cells to injury. A wide range of cell interactions mediated by cytokines and other molecules and the influence of indirect factors such as microglial proliferation or the production of oxidative products resulting from cell destruction may account for the wide variety of lesions observed from a patient to another.

Sequelae of Radiation Therapy to the Brain

ACUTE ENCEPHALOPATHY

Acute encephalopathy usually appears within 2 weeks after the beginning of cranial RT, often a few hours after delivery of the first fraction. The patient presents with nausea and vomiting, drowsiness, headache, dysarthria, and a worsening of preexisting neurological deficits, sometimes associated with fever. The clinical course is usually favorable, but herniation and death have been reported in patients with large tumors who have already presented with intracranial hypertension (e.g., in multiple metastases, posterior fossa tumors, or intraventricular tumors). Large doses per fraction (usually >3 Gy/fraction) are the main risk factor: Young et al.[35] reported acute radiation damage in 50% of patients with brain metastases treated with 15 Gy in two fractions, and Hindo et al.[36] reported four deaths within 48 hours of a 10 Gy RT given in one fraction. As these large doses are no longer in use, this syndrome is rarely seen. However, a minor form of this condition occurs in many patients, consisting of nausea and moderate headache occurring within hours following cranial irradiation. Steroids may help in preventing or limiting the consequences of acute encephalopathy, especially in patients with large primary or secondary brain tumors or with considerable edema, particularly those at risk of herniation. In such patients, daily doses of steroids of at least 16 mg dexamethasone should be prescribed 48 to 72 hr before the first fraction; a limitation of dose per fraction (2 Gy or less per fraction) is also recommended in this situation.[37,38] The pathophysiology of acute complications supposedly results from radiation-induced blood-brain barrier (BBB) disruption, accounting for a rise in intracranial pressure.[39] To prevent this complication, surgical debulking should, ideally, be carried out before starting RT treatment.

EARLY-DELAYED COMPLICATIONS OF RT

Several early-delayed clinical patterns have been described (Table 17-1). They occur 2 weeks to 6 months after RT. The pathophysiology is thought to be due to a transient demyelinating process triggered by BBB disruption and/or selective oligodendrocyte dysfunction.

Somnolence Syndrome

This condition was first described in the late 1920s in children receiving low-dose RT for scalp ringworm. Several studies reported cases of children who developed somnolence syndrome 5 to 8 weeks after prophylactic cranial RT for leukemia[40,41]; other reports have shown that it also occurs in adults. The incidence of somnolence syndrome varies greatly (with figures ranging from 8%[41] to 84%[42]; this difference is related to various factors including tumor types, radiation dose, fractionation, and diagnostic criteria).[43] Prominent symptoms include drowsiness, hypersomnolence, nausea, and anorexia. Headache and/or fever may also be reported. Friends or family often notice irritability, attentional deficits, and short-term memory impairment. The clinical severity of this complication is variable, with extremes ranging from minimal disorders to sleep periods of over 20 hours a day.[41] MRI studies are not contributory. Electroencephalographic abnormalities include nonspecific diffuse slow waves.[43] Most studies report a monophasic course of symptoms, usually with a favorable outcome within a few weeks. However, a prospective study on 19 adults treated for primary brain tumors with cranial RT (45 to 55 Gy) reported a biphasic pattern of symptoms with two critical periods (from the 11th to the 21st day and from the 31st to the 35th day) following RT.[44] Furthermore, in this study, an accelerated fractionation led to significantly more severe drowsiness and fatigue than a conventional scheme. Some authors advocate the use of steroids during and after radiotherapy as prophylactic or symptomatic treatment.[45] A prospective double-blind randomized trial in leukemic children found that a dose of 4 mg/m^2 of dexamethasone during cranial radiotherapy reduced the incidence of somnolence syndrome (17.6% vs. 64.3%) as compared to a dose of 2 mg/m^2.[46]

Worsening of Preexisting Symptoms, or Tumor Pseudoprogression

In patients under treatment for malignant brain tumors, a worsening of preexisting neurological focal deficits leads to concerns over tumor progression, especially when observed in association with features of the somnolence syndrome and with transitory cognitive impairment. This complication arises within 6 weeks to 3 months after RT, and is clinically impossible to differentiate from progressive disease. Neuroimaging may be normal or show edema and contrast enhancement within the tumor bed, a situation that does not allow this syndrome to be differentiated from tumor recurrence and explains why inclusion of patients in experimental regimens for "recurrence" is not indicated during this period[47]; it is worth noting that this radiological pattern can also be associated with no clinical worsening—"pseudoprogression" rates can reach 20% after a concomitant temozolomide and radiotherapy regimen used to treat glioblastoma and may be associated with better tumor response.[48] Improvement usually follows within a few weeks or months and a close followup of CT or MR scan will show spontaneous regression within 4 to 8 weeks. As in the somnolence syndrome, the treatment lies in supportive care with steroids. Improvements in imaging techniques such as magnetic resonance spectroscopy (MRS) may help in distinguishing between pseudoprogression and true progression but are limited by the fact that residual tumor is often still present within the irradiated area.

Transient Cognitive Decline

A transient cognitive decline can be observed within the first 6 months after cranial RT, mainly affecting attention and recent memory, and may sometimes be associated with a somnolence syndrome. Armstrong et al.[49] prospectively followed five patients treated for primary brain tumors: memory impairment was conspicuous in all patients 1.5 months after focal cranial RT (43 to 63 Gy), but complete regression was observed after 2.5 to 10.5 months. In another prospective study by Vigliani et al.[50] comparing 17 patients treated with focal cranial RT (54 Gy) for good-prognosis gliomas and 14 matched control patients who did not undergo RT, 36% of the patients had a significant early-delayed impairment of their reaction test, with a return to normal baseline performance 12 months after RT. This test result was correlated with their occupational status: 69% of the patients could not work at 6 months, whereas 73% had continued or resumed their jobs at 1 year. In our experience, informing patients about this possible difficulty in returning to a normal life (particularly work), at least during the first 6 months following radiotherapy, is useful. Although severe and, in some cases, persistent early-delayed symptoms have been occasionally reported,[51] it is of note that transient cognitive impairment does not appear to be a clear-cut prognostic factor predicting the further development of long-term cognitive disorders.

Subacute Rhombencephalitis

Distinct from brainstem radionecrosis, which occurs later, early-delayed subacute rhombencephalitis may be observed about 1 to 3 months after RT using portals involving the brainstem, as in ocular, pituitary, or head and neck tumors. The clinical picture includes ataxia, dysarthria, diplopia, and/or nystagmus as well as auditory loss. In some cases, the cerebrospinal fluid analysis shows inflammatory changes. MRI may demonstrate white matter abnormalities appearing as grossly round or more extensive T1-weighted hypointensities and T2-weighted hyperintensities affecting the brainstem and the cerebellar peduncles; the lesions may enhance after gadolinium injection.[52,53] The condition usually improves progressively over a few weeks to a few months, either spontaneously or with steroids, but coma and death have been reported in rare cases.[54,55]

LATE-DELAYED COMPLICATIONS OF RT

Two main delayed complications may follow RT, usually after more than 6 months: focal radionecrosis and mild to severe cognitive impairment associated with leukoencephalopathy. These adverse effects may occasionally be delayed by many years.

Focal Brain Radionecrosis

Focal radionecrosis constitutes a challenging complication of radiation therapy because it often mimics tumor recurrence and its functional consequences can be devastating. This complication may occur not only in patients who received local RT for a primary or metastasic brain tumor but also in patients without brain lesions with a history of RT for extraparenchymal lesions, in whom normal brain was included in the radiation field (head and neck or pituitary tumors, meningiomas, skull osteosarcomas). A classical example is the bilateral medial temporal lobe necrosis that results from RT for pituitary or nasopharyngeal tumors. This once frequent complication of conventional RT has become rarer over the last 20 years, as a consequence of the generalized use of safer irradiation protocols. It has been shown that the upper limits of a "safe dose" were defined by a total dose of 55 to 60 Gy administered to a focal field with fractions of 1.8 to 2 Gy per day. Vascular risk factors such as diabetes, old age, and associated chemotherapy may also favor the potential development of radionecrosis. However, patients without any particular risk factors may develop radiation necrosis, probably because of an individual, unpredictable sensitivity to irradiation.[56] The focal delivery of a single large radiation fraction during "radiosurgery" may also lead to focal necrosis of the brain adjacent to the irradiated lesion. In arteriovenous malformations (AVM), the incidence of brain necrosis ranges from less than 5% to 20% of cases, with location and volume found to be the main risk factors.[57–59] After standard RT, radiation necrosis generally occurs within 1 to 2 years,[60] but it has also been observed after several decades. As described above, shorter latencies (as short as 3 months) have also been reported, especially in patients treated with interstitial brachytherapy[61] or radiosurgery. Patients may experience seizures (first symptom in about 50% of cases), intracranial hypertension, and/or focal neurological deficits.[62–64] Such symptoms closely mimic tumor recurrence or progression.

Diagnosing radiation necrosis is often a challenge. In many cases, CT and MR scans show a tumor-like pattern, often indistinguishable from tumor progression or recurrence.[65] As diagnostic assessment based on clinical and standard neuroimaging data is difficult, many studies have tried to address the problem of noninvasive differentiation between tumor recurrence/progression and radionecrosis. Positron emission tomography (PET) with ^{18}F-fluorodeoxyglucose[66] or ^{11}C-methionine, single photon emission computed tomography (SPECT) with ^{201}thallium or marked methoxy-isobutyl-isonitrile (99mTc-MIBI),[67] and, more recently, the use of 3-[^{123}] iodo-alpha-methyl-l-tyrosine (IMT)[68,69] have been used to assess the nature of the lesions. In typical cases, radionecrosis is characterized by hypometabolism and tumoral growth by hypermetabolism. The more recent development of magnetic resonance spectroscopy (MRS) seems promising[70]: spectral analysis of necrosis areas shows an overall, harmonious decrease of metabolite peaks, and a possible increase of lipids corresponding to cellular necrosis; no lactate peak is observed.[71,72] However, none of these techniques offers 100% sensitivity or specificity.[73,74] One of the reasons for limitations is the frequent coexistence of radiation-induced necrosis with viable tumor tissue within the same area, a situation that obviously renders clear cut distinction impossible.[37] In some cases, angiography may provide further information, with an avascular mass seen in patients with radionecrosis; however, the risks and benefits of this procedure must be carefully weighed. While neuropathological examination remains the diagnostic standard (Figure 17-2),[75] even pathological analysis may be difficult because of the frequent mixture of both residual/recurrent tumor and radiation necrosis within the lesion.[13]

Resection of necrotic foci is often the best treatment in symptomatic cases. Steroids are generally used, with possible long-term improvement[37]; however, steroid dependence does occur. Other treatments have been reported in this setting, but their efficacy has not yet been addressed in large studies: anticoagulants have been prescribed by Glantz et al.[76] in eight glioma patients (seven with histological evidence of necrosis) after the failure of steroids, leading to improvement in five patients. In our experience, anticoagulants have been somewhat disappointing. Further assessment of this therapy is required to confirm those results. Some authors have advocated the use of hyperbaric oxygen (HBO), with the rationale that HBO increases the tissue pO_2 and enhances angiogenesis. Chuba et al.[77] treated ten patients with CNS radionecrosis (proved by biopsy in eight cases) with 100% oxygen at 2.0 to 2.4 atm for 90 to 120 minutes/session in at least 20 sessions. All patients were stabilized or improved initially, and the six surviving patients showed durable improvement after 3 to 36 months. However, most patients were given steroids, and the respective effect of each treatment is not clear. HBO treatment was also reported to improve radionecrosis due to radiosurgery.[78,79] The possible role of HBO in radiation-induced neurotoxicity needs to be evaluated in prospective trials.[80] Other drugs or combinations such as pentoxifylline, alpha-tocopherol,[81] low-iron diet, desferrioxamine, and pentobarbital[1] have also been proposed occasionally without definite evidence of efficacy. The usefulness of radioprotective agents such as difluoromethylornithine (DMO),[82] U-74389G (a 21 aminosteroid[83]), or others[84–87] in reducing the risk of necrosis remains to be determined. Preclinical studies have suggested that embryonic stem cell-derived glial precursors could be used as myelinating transplants in demyelinated postradiation experimental lesions.[88]

Several assays have been developed to identify individuals at risk for radiation sensitivity, such as analysis of the survival fraction of cultured skin fibroblasts after 2 Gy irradiation,[56] study of radiation-induced chromosomal aberrations, search for the ataxia-telangectasia mutation, and the G2 cell-cycle phase delay analysis.[1,89] However, to date, such assessments have not reached the clinical setting.

Cognitive Dysfunction and Leukoencephalopathy

Late-delayed cognitive impairment covers a wide continuum of patterns ranging from mild dysfunction to severe (and sometimes fatal) dementia, and has become an important concern over the last 20 years. The impact (and awareness) of this complication has grown partly because of a better assessment of quality-of-life

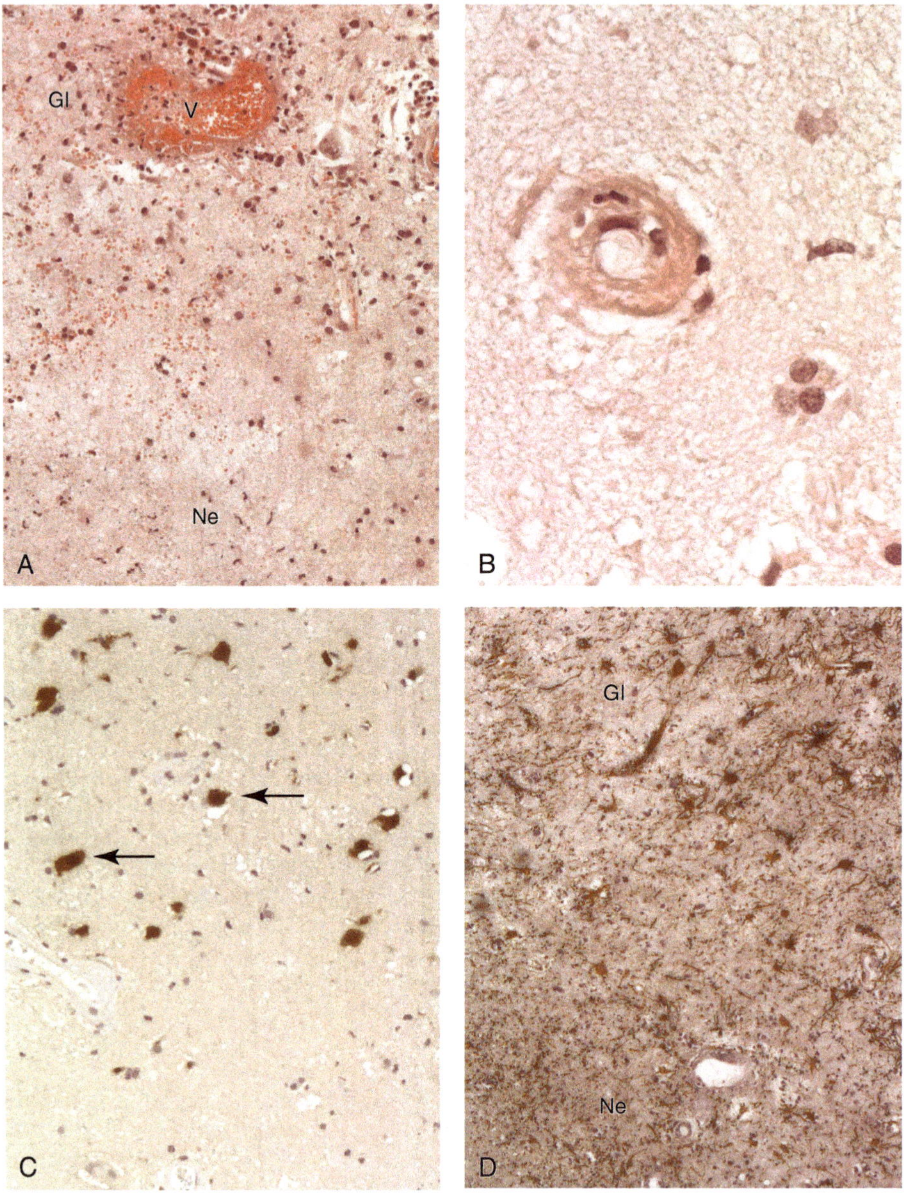

Figure 17-2 **Radionecrosis in the cortex and subcortical white matter in a patient who had received radiation treatment for a high-grade glioma. A,** Border zone between gliotic brain tissue (Gl) and area of radionecrosis, showing loss of cells, rarefaction of the tissue, and occasional foci of necrosis (Ne). **B,** Vascular changes with thickening and hyalinization of vessel walls. This example is from the transition zone between gliotic and rarefied tissue. **C,** Immunohistochemical staining for the neuronal marker NeuN showing occasional neurons labeled in brown (upper part), and in the lower part, the area of rarefaction with an entire loss of neurons. **D,** The same area stained for the astrocyte marker GFAP showing brisk reactive astrocytes on the top, and a transition to an acellular area below, containing only astrocyte processes and hardly any viable cells (Ne). Scale bar 250 μm **(A, C)**, 60 μm **(B)**, and 500 μm **(D)**.

data in clinical practice, but also because of a growing population of long-term survivors with tumor stability or remission.

Considering cognitive dysfunction as a consequence of RT alone would result in a considerable overestimation of the incidence of radiation-induced sequelae. Cognitive impairment may be the consequence of complex interactions[90] between preexisting cognitive abnormalities (especially in the case of brain tumors), brain tumor growth, concomitant treatments (such as chemotherapy, antiepileptic[91] or psychotropic drugs), paraneoplastic encephalomyelitis, and endocrine dysfunction. In practice, this should lead to a precise individual workup in patients with potential radiation-induced cognitive impairment, but also to a careful and critical interpretation of the higher cognitive dysfunction rates found in the literature. Interestingly, a study comparing 195 low-grade glioma patients (104 had undergone RT during the previous years) to low-grade hematological patients and controls, showed that cognitive dysfunction was mostly tumor-related; patients treated with doses per fraction over 2 Gy were the only ones to develop RT-linked memory impairment.[92] A more recent study of these patients followed up for 12 years has shown a progressive cognitive decline in attentional and executive tasks in patients treated with radiotherapy fractions less than 2 Gy/fraction compared with unirradiated patients, which was not apparent after 6 years follow-up.[92a]

Recent studies seem to confirm that RT plays a limited part in cognitive decline when using modern irradiation procedures.[93–95] Nevertheless, several factors have been clearly linked to an increased risk of leukoencephalopathy (Figure 17-3):

(i) *Old age*: several studies have demonstrated that demented patients were clearly older (55 to 60 years) than nondemented patients (less than 45 years old).[96–98]

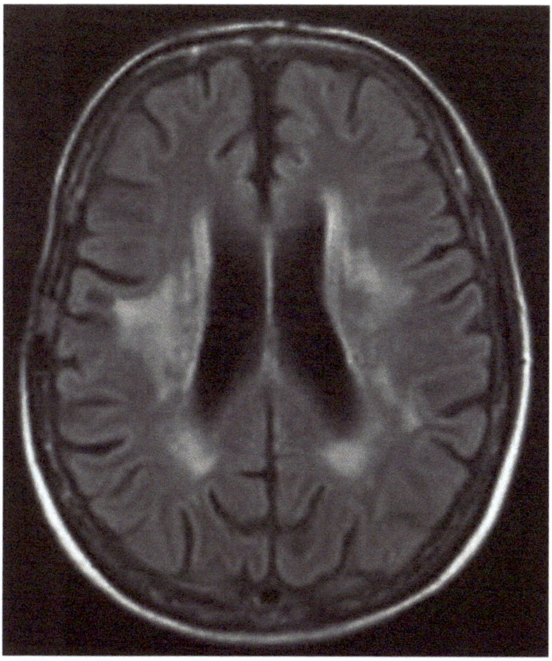

Figure 17-3 Axial FLAIR-weighted MRI of the brain showing a diffuse bilateral hypersignal of the hemispheric white matter compatible with severe radio-induced leukoencephalopathy, in a 52-year-old female patient treated with whole brain radiotherapy for brain metastases of an adenocarcinoma of the breast 15 years ago.

(ii) *Large radiation doses*, particularly when fractions over 2 Gy are used.
(iii) *Large irradiated brain volume*: this factor may also increase the risk of cognitive impairment; the rate of RT-induced cognitive dysfunction[97–100] may be as high as 50% in patients receiving whole brain radiotherapy (WBRT), whereas the precise incidence of cognitive impairment after focal brain radiotherapy is difficult to assess because of contradictory figures in the literature.[101,102]
(iv) *Combined treatment*: the incidence of dementia in patients treated with combined RT and chemotherapy ranges from 4% to 63%.

Methotrexate (MTX) is clearly implicated in combined toxicity; neurotoxic by itself, it is responsible for frequent cognitive dysfunction when associated with RT. In children, most studies to date have concluded that the combination of cranial irradiation and intrathecal MTX was associated with declines in both IQ and achievement scores.[103] In adults treated with WBRT (40 Gy + 14 Gy boost) and a combination of intravenous and intrathecal MTX for CNS lymphoma, the incidence of severe progressive cognitive impairment increases with age, reaching 83% in patients over 60 years.[104,105] The timing of MTX chemotherapy is important, because the cognitive dysfunction rate is higher whenever MTX is prescribed during or after RT. This drug should therefore be given before irradiation. Data about the neurotoxicity of other combinations are sparse, but agents such as nitrosourea, cisplatin, etoposide, cytarabine, or actinomycin D are also suspected to increase radiation-induced cognitive toxicity. Multidrug regimens or high-dose chemotherapy combined with WBRT are probably associated with a higher risk of neurotoxicity.[106] Although there is a progressive continuum between mild to moderate cognitive impairment and severe fatal dementia, we will consider the two conditions separately.

Radiation-Induced Mild to Moderate Cognitive Impairment

A mild to moderate cognitive dysfunction is more frequent in long-term survivors than real dementia. The features of this condition are not perfectly defined, as results greatly vary according to the studies, probably due to neuropsychological evaluation procedures, duration of follow-up, and population discrepancies.[107]

In most reported cases, cognitive impairment affects mainly attention and short-term memory, while intellectual functions are generally preserved as assessed by neuropsychological evaluations. Nevertherless, most patients have to decrease or even discontinue their professional activities. CT scan may be abnormal, showing periventricular hypodensities, an increase in the normal interface between white and gray matter, and ventricular enlargement. However, there seems to be no correlation between CT-scan abnormalities and the degree of cognitive impairment. MRI shows variable degrees of T2-weighted hyperintensities in the white matter, with a gross correlation between neuropsychological status and white matter lesions (Figures 17-3 and 17-4).[108]

The course of the disease is difficult to predict: some patients deteriorate slowly while the majority apparently remains stable. Progression to dementia is seldom reported. There is no recognized treatment for this syndrome although some authors have advocated the use of methylphenidate for symptomatic relief.[109] More recently, anticholinesterase drugs have been used with encouraging results.[110] Data from animal studies have also shown that the administration of erythropoietin (EPO) may prevent cognitive impairment.[111]

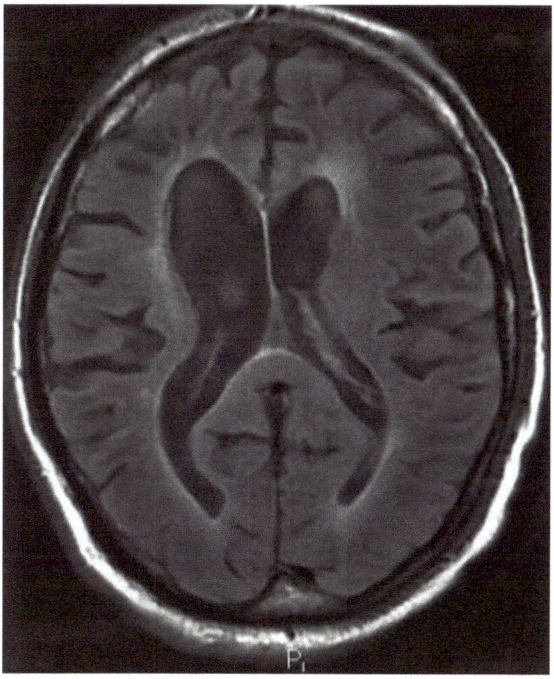

Figure 17-4 Axial FLAIR-weighted MRI of the brain showing a mild difuse white matter hypersignal and severe cortico-subcortical atrophy in a 53-year-old male treated with whole brain radiotherapy and high dose methotrexate chemotherapy 8 years ago for a primary central nervous system lymphoma.

Free-radical scavengers, such as amifostin or angiotensin-converting enzyme inhibitor (ACEi) could have a protective effect.[111b] Amifostin is already under clinical investigation with controversial results,[111c] but to date, despite encouraging preclinical data, no trial has been conducted with ACEi.

Radiation-Induced Dementia

The incidence of this devastating complication varies widely in the literature (from 0% to more than 60%) according to the series. In a large review of several studies comprising 748 adult patients, the incidence of severe cognitive impairment compatible with dementia was at least 12.3%.[112] More recent studies and clinical practice provide less cause for alarm.[30,113]

The clinical picture is characterized by a "subcortical dementia" pattern that probably reflects the consequences of diffuse white matter injury, occuring in 69% of patients within 2 years of radiotherapy.[107]

Patients present with progressive memory and attention deficits, intellectual loss, gait abnormalities, emotional lability, apathy, and fatigue.[114] The absence of hallucinations or delirium and the very unusual occurrence of aphasia, agnosia, or apraxia (deficits suggesting cortical involvement) are important clinical features for narrowing the differential diagnosis, especially in elderly patients. Depression is frequent, but antidepressants do not improve cognitive function. Eventually, patients may develop gait ataxia, incontinence, and sometimes a picture of akinetic mutism. Nonspecific features such as seizures, pyramidal or extrapyramidal signs, or tremor are also frequently encountered in the course of the disease. Neuroimaging always shows diffuse white matter lesions, best seen on MRI as

T2-weighted hyperintensities, associated with cortical and subcortical atrophy as well as ventricular enlargement (Figure 17-4). When performed, the lumbar puncture usually shows normal to moderately elevated (< 1 g/l) CSF protein levels.

No specific treatment is currently able to cure radiation-induced dementia. However, as the clinical features are similar to those of normal-pressure hydrocephalus, some authors have advocated ventriculoperitoneal shunting; this procedure does improve the quality of life in a few selected patients.[30,115,116]

Deterioration occurs in about 80% of cases, leading to the death of the patient; stabilization is possible (18% of cases). Lasting improvement is exceptional. Death generally occurs within 1 to 48 months after the onset of the disorder.[102]

Radiation-Induced Brain Tumors

The precise role of RT in the development of a tumor is difficult to determine and cannot be assessed with certainty, in great part because these tumors have no distinctive features compared to unirradiated patients. However, data from animal and epidemiological studies indicate that irradiated patients or animals are more likely to develop a second brain tumor than would have been expected from the control data.[117]

The relative risk of developing a radiation-induced tumor has been studied in several large studies. A study by Ron et al. of 10,834 patients treated with low-dose cranial and cervical irradiation for *Tinea capitis* (mean dose to neural tissue: 1.5 Gy) showed a relative risk of developing a tumor of 6.9; the risk for glioma was 2.6.[118]

In another study of 10,106 survivors of childhood cancers by the British Childhood Cancer Research Group,[119] the relative risk of developing a secondary CNS tumor was 7. Most other studies have found similar results.[120,121] However, the risk is probably higher in patients treated for acute lymphoblastic leukemia (ALL): a large retrospective cohort study of 9720 children[122] found a relative risk of developing a nervous system tumor as high as 22. In another setting, a large study on second brain tumors in 426 patients with pituitary adenoma treated with surgery and radiotherapy showed a 2.4% risk at 20 years.[121]

Criteria for a radiation-induced tumor include: (a) long interval between radiotherapy and the occurrence of the second tumor (the mean onset delay is 12 years, with cases ranging from 1 to 40 years); (b) tumor growth within the radiation portal or at its margins; (c) a different histological subtype. After stereotactic radiosurgery, radiation-induced neoplasms are extremely rare, with only four reported cases in the literature.[123] Three types of tumors have been reported to be linked with cranial irradiation: meningioma in about 70% of cases, glioma in 20%, and sarcoma in fewer than 10%. More than 300 cases of radiation-induced meningiomas have been reported in the literature; female predominance is less prominent than in spontaneous meningiomas.[124] The risk of occurrence correlates with radiation dose: low-dose RT induced a relative risk of 9.5 in one study,[118] whereas high-dose RT was linked to a relative risk of 37.[120] The tumor emerges after a long latency period: a review found extremes ranging from 2 to 63 years (mean 18.7 years) after high-dose RT.[125]

Most patients (68%) had been irradiated during childhood, and the interval between RT and the onset of the tumor was shorter in younger patients; however, the radiation dose did not influence the latency. Radiation-induced meningiomas are often multiple and recurrent with malignant histological features.[126,127] Unlike sporadic meningiomas, NF2 gene inactivation and chromosome 22q deletions seem to be less frequent in radiation-induced meningiomas, while other chromosomal lesions (especially loss of 1p) possibly induced by irradiation, may be more important in the development of these tumors.[128,129]

Radiation-induced gliomas are much less frequent. Since 1960, about 120 cases have been reported in the English literature;[130,131] fewer than half of them were glioblastomas. In the group of patients treated with RT for acute leukemia, multifocality occurred in 20% of cases. The median delay of onset ranges from 6 to 9 years.[131] The prognosis of these tumors is poor: intrinsic resistance to treatment as well as previously received aggressive therapies considerably limits the applicable therapies.

Molecular alterations are apparently the same in sporadic and radiation-induced gliomas.[132] Fewer than 40 cases of sarcomas have been reported to date, different and they consist of several histological types (e.g., gliosarcomas, meningiosarcomas, neurofibrosarcomas).[117]

Radiation Vasculopathy

Distinct from radionecrosis, in which severe lesions of the arterioles and capillaries constitute a cardinal feature, radiation can induce other types of vascular damage leading to stroke or intracerebral hemorrhage.

Large and Medium Intracranial and Extracranial Arterial Injury

An arteriopathy affecting the large cervical blood vessels, especially the carotid artery,[133] may be a complication of cervical radiation therapy, usually administered for lymphomas or head and neck cancers. Intracranial vessels may also be affected. The main early-delayed vascular complication is carotid rupture,[134,135] which usually follows a few weeks after cervical RT and surgery for head and neck tumors. Associated skin lesions such as necrosis or wound infection are common. The outcome of this exceptional complication is, of course, very poor.

Late-delayed complications are more frequent, and generally occur many years after RT (median time about 20 years for extracranial, 7 years for intracranial artery lesions). The lesions are similar to those induced by atherosclerosis, but are often located in unusual places for common atherosclerosis and occur in an accelerated fashion. It has been observed that the larger the diameter of an irradiated artery, the longer the latency between RT and the onset of vasculopathy, a fact that might explain the shorter latency of RT-induced vasculopathy in children. Shorter latencies have also been reported with interstitial radiotherapy.[136] The dose required to induce vascular lesions usually exceeds 50 Gy, but the type of irradiation, fractionation, and portal differs greatly from one case to another. The lesions consist of one or more stenoses or occlusions in the arteries included within the radiation portal. The diagnosis, suspected when a cervical murmur is heard in the immediate vicinity of radiation-induced skin lesions, relies on magnetic resonance angiography, ultrasound examination and arteriography.

The treatment is similar to that of usual atherosclerotic lesions; in the event of carotid stenoses, endarterectomy may be appropriate. However, surgery may be more difficult than in unirradiated patients because of vascular fibrosis and skin lesions, with higher postoperative risk of infection or healing problems.

In other patients, antiplatelet agents may be prescribed if there is no contraindication. Some authors have advocated lowering serum cholesterol levels to prevent the development of such lesions in patients at risk.[137]

Radiation-Induced Vasculopathy with Moyamoya Pattern

Intracranial vasculopathy leading to a progressive occlusive disease and a moyamoya pattern (characterized by abnormal anastomoses and netlike blood vessels), accounting for focal seizures, strokes, or transient ischemic attacks, may follow intracranial irradiation, especially in very young children. This complication is particularly frequent in children treated for optic chiasm glioma, a condition often associated with neurofibromatosis type 1 (NF-1, which is a risk factor for vasculopathy itself). It may also occur with other tumors such as brainstem glioma and craniopharyngioma.[138] In a series[139] of 69 children (11 with NF-1) treated for optic pathway glioma with RT (median dose 55 Gy), 13 (19%) developed clinical and radiological signs of vasculopathy after a median latency of 36 months. The strong association between NF-1 and moyamoya is one of the reasons why radiation has been replaced with chemotherapy in younger children.[113] The treatment focuses on preventing further strokes through surgical revascularization techniques; calcium blockers such as flunarizine have been advocated by some authors.[140–143] The role of antiplatelet agents has not been defined in this setting.

Silent Lacunar Lesions

One report[144] described a rare pattern of silent cerebral lacunes occurring in children treated for brain tumors. In this study reviewing 524 consecutive children, 5 of 421 treated with RT and chemotherapy had lacunes. Patients were a median of 4.5 years old at the time of the diagnosis and RT, and developed lacunes after a median latency of 2 years (ranging from 0.26 to 6 years). This pattern was associated with no further clinical deficit or neuropsychological impairment when compared to patients without lacunes. This condition is probably linked to delayed radiation-induced capillary and small vessel lesions.

Radiation-Induced Cavernomas, Angiomatous Malformations, and Aneurysms

Brain vascular malformations such as telangiectasias and cavernomas[124,145,146] have been rarely observed following RT. Ocular telangiectasias may also occur.[147] When present, their main risk is intracranial bleeding.

Several cases of multiple radiation-induced cavernous angiomas have also been reported,[148] occurring 18 months to 23 years after RT.

Finally, fewer than 15 cases of radiation-induced intracranial aneurysms have been described in the literature.[149,150] The median age of the patients was 37.5 years (ranging from 11 to 65 years) and a latency of 10 months to 21 years, with no correlation between the onset of aneurysms and the radiation dose. This represents a rare but potentially severe problem, as rupture is always possible; six of nine ruptured aneurysms proved fatal. A growing aneurysm can also mimic tumor recurrence. Aneurysms are sometimes detected preclinically with the usual imaging procedures for tumors (CT scan and MRI), as was stressed by Azzarelli et al.,[151] and particular attention should be drawn to evaluating the onset of such lesions during imaging follow-up. When an aneurysm is detected on CT or MR scan, or if the clinical history strongly suggests its presence, cerebral angiography is required for delineation.

Endocrine Dysfunction

Frequently underestimated,[113,152] endocrine disorders can be the consequence of direct irradiation of a gland (e.g., the thyroid gland, with about 50% of patients developing hypothyroidism within 20 years following radiotherapy for Hodgkin disease or certain head and neck cancers) or result from hypothalamic-pituitary dysfunction secondary to cranial irradiation (several authors believe that the hypothalamus is more radiosensitive than the pituitary gland).[153] We will focus on the second type of disorder, which can be induced by cerebral or nasopharyngeal tumor irradiation.

There is a positive correlation between radiation dose and the incidence of endocrine complications. In a prospective study of 268 patients treated with different RT schemes to the brain, Littley et al. found that, 5 years after RT, the incidence of TSH deficiency was 9% after treatment with 20 Gy, 22% with 35 to 37 Gy, and 52% with 42 to 45 Gy.[154] A hormonal deficit can appear at any time after RT, but may arise more rapidly in patients treated with higher radiation doses.[155]

In children, varied endocrine deficits may result from cranial RT (administered for brain tumors or during prophylactic irradiation in acute lymphoblastic leukemia). Growth hormone (GH) is usually the first, and in many cases the only, anterior pituitary deficit in young patients. This complication affects about 50% of children treated with prophylactic cranial RT for acute lymphoblastic leukemia.[156]

According to a recent Danish study of 73 children treated with RT for a primary brain tumor (not involving the hypothalamo-pituitary axis directly) and with a long follow-up (median 15 years), 80% of patients manifested growth hormone deficiency; the median biological effective dose (BED) in the hypothalamo-pituitary area was higher in GH-deficient children than in patients without GH deficiency.[157] Administration of GH is recommended in children with growth hormone deficiency but, as it has no effects on vertebral bodies, long-term survivors acquire a typical "spiderlike" physical appearance with long extremities and short trunk.[113] A subtle central hypothyroidism is common in children and should be treated with thyroxine replacement therapy in order to limit the potential for thyroid carcinoma as well as to improve longitudinal growth.[158,159]

In adults, a recent study[160] evaluating 31 long-term brain tumor survivors, followed 1.5 to 11 years after RT with a mean total dose of 62.3 ± 2.8 Gy, compared with 31 age- and sex-matched controls, found hypothalamic hypothyroidism in 26% of patients, hypothalamic hypogonadism in 32% of patients, hyperprolactinemia in 29% of patients, and panhypopituitarism in one patient. Low adrenal hormone levels were found in most patients, but without apparent clinical consequence. In the control group, only 6% had a baseline hormonal concentration outside the normal range. None of the controls had two or more hormonal abnormalities, while 42% of the patients had multiple deficits. Only 23% of patients had normal thyroid, gonadal, and adrenal baseline levels; this result is consistent with another earlier study by Taphoorn et al. reporting hypothalamic-pituitary dysfunction in 10 of 13 (77%) long-term survivors irradiated for supratentorial low-grade glioma.[161] Another study of patients treated for nasopharyngeal cancer found secondary hypothyroïdism in 27% of cases (of hypothalamic origin in 19% and pituitary origin in 8%).[162]

The neurological consequences of severe hypothyroidism are well known, including encephalopathy, cerebellar ataxia, pseudo-myotonia, and sometimes peripheral neuropathy. Raised CSF protein is also usual. All these abnormalities may be misleading if the correct diagnosis is not considered.

Secondary hypogonadism is an important concern especially in male patients, responsible for a decrease in libido and sometimes impotence, and impacting negatively on quality of life. Hyperprolactinemia of hypothalamic origin is a notable concern in women who develop oligo-menorrhea and galactorrhea[163]; in men, it may result in gynecomastia and a decrease in libido.

The follow-up consultations are a good place for a regular clinical endocrine evaluation; the precise biological follow-up scheme is debated and is adapted according to the emerging deficits, but long-term assessment should be the rule. The treatment of hormonal deficits lies in replacement therapy, and usually leads to an improvement in the patient's condition. Bromocriptine has been utilized with success in patients with symptomatic hyperprolactinemia.[117]

SEQUELAE OF RADIOTHERAPY TO THE SPINAL CORD

Damage to the spinal cord may be the consequence of RT administered for spinal cord tumors, Hodgkin disease, mediastinal or head and neck cancers. Early descriptions in the 1940s[164] were followed by numerous descriptions of postradiation myelopathy delineating the main clinical patterns, that is, early-delayed myelopathy and several types of late-delayed complications including progressive myelopathy, lower motor neuron disorder, and spinal hemorrhage. There is no clear clinical or experimental evidence of acute spinal cord toxicity due to RT, and a sudden worsening during irradiation should lead to a search for intratumoral hemorrhage or tumor progression.[37]

EARLY-DELAYED (TRANSIENT) RADIATION MYELOPATHY

The onset of this complication occurs from 6 weeks to 6 months after RT, and improvement follows in most cases within 2 to 9 months,[165] though persistence of the symptoms for a longer time is possible in rare cases. It usually follows radiation to the cervical or thoracic spinal cord. After mantle RT for Hodgkin disease, early-delayed myelopathy occurred in 15% of cases.[166] In another study, Fein et al. found a global incidence of 3.6% (40 cases among 1112 patients receiving 30 Gy or more). The incidence was 8% in the group of patients receiving 50 Gy or more, 3% after doses of 45 to 49.9 Gy, 4% after doses of 40 to 44.9 Gy, and 2% after doses of 30 to 39.9 Gy. The risk was also increased with a fraction size over 2 Gy.[167]

The clinical pattern first described by Esik et al.[168] generally consists of Lhermitte phenomenon, triggered by neck flexion, and characterized by brief unpleasant sensations of numbness, tingling, and/or often electric shock–like feelings from the neck to the spine and extremities. There are no MRI changes associated with this condition. This symptom is nonspecific, and other causes should be considered in a patient with cancer,[169] including chemotherapy (cisplatin or docetaxel), spinal tumor, vitamin B12 deficiency, herpes zoster, or even multiple sclerosis (which may be aggravated by irradiation).

The presumed pathophysiology of early-delayed myelopathy is transient demyelination, probably secondary to a loss of oligodendroglial cells following RT.[170,171] There is no specific treatment for this condition, and none is required, as recovery occurs in most cases. Early-delayed spinal cord disorder is not predictive of evolution to the much more serious progressive myelopathy.

LATE-DELAYED RADIATION-INDUCED SPINAL CORD DISORDERS

Spinal radionecrosis (Figure 17-5) (with features similar to its cerebral counterpart), progressive myelopathy, and spinal hemorrhage have been described as late complications of spine radiation.

Progressive Myelopathy, or Delayed Radiation Myelopathy (DRM)

This complication occurs 6 months to 10 years after exposure to RT. Risk factors include advancing age, large radiation doses and fractions, previous irradiation especially in childhood, and large portals involving thoracic or lumbar spinal cord.[165] Chemotherapy may increase the risk of delayed radiation myelopathy,[172] but data are still unclear on this point.

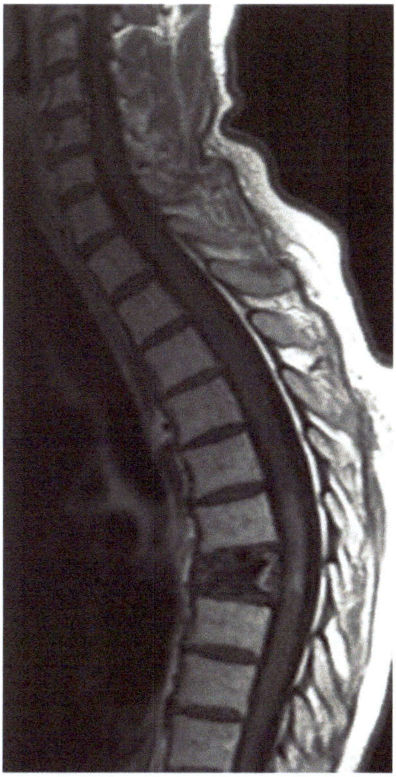

Figure 17-5 Postcontrast sagittal T1-weighted MRI of the spinal cord showing an intramedullary enhancing lesion compatible with spinal cord radionecrosis in a 53-year-old female treated by spinal radiotherapy 6 months ago for a T7 metastasis of lung adenocarcinoma.

The generally accepted tolerance for the spinal cord is 45 Gy in 22 to 25 daily fractions, with a risk of less than 1% for a dose of 50 Gy, increasing to 5% for a dose of 60 Gy delivered in 1.8 to 2 Gy fractions.[173]

Delayed radiation myelopathy may begin abruptly or, more often, in a progressive way; patients complain of sensory and/or motor deficits leading to paraparesis or tetraparesis. A typical initial clinical presentation is a Brown-Séquard syndrome, consisting of a motor deficit associated with ipsilateral sensory loss affecting tactile, vibration, and passive movement sense on one side, and sensory loss affecting mainly temperature and pain modalities on the other side. In some patients, a transverse myelopathy develops with bilateral leg weakness and sensory loss up to the irradiated region. Some patients also experience pain. Bladder and bowel sphincter as well as diaphragmatic dysfunction (in upper cervical spinal cord lesions) are possible. The evolution of delayed radiation myelopathy varies; in some patients the symptoms stabilize, while in others they progress to a complete deficit.

The diagnosis of delayed radiation myelopathy implies—as was underlined as early as 1961 by Pallis et al.[174]—that the site of the main lesion is within the radiation-exposed area of the spinal cord and that all other potential causes of myelopathy have been carefully reviewed and eliminated.

Spinal cord MRI is helpful, though nonspecific. The initial description of Wang et al.[175,176] has been confirmed in several subsequent studies[177–179]: the initial MRI may be normal if performed during the first weeks of the disease, but a slightly delayed examination usually reveals a swollen cord with T1-weighted hypointensity and T2-weighted hyperintensity. Lesions enhance in about 50% of cases after gadolinium injection (Figure 17-5).[180,181] In contrast, late examinations, performed years after the onset of the disease, may show spinal cord atrophy without any signal abnormality; a case of cystic formation in late delayed radiation myelopathy has also been reported.

Moderately elevated protein is the most common finding in the CSF but lacks any specificity. If performed, somatosensory evoked potentials show changes correlated to the extent of the lesions, whereas spinal conduction velocity is decreased.

Neuropathological findings include demyelination, focal necrosis, and axonal loss, together with vascular abnormalities including telangiectasias, endothelial swelling with fibrin exudation, hyaline degeneration, thickening and fibrinoid necrosis of the vessel walls with perivascular fibrosis and sometimes vasculitis.

Corticosteroids may improve some patients, probably because of their action on the inflammatory and edematous components of the disorder; however, patients often become steroid-dependent and only a few experience long-term improvement. There is no current proven long-term treatment for delayed radiation myelopathy. However, Angibaud et al. have reported the efficacy of hyperbaric oxygen in stabilizing or improving six out of nine patients with DRM,[182] and Calabro et al. recently reported a similar case.[183] Anticoagulation has also been tried, with improvement in one patient with myelopathy treated for over 3 months with full anticoagulation, and stabilization in another treated with coumarin.[76]

Late-Delayed Spinal Hematoma

This rare complication has only been described in a few cases, following spinal radiotherapy by 6 to 30 years, and occurring within the radiation portal but outside the location of the primary tumor[184]; acute-onset leg weakness and back pain rapidly lead to paraparesis or tetraparesis. The diagnosis relies on MRI demonstration of hemorrhage.

Spontaneous symptom resolution is possible, but new episodes may occur later. There is no proven effective treatment for this condition. Avoidance of aspirin or NSAIDs is prudent. Radiation-induced telangiectasias with secondary hemorrhage could explain this condition.

Sequelae of Radiotherapy on the Cranial Nerves

Apart from acute reversible radiation toxicity, any of the cranial nerves may be involved in late-delayed radiation-induced complications if included in the radiation portal. These complications are rare, probably arising in fewer than 1% of cases after conventional radiotherapy (60 Gy, 2 Gy per daily fraction). Large daily radiation fractions increase this risk. However, a recent study in brain tumors survivors found that 17% of patients developed neurosensory impairment and that RT exposure greater than 50 Gy to the posterior fossa was associated with a higher likelihood of developing any hearing impairment.[185] The main complications are described below:

OLFACTORY NERVE INJURY

During cranial radiation, patients may describe reversible sensations of smelling an odor.[186] This may be due to direct acute stimulation of the olfactory neurons. Anosmia has also been described in some patients,[187,188] often associated with taste disorders.[189]

OPTIC NEUROPATHY

Probably facilitated by preexisting lesions (e.g., in diabetic patients), optic neuropathy may occur 6 months to 14 years after radiation therapy for a tumor of the orbital, pituitary, or suprasellar regions.[190] In one study, the incidence of retrobulbar optic neuropathy was 3.8% after a conventional radiation scheme for head and neck cancer.[191] Optic neuropathy can also overshadow the prognosis of patients treated with high-energy electron beam therapy for age-related macular degeneration in up to 19% of cases.[192]

Proton beam irradiation, currently proposed in the treatment of several tumors including meningioma and choroidal melanoma, may also induce this complication.[193] The classical pattern consists of progressive or sometimes acute-onset visual loss, leading to monocular or binocular blindness with optic atrophy.[194] This disorder is painless. In the case of anterior lesions, the ocular fundus usually shows papilledema and prepapillary and premacular hemorrhage, sometimes associated with radiation-induced retinal lesions. In contrast, fundoscopy may be normal if the lesions are posterior. In those cases, brain MRI may be useful, demonstrating enlargement of the optic nerve and chiasma, with T2-weighted hyperintensities and contrast enhancement.

Demyelination, axonal loss, gliosis, and modifications of the vessel walls characterize these lesions histologically; endothelial cell loss has recently been stressed in this setting, with more significant abnormalities in patients treated with high-dose (55 to 70 Gy) compared with those treated with low-dose (10 Gy or less) radiation therapy.[195] These lesions are irreversible in many patients. Steroids and anticoagulants[186] have been advocated in chiasmatic lesions, with inconsistent results, while the use of hyperbaric oxygen in optic neuropathy remains controversial.[197–199] Optic nerve sheath fenestration has been attempted with some success in a few patients.[200]

ACEi may have a protective role in the optic nerve independent of its antihypertensive effect. ACEi given 2 weeks after stereotactic brain irradiation of rats significantly reduced radiation-induced optic neuropathy electrophysiologically in terms of the visual evoked-potential response to light and morphologically in terms of quantitative changes in myelin contents and axons in the optic nerves and chiasm.[200b]

OCULAR MOTOR NERVE INJURY

Rarely reported, the involvement of ocular motor nerves may be associated with optic neuropathy. The most frequent of these palsies affects the abducens nerve.[37] Transient ocular motor palsies have been reported following radiation schemes focused on the pituitary tract, but permanent palsies have also been described after radiation therapy of nasopharyngeal carcinoma. Possible regression suggests that a demyelinating process may be involved, rather than progressive fibrosis.

Neuromyotonia is a late-delayed complication following RT to the sella turcica or the cavernous sinus region by several years, and is characterized by spontaneous spasms of the eye muscles responsible for episodes of transitory painless diplopia, usually lasting a few seconds; these episodes can occur up to several times an hour.[201] Membrane stabilizers such as phenytoin or carbamazepine may improve this disorder. Radiation-induced hyperexcitability of the nerve fibers may underlie the pathophysiology.

TRIGEMINAL NERVE DYSFUNCTION

Involvement of the trigeminal nerve is quite rare. Neuromyotonia in the trigeminal distribution is exceptionally encountered; treatment with carbamazepine is effective in this condition.[202,203] After gamma knife radiosurgery for trigeminal neuralgia, the main reported complication to this day is mild facial numbness occuring in 2.7% to 14% of patients.[204–206] Trigeminal neuropathy can also result from radiosurgery for vestibular schwannoma.[207]

FACIAL NERVE INJURY

The different branches of the facial nerve are not equally affected by radiation. Taste dysfunction is usual and many patients complain of aguesia, a symptom that may be permanent in up to 50% of patients irradiated with 50 to 60 Gy for head and neck tumors.[208] However, taste disturbances are a common feature in cancer patients, and chemotherapy may play a part.[209]

Motor deficit is almost never a consequence of fractionated RT and should prompt a search for tumoral invasion.[37] In contrast, radiosurgery has been reported to account for possible facial palsy; however, the relatively high initial figures of facial weakness after treatment for vestibular schwannoma[210,211] seem to have much decreased, being currently under 5% of cases.[206,212]

ACOUSTIC NERVE DYSFUNCTION

Acute damage to the cochlea may be responsible for usually reversible complaints of high-frequency hearing loss and tinnitus. Otitis media can also be responsible for an early-delayed hearing loss. Following RT by a few weeks, this condition results from an obliteration of the eustachian tube by edema and mucosal vasodilatation.

The diagnosis is often easy, as otoscopic examination reveals fluid behind the tympanic membrane. Usually spontaneously regressive, otitis media can, in some cases, require myringotomy for symptom alleviation. In most cases, relief can be obtained by prescribing nasal vasoconstriction agents. Late-delayed hearing loss may result from damage to the organ of Corti with subsequent acoustic nerve atrophy; however, a report underlines the relative resistance of the organ of Corti to radiation. The precise histological pattern of these disorders is not known; however, in previous studies, the labyrinth has been shown to be damaged.[213,214]

The consequences to hearing of radiosurgery for vestibular schwannoma have been better assessed over the last few years.[212,215–218] In a recent report,[219] 14% of patients with measurable hearing before treatment became deaf after radiosurgery, and 42% of patients had an elevation of their pure tone threshold of 20 dB or more. The risk factors for hearing loss in this study included neurofibromatosis type 2 (NF-2), history of prior surgical resection, and tumor size.

LOWER CRANIAL NERVE INVOLVEMENT

These nerves (glossopharyngeal, vagus, spinal accessory, and hypoglossal nerves) can be damaged after head or neck radiation therapy with large doses. Complications occur earlier the larger the radiation dose and typically arise months to years after the treatment. The pathophysiology is likely radiation fibrosis. The hypoglossal nerve is the most commonly involved lower cranial nerve[220]; the patient may present with unilateral, often asymptomatic tongue paralysis,[221–223] or with bilateral and disabling paralysis. This complication may occur many years after RT.[222]

Longstanding paralysis is responsible for tongue atrophy, with asymmetry that may be associated with fatty infiltration or edema-like changes on MRI.[224,225] Paralysis of the vagus nerve leads to unilateral paralysis of the vocal cord and of the palate, responsible for difficulties in swallowing.[226] Horner syndrome may be associated with these disorders, resulting from injury to the sympathetic fibers.[37] Lesions of the spinal accessory nerve lead to shoulder drop which is diagnosed during the clinical examination. Patients may also present with multiple lower cranial nerve palsies.[227] Cranial nerve palsies may occur during skull base osteoradionecrosis after radiotherapy for nasopharyngeal carcinoma.[228]

Consequences of Radiotherapy on the Peripheral Nervous System

Apart from rare peripheral nerve tumors, brachial and lumbosacral plexopathies are the main distressing and disabling complications of RT in the peripheral nervous system. In this situation, differential diagnosis with tumor infiltration of the plexus is often a challenge, even with modern imaging techniques.

DROPPED HEAD SYNDROME

Dropped head syndrome has been recently described as a potential late-delayed complication of RT.[229] These patients usually develop weakness of neck extensors several years after irradiation involving the cervical region, for example, mantle irradiation for Hodgkin lymphoma. Clinical examination reveals an amyotrophic deficit of neck muscles, often extending to other muscles innervated by upper cervical roots, without any impairment of sensation. The differential diagnoses include myasthenia gravis, ALS, and inflammatory myopathies. The mechanism and precise location of the causative lesions are unclear.

BRACHIAL PLEXOPATHY

Brachial plexopathy results from RT to the supraclavicular, infraclavicular, or axillary regions, usually for lung or breast cancers and sometimes for Hodgkin disease. In most cases, the main problem is to differentiate this condition from neoplastic invasion of the plexus.

Early-Delayed Brachial Plexopathy

This complication occurs a median of 4.5 months after RT, with a range of 2 to 14 months. Its incidence is about 1% to 2% after irradiation for breast cancer.[230,231] The clinical pattern includes paresthesia in the hand with a distal motor deficit; amyotrophy and fasciculations may be present at later stages. Axillary pain is reported in about 60% of cases; always moderate, it may be spontaneous or occur with movement. Although a progressive course towards paralysis of the brachial plexus is possible, complete improvement is the rule, in most cases after 3 to 6 months. Electrophysiological investigations show a decrease in nerve conduction velocities. The pathophysiology of this condition is not fully understood; a direct radiation toxicity on the Schwann cells inducing demyelination has been invoked.[232]

Late-Delayed Brachial Plexopathy

Delayed radiation-induced brachial plexopathy appears after a median time of 40 months (up to 20 years).[233] Its incidence varies widely in the literature, with figures ranging from 14% to 73%,[234] the most important risk factors being total radiation dose (> 60 Gy) and fraction size (> 2 Gy). Overlap of radiation fields has also been incriminated as well as combined radio-chemotherapy. For example, Olsen et al. found a definite or probable radiation plexopathy in 42% of patients treated with chemotherapy (cyclophosphamide, tamoxifen, or a combination of cyclophosphamide, methotrexate and 5-fluorouracil) and RT, versus 26% in patients treated with RT alone.[235]

The pathophysiology is unclear and may have biphasic conponents: during the first phase, direct radiation damage to the nerves may cause electrophysiological and histochemical changes; later on, injury to the small vessels and fibrosis around the nerves may account for severe nerve injury.[236]

The disorder is usually progressive. Initial symptoms include distal paresthesias (typically, pins-and-needles or numbness of the thumb and first finger) and mild sensory deficit on clinical examination, often with no clear radicular topography.

The other initial findings consist of some degree of amyotrophy and an early abolition of reflexes. Proximal weakness is found in about a quarter of cases.[237,238] Visible myokymia, when present, is quite suggestive of the diagnosis. The examination may also show local complications of radiotherapy, such as radiation dermatitis, painful induration of the axillary region, and/or lymphedema. During the later course of late-delayed plexopathy, a generally progressive motor deficit may be observed (in a few cases, an apoplectic onset has been reported, sometimes after physical effort). Pain is quite uncommon at diagnosis and is usually a relatively minor feature. The severity of the condition is variable, from a simple discomfort to an almost complete paralysis of the limb.

The differential diagnosis must necessarily eliminate a neoplastic invasion of the brachial plexus. Some clinical signs may be important clues. In a large retrospective study on 100 cases of brachial plexus lesions, including 22 radiation plexopathies and 78 metastatic brachial plexopathies (34 in irradiated patients and 44 in nonirradiated patients), Kori et al.[237] found several factors as indicators of neoplastic invasion: (i) *pain*, especially when severe, is an important feature, present in 89% of irradiated patients with neoplastic infiltration of the plexus (versus 18% of patients with radiation plexopathy); (ii) *Horner's syndrome* was present in 56% of patients with tumor infiltration (versus 14%). On the contrary, the following signs argue for a radiation-induced disorder: (i) *dysesthesia*, present in 55% of radiation plexopathies (versus 6% of plexopathies linked with tumor infiltration); (ii) *lymphedema*, reported in 73% of cases (versus 15%). These results are consistent with those of other authors.[239]

Motor conduction velocities are usually normal or slightly decreased in radiation plexopathies. Sensory conduction velocities are rarely altered. The F waves can be absent or delayed. Electromyography is always abnormal, with fasciculations, fibrillation, and slow denervation potentials. The most important finding in favor of radiation-induced plexopathy is the presence of myokymic discharge, present in about two thirds of patients; this feature is quite rare (< 5%) in patients with an infiltrating tumor. Myokymic discharges are often located in the *abductor pollicis brevis* and *pronator quadratus* muscles.[240]

The main aim of imaging is to differentiate between radiation plexopathy and neoplastic invasion. CT scan was the first noninvasive examination to be useful[241,242]; this imaging technique may show a distortion of the tissue planes and fat or may be normal. MRI is superior to CT scan in this indication[243]; furthermore, bone artifacts do not impair the interpretation of MRI, which also allows a study of the cervical spine in search of epidural or cervical root secondary lesions. Radiation fibrosis is responsible for a thickening of the components of the brachial plexus, sometimes with contrast enhancement.[243] Tumor invasion is diagnosed when a mass lesion is visible along the roots of the branches of the brachial plexus. Nevertheless, a retrospective study at the Mayo Clinic of 71 patients with cancer and brachial plexopathy who had an MRI yielded a 21% (15 patients) discordance rate between imaging and eventual diagnosis.[186,239]

A recent study of 50 breast cancer patients,[244] using an association of body-coil and surface-coil techniques, suggests a major role for MRI to assess neoplastic recurrence. This technique allowed a correct diagnosis of tumor recurrence in 26 of 27 patients, directly related to the brachial plexus in 17 of them, and associated with cervical spine degenerative lesions in seven cases. Exclusion of a malignant disease was accurate in 20 of 21 cases. These results corresponded to a sensitivity of the MR criteria for tumor detection of 96% and a specificity of 95%, with similar positive and negative predictive values. Positron emission tomography using 18-fluoro-2 deoxyglucose (18FDG-PET) may also be helpful to differentiate tumor infiltration from radiation-induced plexopathy.[245]

Sometimes, noninvasive investigations are inconclusive, and a biopsy may be indicated. In radiation plexopathy this reveals fibrosis and the absence of tumor infiltration.

The treatment of pain is often challenging, and includes analgesic drugs, tricyclic antidepressants, and/or anticonvulsants. Steroids can also be helpful. Anticoagulants have also been reported to be beneficial in radiation-induced neuropathies.[246] Techniques such as transdermal electrical nerve stimulation and dorsal column roots stimulation have also been proposed. Neurolysis, with or without omentoplasty, has been performed in radiation-induced brachial plexopathy, but the benefit of this approach is questionable. Prudent physiotherapy may be indicated.[238]

Ischemic Late-Delayed Brachial Plexopathy

Sudden late-delayed plexopathy has been reported following an occlusion of the subclavian artery.[247]

LUMBOSACRAL PLEXOPATHY

Far less common than brachial plexopathy, lumbosacral plexopathy may follow radiotherapy for pelvic or lower abdomen cancer (uterus, ovary, testis, rectum, or lymphoma).

Early-Delayed Lumbosacral Plexopathy

As with brachial plexopathies, an early-delayed, generally transient lumbosacral plexopathy is possible. It usually begins a few months (median 4 months) after RT, with a typical pattern of distal bilateral paresthesias of the lower limbs. Clinical examination is normal in most cases, and improvement follows within 3 to 6 months.

Late-Delayed Lumbosacral Plexopathy

This disorder shares similar features with brachial plexopathy but is much less frequently reported. The onset follows initial RT by 1 to 30 years (median 5 years). The clinical pattern is characterized by a progressive, usually asymmetric, and bilateral motor deficit of the lower limbs associated with less-marked sensory deficits. As in brachial plexopathy, pain is generally mild or absent. The course of the disease leads to a slow worsening of the motor deficit. The patient may stabilize after several months or years.[248]

On electromyography (EMG), motor nerve conduction velocities are normal or moderately decreased in the leg.

The saphenous nerve sensory potential is absent or has a decreased amplitude in about 50% of cases. Detection shows myokymias in the proximal muscles in 60% of cases. Fibrillation potentials in the paravertebral muscles are found in 50%

of patients. Histology, when performed, may show fibrosis tightly hugging the plexus, and in some cases the cauda equina as well.

Treatment of pain is identical to that of brachial plexopathy. Two patients treated with anticoagulation remained stable with an improvement of pain.[76]

LOWER MOTOR NEURON SYNDROME

A lower motor neuron syndrome can be a consequence of pelvic irradiation for testicular tumors, lumbosacral RT, or craniospinal RT for medulloblastoma, and begins 3 months to 25 years after RT. Maier et al.[249] reported 15 cases of this syndrome out of 343 patients who had undergone a lumboaortic irradiation scheme. About 30 cases have been reported since that period with various radiation schemes.

The patient presents with a progressive proximal and distal, often bilateral, and more-or-less symmetrical weakness of the inferior limbs; muscle atrophy and fasciculations may be associated with this deficit. Physical examination confirms a flaccid motor deficit and areflexia, but no sensory loss appears during the early stages. Sensory deficit may appear after several years, as well as sphincter disturbance characterized by lack of bladder sensation and incontinence.[250] Variable patterns of progression and associated disability can be seen. MRI may be normal, but contrast enhancement of the roots of the cauda equina has been described.[250]

The CSF is usually acellular, frequently showing high protein levels. On electromyography, different stages of denervation are identified while sural sensory nerve action potentials are usually preserved.

It is unclear whether the lesions localize to the anterior horn cells of the spinal cord or the proximal part of the nerve roots. Some reports advocate an anterior horn cell disorder, as no sensory signs were reported and electrophysiological data were compatible with pure motor neuron syndrome.[251]

In a study of six patients treated with RT (mean dose 45 Gy) for testicular cancer and including neuropathological examination of one case, Bowen et al.[250] found strong arguments favoring radiculopathy, including (i) the presence of late-delayed sensory and sphincter disturbances, appearing 4 to 8 years after the motor symptoms; (ii) MRI abnormalities showing contrast enhancement of the lumbosacral roots of the cauda equina in two out of three patients; (iii) no lesion in the cord at necropsy but thickening of the roots of the cauda equina with focal areas of hemorrhagic discoloration, fibrosis, and axonal loss; the roots included abnormal dilated vessels with thickened and hyalinized walls. Thus, Wohlgemuth et al.[252] suggest that a better term for this syndrome would be "postirradiation cauda equina syndrome."

There is no recognized treatment of this condition. A patient has been reported to improve while on warfarin and steroids.[253]

RADIATION-INDUCED PERIPHERAL NERVE SHEATH TUMORS

A few dozen cases of radiation-induced nerve sheath tumors have been reported.[254,255] Patients with neurofibromatosis type 1 (NF-1) have an increased risk of developing this complication. In a retrospective study on radiation-induced peripheral nerve sheath tumors, three patients out of nine (33%) had familial and/or clinical signs of NF-1[256]; in this series, the latency between RT and the onset of the secondary tumor ranged from 4 to 41 years.

Pain followed by the development of a sensorimotor deficit typifies the clinical presentation. The differential diagnosis of a local recurrence of the primary tumor generally requires biopsy. The treatment of these nerve sheath tumors relies principally on aggressive surgery with tumor-free margins; amputation of a limb, when performed, does not significantly change overall survival.[257] Neither chemotherapy nor radiotherapy have shown any clear benefit has in terms of survival yet in those tumors.[258]

Conclusions

Radiation therapy remains one of the most efficient treatments of cancer and will probably become, through the development of new irradiation techniques, a standard option for treating some nonmalignant diseases. Familiarity with its potential risks is thus essential, in order to prevent complications when possible, as well as to be able to inform the patients of their possible onset. The development of RT-related neurotoxicity remains largely unpredictable, and seems to depend on yet-to-be-discovered individual predisposition. As progress has been made in understanding the pathophysiology of radiation-induced injury and in determining "safe" doses over the past few decades, many complications have become rarer than a few years ago.

REFERENCES

1. New P. Radiation injury to the nervous system. Curr Opin Neurol 2001;14:725–34.
2. Swennen MH. Delayed radiation toxicity after focal or whole brain radiotherapy for low-grade glioma. J Neurooncol 2004;66:333–9.
3. Lai R, Abrey LE, Rosenblum MK, DeAngelis LM. Treatment-induced leukoencephalopathy in primary CNS lymphoma: a clinical and autopsy study. Neurology 2004;62:451–6.
4. Oi S, Kokunai T, Ijichi A, Matsumoto S, Raimondi AJ. Radiation-induced brain damage in children—histological analysis of sequential tissue changes in 34 autopsy cases. Neurol Med Chir 1990;30:36–42.
5. Panagiotakos G, Alshamy G, Chan B, Abrams R, Greenberg E, Saxena A, et al. Long-term impact of radiation on the stem cell and oligodendrocyte precursors in the brain. PLoS ONE 2007;2:e588.
6. Kamiryo T, Kassell NF, Thai QA, Lopes MB, Lee KS, Steiner L. Histological changes in the normal rat brain after gamma irradiation. Acta Neurochir 1996;138:451–9.
7. Calvo W, Hopewell JW, Reinhold HS, Yeung TK. Radiation induced damage in the choroid plexus of the rat brain: a histological evaluation. Neuropathol Appl Neurobiol 1986;12:47–61.
8. Yoneoka Y, Satoh M, Akiyama K, Sano K, Fujii Y, Tanaka R. An experimental study of radiation-induced cognitive dysfunction in an adult rat model. Br J Radiol 1999;72:1196–201.
9. Nordal RA, Nagy A, Pintilie M, Wong CS. Hypoxia and hypoxia-inducible factor-1 target genes in central nervous system radiation injury: a role for vascular endothelial growth factor. Clin Cancer Res 2004;10:3342–53.
10. Belka C, Budach W, Kortmann RD, et al. Radiation-induced CNS toxicity: molecular and cellular mechanisms. Br J Cancer 2001;85:1233–9.
11. Li YQ, Chen P, Haimovitz-Friedman A, et al. Endothelial apoptosis initiates acute blood-brain barrier disruption after ionizing radiation. Cancer Res 2003;63:5950–6.
12. Lyubimova N, Hopewell JW. Experimental evidence to support the hypothesis that damage to vascular endothelium plays the primary role in the development of late radiation-induced CNS injury. Br J Radiol 2004;77:488–92.
13. Perry A, Schmidt RE. Cancer therapy-associated CNS neuropathology: an update and review of the literature. Acta Neuropathol (Berl) 2006;111:197–212.

14. Coderre JA, Morris GM, Micca PL, et al. Late effects of radiation on the central nervous system: role of vascular endothelial damage and glial stem cell survival. Radiat Res 2006;166:495–503.
15. Tofilon PJ, Fike JR. The radioresponse of the central nervous system: a dynamic process. Radiat Res 2000;153:357–70.
16. Schultheiss TE, Kun LE, Ang KK, et al. Radiation response of the central nervous system. Int J Radiat Oncol Biol Phys 1995;31:1093–112.
17. Quarmby S, Kumar P, Kumar S. Radiation-induced normal tissue injury: role of adhesion molecules in leukocyte-endothelial cell interactions. Int J Cancer 1999;82:385–95.
18. Eissner G, Kohlhuber F, Grell M, et al. Critical involvement of transmembrane tumor necrosis factor-alpha in endothelial programmed cell death mediated by ionizing radiation and bacterial endotoxin. Blood 1995;86:4184–93.
19. Daigle JL, Hong JH, Chiang CS, et al. The role of tumor necrosis factor signaling pathways in the response of murine brain to irradiation. Cancer Res 2001;61:8859–65.
20. Van der Maazen RWM, Berhagen I, Kleiboer BJ, et al. Radiosensitivity of glial progenitor cells of the perinatal and adult rat optic nerve studied by an in vitro clonogenic assay. Radiother Oncol 1991;20:258–64.
21. Van der Maazen RWM, Kleiboer BJ, Berhagen I, et al. Irradiation in vitro discriminates between different O-2A progenitor cell subpopulations in the perinatal central nervous system of rats. Radiat Res 1991;128:64–72 [Abstract].
22. Van der Maazen RWM, Kleiboer BJ, Berhagen I, et al. Repair capacity of adult rat glial progenitor cells determined by an in vitro clonogenic assay after in vitro or in *vivo* fractionated irradiation. Int J Radiat Biol 1993;63:661–6.
23. Chow BM, Li YQ, Wong CS. Radiation-induced apoptosis in the adult central nervous system is p53-dependent. Cell Death Differ 2000;7:712–20.
24. Atkinson SL, Li YQ, Wong CS. Apoptosis and proliferation of oligodendrocyte progenitor cells in the irradiated rodent spinal cord. Int J Radiat Oncol Biol Phys 2005;62:535–44.
25. Hornsey S, Myers R, Coultas PG, et al. Turnover of proliferative cells in the spinal cord after X-irradiation and its relation to time-dependent repair of radiation damage. Br J Radiol 1981;54:1081–5.
26. Enokido Y, Araki T, Tanaka K, et al. Involvement of p53 in DNA strand break-induced apoptosis in postmitotic CNS neurons. Eur J Neurosci 1996;8:1812–21.
27. Gobbel GT, Bellinzona M, Vogt AR, et al. Response of postmitotic neurons to X-irradiation: implications for the role of DNA damage in neuronal apoptosis. J Neurosci 1998;18: 147–55.
28. Chiang CS, McBride WH, Withers HR. Radiation-induced astrocytic and microglial responses in mouse brain. Radiother Oncol 1993;29:60–8.
29. Thomas WE. Brain macrophages: evaluation of microglia and their function. Brain Res Rev 1992;B17:61–74.
30. Omuro AM. Delayed neurotoxicity in primary central nervous system lymphoma. Arch Neurol 2005;62:1595–600.
31. Rola R, Zou Y, Huang TT, Fishman K, Baure J, Rosi S, et al. Lack of extracellular superoxide dismutase (EC-SOD) in the microenvironment impacts radiation-induced changes in neurogenesis. Free Radic Biol Med 2007;42:1133–45.
32. Hopewell JW, Cavanagh JB. Effects of X-irradiation on the mitotic activity of the subependymal plate of rats. Br J Radiol 1972;45:461–5.
33. Tada E, Yang E, Gobbel GT, Lamborn KR, et al. Long-term impairment of subependymal repopulation following damage by ionizing irradiation. Exp Neurol 1999;160:66–77.
34. Bellinzona M, Gobbel GT, Shinohara C, et al. Apoptosis is induced in the subependyma of young adult rats by ionizing irradiation. Neurosci Lett 1996;208:163–6.
35. Young DF, Posner JB, Chu F, et al. Rapid-course radiation therapy of cerebral metastases: results and complications. Cancer 1974;34:1069–76.
36. Hindo WA, DeTrana III FA, Lee MS, et al. Large dose increment irradiation in treatment of cerebral metastases. Cancer 1970;26:138–41.
37. Posner JB. Side effects of radiation therapy. In: Posner JB, editor. Neurologic Complications of Cancer. Philadelphia: F.A. Davis Company; 1995. p. 311–37.
38. Keime-Guibert F, Napolitano M, Delattre JY. Neurological complications of radiotherapy and chemotherapy. J Neurol 1998;245:695–708.

39. Phillips PC, Delattre JY, Berger CA, et al. Early and progressive increases in regional brain capillary permeability following singleand fractionated-dose cranial radiation in rat. Neurology 1987;37(Suppl. 1):301.
40. Freeman JE, Johnston PG, Voke JM. Somnolence after prophylactic cranial irradiation in children with acute lymphoblastic leukaemia. Br Med J 1973;4:523–5.
41. Littman P, Rosenstock J, Gale G, et al. The somnolence syndrome in leukemic children following reduced daily dose fractions of cranial radiation. Int J Radiat Oncol Biol Phys 1984;10:1851–3.
42. Ch'ien LT, Aur RJ, Stagner S, et al. Long-term neurological implications of somnolence syndrome in children with acute lymphocytic leukemia. Ann Neurol 1980;8:273–7.
43. Chow E, Davis L, Holden L, et al. Prospective assessment of patient-rated symptoms following whole brain radiotherapy for brain metastases. J Pain Symptom Manage 2005;30:18–23.
44. Faithfull S, Brada M. Somnolence syndrome in adults following cranial irradiation for primary brain tumours. Clin Oncol 1998;10:250–4.
45. Mandell LR, Walker RW, Steinherz P, et al. Reduced incidence of the somnolence syndrome in leukemic children with steroid coverage during prophylactic cranial radiation therapy: results of a pilot study. Cancer 1989;63:1975–8.
46. Uzal D, Ozyar E, Hayran M, et al. Reduced incidence of the somnolence syndrome after prophylactic cranial irradiation in children with acute lymphoblastic leukemia. Radiother Oncol 1998;48:29–32.
47. De Wit MC, de Bruin HG, Eijkenboom W, et al. Immediate post-radiotherapy changes in malignant glioma can mimic tumor progression. Neurology 2004;63:535–7.
48. Brandes AA, Tosoni A, Spagnolli F, Frezza G, Leonardi M, Calbucci F, Franceschi E. Disease progression or pseudoprogression after concomitant radiochemotherapy treatment: Pitfalls in neurooncology. Neuro Oncol 2008;26:2192–7.
49. Armstrong C, Ruffer J, Corn B, et al. Biphasic patterns of memory deficits following moderate-dose partial-brain irradiation: neuropsychologic outcome and proposed mechanisms. J Clin Oncol 1995;13:2263–71.
50. Vigliani MC, Sichez N, Poisson M, et al. A prospective study of cognitive functions following conventional radiotherapy for supratentorial gliomas in young adults: 4-year results. Int J Radiat Oncol Biol Phys 1996;35:527–33.
51. Chak LY, Zatz LM, Wasserstein P, et al. Neurologic dysfunction in patients treated for small cell carcinoma of the lung: a clinical and radiological study. Int J Radiat Oncol Biol Phys 1986;12:385–9.
52. Creange A, Felten D, Kiesel I, et al. Leucoencéphalopathie subaiguë du rhombencéphale après radiothérapie hypophysaire. Rev Neurol (Paris) 1994;150:704–8.
53. Song T, Liang BL, Huang SQ, et al. Magnetic resonance imaging manifestations of radiation injury in brain stem and cervical spinal cord of nasopharyngeal carcinoma patients after radiotherapy. Ai Zheng 2005;24:357–61 [Abstract].
54. Lampert P, Tom MI, Rider WD. Disseminated demyelination of the brain following Co60 radiation. Arch Pathol 1959;68:322–30.
55. Ochi S, Takahashi Y, Yokoyama S. Fulminating midbrain irradiation injury of pediatric brain tumor. No To Shinke 2005;57:800–5 [Abstract].
56. Malone S, Raaphorst GP, Gray R, et al. Enhanced in vitro radiosensitivity of skin fibroblasts in two patients developing brain necrosis following AVM radiosurgery: a new risk factor with potential for a predictive assay. Int J Radiat Oncol Biol Phys 2000;47:185–9.
57. Flickinger JC, Kondziolka D, Lunsford LD, et al. Development of a model to predict permanent symptomatic postradiosurgery injury for arteriovenous malformation patients. Arteriovenous Malformation Radiosurgery Study Group. Int J Radiat Oncol Biol Phys 2000;46:1143–8.
58. Schlienger M, Atlan D, Lefkopoulos D, et al. Linac radiosurgery for cerebral arteriovenous malformations: results in 169 patients. Int J Radiat Oncol Biol Phys 2000;46:1135–42.
59. Miyawaki L, Dowd C, Wara W, et al. Five-year results of LINAC radiosurgery for arteriovenous malformations: outcome for large AVMS. Int J Radiat Oncol Biol Phys 1999;44:1089–106.
60. Morris GM, Coderre JA, Micca PL, et al. Central nervous system tolerance to boron neutron capture therapy with *p*-boronophenylalanine. Br J Cancer 1997;76:1623–9.
61. Oppenheimer JH, Levy ML, Sinha U, et al. Radionecrosis secondary to interstitial brachytherapy: correlation of magnetic resonance imaging and histopathology. Neurosurgery 1992;31:336–43.
62. Van Effenterre R, Boch AL. Radionécrose du chiasma. Neurochirurgie 1993;39:75–84.
63. Coghlan KM, Magennis P. Cerebral radionecrosis following the treatment of parotid tumours: a case report and review of the literature. Int J Oral Maxillofac Surg 1999;28:50–2.

64. Cirafisi C, Verderame F. Radiation-induced rhombencephalopathy. Ital J Neurol Sci 1999; 20:55–8.
65. Kumar AJ, Leeds NE, Fuller GN, et al. Malignant gliomas: MR imaging spectrum of radiation therapy-and chemotherapy-induced necrosis of the brain after treatment. Radiology 2000;217:377–84.
66. Janus TJ, Kim EE, Tilbury R, et al. Use of [18F] fluorodeoxyglucose positron emission tomography in patients with primary malignant brain tumors. Ann Neurol 1993;33:540–8.
67. Lamy-Lhullier C, Dubois F, Blond S, et al. Intérêt de la tomoscintigraphie cérébrale au sestamibi marqué au technétium dans le diagnostic différentiel récidive tumorale-radionécrose des tumeurs gliales sus-tentorielles de l'adulte. Neurochirurgie 1999;45:110–7.
68. Henze M, Mohammed A, Schlemmer H, et al. Detection of tumour progression in the follow-up of irradiated low-grade astrocytomas: comparison of 3-[123I]-iodo-alpha-methyl-l-tyrosine and 99mTc-MIBI SPET. Eur J Nucl Med Mol Imaging 2002;29:1455–61.
69. Matheja P, Weckesser M, Rickert Ch, et al. I-123-lodo-alpha-methyl tyrosine SPECT in nonparenchymal brain tumours. Nuklearmedizin 2002;41:191–6.
70. Galanaud D, Nicoli F, Figarella-Branger D, et al. MR spectroscopy of brain tumors. J Radiol 2006;87:822–32.
71. Schlemmer HP, Bachert P, Herfarth KK, et al. Proton MR spectroscopic evaluation of suspicious brain lesions after stereotactic radiotherapy. AJNR Am J Neuroradiol 2001;22:1316–24.
72. Lichy MP, Bachert P, Hamprecht F, et al. Application of[1] MR spectroscopic imaging in radiation oncology: choline as a marker for determining the relative probability of tumor progression after radiation of glial brain tumors. Rofo 2006;178:627–33 [Abstract].
73. Ricci PE, Karis JP, Heiserman JE, et al. Differentiating recurrent tumor from radiation necrosis: time for re-evaluation of positron emission tomography?. AJNR Am J Neuroradiol 1998;19:407–13.
74. Matheja P, Rickert C, Weckesser M, et al. Scintigraphic pitfall: delayed radionecrosis: case illustration. J Neurosurg 2000;92:732.
75. Forsyth PA, Kelly PJ, Cascino TL, et al. Radiation necrosis or glioma recurrence: is computer-assisted stereotactic biopsy useful?. J Neurosurg 1995;82:436–44.
76. Glantz MJ, Burger PC, Friedman AH, et al. Treatment of radiation-induced nervous system injury with heparin and warfarin. Neurology 1994;44:2020–7.
77. Chuba PJ, Aronin P, Bhambhani K, et al. Hyperbaric oxygen therapy for radiation-induced brain injury in children. Cancer 1997;80:2005–12.
78. Leber KA, Eder HG, Kovac H, et al. Treatment of cerebral radionecrosis by hyperbaric oxygen therapy. Stereotact Funct Neurosurg 1998;70:229–36.
79. Kohshi K, Imada H, Nomoto S, et al. Successful treatment of radiation-induced brain necrosis by hyperbaric oxygen therapy. J Neurol Sci 2003;209:115–7.
80. Feldmeier JJ, Hampson NB. A systematic review of the literature reporting the application of hyperbaric oxygen prevention and treatment of delayed radiation injuries: an evidence based approach. Undersea Hyperb Med 2002;29:4–30 [Abstract].
81. Chan AS, Cheung MC, Law SC, et al. Phase II study of alpha-tocopherol in improving the cognitive function of patients with temporal lobe radionecrosis. Cancer 2004;100:398–404.
82. Fike JR, Gobbel GT, Marton LJ, et al. Radiation brain injury is reduced by the polyamine inhibitor alpha-difluoromethylornithine. Radiat Res 1994;138:99–106.
83. Kondziolka D, Mori Y, Martinez AJ, et al. Beneficial effects of the radioprotectant 21-aminosteroid U-74389G in a radiosurgery rat malignant glioma model. Int J Radiat Oncol Biol Phys 1999;44:179–84.
84. Guelman LR, Zorrilla Zubilete MA, Rios H, et al. WR-2721 (amifostine, ethyol) prevents motor and morphological changes induced by neonatal X-irradiation. Neurochem Int 2003;42:385–91.
85. Sasse AD, Clark LG, Sasse EC, et al. Amifostine reduces side effects and improves complete response rate during radiotherapy: results of a meta-analysis. Int J Radiat Oncol Biol Phys 2006;64:784–91.
86. Lyubimova N, Coultas P, Yuen K, et al. In vivo radioprotection of mouse brain endothelial cells by Hoechst 33342. Br J Radiol 2001;74:77–82.
87. Guelman L, Zorilla Z, Rios H, et al. GM1 ganglioside treatment protects against long-term neurotoxic effects of neonatal X-irradiation on cerebellarcortex cytoarchitecture and motor functions. Brain Res 2000;858:303–11.
88. Brustle O, Jones KN, Learish RD, et al. Embryonic stem cell-derived glial precursors: a source of myelinating transplants. Science 1999;285:650–1.

89. Christie D, Lavin M, Tan L. Clinical application of in vitro radiohypersensitivity testing. Australas Radiol 2000;44:333–5.
90. Taphoorn MJ, Klein M. Cognitive deficits in adult patients with brain tumours. Lancet Neurol 2004;3:159–68.
91. Klein M, Engelberts NH, van der Ploeg HM, et al. Epilepsy in low-grade gliomas: the impact on cognitive function and quality of life. Ann Neurol 2003;54:514–20.
92. Klein M, Heimans JJ, Aaronson NK, et al. Effect of radiotherapy and other treatment-related factors on mid-term to long-term cognitive sequelae in low-grade gliomas: a comparative study. Lancet 2002;360:1361–8.
92a. Douw L, Klein M, Fagel SSAA, et al. Cognitive and radiological effects of radiotherapy in patients with low-grade glioma: long-term follow-up. Lancet Neurol 2009;8:810–8.
93. Armstrong CL, Hunter JV, Ledakis GE, et al. Late cognitive and radiographic changes related to radiotherapy: initial prospective findings. Neurology 2002;59:40–8.
94. Torres IJ, Mundt AJ, Sweeney PJ, et al. A longitudinal neuropsychological study of partial brain radiation in adults with brain tumors. Neurology 2003;60:1113–8.
95. Klein M, Heimans JJ, Aaronson NK, et al. Impaired cognitive functioning in low-grade glioma patients: relationship to tumor localisation, radiotherapy and the use of anticonvulsants. J Clin Oncol 2004;22:966–7.
96. Asai A, Matsutani M, Kohno T, et al. Subacute brain atrophy after radiation therapy for malignant brain tumor. Cancer 1989;63:1962–74.
97. Imperato JP, Paleologos NA, Vick NA. Effects of treatment on long-term survivors with malignant astrocytomas. Ann Neurol 1990;28:818–22.
98. Vigliani MC, Duyckaerts C, Delattre JY. Radiation-induced cognitive dysfunction in adults. In: Vecht CJ, editor. Handbook of Clinical Neurology, vol. 23. Amsterdam: Elsevier; 1997. p. 371–88.
99. Fisher B, Seiferheld W, Schultz C, et al. Secondary analysis of Radiation Therapy Oncology Group study (RTOG) 9310: an intergroup phase II combined modality treatment of primary central nervous system lymphoma. J Neurooncol 2005;74:201–5.
100. Archibald YM, Lunn D, Ruttan LA, et al. Cognitive functioning in long-term survivors of high-grade glioma. J Neurosurg 1994;80:247–53.
101. Lee PW, Hung BK, Woo EK, et al. Effects of radiation therapy on neuropsychological functioning in patients with nasopharyngeal carcinoma. J Neurol Neurosurg Psychiatry 1989;52:488–92.
102. DeAngelis LM, Delattre JY, Posner JB. Radiation-induced dementia in patients cured of brain metastases. Neurology 1989;39:789–96.
103. Duffner PK. Long-term effects of radiation on cognitive and endocrine function in children with leukemia and brain tumors. Neurologist 2004;10:293–310.
104. DeAngelis LM, Yahalom J, Thaler HT, et al. Combined modality therapy for primary CNS lymphoma. J Clin Oncol 1992;10:635–43.
105. Abrey LE, Yahalom J, DeAngelis LM. Treatment for primary CNS lymphoma: the next step. J Clin Oncol 2000;18:3144–50.
106. Wassenberg MW, Bromberg JE, Witkamp TD, et al. White matter lesions and encephalopathy in patients treated for primary central nervous system lymphoma. J Neurooncol 2001;52:73–80.
107. Armstrong CL, Corn BW, Ruffer JE, et al. Radiotherapeutic effects on brain function: double dissociation of memory systems. Neuropsychiatry Neuropsychol Behav Neurol 2000;13:101–11.
108. Postma TJ, Klein M, Verstappen CC, et al. Radiotherapy-induced cerebral abnormalities in patients with low-grade glioma. Neurology 2002;59:121–3.
109. Meyers CA, Weitzner MA, Valentine AD, et al. Methylphenidate therapy improves cognition, mood, and function of brain tumor patients. J Clin Oncol 1998;16:2522–7.
110. Shaw EG, Rosdhal R, D'Agostino Jr RB, et al. Phase II study of donepezil in irradiated brain tumor patients: effect on cognitive function, mood, and quality of life. J Clin Oncol 2006;24:1415–20 Abstract..
111. Senzer N. Rationale for a phase III study of erythropoietin as a neurocognitive protectant in patients with lung cancer receiving prophylactic cranial irradiation. Semin Oncol 2002;29:47–52.
111b. Robbins ME, Diz DI. Pathogenic role of the renin-angiotensin system in modulating radiation-induced late effects. Int J Radiat Oncol Biol Phys 2006;64:6–12.
111c. Nieder C, Andratschke NH, Wiedenmann N, Molls M. Prevention of radiation-induced central nervous system toxicity: a role for amifostine?. Anticancer Res 2004;24:3803–9.
112. Crossen JR, Garwood D, Glatstein E, et al Neurobehavioral sequelae of cranial irradiation in adults: a review of radiation-induced encephalopathy. J Clin Oncol 1994;12:627–42.

113. Mulhern RK, Merchant TE, Gajjar A, et al. Late neurocognitive sequelae in survivors of brain tumours in childhood. Lancet Oncol 2004;5:399–408.
114. Brown PD, Buckner JC, O'Fallon JR, et al. Effects of radiotherapy on cognitive function in patients with low-grade glioma measured by the Folstein Mini-Mental State Examination. J Clin Oncol 2003;21:2519–24.
115. Thiessen B, DeAngelis LM. Hydrocephalus in radiation leukoencephalopathy: results of ventriculoperitoneal shunting. Arch Neurol 1998;55:705–10.
116. Perrini P, Scollato A, Cioffi F, et al. Radiation leukoencephalopathy associated with moderate hydrocephalus: intracranial pressure monitoring and results of ventriculoperitoneal shunting. Neurol Sci 2002;23:237–41.
117. Kleinschmidt-Demasters BK, Kang JS, Lillehei KO. The burden of radiation-induced central nervous system tumors: a single institutions experience. J Neuropathol Exp Neurol 2006;65:204–16.
118. Ron E, Modan B, Boice Jr JD, et al. Tumors of the brain and nervous system after radiotherapy in childhood. N Engl J Med 1988;319:1033–9.
119. Hawkins MM, Draper GJ, Kingston JE. Incidence of second primary tumours among childhood cancer survivors. Br J Cancer 1987;56:339–47.
120. Brada M, Ford D, Ashley S, et al. Risk of second brain tumour after conservative surgery and radiotherapy for pituitary adenoma. BMJ 1992;304:1343–6.
121. Minniti G, Traish D, Ashley S, et al. Risk of second brain tumor after conservative surgery and radiotherapy for pituitary adenoma: update after further 10 years. J Clin Endocrinol Metab 2005;90:800–4.
122. Neglia JP, Meadows AT, Robison LL, et al. Second neoplasms after acute lymphoblastic leukemia in childhood. N Engl J Med 1991;325:1330–6.
123. Muracciole X, Cowen D, Regis J. Radiosurgery and brain radio-induced carcinogenesis: update. Neurochirurgie 2004;50:414–20.
124. Amirjamshidi A, Abbassioun K. Radiation-induced tumors of the central nervous system occurring in childhood and adolescence: four unusual lesions in three patients and a review of the literature. Childs Nerv Syst 2000;16:390–7.
125. Strojan P, Popovic M, Jereb B. Secondary intracranial meningiomas after high-dose cranial irradiation: report of five cases and review of the literature. Int J Radiat Oncol Biol Phys 2000;48:65–73.
126. Musa BS, Pople IK, Cummins BH. Intracranial meningiomas following irradiation: a growing problem?. Br J Neurosurg 1995;9:629–37.
127. De Tommasi A, Occhiogrosso M, De Tommasi C, et al. Radiation-induced intracranial meningiomas: review of six operated cases. Neurosurg Rev 2005;28:104–14.
128. Shoshan Y, Chernova O, Juen SS, et al. Radiation-induced meningioma: a distinct molecular genetic pattern? J Neuropathol Exp Neurol 2000;59:614–20.
129. Rajcan-Separovic E, Maguire J, Loukianova T, et al. Loss of 1p and 7p in radiation-induced meningiomas identified by comparative genomic hybridization. Cancer Genet Cytogene 2003;144:6–11.
130. Mack EE. Radiation-induced tumors. In: Berger MS, Wilson CB, editors. The Gliomas. Philadelphia: WB Saunders; 1999. p. 724–35.
131. Salvati M, Frati A, Russo N, et al. Radiation-induced gliomas: report of 10 cases and review of the literature. Surg Neurol 2003;60:60–7.
132. Brat DJ, James CD, Jedlicka AE, et al. Molecular genetic alterations in radiation-induced astrocytomas. Am J Pathol 1999;154:1431–8.
133. Murros KE, Toole JF. The effect of radiation on carotid arteries: a review article. Arch Neurol 1989;46:449–55.
134. Gupta S. Radiation-induced carotid artery blow out: a case report. Acta Chir Belg 1994;94:299–300.
135. McCready RA, Hyde GL, Bivins BA, et al. Radiation-induced arterial injuries. Surgery 1983;93:306–12.
136. Bernstein M, Lumley M, Davidson G, et al. Intracranial arterial occlusion associated with high-activity iodine-125 brachytherapy for glioblastoma. J Neurooncol 1993;17:253–60.
137. Werner MH, Burger PC, Heinz ER, et al. Intracranial atherosclerosis following radiotherapy. Neurology 1988;38:1158–60.
138. Bitzer M, Topka H. Progressive cerebral occlusive disease after radiation therapy. Stroke 1995;26:131–6.
139. Grill J, Couanet D, Cappelli C, et al. Radiation-induced cerebral vasculopathy in children with neurofibromatosis and optic pathway glioma. Ann Neurol 1999;45:393–6.

140. Suzuki Y, Negoro M, Shibuya M, et al. Surgical treatment for pediatric moyamoya disease: use of the superficial temporal artery for both areas supplied by the anterior and middle cerebral arteries. Neurosurgery 1997;40:324–9.
141. Dauser RC, Tuite GF, McCluggage CW. Dural inversion procedure for moyamoya disease: technical note. J Neurosurg 1997;86:719–23.
142. Ross IB, Shevell MI, Montes JL, et al. Encephaloduroarteriosynangiosis (EDAS) for the treatment of childhood moyamoya disease. Pediatr Neurol 1994;10:199–204.
143. Kim SK, Wang KC, Kim IO, et al. Combined encephaloduroarteriosynangiosis and bifrontal encephalogaleo(periosteal)synangiosis in pediatric moyamoya disease. Neurosurgery 2002;50:88–96.
144. Fouladi M, Langston J, Mulhern R, et al. Silent lacunar lesions detected by magnetic resonance imaging of children with brain tumors: a late sequela of therapy. J Clin Onco 2000;18:824–31.
145. Baumgartner JE, Ater JL, Ha CS, et al. Pathologically proven cavernous angiomas of the brain following radiation therapy for pediatric brain tumors. Pediatr Neurosurg 2003;39:201–7.
146. Heckl S, Aschoff A, Kunze S. Radiation-induced cavernous hemangiomas of the brain: a late effect predominantly in children. Cancer 2002;94:3285–91.
147. Mauget-Faysse M, Vuillaume M, Quaranta M, et al. Idiopathic and radiation-induced ocular telangiectasia: the involvement of the ATM gene. Invest Ophthalmol Vis Sci 2003;44:3257–62.
148. Novelli PM, Reigel DH, Langham GP, et al. Multiple cavernous angiomas after high-dose whole-brain radiation therapy. Pediatr Neurosurg 1997;26:322–5.
149. Jensen FK, Wagner A. Intracranial aneurysm following radiation therapy for medulloblastoma: a case report and review of the literature. Acta Radiol 1997;38:37–42.
150. Louis E, Martin-Duverneuil N, Carpentier AF, et al. Anévrysme post-radique de la carotide intra-caverneuse. Rev Neurol (Paris) 2003;159:319–22.
151. Azzarelli B, Moore J, Gilmor R, et al. Multiple fusiform intracranial aneurysms following curative radiation therapy for suprasellar germinoma: case report. J Neurosurg 1984;61:1141–5.
152. Constine LS, Woolf PD, Cann D, et al. Hypothalamic-pituitary dysfunction after radiation for brain tumors. N Engl J Med 1993;328:87–94.
153. Littley MD, Shalet SM. Beardwell CG, et al. Radiation and hypothalamic-pituitary function. Baillieres Clin Endocrinol Metab 1990;4:147–75.
154. Littley MD, Shalet SM, Beardwell CG, et al. Radiation-induced hypopituitarism is dose-dependent. Clin Endocrinol (Oxf) 1989;31:363–73.
155. Clayton PE, Shalet SM. Dose dependency of time of onset of radiation-induced growth hormone deficiency. J Pediatr 1991;118:226–8.
156. Rappaport R, Brauner R. Growth and endocrine disorders secondary to cranial irradiation. Pediatr Res 1989;25:561–7.
157. Schmiegelow M, Lassen S, Poulsen HS, et al. Cranial radiotherapy of childhood brain tumours: growth hormone deficiency and its relation to the biological effective dose of irradiation in a large population based study. Clin Endocrinol (Oxf) 2000;53:191–7.
158. Stevens G, Downes S, Ralston A. Thyroid dose in children undergoing prophylactic cranial irradiation. Int J Radiat Oncol Biol Phys 1998;42:385–90.
159. Livesey EA, Hindmarsh PC, Brook CGD, et al. Endocrine disorders following treatment of childhood brain tumours. Br J Cancer 1990;61622–5.
160. Arlt W, Hove U, Muller B, et al. Frequent and frequently overlooked: treatment-induced endocrine dysfunction in adult long-term survivors of primary brain tumors. Neurology 1997;49:498–506.
161. Taphoorn MJ, Heimans JJ, van der Veen EA, et al. Endocrine functions in long-term survivors of low-grade supratentorial glioma treated with radiation therapy. J Neurooncol 1995;25:97–102.
162. Samaan NA, Vieto R, Schultz PN, et al. Hypothalamic, pituitary and thyroid dysfunction after radiotherapy to the head and neck. Int J Radiat Oncol Biol Phys 1982;8:1857–67.
163. Petterson T, MacFarlane IA, Foy PM, et al. Hyperprolactinemia and infertility following cranial irradiation for brain tumours: successful treatment with bromocriptine. Br J Neurosurg 1993;7:571–4.
164. Ahlbom H. Results of radiotherapy of hypopharyngeal cancer at Radium-Hemmet, Stockholm. Acta Radiol 1941;22:155–71.
165. Rampling R, Symonds P. Radiation myelopathy. Curr Opin Neurol 1998;11:627–32.
166. Word JA, Kalokhe UP, Aron BS, et al. Transient radiation myelopathy (L'hermitte's sign) in patients with Hodgkin's disease treated by mantle irradiation. Int J Radiat Oncol Biol Phys 1980;6:1731–3.

167. Fein DA, Marcus Jr RB, Parsons JT, et al. L'hermitte's sign: incidence and treatment variables influencing risk after irradiation of the cervical spinal cord. Int J Radiat Oncol Biol Phys 1993;27:1029–33.
168. Esik O, Csere T, Stefanits K, et al. A review on radiogenic L'hermitte's sign. Pathol Oncol Res 2003;9:115–20.
169. Lewanski CR, Sinclair JA, Stewart JS. L'hermitte's sign following head and neck radiotherapy. Clin Oncol (R Coll Radiol) 2000;12:98–103.
170. Li YQ, Jay V, Wong CS. Oligodendrocytes in the adult rat spinal cord undergo radiation-induced apoptosis. Cancer Res 1996;56:5417–22.
171. Lengyel Z, Reko G, Majtenyi K, et al. Autopsy verifies demyelination and lack of vascular damage in partially reversible radiation myelopathy. Spinal Cord 2003;41:577–85.
172. Chao MW, Wirth A, Ryan G, et al. Radiation myelopathy following transplantation and radiotherapy for non-Hodgkin's lymphoma. Int J Radiat Oncol Biol Phys 1998;41:1057–61.
173. Schultheiss TE, Stephens LC. Invited review: permanent radiation myelopathy. Br J Radiol 1992;65:737–53.
174. Pallis CA, Louis S, Morgan RL. Radiation myelopathy. Brain 1961;84:460–79.
175. Wang PY, Shen WC, Jan JS. MR imaging in radiation myelopathy. AJNR Am J Neuroradiol 1992;13:1049–55.
176. Wang PY, Shen WC, Jan JS. Serial MRI changes in radiation myelopathy. Neuroradiology 1995;37:374–7.
177. Yasui T, Yagura H, Komiyama M, et al. Significance of gadolinium-enhanced magnetic resonance imaging in differentiating spinal cord radiation myelopathy from tumor: case report. J Neurosurg 1992;77:628–31.
178. Komachi H, Tsuchiya K, Ikeda M, et al. Radiation myelopathy: a clinicopathological study with special reference to correlation between MRI findings and neuropathology. J Neurol Sci 1995;132:228–32.
179. Koehler PJ, Verbiest H, Jager J, et al. Delayed radiation myelopathy: serial MR-imaging and pathology. Clin Neurol Neurosurg 1996;98:197–201.
180. Michikawa M, Wada Y, Sano M, et al. Radiation myelopathy: significance of gadolinium-DTPA enhancement in the diagnosis. Neuroradiology 1991;33:286–9.
181. Alfonso ER, De Gregorio MA, Mateo P, et al. Radiation myelopathy in over-irradiated patients: MR imaging findings. Eur Radiol 1997;7:400–4.
182. Angibaud G, Ducasse JL, Baille G, et al. Potential value of hyperbaric oxygenation in the treatment of post-radiation myelopathies. Rev Neurol (Paris) 1995;151:661–6.
183. Calabro F, Jinkins JR. MRI of radiation myelitis: a report of a case treated with hyperbaric oxygen. Eur Radiol 2000;10:1079–84.
184. Allen JC, Miller DC, Budzilovich GN, et al. Brain and spinal cord hemorrhage in long-term survivors of malignant pediatric brain tumors: a possible late effect of therapy. Neurology 1991;41:148–50.
185. Packer RJ, Gurney JG, Punyko JA, et al. Long-term neurologic and neurosensory sequelae in adult survivors of a childhood brain tumor: childhood cancer survivor study. J Clin Oncol 2003;21:3255–61.
186. Sagar SM, Thomas RJ, Loverock LT, et al. Olfactory sensations produced by high-energy photon irradiation of the olfactory receptor mucosa in humans. Int J Radiat Oncol Biol Phys 1991;20:771–6.
187. Carmichael KA, Jennings AS, Doty RL. Reversible anosmia after pituitary irradiation. Ann Intern Med 1984;100:532–3.
188. Ophir D, Guterman A, Gross-Isseroff R. Changes in smell acuity induced by radiation exposure of the olfactory mucosa. Arch Otolaryngol Head Neck Surg 1988;114:853–5.
189. Qiu Q, Chen S, Meng C, et al. Observation on the changes in nasopharyngeal carcinoma patients' olfactory before and after radiotherapy. Lin Chuang Er Bi Yan Hou Ke Za Zhi 2001;15:57–8 [Abstract].
190. Lessell S. Friendly fire: neurogenic visual loss from radiation therapy. J Neuroophthalmol 2004;24:243–50.
191. Parsons JT, Bova FJ, Fitzgerald CR, et al. Radiation optic neuropathy after megavoltage external-beam irradiation: analysis of time-dose factors. Int J Radiat Oncol Biol Phys 1994;30:755–63.
192. Valanconny C, Koenig F, Benchaboune M, et al. Complications de la radiothérapie des néovaisseaux de la dégénérescence maculaire liée à l'âge. J Fr Ophtalmol 2000;23:151–7.

193. Meyer A, Levy C, Blondel J, et al. Neuropathie optique après protonthérapie pour mélanome malin de la choroïde. J Fr Ophtalmol 2000;23:543–53.
194. Piquemal R, Cottier JP, Arsene S, et al. Radiation-induced optic neuropathy 4 years after radiation: report of a case followed up with MRI. Neuroradiology 1998;40:439–41.
195. Levin LA, Gragoudas ES, Lessell S. Endothelial cell loss in irradiated optic nerves. Ophthalmology 2000;107:370–4.
196. Danesh-Meyer HV, Savino PJ, Sergott RC. Visual loss despite anticoagulation in radiation-induced optic neuropathy. Clin Experiment Ophthalmol 2004;32:333–5.
197. Borruat FX, Schatz NJ, Glaser JS, et al. Visual recovery from radiation-induced optic neuropathy. The role of hyperbaric oxygen therapy. J Clin Neuroophthalmol 1993;13:98–101.
198. Roden D, Bosley TM, Fowble B, et al. Delayed radiation injury to the retrobulbar optic nerves and chiasm. Clinical syndrome and treatment with hyperbaric oxygen and corticosteroids. Ophthalmology 1990;97:346–51.
199. Boschetti M, De Lucchi M, Giusti M, et al. Partial visual recovery from radiation-induced optic neuropathy after hyperbaric oxygen therapy in a patient with Cushing disease. Eur J Endocrinol 2006;154:813–8.
200. Mohamed IG, Roa W, Fulton D, et al. Optic nerve sheath fenestration for a reversible optic neuropathy in radiation oncology. Am J Clin Oncol 2000;23:401–5.
200b. Kim JH, Brown SL, Kolozsvary A, Jenrow KA, Ryu S, Rosenblum ML, et al. Modification of radiation injury by ramipril, inhibitor of angiotensin-converting enzyme, on optic neuropathy in the rat. Radiat Res 2004;161:137–42.
201. Lessell S, Lessell IM, Rizzo III JF. Ocular neuromyotonia after radiation therapy. Am J Ophthalmol 1986;102:766–70.
202. Marti-Fabregas J, Montero J, Lopez-Villegas D, et al. Post-irradiation neuromyotonia in bilateral facial and trigeminal nerve distribution. Neurology 1997;48:1107–9.
203. Diaz JM, Urban ES, Schiffman JS, et al. Post-irradiation neuromyotonia affecting trigeminal nerve distribution: an unusual presentation. Neurology 1992;42:1102–4.
204. Maesawa S, Salame C, Flickinger JC, et al. Clinical outcomes after stereotactic radiosurgery for idiopathic trigeminal neuralgia. J Neurosurg 2001;94:14–20.
205. Rogers CL, Shetter AG, Fiedler JA, et al. Gamma knife radiosurgery for trigeminal neuralgia: the initial experience of The Barrow Neurological Institute. Int J Radiat Oncol Biol Phys 2000;47:1013–9.
206. Combs SE, Thilmann C, Debus J, et al. Long-term outcome of stereotactic radiosurgery (SRS) in patients with acoustic neuromas. Int J Radiat Oncol Biol Phys 2006;64:1341–7.
207. McClelland 3rd S, Gerbi BJ, Higgins PD, Orner JB, Hall WA. Safety and efficacy of fractionated stereotactic radiotherapy for acoustic neuromas. J Neurooncol 2008;86:191–4.
208. Giese WL, Kinsella TJ. Radiation injury to peripheral and cranial nerves. In: Gutin PH, Leibel SA, Sheline GE, editors. Radiation Injury to the Nervous System. New York: Raven; 1991. p. 383–403.
209. DeWys WD, Walters K. Abnormalities of taste sensation in cancer patients. Cancer 1975; 36:1888–96.
210. Noren G, Greitz D, Hirsch A, et al. Gamma knife surgery in acoustic tumours. Acta Neurochir Suppl (Wien) 1993;58:104–7.
211. Foote RL, Coffey RJ, Swanson JW, et al. Stereotactic radiosurgery using the gamma knife for acoustic neuromas. Int J Radiat Oncol Biol Phys 1995;32:1153–60.
212. Selch MT, Pedroso A, Lee SP, et al. Stereotactic radiotherapy for the treatment of acoustic neuromas. J Neurosurg 2004;101:362–72.
213. Gibb AG, Loh KS. The role of radiation in delayed hearing loss in nasopharyngeal carcinoma. J Laryngol Otol 2000;114:139–44.
214. McDonald LW, Donovo MP, Plantz RG. Radiosensitivity of the vestibular apparatus of the rabbit. Radiat Res 1966;27:510–1.
215. Kondziolka D, Nathoo N, Flickinger JC, et al. Long-term results after radiosurgery for benign intracranial tumors. Neurosurgery 2003;53:815–21.
216. Kondziolka D, Lunsford LD, McLaughlin MR, et al. Long-term outcomes after radiosurgery for acoustic neuromas. N Engl J Med 1998;339:1426–33.
217. Spiegelmann R, Lidar Z, Gofman J, et al. Linear accelerator radiosurgery for vestibular schwannoma. J Neurosurg 2001;94:7–13.
218. Niranjan A, Lunsford LD, Flickinger JC, et al. Dose reduction improves hearing preservation rates after intracanalicular acoustic tumor radiosurgery. Neurosurgery 1999;45:753–62.

219. Ito K, Shin M, Matsuzaki M, et al. Risk factors for neurological complications after acoustic neurinoma radiosurgery: refinement from further experiences. Int J Radiat Oncol Biol Phys 2000;48:75–80.
220. Berger PS, Bataini JP. Radiation-induced cranial nerve palsy. Cancer 1977;40:152–5.
221. Cheng VS, Schultz MD. Unilateral hypoglossal nerve atrophy as a late complication of radiation therapy of head and neck carcinoma: a report of four cases and a review of the literature on peripheral and cranial nerve damages after radiation therapy. Cancer 1975;35:1537–44.
222. Johnston EF, Hammond AJ, Cairncross JG. Bilateral hypoglossal palsies: a late complication of curative radiotherapy. Can J Neurol Sci 1989;16:198–9.
223. Kang MY, Holland JM, Stevens Jr KR. Cranial neuropathy following curative chemotherapy and radiotherapy for carcinoma of the nasopharynx. J Laryngol Otol 2000;114:308–10.
224. King AD, Ahuja A, Leung SF, et al. MR features of the denervated tongue in radiation-induced neuropathy. Br J Radiol 1999;72:349–53.
225. King AD, Leung SF, Teo P, et al. Hypoglossal nerve palsy in nasopharyngeal carcinoma. Head Neck 1999;21:614–9.
226. Stern Y, Marshak G, Shpitzer T, et al. Vocal cord palsy: possible late complication of radiotherapy for head and neck cancer. Ann Otol Rhinol Laryngol 1995;104:294–6.
227. Takimoto T, Saito Y, Suzuki M, et al. Radiation-induced cranial nerve palsy: hypoglossal nerve and vocal cord palsies. J Laryngol Otol 1991;105:44–5.
228. Huang XM, Zheng YQ, Zhang XM, et al. Diagnosis and management of skull base osteoradionecrosis after radiotherapy for nasopharyngeal carcinoma. Laryngoscope 2006;116:1626–31.
229. Rowin J, Cheng G, Lewis SL, Meriggioli MN. Late appearance of dropped head syndrome after radiotherapy for Hodgkin's disease. Muscle Nerve 2006;34:666–9.
230. Salner AL, Botnick LE, Herzog AG, et al. Reversible brachial plexopathy following primary radiation therapy for breast cancer. Cancer Treat Rep 1981;65:797–802.
231. Pierce SM, Recht A, Lingos TI, et al. Long-term radiation complications following conservative surgery (CS) and radiation therapy (RT) in patients with early stage breast cancer. Int J Radiat Oncol Biol Phys 1992;23:915–23.
232. Vega F, Davila L, Delattre JY, et al. Experimental carcinomatous plexopathy. J Neurol 1993;240:54–8.
233. Pradat PF, Poisson M, Delattre JY. Neuropathies radiques. Rev Neurol (Paris) 1994;150:664–77.
234. Stoll BA, Andrews JT. Radiation-induced peripheral neuropathy. BMJ 1966;11:834–7.
235. Olsen NK, Pfeiffer P, Mondrup K, et al. Radiation-induced brachial plexus neuropathy in breast cancer patients. Acta Oncol 1990;29:885–90.
236. Gillette EL, Mahler PA, Powers BE, et al. Late radiation injury to muscle and peripheral nerves. Int J Radiat Oncol Biol Phys 1995;31:1309–18.
237. Kori SH, Foley KM, Posner JB. Brachial plexus lesions in patients with cancer: 100 cases. Neurology 1981;31:45–50.
238. Kori SH. Diagnosis and management of brachial plexus lesions in cancer patients. Oncology (Huntingt) 1995;9:756–60.
239. Thyagarajan D, Cascino T, Harms G. Magnetic resonance imaging in brachial plexopathy of cancer. Neurology 1995;45:421–7.
240. Harper Jr CM, Thomas JE, Cascino TL, et al. Distinction between neoplastic and radiation-induced brachial plexopathy, with emphasis on the role of EMG. Neurology 1989;39:502–6.
241. Cooke J, Powell S, Parsons C. The diagnosis by computed tomography of brachial plexus lesions following radiotherapy for carcinoma of the breast. Clin Radiol 1988;39:602–6.
242. Fishman EK, Campbell JN, Kuhlman JE, et al. Multiplanar CT evaluation of brachial plexopathy in breast cancer. J Comput Assist Tomogr 1991;15:790–5.
243. Wouter van Es H, Engelen AM, Witkamp TD, et al. Radiation-induced brachial plexopathy: MR imaging. Skeletal Radiol 1997;26:284–8.
244. Qayyum A, MacVicar AD, Padhani AR, et al. Symptomatic brachial plexopathy following treatment for breast cancer: utility of MR imaging with surface-coil techniques. Radiology 2000;214:837–42.
245. Ahmad A, Barrington S, Maisey M, et al. Use of positron emission tomography in evaluation of brachial plexopathy in breast cancer patients. Br J Cancer 1999;79:478–82.
246. Soto O. Radiation-induced conduction block: resolution following anticoagulant therapy. Muscle Nerve 2005;31:642–5.
247. Gerard JM, Franck N, Moussa Z, et al. Acute ischemic brachial plexus neuropathy following radiation therapy. Neurology 1989;39:450–1.

248. Thomas JE, Cascino TL, Earle JD. Differential diagnosis between radiation and tumor plexopathy of the pelvis. Neurology 1985;35:1–7.
249. Maier JG, Perry RH, Saylor W, et al. Radiation myelitis of the dorsolumbar spinal cord. Radiology 1969;93:153–60.
250. Bowen J, Gregory R, Squier M, et al. The post-irradiation lower motor neuron syndrome neuronopathy or radiculopathy?. Brain 1996;119(Pt 5):1429–39.
251. Lamy C, Mas JL, Varet B, et al. Post-radiation lower motor neuron syndrome presenting as monomelic amyotrophy. J Neurol Neurosurg Psychiatry 1991;54:648–9.
252. Wohlgemuth WA, Rottach K, Jaenke G, et al. Radiogenic amyotrophy: cauda equina lesion as a late radiation sequel. Nervenarzt 1998;69:1061–5 [Abstract].
253. Anezaki T, Harada T, Kawachi I, et al. A case of post-irradiation lumbosacral radiculopathy successfully treated with corticosteroid and warfarin. Rinsho Shinkeigaku 1999;39:825–9 [Abstract].
254. Hussussian CJ, Mackinnon SE. Post-radiation neural sheath sarcoma of the brachial plexus: a case report. Ann Plast Surg 1999;43:313–7.
255. Adamson DC, Cummings TJ, Friedman AH. Malignant peripheral nerve sheath tumor of the spine after radiation therapy for Hodgkin's lymphoma. Clin Neuropathol 2004;23:245–55.
256. Foley KM, Woodruff JM, Ellis FT, et al. Radiation-induced malignant and atypical peripheral nerve sheath tumors. Ann Neurol 1980;7:311–8.
257. Shiu MH, Hilaris BS, Harrison LB, et al. Brachytherapy and function-saving resection of soft tissue sarcoma arising in the limb. Int J Radiat Oncol Biol Phys 1991;21:1485–92.
258. Wanebo JE, Malik JM, VandenBerg SR, et al. Malignant peripheral nerve sheath tumors: a clinicopathologic study of 28 cases. Cancer 1993;71:1247–53.

18 Paraneoplastic Disorders

MYRNA R. ROSENFELD • JOSEP DALMAU

Introduction

Paraneoplastic neurological disorders (PND) are a heterogeneous group of disorders that can affect any part of the neuraxis, including the retina and muscle.[1] Unlike other neurological complications that occur in patients with cancer, many PNDs are believed to be mediated by immune mechanisms. The current concept is that the expression of normal neuronal proteins by a cancer induces an immune response that targets the nervous system, resulting in neuronal dysfunction and/or neuronal cell death.[2] These immune responses are often associated with the presence of specific antineuronal serum and cerebrospinal fluid antibodies.

Antineuronal antibodies play a direct pathogenic role in three PNDs that affect the peripheral nervous system. These include antibodies to P/Q-type voltage-gated calcium channels (VGCC) in patients with the Lambert-Eaton myasthenic syndrome (LEMS),[3] antibodies to acetylcholine receptor in patients with myasthenia gravis, and antibodies to voltage-gated potassium channels (VGKC) in some patients with peripheral nerve hyperexcitability (neuromyotonia).[4] A common feature of these antibodies is that they target cell surface antigens and the associated disorders can occur without cancer; therefore, detection of these antibodies does not predict the presence of cancer. Antibodies to P/Q type VGCC are also found in a subgroup of patients with paraneoplastic cerebellar degeneration (PCD)[5] and antibodies to VGKC-related proteins can be found in some patients with cancer-associated or non–cancer-associated limbic encephalitis (LE) and Morvan syndrome.[6,7] In these cases, the antibodies are believed to be pathogenic, but this has not yet been proven. Similarly, there is recent evidence that antibodies to the N-methyl-D-aspartate (NMDA) receptor located on the cell surface are associated with a severe form of encephalitis and are likely pathogenic (Figure 18-1).[8] An antibody-mediated immunopathogenesis is also strongly suggested for the cerebellar and stiff-person syndromes associated with antibodies to glutamic-acid decarboxylase (GAD), and the paraneoplastic stiff-person

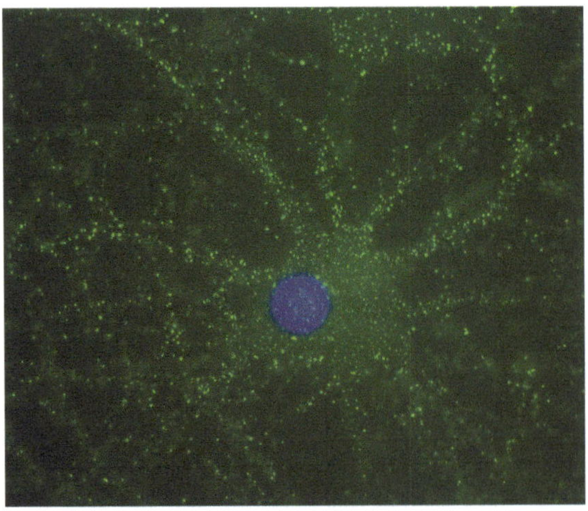

Figure 18-1 Anti-NMDA receptor antibody. Reactivity of the CSF of a patient with antibodies to NR1/NR2 heteromers of the NMDA receptor with cultures of rat hippocampal neurons. Note the intense reactivity of the antibodies with the cell surface of neurons. *×900 oil lens.*

syndrome related to antiamphiphysin antibodies. These two antigens are intracellular, close to the synaptic membrane, and the patients' antibodies appear to have a functional effect in vivo.[9,10]

For other PNDs, usually those that affect the central nervous system, more complex immune mechanisms appear to exist. In addition to the presence of antineuronal antibodies, PNDs of the central nervous system are associated with infiltrates of CD4+ and CD8+ T cells, microglial activation, gliosis, and variable neuronal loss.[11–13] The infiltrating T cells are often in close contact with neurons undergoing degeneration, suggesting a primary pathogenic role. The interaction of B- and T-cell mechanisms and the subacute development of extensive inflammatory abnormalities and neuronal degeneration could explain the difficulty in treating these disorders as well as their poor response to plasma exchange or intravenous immunoglobulins (IVIg).

Although they are increasingly becoming recognized, significant diagnostic delays are frequent even for well-described syndromes. In a series of 50 patients with LEMS, about half of the patients were initially misdiagnosed, usually with myasthenia gravis.[14] Another study noted an inverse correlation between the severity of the neurologic symptoms and the time to the diagnosis of the PND.[15] For patients who develop a syndrome that is typically associated with cancer and are found to have well-characterized paraneoplastic antibodies, the diagnosis of PND is relatively straightforward. The diagnosis of PND is more difficult in patients who develop less characteristic symptoms, especially if no antibodies are found in the serum or CSF. Features that suggest a paraneoplastic origin include an acute or subacute onset, and, if the central nervous system is involved, the CSF will often suggest an inflammatory process. If the patient is known to have cancer, metastastic or other nonmetastatic complications of cancer should be ruled out. For a patient in cancer remission, a recurrence should be suspected if symptoms of PND develop. For patients without a known cancer, if a PND is suspected, a detailed search for an underlying neoplasm is mandated. Whole body FDG-PET scans may detect tumors that escape detection by other standard imaging methods.[16–18] Features of individual syndromes that may aid in diagnosis (e.g., by neuroimaging) are noted in the following descriptions of individual syndromes.

Paraneoplastic Syndromes of the Brain

PARANEOPLASTIC CEREBELLAR DEGENERATION (PCD)

Paraneoplastic cerebellar degeneration is characterized by the rapid development of severe pancerebellar dysfunction that may be preceded by prodromic symptoms including dizziness, oscillopsia, blurry or double vision, nausea, and vomiting. Eventually, symptoms progress to truncal and appendicular ataxia, dysarthria, and downbeating nystagmus.[19] Symptoms of brainstem dysfunction, upgoing toes, or a mild neuropathy may occur. The subacute onset of PCD differentiates it from chronic degenerative diseases involving the cerebellum. Early MRI studies are usually normal; in some patients, transient enhancement of the cerebellar cortex has been noted. MRI studies late in the course usually show cerebellar atrophy.

The tumors more frequently involved are small cell lung cancer (SCLC), cancer of the breast and ovary, and Hodgkin lymphoma.[20] The paraneoplastic antibodies typically associated with prominent or pure cerebellar degeneration are anti-Yo antibodies in patients with breast and gynecologic cancers, and anti-Tr antibodies in patients with Hodgkin lymphoma. When PCD occurs in association with paraneoplastic encephalomyelitis (PEM), anti-Hu antibodies are almost always present.[21] When neoplasms other than breast and gynecological tumors are involved, patients are usually anti-Yo negative. Anti-Yo antibodies have been identified in a few male patients with PCD and cancer of the salivary gland, lung, and esophagus.[22,23] Patients with predominant truncal ataxia and opsoclonus or other ocular movement abnormalities may have anti-Ri antibodies, in which case the tumor is usually a breast carcinoma or, less frequently, gynecologic, bladder, or SCLC.[24,25] Antibodies to P/Q-type VGCC occur in some patients with SCLC and cerebellar dysfunction, although only some of these patients develop LEMS.[5] There is a group of patients, usually with SCLC, who harbor two or more antibodies, such as Zic4 and Hu or CRMP5 or all three. Patients who harbor only Zic4 antibodies are more likely to develop cerebellar dysfunction than patients with several antibodies.[26]

Prompt tumor control, immunosuppressive intervention, or perhaps different pathogenic mechanisms, may explain a number of single case reports describing neurologic improvement after tumor treatment, plasma exchange, IVIg, cyclophosphamide, or steroids.[27–29] However, large series of patients with well-defined antibody-positive PCD show that, in general, there is only rare improvement with treatment, if any.

PARANEOPLASTIC ENCEPHALOMYELITIS

Patients with paraneoplastic encephalomyelitis (PEM) develop multifocal involvement of the nervous system, including brain, brainstem, cerebellum, or spinal cord.[15,21] Many patients with PEM also have paraneoplastic sensory neuropathy. The clinical features depend on the area(s) predominantly involved, but pathology studies almost always show abnormalities (inflammatory infiltrates, neuronal loss, gliosis) in asymptomatic regions. Several syndromes have been described that may occur alone or in combination. These include *cortical encephalitis*, that may present as epilepsia partialis continua; *limbic and/or brainstem encephalitis*, which is discussed in further detail later; *cerebellar* gait and limb ataxia; *myelitis* that may cause lower or upper motor neuron symptoms, myoclonus, muscle rigidity, and spasms; and *autonomic dysfunction*.

Paraneoplastic encephalomyelitis with or without PSN has been reported in association with almost all types of tumors, but the most common is lung carcinoma, particularly SCLC. The most frequently associated antibodies are anti-Hu and anti-CRMP5/CV2; antibodies to amphiphysin and Zic proteins are less frequently reported.[15,26,30]

All types of PEM except LE respond poorly to treatment. Stabilization or partial neurologic improvement may occur and usually correlates with tumor response to treatment. In a large series of patients with anti-Hu–associated PEM, treatment of the tumor with or without associated immunotherapy was an independent predictor of neurologic improvement or stabilization.[15] The roles of plasma exchange, IVIg, and immunosuppression have not been established. Some patients with LE show marked improvement after tumor treatment and immunomodulatory therapies.[31,32]

LIMBIC ENCEPHALITIS

Limbic encephalitis is characterized by confusion, depression, agitation, severe short-term memory deficits, partial-complex seizures, sleep disturbances, and dementia.[31] The EEG usually reveals foci of epileptic activity in one or both temporal lobes, or focal or generalized slow activity. About 80% of patients have MRI fluid-attenuated inversion recovery (FLAIR) or, in T2 sequences, hyperintense signal abnormality in the medial aspect of one or both temporal lobes (Figure 18-2). FDG-PET may show hypermetabolism in one or both temporal lobes even when the MRI is normal.[33] Recent studies have shown that immune-mediated LE can be categorized into four groups based on the type and location of the target antigens.

Limbic Encephalitis Associated with Antibodies to Intracellular Antigens

The main intracellular antigens related to LE are Hu, Ma2, and, less frequently, CV2/CRMP5 and amphiphysin. In these immune responses, cytotoxic T cell mechanisms are considered the main pathogenic effectors. Patients with Hu antibodies have PEM, although the disorder may initially present as a focal syndrome; the associated tumor is almost always a SCLC.[15,21]

Antibodies to Ma proteins are associated with limbic and brainstem encephalitis and occasionally with cerebellar symptoms; prominent hypothalamic dysfunction, hypersomnia, and cataplexy can occur.[32,34] Patients less than 50 years of age with limbic dysfunction and antibodies to Ma proteins usually have an underlying germ cell tumor of the testis.[35] These patients often benefit from orchiectomy and from immunotherapy that may include corticosteroids and IVIg. Overall, 35% of patients with anti-Ma2 encephalitis have neurological responses to treatment.[36] One case of spontaneous neurological improvement has recently been reported.[37]

Anti-CV2 or CRMP5 antibodies associate with encephalomyelitis, sensorimotor neuropathy, and, more distinctively, with cerebellar ataxia, chorea, uveitis, and optic neuritis.[30,38,39] The development of myelitis and optic neuritis may resemble Devic syndrome.[40] SCLC and thymoma are the tumors more

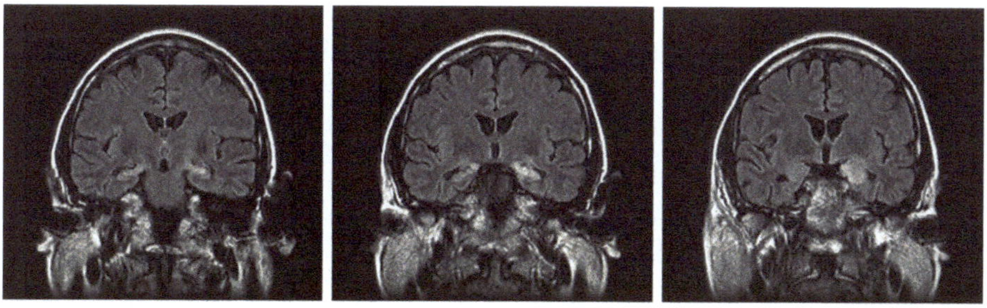

Figure 18-2 Brain MR of a patient with limbic encephalitis. This patient had limbic encephalitis that preceded by 6 months the diagnosis of a thyroid cancer. The MRI shows bilateral medial temporal lobe hyperintensities in FLAIR sequences, associated with hippocampal atrophy. By the time the MRI was obtained, the patient had progressive neurological symptoms and inflammatory abnormalities in the CSF.

frequently involved. In patients with SCLC, anti-CV2/CRMP5 may coexist with anti-Hu or Zic antibodies; these patients usually have multifocal deficits or encephalomyelitis.[26]

Anti-N-Methyl-D-Aspartate (NMDA) Receptor-Associated Encephalitis

Anti-NMDA receptor-associated encephalitis is a recently described disorder that usually affects young women.[8] About 65% of patients have an underlying tumor, usually a cystic teratoma of the ovary. After prodromal symptoms that may include headache, fever, or a viral-like illness, patients develop severe psychiatric symptoms or memory loss, seizures, and decreased level of consciousness, accompanied by dyskinesias, hypoventilation, or autonomic instability. Intensive care support and ventilation may be required for several weeks or many months. Although the disorder is potentially lethal, most patients recover after immunotherapy; when a tumor is found, removal expedites recovery and decreases relapses.[41] The disorder can also occur in men or women without a detectable tumor.[42] Due to the location of the target antigens on the cell surface (Figure 18-1) and the dramatic response to immunotherapy, it is likely that these antibodies play a direct pathogenic role.

Encephalitis and Antibodies to Voltage-Gated Potassium Channels

Recent evidence suggests that the target of these antibodies is not in fact the VGKC but other related proteins. The two main syndromes associated with these antibodies include typical LE and a lesser focal encephalitis that is associated with psychiatric symptoms, hallucinations, peripheral nerve hyperexcitability, hyperhydrosis, and other symptoms of autonomic dysfunction (Morvan syndrome). REM sleep disturbances and hyponatremia are common in both, and some patients may develop hypothermia, hypersalivation, pain, and disorders of appetite.[43] About 20% of patients with antibodies to VGKC-related proteins have a tumor, often SCLC or thymoma. About 80% of patients will respond to treatment that includes corticosteroids, plasma exchange, or IVIg.

Antibodies to Other Cell Membrane Antigens

There are other antibodies to cell surface antigens that have not been fully characterized. Some of these antibodies occur along with other well-characterized immune responses, such as GAD antibodies, and the associated disorders respond differently to immunotherapy.[33] It is unclear whether these novel antibodies have one or several target antigens. Tumors found in association with these antibodies include thymoma, SCLC, and Hodgkin lymphoma.

PARANEOPLASTIC OPSOCLONUS-MYOCLONUS

Opsoclonus is a disorder of eye movement characterized by spontaneous, arrhythmic, large-amplitude conjugate saccades occurring in all directions of gaze. Opsoclonus frequently associates with myoclonus and ataxia of the head, trunk, or limbs. When paraneoplastic in adults, symptoms can range from opsoclonus with mild truncal ataxia to a severe syndrome associated with encephalopathy that can lead to stupor and death. A number of associated tumors have been reported, but the most common is SCLC.[44] Paraneoplastic opsoclonus-myoclonus in children usually has a subacute onset with frequent fluctuations and is accompanied by ataxia, hypotonia, and irritability.[45] Almost 50% of children with paraneoplastic opsoclonus-myoclonus have neuroblastoma, and in half of the patients, the neurologic symptoms precede the diagnosis of the tumor. Children with neuroblastoma and opsoclonus have a better tumor prognosis than those without paraneoplastic symptoms.

Some adult patients, in particular those with SCLC, and 5% to 10% of children with neuroblastoma have anti-Hu antibodies.[46] Patients with breast and gynecologic cancers may harbor anti-Ri antibodies;[25] some of these patients develop muscle rigidity, autonomic dysfunction, and dementia. A small number of patients have been reported with other antibodies including antibodies to CRMP5/CV2, Zic2, amphiphysin, Yo, and Ma2.[30,47,48] However, in many adults and children with neuroblastoma, no paraneoplastic antibodies are found.

When associated with neuroblastoma, the disorder frequently responds to treatment of the tumor, steroids, ACTH, IVIg, plasma exchange, or rituximab;[49,50] however, developmental and neurologic sequelae are frequent.[45] Paraneoplastic opsoclonus-myoclonus in adults may respond to immunosuppression and IVIg. Patients whose tumors are treated promptly appear to have a better prognosis than those whose tumors are not treated.[51]

Paraneoplastic Disorders of the Visual System

Paraneoplastic retinopathy is characterized by photosensitivity, progressive loss of vision and color perception, central or ring scotomas, and night blindness.[52] The fundoscopic examination is normal or demonstrates arteriolar narrowing, and the electroretinogram (ERG) shows attenuation of photopic and scotopic responses. Paraneoplastic retinopathy associated with antibodies to recoverin is known as cancer-associated retinopathy (CAR).[53] Patients with CAR usually have SCLC, but cases have been reported associated with breast or gynecological cancers. Other target antigens that have been described include the tubby-like protein, photoreceptor cell-specific nuclear receptor, and the polypyrimidine tract binding-like protein.[54,55] Retinopathy in association with metastatic cutaneous melanoma is known as melanoma-associated retinopathy (MAR).[56] As opposed to CAR, these patients present with acute visual loss years or months after the diagnosis of the metastatic disease. The ERG shows reduced or absent b-waves with normal dark-adapted a-waves indicating bipolar cell dysfunction. Some of these patients have antibodies that target unknown antigens in the retinal bipolar cells.[57]

Optic neuritis has been described in some patients with paraneoplastic syndromes of the central nervous system in association with several antibodies including anti-Hu, anti-Tr, anti-Yo, and, more frequently, anti-CV2/CRMP5.[39,58] Patients present with sudden bilateral loss of vision, swollen optic discs, and field defects; the majority have SCLC.

Bilateral diffuse uveal melanocytic proliferation is a rare paraneoplastic entity in which an underlying tumor causes diffuse bilateral proliferation of melanocytes in the uveal tract, leading to bilateral visual loss.[59,60] The visual symptoms precede the diagnosis of a systemic malignancy. Carcinoma of the reproductive tract in women and carcinomas of the lung and pancreas in men appear to be the more commonly-associated tumors. Patients present with abrupt bilateral visual loss and few or no findings on examination of the fundus. Nearly all patients described have had rapid cataract progression, and all have had retinal detachment.[59] One case ascribed improvement in vision to treatment with external beam irradiation and subretinal fluid drainage.

In general, paraneoplastic visual loss is usually irreversible. Immunosuppression, plasma exchange, or steroids is mostly ineffective but in rare cases may result in symptom stabilization.[61]

Paraneoplastic Syndromes of the Spinal Cord and Dorsal Root Ganglia

PARANEOPLASTIC MOTOR NEURON SYNDROMES

A wide range of spinal cord syndromes including upper or lower motor neuron dysfunction, myelitis, myelopathy, and sensory and motor neuronopathies have been described in patients with cancer, and it is unclear if these are truly paraneoplastic or simply represent a coincidental association with cancer. Furthermore no specific paraneoplastic antibodies have been found in these patients. A recent study examined the sera of 145 patients with motor neuron disease for well characterized paraneoplastic antibodies (Hu, Yo, Ri, CV2/CRMP5, Ma2 and amphiphysin) and found only low reactivity in five sera that likely represented background activity.[62] For some syndromes, such necrotizing myelopathy, the identification of non-paraneoplastic causes such as human herpesvirus has, in many instances, clarified the nature of the disorder.[63]

The existence of paraneoplastic motor neuron dysfunction is based on reports of patients with typical amyotrophic lateral sclerosis (ALS) who improved after treatment of the underlying tumor (usually renal cell cancer and carcinoma of the lung or breast) suggesting more than a coincidental relationship.[64–66] A patient with renal cell carcinoma, neuromyotonia, and lower motor neuron syndrome had recovery of neurological deficits after tumor removal.[67] For these patients the neurologic syndrome and laboratory studies are similar to those seen in typical ALS patients. A more-than-coincidental association has been suggested between lymphoproliferative disorders with motor neuron dysfunction.[64,68] Patients with PEM may develop symptoms resembling motor neuron disease.[21,69] These patients almost always develop signs of involvement of other areas of the nervous system, which, along with the presence of the anti-Hu antibody, helps to rule out typical ALS.

Some patients with cancer develop a subacute lower motor neuronopathy characterized by subacute, progressive, painless, and asymmetrical muscle weakness that is more prominent in the lower extremities.[70] Reflexes are decreased or abolished, and, in contrast to typical ALS, bulbar muscles are usually spared, fasciculations are rare, and upper motor neuron signs are absent. Sensory symptoms, if any, are mild and transitory. The neurologic symptoms may have a benign course, independent of the activity of the neoplasm. The associated tumors are Hodgkin lymphoma and less frequently non-Hodgkin lymphoma. This disorder needs to be differentiated from the lower motor neuron syndrome that patients may develop secondary to radiation therapy of the spinal cord.[71] In these patients, the distribution of muscle weakness is more distal and, although symptoms stabilize, they do not improve. Patients with Hodgkin lymphoma treated with mantle radiation may develop slowly progressive (over years) weakness and atrophy involving neck flexors and extensors and proximal muscles of the upper extremities. Characteristically, a strip of atrophy involving paraspinal muscles is also observed. Distal reflexes are usually preserved; sensation is normal. No effective therapies have been described.

A disorder with prominent upper motor neuron dysfunction that mimics primary lateral sclerosis has been reported in a few patients with breast cancer. Because no specific paraneoplastic markers have been identified, the association of these disorders may be coincidental.[72]

PARANEOPLASTIC STIFF-PERSON SYNDROME

This disorder is characterized by progressive muscle rigidity, stiffness, and painful spasms triggered by auditory, sensory, or emotional stimuli. Rigidity mainly involves the lower trunk and legs, but it can affect the upper extremities, shoulders and neck. Symptoms improve with sleep and general anesthetics. Electrophysiologic studies demonstrate continuous motor unit activity at rest that improves with diazepam. The paraneoplastic form of stiff-person syndrome is usually associated with breast and lung cancers and Hodgkin lymphoma. Several antibodies, indicating different immune mechanisms, have been described. The main autoantigen of the paraneoplastic form of the disorder is amphiphysin, which commonly associates with breast and lung cancer.[73,74] Antibodies to GAD may occur in some patients with thymoma or cancer,[75,76] but these antibodies are far more common in the nonparaneoplastic disorder.[74,77] Treatment of the tumor, steroids, and drugs that enhance GABA-ergic function (diazepam, baclofen, sodium valproate, vigabatrin) usually improve symptoms. The benefit of IVIg has been demonstrated for the nonparaneoplastic disorder.[78]

PARANEOPLASTIC MYELITIS (PROGRESSIVE ENCEPHALOMYELITIS WITH RIGIDITY)

This disorder may present with either upper or lower motor neuron symptoms, segmental myoclonus and rigidity. Autopsy studies have demonstrated perivascular inflammatory infiltrates and neuronal degeneration, mainly involving the cervical portion of the spinal cord. It often forms part of, or evolves to, encephalomyelitis, and may associate with SCLC. Some patients harbor anti-amphiphysin antibodies or, less frequently, anti-Ri, CV2/CRMP5, or anti-Hu. This disorder has a poor prognosis and often results in death.

PARANEOPLASTIC SENSORY NEURONOPATHY (PSN) OR DORSAL ROOT GANGLIONOPATHY

This syndrome is characterized by symmetric or asymmetric sensory deficits, painful dysesthesias, radicular pain, and decreased or absent reflexes. All modalities of sensation, including taste and hearing, can be affected. With symptom

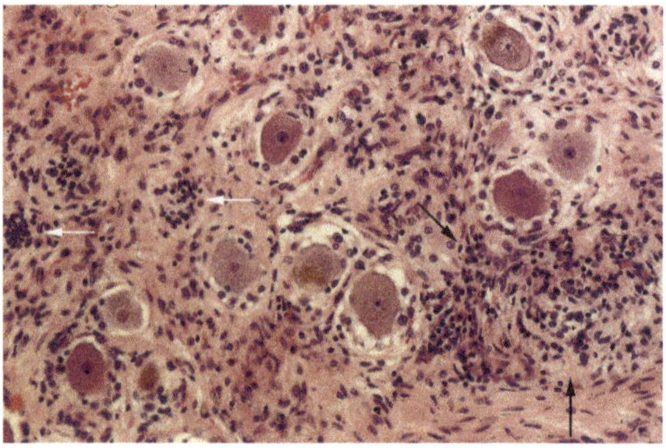

Figure 18-3 Dorsal root ganglia of a patient with paraneoplastic sensory neuronopathy. Dorsal root ganglia obtained at autopsy of a patient with paraneoplastic sensory neuronopathy and anti-Hu antibodies. Note the infiltrates of mononuclear cells (indicated with black arrows), and the presence of Nageotte nodules (white arrows). *Hematoxylin-eosin, ×400.*

progression, the sensory deficits result in ataxia, gait difficulty, and pseudoathetoid movements. Electrophysiologic studies show decreased or absent sensory nerve potentials with normal or near-normal motor conduction velocities and normal F-wave studies.[79] Some patients also have electrophysiological evidence of axonal and demyelinating neuropathy.[79,80] Autopsy studies demonstrate inflammation in the dorsal root ganglia characterized by infiltrates of mononuclear cells, neuronal degeneration, and proliferation of the satellite cells (Nageotte nodules) (Figure 18-3). Almost any cancer may be found associated with PSN. In about 70% of patients, PSN precedes or associates with PEM and autonomic dysfunction and has the same immunologic and oncologic associations, mainly anti-Hu antibodies and SCLC.[81] Fewer patients with PSN have antibodies to amphiphysin and CV2/CRMP5.[47,82] Some patients harbor both anti-Hu and CV2/CRMP5 antibodies. The therapeutic approach focuses on prompt treatment of the tumor. Studies of patients with SCLC and anti-Hu associated PSN and PEM indicate that patients whose tumors had a complete response to therapy were more likely to have stabilization or improvement of neurological symptoms compared to patients whose tumors were not treated or did not respond well to therapy.[15,83] In some patients, prompt treatment with steroids may result in partial improvement of the sensory deficits.[83,84] The benefit of IVIg and plasma exchange is not proven.

Paraneoplastic Syndromes of the Nerves and Neuromuscular Junction

AUTONOMIC NEUROPATHY

Paraneoplastic autonomic neuropathy usually develops as a component of other disorders, such as LEMS and PEM. It may rarely occur as a pure or predominant autonomic neuropathy with adrenergic or cholinergic dysfunction at the preganglionic or postganglionic levels. Patients can develop several life-threatening complications, such as gastrointestinal paresis with pseudoobstruction, cardiac dysrhythmias, and postural hypotension. Other symptoms include hypoventilation, dry mouth, erectile dysfunction, anhidrosis, and sphincter dysfunction. The disorder has been reported in association with several tumors, including

SCLC, cancer of the pancreas, testis, carcinoid tumors, and lymphoma. When it develops as a component of PEM, serum anti-Hu and anti-CV2/CRMP5 antibodies may be present.[21] Serum antibodies to ganglionic acetylcholine receptors have been reported, but they can occur also without a cancer association.[85] In some patients, treatment of the tumor may stabilize or improve the autonomic symptoms. A recent study showed that combined immunomodulatory treatment, including prednisone, mycophenolate mofetil, and plasma exchange, was effective in patients with nonparaneoplastic autoimmune autonomic ganglionopathy associated with antibodies to ganglionic acetylcholine receptors.[86]

PERIPHERAL NERVE HYPEREXCITABILITY (PNH)

Also known as neuromyotonia, undulating myokymia, and Isaacs syndrome, PNH is characterized by spontaneous and continuous muscle fiber activity of peripheral nerve origin triggered by voluntary muscle contraction. Patients develop cramps, stiffness, delayed muscle relaxation, and spontaneous or evoked muscle spasms. PNH is often associated with motor weakness and hyperhidrosis and, less commonly, a sensorimotor neuropathy. The electromyogram may show fibrillation, fasciculation, and doublet, triplet or multiplet single-unit discharges that have a high intraburst frequency.[4] The motor discharges can continue during sleep, general anesthesia, and proximal nerve block and are abolished by blocking the neuromuscular junction. PNH can develop without cancer; when paraneoplastic, thymoma and lung cancers are more commonly involved. Patients with thymoma may also have myasthenia gravis.[4] Many patients have antibodies to VGKCs that contribute to the nerve hyperexcitability.[87,88] Patients with PNH and thymoma, with or without myasthenia gravis, may also harbor antibodies to acetylcholine receptors.[4] Symptomatic improvement has been reported with phenytoin, carbamazepine, and plasma exchange.[87,89] The cramp-fasciculation syndrome resembles PNH, but the electromyogram does not show myokymic discharges. It may occur in association with cancer (usually thymoma or lung cancer) and antibodies to VGKC.

VASCULITIS OF THE NERVE AND MUSCLE

Patients with this disorder develop a painful symmetric or asymmetric subacute distal sensorimotor neuropathy with variable proximal weakness or, less frequently, a multiple mononeuropathy.[90] It predominantly affects elderly men, and is associated with an elevated erythrocyte sedimentation rate and increased CSF protein concentration. Electrophysiological findings are compatible with axonal degeneration involving motor and sensory nerves. Lymphoma and SCLC are the main tumors involved.[90] Pathology studies show axonal degeneration and T cell infiltrates involving the small vessels of the nerve and muscle.[91,92] Most patients do not have paraneoplastic antibodies, although anti-Hu antibodies can be found in some patients with SCLC. Immunosuppressants (steroids and cyclophosphamide) often result in neurologic improvement.[90,93]

SENSORIMOTOR NEUROPATHIES

Patients with cancer commonly develop a mild peripheral sensorimotor neuropathy, most often in the later stages of the disease. The cause is often multifactorial, including metabolic and nutritional deficits and treatment-related toxicity. In contrast, the paraneoplastic neuropathies that develop in the early stages of cancer often show a rapid progression and evidence of inflammatory infiltrates and axonal loss or demyelination in biopsy studies.

Paraneoplastic sensorimotor neuropathy may develop before or after the cancer diagnosis. The presentation is usually subacute followed by continued progression, although some patients have a relapsing and remitting course.[94] The most commonly associated tumors are lung and breast cancers. There are usually no serum antineuronal antibodies, although some patients with lung cancer and thymoma may harbor CV2/CRMP5 antibodies.[82] The detection of anti-Hu suggests concurrent dorsal root ganglionitis.[81]

An acute neuropathy identical to Guillain-Barré syndrome (GBS) has been reported in patients with lymphoma, usually Hodgkin lymphoma. In one series of 435 patients with GBS, nine developed cancer in the 6 months preceding or following the onset of the GBS.[95] In general, patients with cancer and GBS appear to have higher mortality than those with GBS alone. For brachial neuritis, the differential diagnosis should include more common causes of brachial plexopathy in cancer patients, including tumor infiltration, radiation injury, ischemic neuropathy, and traumatic injury of the plexus.

Monoclonal gammopathy of uncertain significance (MGUS), multiple myeloma, Waldenström macroglobulinemia, Castleman disease, and osteosclerotic myeloma may be associated with a peripheral neuropathy. In some cases, the neuropathy is due to compression of roots and plexuses by metastasis to the vertebral bodies and pelvis or deposits of amyloid in peripheral nerves.

About 50% of patients with osteosclerotic myeloma develop a symmetric, distal, sensorimotor neuropathy with predominant motor deficits resembling a chronic inflammatory demyelinating neuropathy. Some patients develop additional symptoms of the POEMS syndrome (*p*olyneuropathy, *o*rganomegaly, *e*ndocrinopathy, *m*onoclonal proteinemia and *s*kin changes). If there is a solitary sclerotic lesion, radiation is the most effective and least toxic therapy.[96] Systemic chemotherapy with or without corticosteroid therapy should be considered for patients with diffuse sclerotic lesions or those with no obvious bone lesions.

About 5% to 10% of patients with Waldenström macroglobulinemia develop a neuropathy. The neuropathy may be a distal symmetric demyelinating sensorimotor neuropathy that is often associated with IgM antibodies to myelin-associated glycoprotein or gangliosides, including GD1b and GM1. Other neuropathies include an axonal neuropathy, neuropathy associated with amyloid deposition, and a cryoglobulinemic vasculitis. In addition to treating the Waldenström macroglobulinemia, the use of plasma exchange, IVIg, chlorambucil, cyclophosphamide, fludarabine, or rituximab may result in improvement.[97,98]

Castleman disease, or angiofollicular lymph node hyperplasia, represents a group of lymphoproliferative disorders that are often accompanied by a marked systemic inflammatory response and acquired systemic amyloidosis. Patients may develop a painful sensorimotor neuropathy, a chronic relapsing sensorimotor neuropathy, and a predominant motor neuropathy.[99] Additional symptoms indicative of POEMS syndrome are common as there is considerable overlap between the syndromes.[100,101] There are reports of neurological improvement with cyclophosphamide and prednisolone or immunosuppression.[102,103]

Paraneoplastic Syndromes of the Neuromuscular Junction

LAMBERT-EATON MYASTHENIC SYNDROME (LEMS)

LEMS is characterized by the development of proximal muscle weakness in the lower and upper extremities.[14] Symptoms usually develop gradually over a period of weeks or months but can develop acutely. The frequency of ocular symptoms including diplopia and ptosis is low at symptom presentation, but eventually about 50% of patients became affected.[104] In a few reported cases, ocular symptoms were the only clinical manifestation of LEMS.[105] More than 50% of patients also develop autonomic dysfunction including dry mouth, erectile dysfunction and blurring of vision.[106] Reflexes are decreased or abolished but may increase after a brief muscle contraction. The diagnosis of LEMS is based on electrophysiological studies. Nerve conduction studies show small-amplitude compound muscle action potentials (CMAP). At slow rates of repetitive nerve stimulation (2 to 5 Hz) there is a decremental response, while at fast rates (20 Hz or greater) or after maximal voluntary muscle contraction, facilitation occurs with an incremental response of at least 100%.

Approximately 60% of patients with LEMS have SCLC or lymphoma; other cancers have rarely been reported. The neurologic symptoms usually precede the cancer diagnosis. LEMS can develop in association with other paraneoplastic syndromes such as PCD and PEM, and recurrence of LEMS after a remission often heralds tumor recurrence.[107,108] Most patients with LEMS have serum antibodies against P/Q type VGCCs.[109] When LEMS develops in association with PEM, patients often have anti-Hu antibodies. Treatment of the tumor and medication that enhances acetylcholine release (3,4-diaminopyridine, or the combination of pyridostigmine and guanidine) usually control the disorder.[84,110] Plasma exchange and IVIg improve symptoms within 2 to 4 weeks but the benefit is transient.[111,112] Long-term immunosuppression with prednisone or azathioprine is an alternative for patients who do not improve with 3,4-diaminopyridine.

MYASTHENIA GRAVIS

The main features of MG are weakness and fatigability of skeletal muscles that improve with rest and increase with activity. Ptosis and diplopia occur in most patients and, in about 15% of cases, symptoms remain localized to the extraocular and eyelid muscles. In contrast to LEMS, reflexes and sensation are spared. Approximately 10% of patients have thymoma or a thymic carcinoma; one third of thymoma patients develop myasthenia gravis.[113] In a few instances, MG has been reported in association with other tumors, including thyroid gland tumors, SCLC, breast cancer, and lymphoma. Whether the underlying disorder is thymoma or thymic hyperplasia, about 80% to 90% of the patients have antibodies to acetylcholine receptors. About 70% of patients with symptoms restricted to the eyes also have these antibodies. A group of patients without acetylcholine receptor antibodies develop antibodies to MusK, a muscle tyrosine kinase receptor.[114] Patients with MusK antibodies predominantly develop cranial and bulbar symptoms and respiratory crises. Most of these patients do not have tumors. A case with overlapping acetylcholine, MusK, and VGKC antibodies has recently been reported without an association with cancer.[115] High-titer neutralizing antibodies to IL-12 and interferon-α are frequently detected in patients with MG and thymoma, but not in patients without thymoma.[116] The first approach to treatment is directed at the underlying tumor. Additional therapeutic strategies, including symptomatic treatment (e.g., anticholinesterase drugs), immunomodulation (plasma exchange, IVIg), and immunosuppression (steroids, azathioprine, mycophenolate mofetil) are similar for patients with and without cancer.[112]

Paraneoplastic Disorders of the Muscle

DERMATOMYOSITIS

Most epidemiological studies indicate a clear association between dermatomyositis and cancer, particularly in older patients.[117] The symptoms of paraneoplastic dermatomyositis are the same as those in patients without cancer. Patients usually present with the subacute onset of proximal muscle weakness. Neck flexors, pharyngeal muscles, and respiratory muscles are commonly involved, which may lead to aspiration and hypoventilation. Reflexes and sensory exam are normal. Cutaneous changes include purplish discoloration of the eyelids (heliotrope rash) with edema and erythematous lesions over the knuckles. The presence of necrotic skin ulcerations and pruritis are felt to be indicators of an underlying cancer.[118,119] Life-threatening complications of dermatomyositis include respiratory muscle weakness, myocarditis, and interstitial lung disease; serum muscle enzymes are usually elevated. The electromyogram shows increased spontaneous activity (fibrillations, positive sharp waves, and complex repetitive discharges), and short duration, low-amplitude polyphasic units on voluntary activation.

When associated with cancer, the tumors more frequently involved are cancer of the breast, lung, ovary, and stomach. Less frequently associated are cancer of the pancreas, thymoma, germ cell tumors, melanoma, nasopharyngeal cancer, and lymphoma. There are no distinctive serologic markers of paraneoplastic or nonparaneoplastic dermatomysositis. Interstitial lung disease is less frequent in paraneoplastic dermatomyositis than in patients without cancer.[120] After treating the tumor, the therapy of paraneoplastic dermatomyositis does not differ from cases not associated with cancer and consists of steroids and long-term immunosuppression (e.g., azathioprine).[121,122] IVIg has been reported useful in refractory dermatomyositis.

ACUTE NECROTIZING MYOPATHY

This rare disorder is characterized by the acute onset of painful proximal muscle weakness with rapid generalization and involvement of respiratory and pharyngeal muscles. Serum muscle enzymes are markedly elevated and electrophysiological studies demonstrate myopathic findings. Muscle biopsy shows extensive necrosis with minimal or absent inflammation. In patients with cancer, the differential diagnosis of an acute necrotizing myopathy should include chemotherapy-induced and cytokine-induced rhabdomyolysis.[123] The disorder has been reported in association with a variety of solid tumors, including carcinomas of the lung, bladder, breast, prostate, and gastrointestinal tract.[124] No specific immune responses have been identified. Treatment of the tumor may result in neurologic improvement.

GENERAL TREATMENT APPROACH

For PNDs of the peripheral nervous system such as LEMS, myasthenia gravis, PNH and some types of autonomic neuropathy, the associated serum antibodies directly block the function of ion channels or membrane receptors. These disorders usually respond to plasma exchange, IVIg, and immunosuppressive therapies.[125] Most patients with paraneoplastic neuropathies do not harbor antineuronal antibodies, but an immune-mediated etiology is inferred by the subacute development of symptoms, pleocytosis or increased proteins in the CSF, or presence of inflammatory infiltrates on nerve biopsy. For these disorders, and particularly those with predominant demyelinating features, plasmapheresis, IVIg, and immunosuppression can be effective. Paraneoplastic axonal neuropathies are poorly responsive to immunotherapy; treatment is largely symptomatic or supportive, along with treatment of the tumor.

In adults, there are several PNDs of the CNS that are responsive or more likely to respond to treatment of the tumor and immunomodulatory therapies. These include anti-NMDAR encephalitis and limbic encephalitis in patients without anti-Hu antibodies (some of whom may have antibodies to VGKC-related proteins)[126]; opsoclonus-myoclonus; limbic encephalitis in young patients with testicular tumors and anti-Ma2 antibodies; and stiff-person syndrome associated with anti-amphiphysin antibodies.[36,51]

For other PNDs, the first therapeutic step is the early diagnosis and treatment of the tumor.[29,125] For many PNDs affecting the CNS, there is recent data that demonstrates the importance of the early institution of immunologic therapies (immunomodulation, immunosuppression) when the neurologic deficits are not fully established or still partially reversible.[127,128] Since the combination of oncologic and immunosuppressive therapies may have significant toxicity, it is recommended that immunologic treatments be stratified accordingly. For patients with progressive PNDs who are receiving chemotherapy, immunosuppression or immunomodulation may include oral or intravenous corticosteroids and IVIg; anecdotal experience suggests that plasma exchange is rarely effective in PNDs of the CNS. Patients with progressive PNDs, who are not receiving chemotherapy, should be considered for more aggressive immunosuppression that may include oral or intravenous cyclophosphamide, tacrolimus, or cyclosporine.

REFERENCES

1. Bataller L, Dalmau JO. Paraneoplastic disorders of the central nervous system: update on diagnostic criteria and treatment. Semin Neurol 2004;24:461–71.
2. Dalmau J, Gultekin HS, Posner JB. Paraneoplastic neurologic syndromes: pathogenesis and physiopathology. Brain Pathol 1999;9:275–84.
3. Motomura M, Johnston I, Lang B, Vincent A, Newsom-Davis J. An improved diagnostic assay for Lambert-Eaton myasthenic syndrome. J Neurol Neurosurg Psychiatry 1995;58:85–7.
4. Hart IK, Maddison P, Newsom-Davis J, Vincent A, Mills KR. Phenotypic variants of autoimmune peripheral nerve hyperexcitability. Brain 2002;125:1887–95.
5. Graus F, Lang B, Pozo-Rosich P, Saiz A, Casamitjana R, Vincent A. P/Q type calcium-channel antibodies in paraneoplastic cerebellar degeneration with lung cancer. Neurology 2002;59:764–6.
6. Vincent A, Buckley C, Schott JM, et al. Potassium channel antibody-associated encephalopathy: a potentially immunotherapy-responsive form of limbic encephalitis. Brain 2004;127:701–12.
7. Liguori R, Vincent A, Clover L, et al. Morvan's syndrome: peripheral and central nervous system and cardiac involvement with antibodies to voltage-gated potassium channels. Brain 2001;124:2417–26.

8. Dalmau J, Tuzun E, Wu HY, et al. Paraneoplastic anti-N-methyl-D-aspartate receptor encephalitis associated with ovarian teratoma. Ann Neurol 2007;61:25–36.
9. Sommer C, Weishaupt A, Brinkhoff J, et al. Paraneoplastic stiff-person syndrome: passive transfer to rats by means of IgG antibodies to amphiphysin. Lancet 2005;365:1406–11.
10. Manto MU, Laute MA, Aguera M, Rogemond V, Pandolfo M, Honnorat J. Effects of anti-glutamic acid decarboxylase antibodies associated with neurological diseases. Ann Neurol 2007;61:544–51.
11. Benyahia B, Liblau R, Merle-Béral H, Tourani JM, Dalmau J, Delattre J-Y. Cell-mediated autoimmunity in paraneoplastic neurologic syndromes with anti-Hu antibodies. Ann Neurol 1999;45:162–7.
12. Tanaka K, Tanaka M, Inuzuka T, Nakano R, Tsuji S. Cytotoxic T lymphocyte-mediated cell death in paraneoplastic sensory neuronopathy with anti-Hu antibody. J Neurol Sci 1999;163:159–62.
13. Albert ML, Darnell JC, Bender A, Francisco LM, Bhardwaj N, Darnell RB. Tumor-specific killer cells in paraneoplastic cerebellar degeneration. Nat Med 1998;4:1321–4.
14. O'Neill JH, Murray NM, Newsom-Davis J. The Lambert-Eaton myasthenic syndrome. A review of 50 cases. Brain 1988;111:577–96.
15. Graus F, Keime-Guibert F, Rene R, et al. Anti-Hu-associated paraneoplastic encephalomyelitis: analysis of 200 patients. Brain 2001;124:1138–48.
16. Younes-Mhenni S, Janier MF, Cinotti L, et al. FDG-PET improves tumour detection in patients with paraneoplastic neurological syndromes. Brain 2004;127:2331–8.
17. Rees JH, Hain SF, Johnson MR, et al. The role of 18F.fluoro-2-deoxyglucose-PET scanning in the diagnosis of paraneoplastic neurological disorders. Brain 2001;124:2223–31.
18. Linke R, Schroeder M, Helmberger T, Voltz R. Antibody-positive paraneoplastic neurologic syndromes: value of CT and PET for tumor diagnosis. Neurology 2004;63:282–6.
19. Peterson K, Rosenblum MK, Kotanides H, Posner JB. Paraneoplastic cerebellar degeneration. I. A clinical analysis of 55 anti-Yo antibody-positive patients. Neurology 1992;42:1931–7.
20. Shams'ili S, Grefkens J, De Leeuw B, et al. Paraneoplastic cerebellar degeneration associated with antineuronal antibodies: analysis of 50 patients. Brain 2003;126:1409–18.
21. Dalmau J, Graus F, Rosenblum MK, Posner JB. Anti-Hu—associated paraneoplastic encephalomyelitis/sensory neuronopathy. A clinical study of 71 patients. Medicine (Baltimore) 1992;71:59–72.
22. Felician O, Renard JL, Vega F, et al. Paraneoplastic cerebellar degeneration with anti-Yo antibody in a man. Neurology 1995;45:1226–7.
23. Krakauer J, Balmaceda C, Gluck JT, Posner JB, Fetell MR, Dalmau J. Anti-Yo-associated paraneoplastic cerebellar degeneration in a man with adenocarcinoma of unknown origin. Neurology 1996;46:1486–7.
24. Budde-Steffen C, Anderson NE, Rosenblum MK, et al. An antineuronal autoantibody in paraneoplastic opsoclonus. Ann Neurol 1988;23:528–31.
25. Luque FA, Furneaux HM, Ferziger R, et al. Anti-Ri: an antibody associated with paraneoplastic opsoclonus and breast cancer. Ann Neurol 1991;29:241–51.
26. Bataller L, Wade DF, Graus F, Stacey HD, Rosenfeld MR, Dalmau J. Antibodies to Zic4 in paraneoplastic neurologic disorders and small-cell lung cancer. Neurology 2004;62:778–82.
27. Shams'ili S, de Beukelaar J, Gratama JW, et al. An uncontrolled trial of rituximab for antibody associated paraneoplastic neurological syndromes. J Neurol 2006;253:16–20.
28. Blaes F, Strittmatter M, Merkelbach S, et al. Intravenous immunoglobulins in the therapy of paraneoplastic neurological disorders. J Neurol 1999;246:299–303.
29. David YB, Warner E, Levitan M, Sutton DM, Malkin MG, Dalmau JO. Autoimmune paraneoplastic cerebellar degeneration in ovarian carcinoma patients treated with plasmapheresis and immunoglobulin. A case report. Cancer 1996;78:2153–6.
30. Yu Z, Kryzer TJ, Griesmann GE, Kim KK, Benarroch EE, Lennon VA. CRMP-5 neuronal autoantibody: Marker of lung cancer and thymoma related autoimmunity. Ann Neurol 2001;49:146–54.
31. Gultekin SH, Rosenfeld MR, Voltz R, Eichen J, Posner JB, Dalmau J. Paraneoplastic limbic encephalitis: Neurological symptoms, immunological findings, and tumor association in 50 patients. Brain 2000;123:1481–94.
32. Rosenfeld MR, Eichen J, Wade D, Posner JB, Dalmau J. Molecular and clinical diversity in paraneoplastic immunity to Ma proteins. Ann Neurol 2001;50:339–48.
33. Ances BM, Vitaliani R, Taylor RA, et al. Treatment-responsive limbic encephalitis identified by neuropil antibodies: MRI and PET correlates. Brain 2005;128:1764–77.
34. Dalmau J, Gultekin SH, Voltz R, et al. Ma1, a novel neuronal and testis specific protein, is recognized by the serum of patients with paraneoplastic neurologic disorders. Brain 1999;122:27–39.

35. Mathew RM, Vandenberghe R, Garcia-Merino A, et al. Orchiectomy for suspected microscopic tumor in patients with anti-Ma2-associated encephalitis. Neurology 2007;68:900–5.
36. Dalmau J, Graus F, Villarejo A, et al. Clinical analysis of anti-Ma2-associated encephalitis. Brain 2004;127:1831–44.
37. Pruss H, Voltz R, Gelderblom H, et al. Spontaneous remission of anti-Ma associated paraneoplastic mesodiencephalic and brainstem encephalitis. J Neurol 2008;255:292–4.
38. Vernino S, Tuite P, Adler CH, et al. Paraneoplastic chorea associated with CRMP-5 neuronal antibody and lung carcinoma. Ann Neurol 2002;51:625–30.
39. Antoine JC, Honnorat J, Vocanson C, et al. Posterior uveitis, paraneoplastic encephalomyelitis and auto- antibodies reacting with developmental protein of brain and retina. J Neurol Sci 1993;117:215–23.
40. Ducray F, Roos-Weil R, Garcia PY, et al. Devic's syndrome-like phenotype associated with thymoma and anti-CV2/CRMP5 antibodies. J Neurol Neurosurg Psychiatry 2007;78:325–7.
41. Seki M, Suzuki S, Iizuka T, et al. Neurological response to early removal of ovarian teratoma in anti-NMDAR encephalitis. J Neurol Neurosurg Psychiatry 2008;79:324–6.
42. Novillo-Lopez ME, Rossi J, Dalmau J, Masjuan J. Treatment-responsive subacute limbic encephalitis and NMDA receptor antibodies in a man. Neurology 2008;70:728–9.
43. Jacob S, Irani SR, Rajabally YA, et al. Hypothermia in VGKC antibody-associated limbic encephalitis. J Neurol Neurosurg Psychiatry 2008;79:202–4.
44. Anderson NE, Rosenblum MK, Posner JB. Paraneoplastic cerebellar degeneration: clinical-immunological correlations. Ann Neurol 1988;24:559–67.
45. Russo C, Cohn SL, Petruzzi MJ, de Alarcon PA. Long-term neurologic outcome in children with opsoclonus-myoclonus associated with neuroblastoma: a report from the Pediatric Oncology Group. Med Pediatr Oncol 1997;28:284–8.
46. Hersh B, Dalmau J, Dangond F, Gultekin S, Geller E, Wen PY. Paraneoplastic opsoclonus-myoclonus associated with anti-Hu antibody. Neurology 1994;44:1754–5.
47. Saiz A, Dalmau J, Butler MH, et al. Anti-amphiphysin I antibodies in patients with paraneoplastic neurological disorders associated with small cell lung carcinoma. J Neurol Neurosurg Psychiatry 1999;66:214–7.
48. Bataller L, Rosenfeld MR, Graus F, Vilchez JJ, Cheung NK, Dalmau J. Autoantigen diversity in the opsoclonus-myoclonus syndrome. Ann Neurol 2003;53:347–53.
49. Tate ED, Allison TJ, Pranzatelli MR, Verhulst SJ. Neuroepidemiologic trends in 105 US cases of pediatric opsoclonus-myoclonus syndrome. J Pediatr Oncol Nurs 2005;22:8–19.
50. Bell J, Moran C, Blatt J. Response to rituximab in a child with neuroblastoma and opsoclonus-myoclonus. Pediatr Blood Cancer 2008;50:370–1.
51. Bataller L, Graus F, Saiz A, Vilchez JJ. Clinical outcome in adult onset idiopathic or paraneoplastic opsoclonus-myoclonus. Brain 2001;124:437–43.
52. Thirkill CE. Cancer-induced, immune-mediated ocular degenerations. Ocul Immunol Inflamm 2005;13:119–31.
53. Thirkill CE, Tait RC, Tyler NK, Roth AM, Keltner JL. The cancer-associated retinopathy antigen is a recoverin-like protein. Invest Ophthalmol Vis Sci 1992;33:2768–72.
54. Kikuchi T, Arai J, Shibuki H, Kawashima H, Yoshimura N. Tubby-like protein 1 as an autoantigen in cancer-associated retinopathy. J Neuroimmunol 2000;103:26–33.
55. Eichen JG, Dalmau J, Demopoulos A, Wade D, Posner JB, Rosenfeld MR. The photoreceptor cell-specific nuclear receptor is an autoantigen of paraneoplastic retinopathy. J Neuroophthalmol 2001;21:168–72.
56. Boeck K, Hofmann S, Klopfer M, et al. Melanoma-associated paraneoplastic retinopathy: case report and review of the literature. Br J Dermatol 1997;137:457–60.
57. Milam AH, Saari CJ, Jacobson SG, et al. Autoantibodies against retinal bipolar cells in cutaneous melanoma-associated retinopathy. Invest Ophthalmol Visual Sci 1993;34:91–100.
58. Cross SA, Salomao DR, Parisi JE, et al. Paraneoplastic autoimmune optic neuritis with retinitis defined by CRMP-5-IgG. Ann Neurol 2003;54:38–50.
59. O'Neal KD, Butnor KJ, Perkinson KR, Proia AD. Bilateral diffuse uveal melanocytic proliferation associated with pancreatic carcinoma: a case report and literature review of this paraneoplastic syndrome. Surv Ophthalmol 2003;48:613–25.
60. Saito W, Kase S, Yoshida K, et al. Bilateral diffuse uveal melanocytic proliferation in a patient with cancer-associated retinopathy. Am J Ophthalmol 2005;140:942–5.
61. Keltner JL, Thirkill CE, Yip PT. Clinical and immunologic characteristics of melanoma-associated retinopathy syndrome: eleven new cases and a review of 51 previously published cases. J Neuroophthalmol 2001;21:173–87.

62. Stich O, Kleer B, Rauer S. Absence of paraneoplastic antineuronal antibodies in sera of 145 patients with motor neuron disease. J Neurol Neurosurg Psychiatry 2007;78:883–5.
63. Iwamasa T, Utsumi Y, Sakuda H, et al. Two cases of necrotizing myelopathy associated with malignancy caused by herpes simplex virus type 2. Acta Neuropathol (Berl) 1989;78:252–7.
64. Gordon PH, Rowland LP, Younger DS, et al. Lymphoproliferative disorders and motor neuron disease: an update. Neurology 1997;48:1671–8.
65. Rosenfeld MR, Posner JB. Paraneoplastic motor neuron disease. In: Rowland LP, editor. Advances in Neurology, Volume 56: Amyotrophic Lateral Sclerosis and Other Motor Neuron Diseases. New York: Raven Press; 1991. p. 445–59.
66. Evans BK, Fagan C, Arnold T, Dropcho EJ, Oh SJ. Paraneoplastic motor neuron disease and renal cell carcinoma: improvement after nephrectomy. Neurology 1990;40:960–2.
67. Canovas D, Martinez JM, Viguera M, Ribera G. Association of renal carcinoma with neuromyotonia and involvement of inferior motor neuron. Neurologia 2007;22:399–400.
68. Louis ED, Hanley AE, Brannagan TH, et al. Motor neuron disease, lymphoproliferative disease, and bone marrow biopsy. Muscle Nerve 1996;19:1334–7.
69. Verma A, Berger JR, Snodgrass S, Petito C. Motor neuron disease: a paraneoplastic process associated with anti-hu antibody and small-cell lung carcinoma. Ann Neurol 1996;40:112–6.
70. Schold SC, Cho ES, Somasundaram M, Posner JB. Subacute motor neuronopathy: a remote effect of lymphoma. Ann Neurol 1979;5:271–87.
71. Sadowsky CH, Sachs Jr E, Ochoa J. Postradiation motor neuron syndrome. Arch Neurol 1976;33:786–7.
72. Forsyth PA, Dalmau J, Graus F, Cwik V, Rosenblum MK, Posner JB. Motor neuron syndromes in cancer patients. Ann Neurol 1997;41:722–30.
73. De Camilli P, Thomas A, Cofiell R, et al. The synaptic vesicle-associated protein amphiphysin is the 128- kD autoantigen of Stiff-Man syndrome with breast cancer. J Exp Med 1993;178:2219–23.
74. Folli F, Solimena M, Cofiell R, et al. Autoantibodies to a 128-kd synaptic protein in three women with the stiff-man syndrome and breast cancer. N Engl J Med 1993;328:546–51.
75. Hernandez-Echebarria L, Saiz A, Ares A, et al. Paraneoplastic encephalomyelitis associated with pancreatic tumor and anti-GAD antibodies. Neurology 2006;66:450–1.
76. McHugh JC, Murray B, Renganathan R, Connolly S, Lynch T. GAD antibody positive paraneoplastic stiff person syndrome in a patient with renal cell carcinoma. Mov Disord 2007;22:1343–6.
77. Brown P, Marsden CD. The stiff man and stiff man plus syndromes. J Neurol 1999;246:648–52.
78. Vasconcelos OM, Dalakas MC. Stiff-person Syndrome. Curr Treat Options Neurol 2003;5:79–90.
79. Camdessanche JP, Antoine JC, Honnorat J, et al. Paraneoplastic peripheral neuropathy associated with anti-Hu antibodies. A clinical and electrophysiological study of 20 patients. Brain 2002;125:166–75.
80. Oh SJ, Gurtekin Y, Dropcho EJ, King P, Claussen GC. Anti-Hu antibody neuropathy: a clinical, electrophysiological, and pathological study. Clin Neurophysiol 2005;116:28–34.
81. Molinuevo JL, Graus F, Rene R, Guerrero A, Illa I. Utility of anti-Hu antibodies in the diagnosis of paraneoplastic sensory neuropathy. Ann Neurol 1998;44:976–80.
82. Antoine JC, Honnorat J, Camdessanche JP, et al. Paraneoplastic anti-CV2 antibodies react with peripheral nerve and are associated with a mixed axonal and demyelinating peripheral neuropathy. Ann Neurol 2001;49:214–21.
83. Sillevis SP, Grefkens J, De Leeuw B, et al. Survival and outcome in 73 anti-Hu positive patients with paraneoplastic encephalomyelitis/sensory neuronopathy. J Neurol 2002;249:745–53.
84. Oh SJ, Kim DS, Head TC, Claussen GC. Low-dose guanidine and pyridostigmine: Relatively safe and effective long-term symptomatic therapy in Lambert-Eaton myasthenic syndrome. Muscle Nerve 1997;20:1146–52.
85. Vernino S, Low PA, Fealey RD, Stewart JD, Farrugia G, Lennon VA. Autoantibodies to ganglionic acetylcholine receptors in autoimmune autonomic neuropathies. N Engl J Med 2000;343:847–55.
86. Gibbons CH, Vernino SA, Freeman R. Combined immunomodulatory therapy in autoimmune autonomic ganglionopathy. Arch Neurol 2008;65:213–7.
87. Newsom-Davis J, Mills KR. Immunological associations of acquired neuromyotonia (Isaac's syndrome). Report of five cases and literature review. Brain 1993;116:453–69.
88. Shillito P, Molenaar PC, Vincent A, et al. Acquired neuromyotonia: evidence for autoantibodies directed against K+ channels of peripheral nerves. Ann Neurol 1995;38:714–22.

89. van den Berg JS, Van Engelen BG, Boerman RH, De Baets MH. Acquired neuromyotonia: superiority of plasma exchange over high-dose intravenous human immunoglobulin. J Neurol 1999;246:623–5.
90. Oh SJ. Paraneoplastic vasculitis of the peripheral nervous system. Neurol Clin 1997;15:849–63.
91. Matsumuro K, Izumo S, Umehara F, et al. Paraneoplastic vasculitic neuropathy: immunohistochemical studies on a biopsied nerve and post-mortem examination. J Intern Med 1994;236:225–30.
92. Vincent D, Dubas F, Hauw JJ, et al. Nerve and muscle microvasculitis in peripheral neuropathy: a remote effect of cancer?. J Neurol Neurosurg Psychiatry 1986;49:1007–10.
93. Oh SJ, Slaughter R, Harrell L. Paraneoplastic vasculitic neuropathy: a treatable neuropathy. Muscle Nerve 1991;14:152–6.
94. Antoine JC, Mosnier JF, Absi L, Convers P, Honnorat J, Michel D. Carcinoma associated paraneoplastic peripheral neuropathies in patients with and without anti-onconeural antibodies. J Neurol Neurosurg Psychiatry 1999;67:7–14.
95. Vigliani MC, Magistrello M, Polo P, Mutani R, Chio A. Risk of cancer in patients with Guillain-Barré syndrome (GBS). A population-based study. J Neurol 2004;251:321–6.
96. Rotta FT, Bradley WG. Marked improvement of severe polyneuropathy associated with multifocal osteosclerotic myeloma following surgery, radiation, and chemotherapy. Muscle Nerve 1997;20:1035–7.
97. Latov N. Prognosis of neuropathy with monoclonal gammopathy. Muscle Nerve 2000;23: 150–222.
98. Weide R, Heymanns J, Koppler H. The polyneuropathy associated with Waldenstrom's macroglobulinaemia can be treated effectively with chemotherapy and the anti-CD20 monoclonal antibody rituximab. Br J Haematol 2000;109:838–41.
99. Bowne WB, Lewis JJ, Filippa DA, et al. The management of unicentric and multicentric Castleman's disease: a report of 16 cases and a review of the literature. Cancer 1999;85:706–17.
100. Dispenzieri A, Kyle RA, Lacy MQ, et al. POEMS syndrome: definitions and long-term outcome. Blood 2003;101:2496–506.
101. Ku A, Lachmann E, Tunkel R, Nagler W. Severe polyneuropathy: initial manifestation of Castleman's disease associated with POEMS syndrome. Arch Phys Med Rehabil 1995;76:692–4.
102. Donaghy M, Hall P, Gawler J, et al. Peripheral neuropathy associated with Castleman's disease. J Neurol Sci 1989;89:253–67.
103. Fernandez-Torre JL, Polo JM, Calleja J, Berciano J. Castleman's disease associated with chronic inflammatory demyelinating polyradiculoneuropathy: a clinical and electrophysiological follow-up study. Clin Neurophysiol 1999;110:1133–8.
104. Titulaer MJ, Wirtz PW, Wintzen AR, Verschuuren JJ. Re: Lambert-Eaton myasthenic syndrome with pure ocular weakness. Neurology 2008;70:86–7.
105. Rudnicki SA. Lambert-Eaton myasthenic syndrome with pure ocular weakness. Neurology 2007;68:1863–4.
106. O'suilleabhain P, Low PA, Lennon VA. Autonomic dysfunction in the Lambert-Eaton myasthenic syndrome: serologic and clinical correlates. Neurology 1998;50:88–93.
107. Clouston PD, Saper CB, Arbizu T, et al. Paraneoplastic cerebellar degeneration. III. Cerebellar degeneration, cancer, and the Lambert-Eaton myasthenic syndrome. Neurology 1992;42: 1944–50.
108. Mason WP, Graus F, Lang B, et al. Small-cell lung cancer, paraneoplastic cerebellar degeneration and the Lambert-Eaton myasthenic syndrome. Brain 1997;120:1279–300.
109. Motomura M, Lang B, Johnston I, Palace J, Vincent A, Newsom-Davis J. Incidence of serum anti-P/O-type and anti-N-type calcium channel autoantibodies in the Lambert-Eaton myasthenic syndrome. J Neurol Sci 1997;147:35–42.
110. Sanders DB, Massey JM, Sanders LL, Edwards LJ. A randomized trial of 3,4-diaminopyridine in Lambert-Eaton myasthenic syndrome. Neurology 2000;54:603–7.
111. Bain PG, Motomura M, Newsom-Davis J, et al. Effects of intravenous immunoglobulin on muscle weakness and calcium-channel autoantibodies in the Lambert-Eaton myasthenic syndrome. Neurology 1996;47:678–83.
112. Newsom-Davis J. Therapy in myasthenia gravis and Lambert-Eaton myasthenic syndrome. Semin Neurol 2003;23:191–8.
113. Wirtz PW, Nijnuis MG, Sotodeh M, et al. The epidemiology of myasthenia gravis, Lambert-Eaton myasthenic syndrome and their associated tumours in the northern part of the province of South Holland. J Neurol 2003;250:698–701.

114. Sanders DB, El Salem K, Massey JM, McConville J, Vincent A. Clinical aspects of MuSK antibody positive seronegative MG. Neurology 2003;60:1978–80.
115. Diaz-Manera J, Rojas-Garcia R, Gallardo E, et al. Antibodies to AChR, MuSK and VGKC in a patient with myasthenia gravis and Morvan's syndrome. Nat Clin Pract Neurol 2007;3:405–10.
116. Buckley C, Newsom-Davis J, Willcox N, Vincent A. Do titin and cytokine antibodies in MG patients predict thymoma or thymoma recurrence?. Neurology 2001;57:1579–82.
117. Leow YH, Goh CL. Malignancy in adult dermatomyositis. Int J Dermatol 1997;36:904–7.
118. Mautner GH, Grossman ME, Silvers DN, Rabinowitz A, Mowad CM, Johnson Jr BL. Epidermal necrosis as a predictive sign of malignancy in adult dermatomyositis. Cutis 1998;61:190–4.
119. Mahe E, Descamps V, Burnouf M, Crickx B. A helpful clinical sign predictive of cancer in adult dermatomyositis: cutaneous necrosis. Arch Dermatol 2003;139:539.
120. Chen YJ, Wu CY, Shen JL. Predicting factors of malignancy in dermatomyositis and polymyositis: a case-control study. Br J Dermatol 2001;144:825–31.
121. Amato AA, Barohn RJ. Idiopathic inflammatory myopathies. Neurol Clin 1997;15:615–48.
122. Dalakas MC, Illa I, Dambrosia JM, et al. A controlled trial of high-dose intravenous immune globulin infusions as treatment for dermatomyositis. N Engl J Med 1993;329:1993–2000.
123. Anderlini P, Buzaid AC, Legha SS. Acute rhabdomyolysis after concurrent administration of interleukin-2, interferon-alfa, and chemotherapy for metastatic melanoma. Cancer 1995;76:678–9.
124. Levin MI, Mozaffar T, Al-Lozi MT, Pestronk A. Paraneoplastic necrotizing myopathy: clinical and pathological features. Neurology 1998;50:764–7.
125. Rosenfeld MR, Dalmau J. Current therapies for paraneoplastic neurologic syndromes. Curr Treat Options Neurol 2003;5:69–77.
126. Bataller L, Kleopa KA, Wu GF, Rossi JE, Rosenfeld MR, Dalmau J. Autoimmune limbic encephalitis in 39 patients: immunophenotypes and outcomes. J Neurol Neurosurg Psychiatry 2007;78:381–5.
127. Keime-Guibert F, Graus F, Fleury A, et al. Treatment of paraneoplastic neurological syndromes with antineuronal antibodies (Anti-Hu, anti-Yo) with a combination of immunoglobulins, cyclophosphamide, and methylprednisolone. J Neurol Neurosurg Psychiatry 2000;68:479–82.
128. Vernino S, O'Neill BP, Marks RS, O'Fallon JR, Kimmel DW. Immunomodulatory treatment trial for paraneoplastic neurological disorders. Neuro-oncol 2004;6:55–62.

19 Neurological Complications of Bone Marrow and Organ Transplantation

CLAUDIO S. PADOVAN • ANDREAS STRAUBE

Introduction

Organ transplantation is the only curative treatment for advanced cases of kidney, heart, liver, or lung failure. Bone marrow transplantation is performed in patients with otherwise untreatable leukemias, lymphomas, or storage disorders. Following transplantation, 30% to 60% of patients develop neurological complications.[1] The differential diagnosis includes preexisting complications of the underlying disease, intraoperative complications, metabolic disorders, and side effects of the necessary immunosuppressive medication. Immunosuppressants may either directly cause neurotoxicity or indirectly promote an increased rate of central nervous system (CNS) infections and secondary CNS malignancies. Although the rate of metabolic encephalopathies or opportunistic CNS infections is quite similar for all posttransplantation patients, certain neurological syndromes are typical to transplantation of specific organs (see Table 19-1).

TABLE 19-1 Specific and Common Complications Following Organ Transplantation

Transplantation	Complication
Bone marrow	Intracerebral hemorrhage due to thrombocytopenia
	Bacterial CNS infection (early period after transplantation)
	Viral CNS infection (especially herpes viruses)
	Leukoencephalopathy
	Neurologic manifestations of graft-versus host disease: myasthenia, myositis, polyneuropathy, central nervous system involvement
Liver	Brain edema/elevated intracranial pressure due to acute liver failure
	Intracerebral hemorrhage due to coagulation disorders
	Central pontine or extrapontine myelinolysis
	Brachial plexus lesion (pulmonary and cerebral aspergillosis)
Kidney	Femoral nerve lesion (lateral cutaneous femoral nerve)
	Hypertensive encephalopathy
	Encephalopathy due to acute organ rejection
Heart	Perioperative cerebral emboli
	Hypoxic-ischemic brain damage
	Phrenic nerve or brachial plexus lesion
	Aseptic meningitis following OKT3 (CNS lymphoma)
Lung	Air embolism (see heart transplantation)
Pancreas	Angiopathy
	Carpal tunnel syndrome

Clinical Syndromes

Clinical evaluation is limited in the acute phase following organ transplantation by the necessity of treatment with analgesics and sedative drugs as well as by the severe illness of the patients. The unconscious patient in the intensive care unit (e.g., due to drugs or metabolic encephalopathy) may develop increased depth of coma, focal or generalized epileptic seizures, asymmetric reactions to pain stimuli, pupillary abnormalities, or specific oculomotor findings (e.g., vertical divergence), that indicate a CNS complication. After organ transplantation, conscious patients may experience nonspecific symptoms such as headaches, visual disturbances, delirium, psychosis, somnolence, or epileptic seizures. These symptoms may be caused by cerebrovascular complications, CNS infections, metabolic disturbances, or pharmacological neurotoxicity. An overview of the neurological differential diagnosis following organ transplantation, according to clinical syndromes, is given in Table 19-2.

Investigations

The classification of clinical syndromes occurring after transplantation requires neuroradiological, laboratory, microbiological, and electrophysiological investigation. Computed tomography or magnetic resonance imaging (MRI) can identify ischemic infarction, intracerebral bleeding, brain abscess, granuloma, white

TABLE 19-2 Differential Diagnosis of Neurological Syndromes Following Organ Transplantation

Symptom	Etiology	Risk factor (transplantation)
Acute coma	Intracerebral hemorrhage	Thrombocytopenia (BMT, LTX), coagulation disorder (LTX, BMT)
	Cerebral ischemia	Cardiac emboli (HTX), endocarditis (BMT), air embolism (HTX, LuTX)
	Status epilepticus	Metabolic disorder, neurotoxicity, CNS infection
Impaired consciousness	Metabolic	Hepatic encephalopathy (LTX, organ failure), uremia (KTX), hypomagnesemia
	Neurotoxicity	Cyclosporine/tacrolimus (LTX, HTX)
	CNS infection	Meningitis: *Listeria*, *Cryptococcus*; Encephalitis: CMV, HSV, VZV; Cerebritis/abscess: *Aspergillus*, *Toxoplasma*, *Nocardia*
	Myelinolysis	Hyponatremia (LTX)
Postoperative coma	Cerebral hypoxia	Intraoperative complication (HTX, LuTX),
	Increased intracranial pressure	Brain edema (LTX)
		Sedatives/anesthetics
	Pharmacogenic	See above
	Myelinolysis	See above
	Ischemia/hemorrhage	
Focal neurological signs	Ischemia/hemorrhage	See above
	CNS infection	Abscess: *Aspergillus*, *Nocardia*, *Toxoplasma*, PML
	Neurotoxicity	Cyclosporine/tacrolimus (cortical blindness)
Seizures	Neurotoxicity	Cyclosporine/tacrolimus
	Metabolic	Uremia, liver failure, hypo/hypernatremia, hypomagnesemia, hypocalcemia, hypo/hyperglycemia
	Ischemia/hemorrhage	See above
	CNS infection	See above
Neck stiffness	Meningitis (infectious agent)	Immunosuppression (BMT): *Listeria*, *Cryptococcus*
	Aseptic meningitis	OKT3 (HTX)
Headache	Pharmacogenic	Cyclosporine, tacrolimus, OKT3
	Meningitis	See above
Tetraparesis	Pharmacogenic	Muscle relaxants, steroid myopathy
	Neuropathy	Critical illness polyneuropathy, Guillain-Barré syndrome
	Myopathy	Critical illness myopathy, myositis (BMT)
Tremor (ataxia)	Neurotoxicity	Cyclosporine/tacrolimus
	Encephalopathy	Organ failure (LTX, KTX)
	CNS infection	Viral encephalitis, *Legionella*

BMT = bone marrow transplantation, LTX = liver transplantation, HTX = heart transplantation, KTX = kidney transplantation, LuTX = lung transplantation, CMV = cytomegalovirus, HSV = herpes simplex virus, VZV = varizella zoster virus, PML = progressive multifocal leukencephalopathy (JC virus encephalitis) matter abnormalities, or brain edema.[2] Laboratory parameters should include electrolytes, glucose, ammonia, renal function, coagulation status, and concentration of immunosuppressants (cyclosporine or tacrolimus). The examination of the cerebrospinal fluid (CSF) should include testing for routine parameters, and microbiological or serological testing for bacteria and fungi, including specific antigen testing as well as cytological examination and culture. In cases of a suspected viral etiology, PCR and serological CSF/serum antibody index have to be determined. Systemic infections, mainly pulmonary infection with *Aspergillus*, *Nocardia*, and cryptococci, are potential sources of secondary CNS infections and must be diagnosed, or ruled out if suspected. Electroencephalography is necessary for patients with epileptic seizures or suspected nonconvulsive status epilepticus.

Nonspecific Neurological Complications Following Organ Transplantation

Posttransplantation patients require lifelong immunosuppression to prevent organ rejection, except in cases of organ transplantation between identical twins, and in some patients following bone marrow transplantation (who may develop immunological tolerance 1 to 2 years following the transplantation). Thus, regardless of the transplanted organ, several neurological complications may arise from immunosuppressive treatment due to its direct neurotoxicity or because of increased occurrence of CNS infections and epileptic seizures, or, in rare cases, induction of CNS malignancies.

Neurotoxicity of Immunosuppressants

Cyclosporine

Cyclosporin A has been used for many years for chronic immunosuppression following transplantation and also for the treatment of acute organ rejection. Cyclosporine suppresses T-helper cells and cytotoxic T cells by reducing their release of interleukin-2 and other cytokines. It is associated with systemic side effects, such as nephrotoxicity, hepatotoxicity, and arterial hypertension.

Neurological complications following cyclosporin A occur in 15% to 30% of patients.[3] The most common complications are isolated tremor (40%), headache (10% to 20%), and distal sensory deficits (electrophysiological examination shows a combined demyelinating and axonal neuropathy only in severe cases). About 5% of patients develop severe neurological side effects, with predominantly two distinct clinical syndromes: (1) Acute neurotoxicity may occur within the first weeks after transplantation as an encephalopathy combined with headache, dysarthria, depressive or manic symptoms, visual hallucinations, cortical blindness, seizures, or impaired consciousness, and (2) weeks to months after transplantation, cyclosporine neurotoxicity can manifest as a subacute motor syndrome with hemiparesis, paraparesis, or tetraparesis, possibly accompanied by cerebellar tremor, ataxia, and cognitive impairment. Cyclosporine is epileptogenic, and 2% to 6% of patients develop focal or generalized seizures. Status epilepticus may occur in patients with high cyclosporine serum levels.

It has been suggested that activation of the sympathetic system causes cyclosporine-induced tremor. Headache may result from the release of nitric oxide.

In cases with severe neurotoxicity syndromes, there may be impairment of the blood-brain barrier. Cyclosporine serum concentrations in patients with neurotoxicity are generally in the upper range of therapeutic levels. Higher cyclosporine concentrations always cause neurological side effects.

The neurotoxicity of cyclosporine is exacerbated by low cholesterol or magnesium levels, concomitant ß-lactam-antibiotic treatment, high-dose steroid medication, hypertension, and uremia, previous irradiation, or microangiopathy, which might occur after bone marrow transplantation.

Magnetic resonance imaging using FLAIR sequences typically shows confluent parieto-occipital white matter lesions without contrast enhancement.[4] CSF analysis shows elevated CSF albumin concentrations in almost all patients with cyclosporine neurotoxicity because of impaired blood-brain barrier function.

The treatment of cyclosporine-induced neurological side effects consists of dose reduction for patients with mild symptoms. Patients with severe neurotoxicity have to be switched to tacrolimus or to mycophenolate mofetil (see below).

Concomitantly, elevated blood pressure and metabolic disturbances (e.g., impaired creatinine clearance, magnesium or cholesterol levels) must be normalized. Epileptic seizures should be treated with valproic acid or gabapentin because they do not induce hepatic enzymes. Patients with isolated headache should be treated with propanolol. Most of the cyclosporine-induced neurological side effects are reversible if the drug is discontinued in time.

Tacrolimus

Tacrolimus is increasingly being used instead of cyclosporine because of its more pronounced immunosuppressive effects in renal, liver, or heart transplantation. Although the pharmacological mechanism of tacrolimus is similar to that of cyclosporine, less frequent rejection episodes have occurred, and arterial hypertension is rare. However, systemic side effects such as nephrotoxicity or hepatotoxicity and also neurologic complications are slightly more frequent than with cyclosporine.

Neurotoxicity is observed in 30% to 50% of patients following organ transplantation. Symptoms include headache, sensory deficits, tremor, anxiety, nightmares, and sleep disorders. Severe neurologic complications include disorientation, dysarthria, epileptic seizures, encephalopathy, apraxia, akinetic mutism, and impaired consciousness and occur in about 5% of patients, mainly during the initial treatment.[5] Tacrolimus has been reported to cause a severe demyelinating polyneuropathy, which responds to treatment with corticosteroids or immunoglobulins, as well as a changeover to cyclosporine.[6] In such cases, however, polyradiculitis due to cytomegalovirus infection (CMV) has to be ruled out.

Patients with tacrolimus neurotoxicity may have multifocal white matter lesions on magnetic resonance imaging, but radiographic abnormalities generally develop with some latency after clinical symptoms. In contrast to cyclosporine neurotoxicity, the lesions may show contrast enhancement, and are not typically distributed like a posterior leukoencephalopathy. Tacrolimus neurotoxicity may result in both subcortical and cortical lesions. In these patients, however, neurovascular diseases of other etiology, CNS infections, or an extrapontine myelinolysis (e.g., following liver transplantation) have to be ruled out. The majority of tacrolimus-associated neurological symptoms are reversible if the dosage is reduced or if the immunosuppressive drug is changed. White matter lesions, however, may persist even after clinical symptoms have resolved.

Mycophenolate mofetil

Mycophenolate mofetil is generally used after organ transplantation in addition to other immunosuppressive drugs to reduce the rejection rate. It acts as an antimetabolite and suppresses T cells, the proliferation of B cells, and the antibody production of plasma cells. Systemic side effects consist of reduced leukocyte counts, gastrointestinal disorders, and possibly an increased rate of viral infections (especially CMV). Neurotoxic side effects have been reported for single patients, but in general there is a possible association only with headache, tremor, vertigo, sleep disorders, depression, and sensory deficits.

Steroids

Corticosteroids are used after transplantation as treatment for chronic immunosuppression and for acute organ rejection. Because of their nonselective effect on cellular and humoral immunity, steroids increase the risk of opportunistic infections. Other systemic steroid side effects (e.g., osteoporosis, diabetes mellitus) are well known and therefore not reported on in detail.

Common neurological side effects of steroids include myopathies and psychiatric symptoms.[7] It is probable that 50% of patients treated with medium to high doses of steroids for more than 3 weeks will develop a proximal myopathy (manifesting initially in the hip muscles). Because it is seldom possible to reduce the dosage in symptomatic patients, a nonfluorized steroid should be tried instead. Steroid myopathy usually resolves only after 2 to 8 months following discontinuation.[8,9] Mood impairment occurs in almost all patients taking steroids, and some develop mild psychiatric symptoms such as anxiety, sleeplessness, and reduced concentration. Steroid-induced psychosis has been reported in about 3% of patients, but affective disorders, schizophrenic syndromes or delirium have also been described. Symptomatic treatment with neuroleptic drugs, valproic acid (in patients with manic syndromes), or sedatives will also be necessary. Epidural lipomatosis with compression of the cord or cauda equina may occur rarely in patients who receive more than 30 mg prednisolone daily (or equivalent doses of another steroid). Epidural lipomatosis manifests with thoracic or lumbar pain, radicular syndromes, or myelopathy. Neurosurgical treatment (decompression and resection) may be necessary, but the discontinuation of steroids has also been reported to cause improvement.[10]

OKT3

OKT3 is a monoclonal anti-T-cell antibody used to initially induce immunosuppression and to treat acute organ rejection episodes. It binds at the CD3 antigen, leading to suppression of T cell function but also to the release of cytokines (e.g., TNF-alpha). This may cause systemic OKT3 side effects, which include fever, cough, and gastrointestinal disorders.

Neurologic side effects occur in 2% to 14% of patients,with a latency of 24 to 72 hours after OKT3 treatment, and include aseptic meningitis with fever, headache, neck stiffness, and CSF pleocytosis. Meningitis rarely occurs after pretreatment with steroids, and resolves—when CSF microbiological cultures are negative—within days, even when OKT3 treatment is continued.[11] Patients on OKT3 in rare instances develop an encephalopathic syndrome with fever, apathy, increased muscle rigidity, CSF pleocytosis, and brain edema. Single patients with potentially reversible, subcortical, contrast-enhancing MRI lesions have also been described.[12]

ATG and ALG

Polyclonal anti-thymocyte globulin (ATG) or anti-lymphocyte globulin (ALG) from horse, goat, or rabbit is rarely used in the initial induction of immunosuppression and in cases of acute organ rejection. This treatment may cause serum sickness as a systemic side effect. ATG- or ALG-induced cytokine release may lead to symptoms mimicking OKT3 neurotoxicity.

Azathioprine

Azathioprine is used as an antimetabolite drug for chronic immunosuppression to suppress cellular and humoral immunity. Its major side effects are myelosuppression and hepatotoxicity. Direct neurotoxic side effects have not been reported.

Sirolimus

Sirolimus has been recently developed for use in immunosuppression. It is especially effective after renal transplantation, since it has no nephrotoxicity. Sirolimus may induce secondary malignancies less frequently compared to other immunosuppressive drugs because of its antiangiogenic effect. Systemic side effects include diarrhea, anemia, thrombocytopenia, hyperlipidemia, and lowered potassium concentrations. Neurologic complications during sirolimus treatment have rarely been reported.

Thalidomide

Thalidomide is used in patients with chronic graft-versus-host disease (GvHD) following bone marrow transplantation as an add-on immunosuppressant. It may lead to a severe painful, and possibly irreversible, polyneuropathy. In addition, it is sedating and, rarely, can cause impaired consciousness.

CNS INFECTIONS

Patients who undergo organ transplantation are at increased risk of acquiring systemic and CNS infections because of immunosuppression, implanted foreign materials during the perioperative period (central venous cannula, ventilation tube, port system), and an impaired immune system due to the underlying disease (e.g., diabetes mellitus, uremia). The rate of infectious complications following transplantation has been reduced since introduction of lymphocyte-specific immunosuppressants (cyclosporine or tacrolimus) and antimicrobial prophylaxis (e.g., perioperative gut decontamination, treatment with fluconazole, acyclovir, CMV-hyperimmunoglobulin).

After organ transplantation, CNS infections occur in about 5% to 10% of patients, with a death rate of 44% to 77%.[13] Otherwise-typical clinical signs like fever or neck stiffness may be absent in these patients, and the initial clinical examination may be obscured by the postoperative status (use of analgesics and sedatives) and organ failure. The presence of a systemic infection, possibly with secondary CNS involvement, is of diagnostic relevance. Most patients with cerebral *Aspergillus* or *Nocardia asteroides* infection have a primary pulmonary infection, and in many patients with *Cryptococcus neoformans* meningitis, primary infection of the skin or the lung can be shown. The clinical syndrome also helps in the differential diagnosis, since an acute meningitis is often caused by *Listeria monocytogenes*, whereas in patients with subacute or chronic meningitis, *Cryptococcus* or other fungi are generally found. Encephalitis can be caused by many viruses (e.g., herpes simplex, varicella-zoster, cytomegalovirus, human herpesvirus types 6–8, BK virus, and adenovirus) and, rarely, by bacteria. Slowly deteriorating cognitive impairment with additional focal neurological signs is typically caused by a JC papovavirus infection (progressive multifocal leukoencephalopathy). Focal space-occupying infectious lesions or abscesses are caused by *Aspergillus*, *Toxoplasma gondii*, *Listeria*, or *Nocardia* infections.[14]

The time interval between organ transplantation and the appearance of CNS infection may give information about the putative infective organism. Within the first month following transplantation, common perioperative wound or catheter infections as well as pulmonary and urogenital infections (caused by bacteria or *Candida*) predominate; only rare cases of CNS involvement in the form of septic encephalitis have been reported. Reactivated or transmitted (through the transplanted organ) viral CNS infections occur in some patients during this early period. A high risk of CNS infections persists between 1 to 6 months after transplantation, because of the intensive pharmacological immunosuppression. In this period, *Listeria*, *Aspergillus*, and *Nocardia* are the most common opportunistic infections. Latent CNS infections may become manifest in patients who survive organ transplantation for more than 6 months, e.g., as CMV chorioretinitis with additional CNS involvement or as Epstein-Barr virus (EBV)-associated CNS lymphoma. In addition, opportunistic infections with *Cryptococcus*, *Listeria*, and *Nocardia* may occur.

The highest risk of CNS infections is found in patients who are on extensive immunosuppression including steroids and who have received additional rejection treatment (OKT3, ATG or ALG). A medium risk is found in patients with systemic viral infections (e.g., hepatitis, CMV, EBV) that cause the impaired immune system to further deteriorate. In contrast, patients with an uncomplicated course following transplantation and on minimal immunosuppression have only a slightly elevated risk of CNS infections. In such patients, the spectrum of infectious agents is similar to that of immunocompetent persons.

Treatment recommendations for CNS infections following organ transplantation are given in Table 19-3. The additive nephrotoxicity of immunosuppressive medication (cyclosporine, tacrolimus) and others such as acyclovir, aminoglycosides, fluconazole, or amphotericin B has to be considered, and the dosage of antibiotic/antiviral drugs has to be adjusted to actual renal clearance function.

TABLE 19-3 Treatment of Common CNS Infections Following Transplantation

CNS Infection	Infectious Agent	Syndrome/Localization	Treatment
Protozoan	*Toxoplasma*	Focal encephalitis	Pyrimethamine + sulfadiazine (+ folic acid) or pyrimethamine + clindamycin (+ folic acid)
Fungal	*Candida* spp.	Acute meningitis, brain abscess	Fluconazole or amphotericin B + flucytosine (or following antibiogram)
	Aspergillus spp.	Brain abscess, hemorrhagic focal encephalitis	Amphotericin B + flucytosine, voriconazole
	Cryptococcus	Subacute/chronic meningitis	Initial amphotericin B + flucytosine, thereafter fluconazole (long-term treatment)
Bacterial	Gram-negative bacteria	Acute meningitis, brain abscess	Meropenem, following antibiogram
	Listeria monocytogenes	Acute meningitis, encephalitis (brainstem), brain abscess	Ampicillin + gentamicin, alternatively trimethoprim-sulfamethoxazole
	Nocardia	Multiple brain abscesses	Trimethoprim-sulfamethoxazole, cefotaxime (or following antibiogram), surgical drainage
Viral	Varicella-zoster virus	Encephalitis, vasculitis	Aciclovir
	Cytomegalovirus	Encephalitis	Ganciclovir
	Herpes simplex virus	Encephalitis (atypical encephalitis)	Aciclovir
	Human herpesvirus (HHV) 6	Encephalitis (limbic encephalitis)	Ganciclovir, foscarnet
	JC virus (PML)	Subacute encephalitis	Reduction of immunosuppression (cytosine arabinoside without benefit)

SEIZURES

Epileptic seizures, which occur in 4% to 16% of organ recipients, are generally caused by neurotoxicity (cyclosporine, tacrolimus), metabolic disturbances, or hypoxic-ischemic CNS lesions. Hypoxia-induced seizures, in general, manifest within the first week after heart or liver transplantation. CNS infections or cerebral neoplasms are less likely to cause seizures. Since epileptic seizures often disappear following a reduction of immunosuppression, the normalization of metabolic disorders, or the treatment of CNS infections, a continuous antiepileptic medication is not necessary in all patients.[15] Patients with repeated seizures or with status epilepticus should, however, be given benzodiazepines (e.g., lorazepam 1 to 2 mg IV, respiratory depression has to be considered with higher doses) and anticonvulsants.

If continuous antiepileptic treatment with phenytoin or carbamazepine is started, higher doses of cyclosporine or tacrolimus are necessary because of hepatic induction of cytochrome P450 oxygenase. Although epileptic seizures are, in some centers, primarily treated with phenytoin, valproic acid is accepted as the first choice for seizure control, because it does not induce hepatic cyclosporine metabolism and because it can also be administered intravenously.

Valproic acid, however, has the potential to cause encephalopathy in the initial treatment phase and may be also hepatotoxic, which limits its use following liver transplantation. Gabapentin and levetiracetam may be promising alternative drugs, because they do not induce hepatic metabolism of immunosuppressants, rarely have side effects, and are effective in the treatment of focal and secondary generalized epileptic seizures. However, treatment with these newer anticonvulsant drugs has been reported only for single patients after organ transplantation.

SECONDARY LYMPHOPROLIFERATIVE DISEASE

Systemic lymphoproliferative diseases occur in 0.5% to 4% of patients following organ transplantation. This heterogeneous group contains patients with "benign" polyclonal lymphoid hyperplasia as well as patients with malignant lymphoma. In the majority of cases, transformed lymphoid cells contain EBV-DNA or EBV-transcribed proteins. Thus, viral B-cell transformation is suspected to occur after EBV infection, and the malignant development of transformed cells occurs because of chronic immunosuppression. Infection with CMV is possibly an additional risk factor.

CNS involvement occurs in 15% to 25% of patients with lymphoproliferative disease following organ transplantation, but the majority of patients have primary isolated CNS lymphoma.[16,17] The high frequency of CNS lymphoma might be due to the particular immunologic situation of the brain, where transformed viral B cells are more likely to survive. Clinical symptoms of lymphoproliferative CNS disease consist of cognitive disturbances and focal neurological signs. CT and MRI imaging show hyperintense lesions (T2-weighted images) with contrast enhancement most often in the periventricular areas, in the deep white matter, or in the basal ganglia, but multifocal or meningeal involvement may also occur. The presence of CNS lymphoma must be proven histologically by stereotactic biopsy.

Treatment of CNS lymphoma usually consists of systemic chemotherapy, but the reduction of immunosuppression and administration of acyclovir (or alpha-interferon) have been discussed.[18] Although patients with CNS lymphoma after organ transplantation have not been included in clinical trials, treatment recommendations, by analogy to immunocompetent patients with primary CNS lymphoma, consist of initial systemic chemotherapy followed by irradiation when necessary (see chapter on primary CNS lymphoma).[19] Systemic treatment with anti-B-cell antibody has no beneficial effect on CNS lymphoma, but single patients with complete remission have been described after intrathecal anti-B-cell antibody treatment. These data, however, must be confirmed in a larger, blinded study. In general, prognosis of CNS lymphoma after organ transplantation is poor, and the death rate exceeds that of systemic lymphoproliferative diseases (36% to 72%).

Neurological Complications Following Transplantation of a Specific Organ

The syndromes and diseases described in the previous sections are nonspecific complications that can occur in all organ recipients. Patients may, however, also develop organ-specific neurologic complications, that are caused either by problems associated with the surgical procedure or by a particular metabolic or immunologic situation, e.g., following liver or bone marrow transplantation.

BONE MARROW TRANSPLANTATION

Bone marrow or peripheral stem cell transplantation is generally performed in patients with hematologic malignancies (leukemia, lymphoma), less often in those with other malignancies following high-dose chemotherapy (for reconstitution of hematopoiesis), and rarely in patients with metabolic (adrenoleukodystrophy, metachromatic leukodystrophy) or autoimmune disease (systemic lupus erythematosus, rheumatoid arthritis).

Depending on the underlying illness, autologous, syngeneic, or allogeneic transplantation is performed. Because autologous transplantation entails the reinfusion of the patient's own bone marrow or peripheral blood stem cells, the subsequent course of the patient is in general uncomplicated, and immunosuppression is not necessary. Neurological complications occur in the form of intracerebral bleeding during the thrombocytopenic period and as metabolic encephalopathy following organ failure.[20] Syngeneic transplantation is performed between homozygotic twins, and is thus based on an immunological situation identical to that of autologous transplantation. Conversely, in allogeneic transplantation, bone marrow (or peripheral blood stem cells) from an HLA-identical family member or from an unrelated donor is transferred. These patients require prophylactic immunosuppression with cyclosporine, due to the mismatch of minor histocompatibility antigens. Despite treatment, 40% to 60% of them develop graft-versus-host disease (GvHD). After allogeneic bone marrow transplantation, patients are exposed to various types of primary and secondary CNS damage.[21,22] Depending on the study design, neurological complications develop in 11% to 77%, and lead to death in 6% to 26%.[23] Cerebral ischemia occurs in 3% to 9% of the patients, 2% to 7% of the patients develop intracranial hemorrhage, and 7% to 37% suffer from usually-reversible metabolic encephalopathy.[24,25] Immunosuppression causes neurotoxicity in up to 15% (see section on neurotoxicity of immunosuppressants), and 5% to 15% of the patients acquire CNS infections after allogeneic bone marrow transplantation. Cerebral relapse of the original hematologic malignancy is observed in mixed study populations in 2% to 5% of the patients. With acute lymphatic leukemia, the risk of CNS relapse is about 7%, despite prophylactic intrathecal methotrexate treatment.[26] Buffy coat treatment (infusion of mononuclear cells from the initial donor) can be performed in patients with leukemia recurrence in an attempt to utilize the graft-versus-leukemia effect, but this may lead to severe GvHD.

The etiology of cerebral ischemic infarctions includes nonbacterial thrombotic endocarditis, a hypercoagulability state, or thrombotic thrombocytopenic purpura. Intracranial bleeding (i.e., subdural hematoma or parenchymal bleeding) is most often due to thrombocytopenia. CNS infections are more frequent after bone marrow transplantation than after other organ transplants, because of the severe immunosuppression required and the initial leukopenia.[27] During the early phase after transplantation, patients are at high risk for infections with gram-negative bacteria, viuses (especially herpes viruses) and fungi. Cellular and humoral immunity is still reduced during the first year after bone marrow transplantation despite hematologic reconstitution. Viral (e.g., CMV) and protozoan (e.g., *Toxoplasma gondii*) infections are particularly frequent in patients with chronic GvHD.

Severe leukencephalopathy of unknown etiology may occur years after bone marrow transplantation. It can manifest as cognitive impairment, tetraparesis, or as a cerebellar syndrome. Chronic GvHD and the resulting immunosuppression have been identified as risk factors for clinical, neuropsychological, and MRI abnormalities in long-term survivors. Neurological complications of chronic GvHD, which may cause scleroderma-like skin changes and liver or gut involvement, include polymyositis, myasthenia gravis, and polyneuropathy syndromes (also described in patients with acute GvHD). In these patients, treatment does not differ from that for other GvHD manifestation (immunosuppression, i.e., with steroids). Patients with myasthenia require additional medication with cholinesterase inhibitors (e.g., pyridostigmine). Possible CNS involvement during chronic GvHD, which has been described in case reports and animal experiments, should be suspected in patients with vasculitis-like or encephalitis-like disease.[28] Stereotactic brain biopsy is recommended, if endocarditis and CNS infections have been ruled out. If the neuropathological findings are positive, trial treatment with steroids (500 to 1000 mg IV daily for 5 days) and cyclophosphamide (750 mg/m^2 every 4 weeks for 2 to 4 months) is justified, despite the considerable risks (marrow toxicity, immunosuppression).

LIVER TRANSPLANTATION

Liver transplantation is performed in patients with advanced organ failure, some causes of which include viral hepatitis, alcoholic cirrhosis, primary biliary cirrhosis, hepatocellular carcinoma, Wilson disease, and congenital liver disorders. At the time of transplantation, most patients have metabolic encephalopathy and polyneuropathy. Approximately 50% of the patients with hepatic encephalopathy grade III or IV develop diffuse brain edema with a possible increase in intracranial pressure. This may be temporarily reversed by aggressive treatment with osmotic therapy and barbiturate anesthesia, thus in some cases making emergency transplantation possible. Perioperative intracranial pressure monitoring with implanted devices cannot be recommended because of the frequency of bleeding complications.[29] During liver transplantation surgery, extensive intraoperative blood loss may cause episodes of hypotension, during which the necessary replacement with blood products and crystalloid infusions may lead to electrolyte imbalance.

Neurological complications following liver transplantation occur in 20% to 30% of patients.[30] Encephalopathy due to metabolic disorders and neurotoxicity of immunosuppressants are most frequent. Other complications include epileptic seizures, plexus or peripheral nerve lesions, ischemic brain infarctions, and CNS infections. Because of hepatic encephalopathy in the early transplantation phase, neurological complications may be difficult to recognize. Autopsy studies have reported neuropathological abnormalities in 70% to 90% of patients.[31] Of these, the most frequent are anoxic-ischemic brain damage, cerebral infarctions, intracerebral bleeding, and opportunistic CNS infections. Pontine or extrapontine myelinolysis, which is caused by intraoperative electrolyte and osmolarity changes due to mass transfusions, manifests clinically in approximately 2% of the patients, but is found in 10% of neuropathologically examined patients. Patients with liver transplantation develop neurotoxicity due to immunosuppressants more frequently than patients with other organ transplantations. This can be attributed to the extensive immunosuppression required, as well as the frequent presence of risk factors, e.g., hypocholesterolemia and hypertension. In general, the neurological outcome after transplantation is worse in patients with alcohol-toxic liver cirrhosis or with acute liver failure (who more frequently have severe hepatic encephalopathy) than in patients with chronic liver failure of other etiology.

KIDNEY TRANSPLANTATION

Kidney transplantation is performed in patients requiring hemodialysis due to kidney failure, some causes of which include glomerulonephritis, diabetic nephropathy, and hypertensive kidney disease. The transplantation procedure itself does not pose any neurological risks, with the exception of occasionally occurring lesions of the femoral or lateral cutaneous femoral nerve (both with a favorable prognosis).[32] Individual patients, however, have been reported to have spinal ischemia due to a vascular variant.[33] Due to the frequently preexisting angiopathy, approximately 6% of patients develop cerebral ischemia and 1% intracerebral bleeding after kidney transplantation. As a result of the necessary immunosuppression, CNS infections and secondary lymphoproliferative diseases can occur. Specifically, patients who undergo a kidney transplantation can develop an encephalopathic syndrome with headache and epileptic seizures during acute organ rejection.[34] This may be caused by a cytokine-mediated reaction just like the OKT3 side effects, but hypertensive encephalopathy must be excluded. In general, a preexisting or relapsing uremia is a risk factor for transplantation-associated CNS disease, but metabolic encephalopathy may also occur in isolated instances.

HEART TRANSPLANTATION

Heart transplantation is usually performed in patients with cardiomyopathy or severe coronary heart disease, more rarely in patients with heart valve disorders or congenital cardiac abnormalities. Cerebral ischemia often preexists, or can occur independently of the transplantation procedure because of generalized arteriosclerosis. Extracorporeal circulation with a heart-lung device is necessary during heart transplantation surgery, and the aorta and central veins must be cannulated and clamped. This may rarely cause cerebral emboli (plaque or thrombotic material, air) or cerebral hypoxia due to hypoperfusion. Such intraoperative cerebrovascular complications have become less frequent in recent years due to improvements in surgical technique.

Neurological complications are observed in up to 60% of the patients who undergo heart transplantation.[35] Cerebral ischemic infarctions (which may often cause epileptic seizures) or intracerebral hemorrhage were found in clinical studies in 5% to 7% of the patients. Autopsy studies found cerebral ischemia or hypoxia in approximately 50% of the patients following heart transplantation. Rarely, intraoperative lesions of the brachial plexus or the phrenic nerve occur. Due to the extensive immunosuppression required, the rate of CNS infections (especially *Toxoplasma*) and the risk of a secondary lymphoproliferative disease are somewhat higher than after other organ transplantations.

LUNG TRANSPLANTATION

Neurological complications following lung transplantation have rarely been studied in detail. Aside from the possible sequelae due to extracorporeal circulation and immunosuppression (see sections on neurotoxicity of immunosuppressants and heart transplantation), cerebral air emboli have been described as a specific complication following lung transplantation in patients with bronchial fistulas.[36] In general, the risk of hematogeneous CNS infection is elevated, due to the high rate of bacterial, viral (especially CMV), and fungal infections of the transplanted lung.

PANCREAS TRANSPLANTATION

Pancreas transplantation is usually performed in combination with kidney transplantation in patients with severe complications due to insulin-dependent diabetes mellitus type I. These patients almost always have nephropathy, retinopathy, and polyneuropathy. Thus, following transplantation, cerebral ischemia may occur because of a preexisting diabetic angiopathy, or renal insufficiency may cause metabolic encephalopathy. The pancreatic transplantation itself usually does not cause any neurological complications. Although one study reported an increased occurrence of carpal tunnel syndrome following transplantation, polyneuropathy syndromes as well as autonomic neuropathy generally improve after combined pancreas and kidney transplantation.[37]

REFERENCES

1. Adair JC, Woodley SL, O'Connell JB, et al. Aseptic meningitis following cardiac transplantation: clinical characteristics and relationship to immunosuppressive regimen. Neurology 1991;41:249–52.
2. Adams Jr HP, Dawson G, Coffman TJ, et al. Stroke in renal transplant recipients. Arch Neurol 1986;43:113–5.

3. Antonini G, Ceschin V, Morino S, et al. Early neurologic complications following allogeneic bone marrow transplant for leukemia: A prospective study. Neurology 1998;50:1441–5.
4. Benkerrou M, Durandy A, Fischer A. Therapy for transplant-related lymphoproliferative diseases. Hematol Oncol Clin North Am 1993;7:467–75.
5. Blanco R, De Girolami U, Jenkins RL, et al. Neuropathology of liver transplantation. Clin Neuropathol 1995;14:109–17.
6. Bleggi-Torres LF, de Medeiros BC, Werner B, et al. Neuropathological findings after bone marrow transplantation: an autopsy study of 180 cases. Bone Marrow Transplant 2000;25:301–7.
7. Bowyer SL, LaMothe MP, Hollister JR. Steroid myopathy: incidence and detection in a population with asthma. J Allergy Clin Immunol 1985;76:234–42.
8. Campellone JV, Lacomis D. Neuromuscular disorders. In: Wijdicks EFM (Hrsg), Neurologic complications in organ transplant recipients. Boston: Butterworth Heinemann; 1999. p. 169–92.
9. Conti DJ, Rubin RH. Infection of the central nervous system in organ transplant recipients. Neurol Clin 1988;6:241–60.
10. Coplin WM, Cochran MS, Levine SR, et al. Stroke after bone marrow transplantation: frequency, aetiology and outcome. Brain 2001;124:1043–51.
11. de Brabander C, Cornelissen J, Smitt PA, et al. Increased incidence of neurological complications in patients receiving an allogenic bone marrow transplantation from alternative donors. J Neurol Neurosurg Psychiatry 2000;68:36–40.
12. Faraci M, Lanino E, Dini G, et al. Severe neurologic complications after hematopoietic stem cell transplantation in children. Neurology 2002;59:1895–904.
13. Fishman JA, Rubin RH. Infection in organ-transplant recipients. N Engl J Med 1998; 338:1741–51.
14. Gallardo D, Ferra C, Berlanga JJ, et al. Neurologic complications after allogeneic bone marrow transplantation. Bone Marrow Transplant 1996;18:1135–9.
15. Gilmore RL. Seizures and antiepileptic drug use in transplant patients. Neurol Clin 1988;6:279–96.
16. Goldstein LS, Haug MT, Perl J, et al. Central nervous system complications after lung transplantation. J Heart Lung Transplant 1998;17:185–91.
17. Graus F, Saiz A, Sierra J, et al. Neurologic complications of autologous and allogeneic bone marrow transplantation in patients with leukemia: a comparative study. Neurology 1996;46:1004–9.
18. Gross ML, Sweny P, Pearson RM, et al. Rejection encephalopathy. An acute neurological syndrome complicating renal transplantation. J Neurol Sci 1982;56:23–34.
19. Guarino M, Stracciari A, Pazzaglia P, et al. Neurological complications of liver transplantation. J Neurol 1996;243:137–42.
20. Jog MS, Turley JE, Berry H. Femoral neuropathy in renal transplantation. Can J Neurol Sci 1994;21:38–42.
21. Lidofsky SD, Bass NM, Prager MC, et al. Intracranial pressure monitoring and liver transplantation for fulminant hepatic failure. Hepatology 1992;16:1–7.
22. Niedobitek G, Mutimer DJ, Williams A, et al. Epstein-Barr virus infection and malignant lymphomas in liver transplant recipients. Int J Cancer 1997;73:514–20.
23. Nymann T, Hathaway DK, Bertorini TE, et al. Studies of the impact of pancreas-kidney and kidney transplantation on peripheral nerve conduction in diabetic patients. Transplant Proc 1998;30:323–4.
24. Pace MT, Slovis TL, Kelly JK, et al. Cyclosporin A toxicity: MRI appearance of the brain. Pediatr Radiol 1995;25:180–3.
25. Padovan CS, Yousry TA, Schleuning M, et al. Neurological and neuroradiological findings in long-term survivors of allogeneic bone marrow transplantation. Ann Neurol 1998;43:627–33.
26. Parizel PM, Snoeck HW, van den Hauwe L, et al. Cerebral complications of murine monoclonal CD3 antibody (OKT3): CT and MR findings. Am J Neuroradiol 1997;18:1935–8.
27. Patchell RA. Primary central nervous system lymphoma in the transplant patient. Neurol Clin 1988;6:297–303.
28. Patchell RA. Neurological complications of organ transplantation. Ann Neurol 1994;36:688–703.
29. Pomeranz S, Naparstek E, Ashkenazi E, et al. Intracranial haematomas following bone marrow transplantation. J Neurol 1994;241:252–6.
30. Swinnen LJ. Durable remission after aggressive chemotherapy for post-cardiac transplant lymphoproliferation. Leuk Lymphoma 1997;28:89–101.
31. van de Beek D, Kremers W, Daly RC, et al. Effect of neurologic complications on outcome after heart transplant. Arch Neurol 2008;65:226–31.

32. Wijdicks EF, Wiesner RH, Dahlke LJ, et al. FK506-induced neurotoxicity in liver transplantation. Ann Neurol 1994;35:498–501.
33. Wijdicks EF, Wiesner RH, Krom RA. Neurotoxicity in liver transplant recipients with cyclosporine immunosuppression. Neurology 1995;45:1962–4.
34. Wilson JR, Conwit RA, Eidelman BH, et al. Sensorimotor neuropathy resembling CIDP in patients receiving FK506. Muscle Nerve 1994;17:528–32.
35. Wolkowitz OM, Reus VI, Canick J, et al. Glucocorticoid medication, memory and steroid psychosis in medical illness. Ann N Y Acad Sci 1997;823:81–96.
36. Zentner J, Buchbender K, Vahlensieck M. Spinal epidural lipomatosis as a complication of prolonged corticosteroid therapy. J Neurosurg Sci 1995;39:81–5.
37. Zivkovi S. Neuroimaging and neurologic complications after organ transplantation. J Neuroimaging 2007;17:110–23.

INDEX

Note: Page numbers followed by *f* refer to figures; those followed by *t* refer to tables.

B

C

D

J

K

L

N

O

T